Choroidal Neovascularization

Jay Chhablani
Editor

Choroidal Neovascularization

Springer

Editor
Jay Chhablani
Department of Ophthalmology
University of Pittsburgh Medical Center
Pittsburgh, PA
USA

ISBN 978-981-15-2212-3 ISBN 978-981-15-2213-0 (eBook)
https://doi.org/10.1007/978-981-15-2213-0

This Springer imprint is published by the registered company Springer Nature Singapore Pte Ltd.
The registered company address is: 152 Beach Road, #21-01/04 Gateway East, Singapore 189721, Singapore

To my family, for standing by me, through everything
To my mentors, for showing me the right path
To my fellows, for asking the right questions

GPSR Compliance

The European Union's (EU) General Product Safety Regulation (GPSR) is a set of rules that requires consumer products to be safe and our obligations to ensure this.

If you have any concerns about our products, you can contact us on ProductSafety@springernature.com

In case Publisher is established outside the EU, the EU authorized representative is:

Springer Nature Customer Service Center GmbH
Europaplatz 3
69115 Heidelberg, Germany

Batch number: 10756355

Printed by Printforce, the Netherlands

Foreword

Nearly two decades ago, I read a fascinating and illustrated book *The Hole in My Vision* (Penfield Press, 2000) authored by the University of Iowa ophthalmic artist and photographer Lee Allen. This book is an illustrative documentation of how a patient sees the world with progression of age-related macular degeneration (AMD), from the stage of drusen to formation of the choroidal neovascular membrane (CNVM), and the response to repeated laser treatment, including the entopic phenomenon.

CNVM is classically described in AMD, but there are other causes, and some of the important ones include the polypoid choroidal vasculopathy (PCV; also called Asian AMD) and pathological myopia. Today, CNVM associated with any retinal disease has several treatment options other than laser suggested by the Macular Photocoagulation Study (MPS) in the 1980s. Our understanding of the disease pathology and natural history have expanded with new knowledge of underlying biological mechanism (vascular endothelial growth factor, VEGF, and several complement factors), improved imaging modalities (indocyanine angiography, optical coherence tomography, and OCT angiography), and newer treatment options directed from mere preservation of residual vision to possible improvement of vision (photodynamic therapy, intravitreal anti-VEGF therapy, and vitreoretinal surgery). Pharmaceutical companies and regulatory authority sponsored clinical trials have increased the opportunity and confidence of the treating physicians to practice evidence-based medicine.

The book, *Choroidal neovascularization*, captures it all from history to basics, from clinical entities to lessons from clinical trials, and from treatment to rehabilitation. Have we reached the last mile in understanding and care of CNVMs?

Not yet.

One of the hurdles with the current standard of care with the intravitreal anti-VEGF is the need for repeat injection, nearly every month, due to short half-life of the currently used molecules. This reduces patient compliance, increases both direct and indirect costs of care, and exposes the patient to some of the injection-related adverse events, such as endophthalmitis. Thus, there is a need for a longer duration anti-VEGF molecule or a surgically placed depot device with slow and pulsed release of the anti-VEGF molecule. But would blocking of VEGF-A, as done by ranibizumab, suffice? Scientists have already identified the role of VEGF-B and placental growth factor, and there are molecules, such as aflibercept, that block these substances. Current research is also directed to block the complement factors, and lampalizumab (blocks Complement Factor D) is one such monoclonal antibody currently under trial. Unfortunately, there is a ceiling effect of all these pharmacological treatments. In such a situation, visual rehabilitation with a variety of magnifying system helps. While most times the magnifying systems are external devices, hand-held or table-top magnifiers, an implantable miniature telescope (IMT) in the capsular bag after a standard cataract extraction is also a distinct possibility to improving the near vision.

Randomized control trial (RCT) is the gold standard to create evidence-based practice guidelines. But it is expensive and does not necessarily adhere to the real-world patient criteria. Hence clubbing the RCT information with the patient's preferences and the clinician's expertise creates a new standard of care that is closer to the real-world medicine and meets patient's medical and social need. The pro re nata (PNR) strategy of intravitreal anti-VEGF in CNVM is a step close to the real-world patient care. The scientific way of reaching a consensus of treatment decision that is between the RCT and the clinical expertise is to answer PICO (Patient, Intervention, Comparison, Outcome) questions of any specific disease. This is more than necessary in care of CNVMs.

Two important chapters in the book are the "Future Therapy" and "Rehabilitation." The future of care for CNVM is promising with newer imaging technology, with newer drugs to block choroidal bleeding, and with the possibility of stem cell therapy to reverse the disease process. And where these medical strategies stop, visual rehabilitation begins so that the quality of life is not decreased to depression.

This book, *Choroidal Neovascularization*, would be an excellent comprehensive treatise on the subject and would fulfill a long-felt need of ophthalmologists at all levels of training and practice.

Taraprasad Das
L V Prasad Eye Institute, Hyderabad, India

Foreword

The most exciting advances in ophthalmology over the past two decades are those that have advanced the diagnosis and management of chorioretinal vascular diseases. These have been driven by the invention of laser-based imaging technology, particularly optical coherence tomography (OCT), and the concomitant development of retinal pharmacotherapy, especially those drugs that inhibit the actions of vascular endothelial growth factor (VEGF). Together these technologies have revolutionized the management of a variety of chorioretinal vascular diseases, but most importantly they enable us to successfully treat choroidal neovascularization. This breakthrough comes none too soon since neovascular age-related macular degeneration (nAMD) is the leading cause of blindness in the industrialized world, and the post-World War 2 baby boomers of North America and Europe continue to swell the at-risk populations.

Laser photocoagulation was introduced in the late 1960s to treat choroidal neovascular membranes (CNVM), but after 30 years of disappointing results physicians clamored for more effective therapy. Photodynamic therapy was greeted with great fanfare (2000), but it only served to bridge the gap between laser and the soon-to-be introduced, much more effective, pharmacotherapy.

The pathway to anti-VEGF therapy began (1983) with the little heralded discovery of vasopermeability factor (VPF) and the subsequent (1989) identification and sequencing of vascular endothelial growth factor, which turned out to be the previously described VPF. After 15 additional years of prodigious basic science discoveries and elegant drug development, the anti-VEGF drugs pegaptanib and bevacizumab were approved (2004). The subsequent 15 years have featured successful pivotal trials for the treatment of CNVM due to both nAMD and myopia, parallel advances in OCT, and approval of new anti-VEGF drugs.

Into this rapidly changing field enters an ambitious text by Dr. Chhablani and colleagues. The authors have jumped head first into one of the most intensively researched areas of ophthalmology with a comprehensive work, the likes of which we have not previously seen. Other texts have discussed CNVM within the broader context of conditions such as nAMD, but none have been written with a focus on CNVM itself.

Senior ophthalmologists will enjoy revisiting the history of CNVM, while their younger, less seasoned colleagues will benefit from learning what patients and physicians faced in the past few decades. Appreciating those past medical successes and failures is one of the best ways to both understand the present and prepare oneself for the future. I am pleased that the authors have devoted considerable space to the pathophysiology of CNVM since both basic scientists and research-oriented medical retina specialists will appreciate the detailed discussion of CNVM biology.

The main body of this book discusses CNVM within the context of several important retinal diseases. Readers will be treated to state-of-the-art discussions of AMD and a variety of other macular conditions, with neovascularization from the choriocapillaris serving as their common thread.

The release of this book is particularly well timed since we are entering a period of accelerated drug development for the treatment of CNVM. For the first time, investigational drugs promise extended duration anti-VEGF therapy and true combination therapy for CNVM. The latter resembles the strategies commonly employed by oncologists, an approach that has been anticipated by retina specialists for several years.

The book will appeal to a broad group of medical professionals since it contains useful information for everyone. Medical students taking ophthalmology rotations will find important clinical information upon which to build their knowledge bases; ophthalmology residents will acquire principles of patient management and understand the needs for referral; retina fellows will use this to manage a broad spectrum of medical retina conditions; general ophthalmologists will familiarize themselves with the latest research; and retina specialists will enjoy the detailed coverage of pivotal clinical trials and important pathophysiology.

My only concern about this volume, which has nothing to do with the quality and scope of the work, is its durability within the rapidly changing CNVM landscape. If this book receives the accolades it deserves, the authors may need to publish frequent updates to keep us up to date.

Finally, I have known Dr. Chhablani for the past seven years and I am honored to write this foreword. Dr. Chhablani has established himself as one of the rising stars in ophthalmology, and this book adds to the volume of quality work he has produced in his brief academic career. I look forward to the success of this book and I eagerly await future publications by this talented, industrious, young physician.

Michael W. Stewart
Mayo Clinic Florida, Jacksonville, FL, USA

Preface

In the last three decades, with advanced imaging, the understanding and management of choroidal neovascularization (CNV) has been transformed. Through extensive basic research, several pathomechanisms have been established over the years, and subsequently various therapeutic approaches have been developed toward these molecules and/or biological steps. A recent surge in newer therapeutic approaches to prevent, stop, or slow the CNV progression has brought hope for the patients. Advancement in monitoring, rehabilitation, and use of peripheral vision is a new dimension in this field. CNV has been part of many comprehensive books on the retina; however, there is no book which focuses on this specific entity.

Book titled *Choroidal neovascularization* includes sections on basics, clinical conditions associated with choroidal neovascularization (CNV), clinical trials related to CNV in various conditions, future directions, and rehabilitation. The section on "Basics" includes chapters on pathogenesis, proposed mechanisms, disease models, histopathology, and electron microscopy. The section on "Clinical conditions" includes CNV secondary to various clinical conditions including common conditions such as age-related macular degeneration, myopia, and uncommon conditions such as choroidal osteoma. This section includes various clinical features, imaging characteristics, treatment approach, and prognosis. The section on "Clinical trials" describes clinical trials in various CNV conditions with recent updates. The section on "Future directions" includes stem cell therapy, gene therapy, newer molecules, and lasers. Rehabilitation is an important aspect of the management of this disease; a focused section on "Rehabilitation" includes home monitoring and low vision aids.

This is a comprehensive unique book on "CNV." Unlike other books, this book comprises all aspects of "CNV" from bench to bedside including future directions and rehabilitation, with updated information on clinical trials. All clinical chapters cover the latest evidence-based approach in the diagnosis and management of CNV and supplemented with many illustrations and figures.

I would like to thank all the authors who are experts in this field and have contributed their best work to make this book very comprehensive, up-to-date, and state of the art. I hope the readers would enjoy reading this book and this helps in better patient management.

Pittsburgh, PA — Jay Chhablani

Contents

Part IV Therapy and Rehabilitation

About the Editor

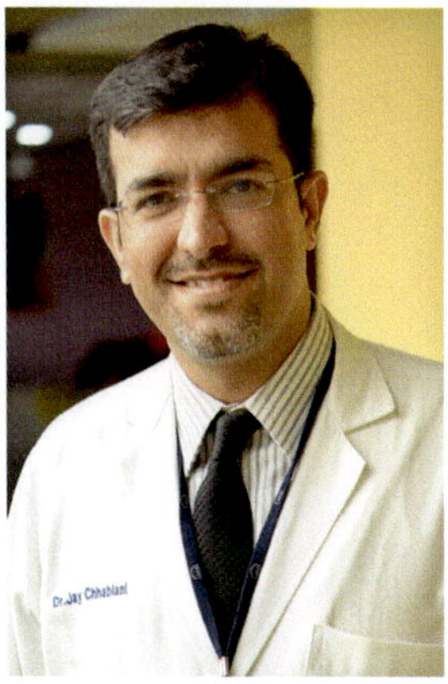

Jay Chhablani is a Vitreo-Retina Specialist at the University of Pittsburgh Eye Center. He completed a clinical vitreo-retina fellowship at Sankara Nethralaya, Chennai, India, and was an International Council of Ophthalmology (ICO) fellow at Jules Gonin Eye Hospital, Switzerland, in 2009. He was a Clinical Instructor at the Jacobs Retina Center at Shiley Eye Center, University of California, San Diego, USA (2010–2012), before joining the faculty at L V Prasad Eye Institute, Hyderabad, India (2012–2019). His areas of interest are macular disorders and recent imaging techniques. He has published more than 300 articles in peer-reviewed journals with a focus on the field of the choroid. He is the editor of the books *Choroidal Disorders* and *Central Serous Chorioretinopathy*, and he is on the review boards of all the high-impact ophthalmology journals. He is also on the editorial board of several specialty journals, including the *American Journal of Ophthalmology*. He is a member of the American Academy of Ophthalmology's Global ONE network committee. He has won several national and international awards and delivered the inaugural Ian Constable lecture at the Asia-Pacific Vitreo-Retina Society in 2016. He received the Inaugural Namperumalsamy Young Researcher Award in 2018, presented by the Vitreo-Retina Society of India.

Choroidal Neovascular Membrane: Historical Perspectives

1

Aniruddha Agarwal and Krinjeela Bazgain

1.1 Introduction

Choroidal neovascular membranes (CNV) represent the pathological growth of blood vessels that can result in loss of vision [1]. Age-related macular degeneration (AMD) is the leading cause of central visual loss and legal blindness in patients over the age of 65 years. As many as 30% of adults over the age of 75 develop signs of senile retinal degeneration. The prevalence of AMD is on the rise worldwide due to an aging population. The exudative or neovascular form of AMD, which is characterized by choroidal neovascular membrane (CNV) growth and/or serous retinal pigment epithelial (RPE) detachments, accounts for over 90% of the cases with severe visual loss.

Since the initial descriptions of AMD-related CNV more than 100 years ago, there has been a complete paradigm shift in the diagnosis and management of this condition. From a near-certain blindness in these patients in the past, the current management strategies ensure stabilization and improvement of vision over a long term period. In this chapter, historical perspectives that led to the discovery of CNV have been highlighted. In addition, early epidemiological trials that established the worldwide significance of this condition have been briefly described.

1.2 Historical Perspectives of Choroidal Neovascularization

In the year 1876, Sattler first noted blood vessels in between the RPE and the Bruch's membrane in the fundus periphery [2]. Reichling and Klemans, Friedman et al., and Daicker noted similar patterns of neovascularization in their studies of the fundus [3–5]. Very few of these vessels have shown continuity with the choroid, leading to speculation of their origin [6]. Spitnaz suggested that an additional vascular layer is present in between the Bruch's membrane and the RPE, anterior to the equator that results in these pathological changes [7]. He suggested that this is a physiologic process rather than an aging pathology [7].

Oeller [8] in 1905 coined the term "disciform degeneration of the macula." Junius and Khunt [9] in 1928 described disc-shaped lesions in the macula associated with significant vision loss. Holloway and Verhoeff [10] reported eight cases of similar appearance in the macula with disciform lesions. In one of the eyes they noted few blood vessels with a small amount of connective tissue extending from choroid through breaks in Bruch's membrane [10]. Verhoeff and Grossman

A. Agarwal (✉) · K. Bazgain
Department of Ophthalmology, Advanced Eye Centre, Postgraduate Institute of Medical Education and Research (PGIMER), Chandigarh, India

J. Chhablani (ed.), *Choroidal Neovascularization*, https://doi.org/10.1007/978-981-15-2213-0_1

[11] said that the disciform lesion was secondary to a reparative process and also termed the lesion "juvenile disciform macular degeneration" as they found it in a 29-year-old patient. Sorsby and Mason postulated that a breach in the elastic lamina of Bruch's membrane results in capillary herniation with subsequent subretinal hemorrhage [12, 13]. They also suggested that wandering histiocytes and fibroblasts from the choroid form connective tissue in the subepithelial coagulated transudate [12, 13].

Gass in 1967 said that loss of normal adhesion of the RPE to Bruch's membrane, breach in Bruch's membrane, and neovascular invasion of the sub-pigment epithelial space from the choroid predisposes the eye to hemorrhagic disciform detachment [14]. He also said that fundus fluorescein angiography helps in differentiating the disciform stage of the disease from intraocular neoplasms [15]. Sarks noted new vessel proliferation through Bruch's membrane in the vicinity of the macula on histological examination [16]. She also described basal linear deposits between the plasma infoldings and the basement membrane of RPE [17]. These deposits were suggested to be secondary to RPE failure. They consist of banded fibers embedded in granular material [17].

Various experimental models have employed various methods in producing choroidal neovascularization. However, Heriot et al. [18] in 1984 proposed that phototoxicity damages the RPE cells and promotes choriocapillaris budding. The adjacent healthy RPE slides forming a bridge over the vessels [18]. Hence, an antecedent break in the RPE is not needed for the formation of CNV [18]. The budding capillary forms a lytic hole secondary to RPE damage [18]. In the same year, Penfold et al. suggested that lymphocytes, monocytes, mast cells, and fibroblasts may have a role to play in the formation of a hole in Bruch's membrane and subsequent choroidal neovascularization [19, 20]. In the past three decades, the knowledge of the patho-anatomy of CNV and its natural history is still evolving. However, the scientific contributions by various researchers in the past century is truly extraordinary.

1.3 Early Epidemiological Studies of Choroidal Neovascularization

The large body of literature on AMD-related CNV is due to the strong foundations laid by large studies focusing on the epidemiology and natural history of the disease. Two of the most significant studies include Beaver Dam Eye Study and Blue Mountain Eye Study.

1.4 Beaver Dam Eye Study

The Beaver Dam Eye Study was conducted in 1987 [21]. The study consisted of more than 5000 patients from the Beaver Dam area of Wisconsin. Follow-up data of these patients were also included. Fundus photography and standardized macular grading were performed for all the eyes. This study was significant because it provided the first ever evidence of high prevalence of AMD and CNV in the elderly Caucasian population. In addition, the study suggested genetic linkage to the development of CNV as well as a potential link between cigarette smoking and advanced forms of AMD. Other risk factors identified included sunlight exposure and cardiovascular risk factors [21].

1.5 Blue Mountain Eye Study

The Blue Mountain Eye Study was performed in Australia in 1992 [22]. The study evaluated baseline and follow-up clinical data of more than 3500 individuals aged 49 years and above. The investigators used fundus photographs and standardized macular grading protocols similar to the Beaver Dam Study and observed a strong correlation between age and AMD. Patients with pigmentary fundus changes and drusen were linked to the progression of AMD. Other risk factors identified by the Blue Mountain Eye Study were smoking, plasma fibrinogen levels, and family history [22].

1.6 Summary

Since the initial descriptions of CNV, there has been a significant advancement of knowledge in the field of choroidal imaging, and diagnosis and management of CNV. CNV has been associated with a number of conditions, AMD and myopia being the leading causes, ocular inflammation being the next most frequently implicated etiology of development of CNV. Irrespective of the cause, the novel treatments available for this condition have greatly impacted the visual and anatomical outcomes of patients, and contributed in reducing the blinding complications of CNV.

References

1. Agarwal A, Invernizzi A, Singh RB, et al. An update on inflammatory choroidal neovascularization: epidemiology, multimodal imaging, and management. J Ophthalmic Inflamm Infect. 2018;8:13.
2. Sattler H. Ueber den feineren Bau der Choroidea des Menschen nebst Beitra¨gen zur pathologischen und vergleichenden Anatomie der Aderhaut. Albrecht von Graefes Arch Ophthalmol. 1976;22(Pt 2):1–100.
3. Reichling W, Klemens F. Uber eine gefassfilhrende Bindegew·ebsschicht zwischen dem Pigmentepithel der Retina und der Lamina vitrea. Albrecht von Graefes Arch Ophthalmol. 1940;141:500–12.
4. Friedman E, Smith TR, Kuwabara T. Senile choroidal vascular patterns and drusen. Arch Ophthalmol. 1963;69:220–30.
5. Daicker B. Lineare Degenerationen des peripheren retinalen Pig· mentepithels; eine pathologisch·anatomische Studie. Albrecht von Graefes Arch Klin Exp Ophthalmol. 1973;186:1–12.
6. Bec P, Secheyron P, Arne JL, et al. La neovascularisation sous·retinienne peripherique et ses consequences pathologiques. J Fr Ophtalmol. 1979;2:329–36.
7. Spitznas M, Bomfeld N. Development and ultrastructure of peripheral subretinal neovascularizations. Albrecht von Graefes Arch Klin Exp Ophthalmol. 1978;208:125–33.
8. Oeller JN. Atlas Seltener Ophthalmoskopischer Befunde. Zugleich Evga¨nzungstateln zu dem Atlas der Ophthalmoskopie. Wiesbaden: JF Bergeman; 1900–1905.
9. Junius P, Kuhnt H. Die scheibenfo¨rmige Entargung der Netzhautmitte (Degeneratio maculae luteae disciformis). Berlin: Karger; 1926. p. 132.
10. Holloway TB, Verhoeff FH. Disc·like degeneration of the macula with microscopic report concerning a tumor·like mass in the macular region. Trans Am Ophthalmol Soc. 1928;26:206–28.
11. Verhoeff FH. Histological findings in a case of angioid streaks. Br J Ophthalmol. 1948;32: 531–44.
12. Ashton N, Sorsby A. Fundus dystrophy with unusual features: a histological study. Br J Ophthalmol. 1951;35:751–64.
13. Sorsby A, Mason MEJ. A fundus dystrophy with unusual features (late onset and dominant inheritance of a central retinal lesion showing oedema, haemorrhage and exudates developing into generalised choroidal atrophy with massive pigment proliferation). Br J Ophthalmol. 1949;33:67–97.
14. Gass JDM. Pathogenesis of disciform detachment of the neuroepithelium. III. Senile disciform macular degeneration. Am J Ophthalmol. 1967;63:617–44.
15. Gass JDM. Pathogenesis of disciform detachment of the neuroepithelium. IV. Fluorescein angiographic study of senile disciform mac·ular degeneration. Am J Ophthalmol. 1967;63:645–59.
16. Sarks SH. New vessel formation beneath the retinal pigment epithelium in senile eyes. Br J Ophthalmol. 1973;57:951–65.
17. Sarks SH. Ageing and degeneration in the macular region: a clinicopathological study. Br J Ophthalmol. 1976;60:324–41.
18. Heriot WJ, Henkind P, Bellhorn RW, Burns MS. Choroidal neovascularization can digest Bruch's membrane: a prior break is not essential. Ophthalmology. 1984;91:1603–8.
19. Penfold P, Killingsworth M, Sarks S. An ultrastructural study of the role of leucocytes and fibroblasts in the breakdown of Bruch's membrane. Aust J Ophthalmol. 1984;12:23–31.
20. Penfold PL, Killingsworth MC, Sarks SH. Senile macular degeneration: the involvement of immunocompetent cells. Graefes Arch Clin Exp Ophthalmol. 1985;223:69–76.
21. Klein R, Klein BE, Linton KL. Prevalence of age-related maculopathy. The Beaver Dam Eye Study. Ophthalmology. 1992;99(6):933–43.
22. Mitchell P, Smith W, Attebo K, Wang JJ. Prevalence of age-related maculopathy in Australia. The Blue Mountains Eye Study. Ophthalmology. 1995;102(10):1450–60.

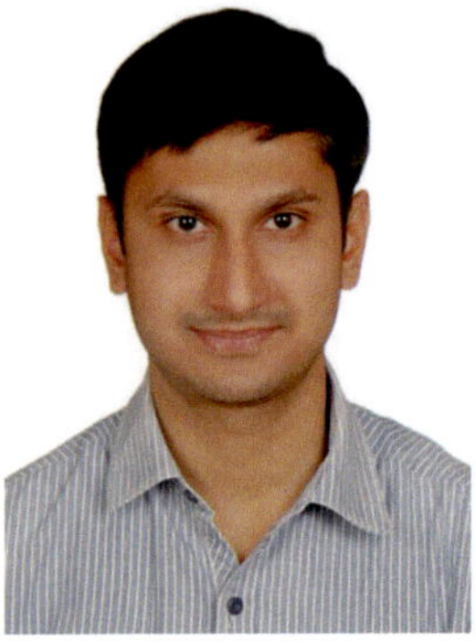

Aniruddha Agarwal is currently working as an Assistant Professor in Vitreoretina and Uveitis in the Department of Ophthalmology, Postgraduate Institute of Medical Education and Research (PGIMER), Chandigarh, India. He has completed his Clinical Research Fellowship (subspecialty of vitreoretina and uveitis) in the Ocular Imaging Research and Reading Center, Stanley M. Truhlsen Eye Institute, Omaha, Nebraska, USA between 2014 and 2016. He did his ophthalmology residency and Surgical Vitreoretina and Uveitis Fellowship at the PGIMER, Chandigarh, India. He is the recipient of prestigious awards such as the Bayer Global Ophthalmology Association Project (GOAP) Fellowship, Carl Camras Best Researcher Award, J. M. Pahwa Award by Vitreoretina Society of India (VRSI), Narsing Rao Award by Uveitis Society of India (USI), and the Carl Herbort Award by the USI. In 2015, he was felicitated by the Hon. Prime Minister of India for his excellent contribution. He has authored more than 150 publications and 36 book chapters. His areas of interest include uveitis, as well as medical and surgical diseases of the retina. He is an expert in ocular imaging and has numerous international presentations and collaborations for the same.

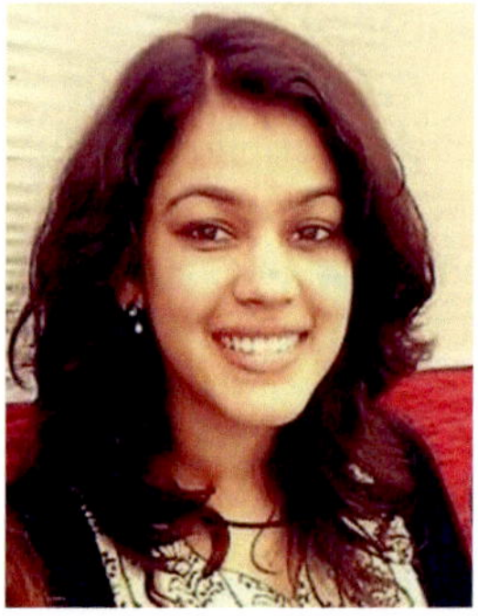

Krinjeela Bazgain is currently pursuing her M.Ch. in Vitreoretinal surgery in the Postgraduate Institute of Medical Education and Research (PGIMER), Chandigarh, India. She did her Ophthalmology residency from PGIMER, Chandigarh, India.

Part I

Basic Science

Pathogenesis of Choroidal Neovascularization

2

Mayss Al-Sheikh and Daniel Barthelmes

Choroidal neovascularization (CNV) is a major cause of severe vision loss in patients with age-related macular degeneration (AMD) [1]. Neovascular AMD is characterized by the development of a neovascular membrane, emerging from the choroid, which may remain underneath the retinal pigment epithelium (RPE) or extend through the Bruch's membrane and the RPE to the subretinal space [2]. Early signs of CNV are hemorrhage, macular edema, lipid deposition, or detachment of the retinal pigment epithelium. End stages are characterized by a scar formation [3]. For the localization of CNV in the central macula, the thinning of the Bruch's membrane with its elastic and collagenous laminae in the foveal region has been proposed to play a role [4]. The lamina elastica of Bruch's membrane is described to be 3–6 times thinner and 2–5 times more porous in the macular region than it is in the peripheral region at all ages, especially in elderly. This large discontinuities within the macular lamina elastica may explain the predilection toward CNV formation in the macular region since for a neovessel to grow from the choroid into the sub-RPE space, its cells must be able to pass physically through Bruch's membrane.

The exact pathophysiology of CNV is not yet understood. There is an evidence that *choroidal blood flow* decreases in patients with AMD; however, the exact nature of impairment remains unclear. Interestingly, eyes with neovascular AMD showed CNV development in areas of hypofluorescence in the macula and areas of watershed zone [5]. For decades, different modalities were used to investigate blood flow in patients with neovascular AMD [6–8]. Using fundus fluorescence angiography, a prolonged choroidal filling phase was identified in many patients [6]. Using indocyaningreen dye angiography, an attenuation of choriocapillaris blood flow was revealed [7]. Recently, using optical coherence tomography angiography, an impairment of the perfusion of the choriocapillaris around the CNV lesion was described [9]. Those observations led to the hypothesis that abnormalities of the choriocapillaris may reduce diffusion of debris material derived from the RPE into the intravascular space leading to accumulating into the Bruch's membrane and consecutively to its thickening.

Friedman reported that the development of CNV is associated with *hemodynamic changes* in the ocular vessels [10, 11]. Accumulation of lipids in the sclera and the Bruch's membrane, which leads to a stiffening of the tissue, increases the resistance of choroidal blood flow. This, in turn, results in decreased choroidal perfusion and impaired RPE transport function, which leads to the formation of drusen, RPE atrophy, and lipid infiltration of the Bruch's membrane, while

M. Al-Sheikh (✉) · D. Barthelmes
University Hospital Zurich, University of Zurich, Zurich, Switzerland

J. Chhablani (ed.), *Choroidal Neovascularization*, https://doi.org/10.1007/978-981-15-2213-0_2

increased intravascular pressure is suggested to lead to RPE detachment and CNV formation [5, 8, 12, 13].

Regardless of what is the initial cause of CNV, angiogenic factors are critically involved in the development of CNV. *Angiogenesis* is defined as the development of new capillaries from preexisting networks. Angiogenesis is a critical process in the embryologic phase, somatic growth as well as in tissue and wound repair. An important factor in the angiogenesis process is the balance between pro-angiogenic and antiangiogenic factors; however, if there is an excessive stimulus and/or reduced inhibitory effects, then pathologies such as CNV may result. Another important factor in angiogenesis is the extracellular matrix (ECM) molecules that are involved in several ways in the regulation of the growth of new blood vessels.

Vascular endothelial growth factor (VEGF) was initially discovered as a peptide secreted by tumor cells that leads to increased vascular permeability [14]. Later it was explained to be an angiogenic growth factor with high specificity for vascular endothelial cells [15, 16]. The synthesis of VEGF is driven by hypoxia [17] where the concentration is increased in the retina and vitreous [18, 19].

In contrast to CNV, we better understand neovascularization development in the retina and the iris [20–23]. Many studies have reported a central role of *hypoxia* or *ischemia* in the development of retinal neovascularization in ischemic diseases like diabetic retinopathy, retinal vein occlusion, and neovascular glaucoma [24, 25]. In contrast, the role of hypoxia and ischemia in CNV is not completely clear [8]. The VEGF secretion of RPE is described to be polarized with a higher secretion toward the Bruch's membrane and a lower secretion rate toward the photoreceptors [26]. Under abnormal conditions, specifically hypoxia, this disparity may exaggerate. Since VEGF has a trophic function for the choriocapillaris by its ability to induce endothelial fenestration [27], it is conceivable that thickening of the Bruch's membrane with lipophilic material deposition may prevent VEGF from reaching the choriocapillaris causing its atrophy—which in its turn decreases diffusion of oxygen from the choroid to the RPE and outer retina in aging patients as well as reduce the clearance of debris from RPE and Bruch's membrane. Those two factors, hypoxia and Bruch's membrane degradation, induce VEGF secretion and promote CNV development. On the other hand, this hypothesis is less likely to occur in other types of CNV that are not age-related, such as those associated with young myopic patients and patients with ocular histoplasmosis.

While VEGF is crucial, especially in the early stages of development of blood vessels, *angiopoietins* are involved in stabilization and maturation of vessels in later stages. Angiopoietin-1, produced by pericytes, induces endothelial cells to recruit periendothelial support cells and associate with the extracellular matrix and mesenchyme, promoting vascular integrity and maintenance of adult vasculature and affects vascular tight junctions [28–30]. In contrast to VEGF, which its overexpression leads to the development of leaky vessels due to a disturbance of the blood–retina barrier, overexpression of angiopoietin-1 leads to an increased density and caliber of non-leaky vessels, and modulate VEGF-induced growing and existing vessels [31–33]. In other words, angiopoietin-1 promotes the maturation of the immature vessels induced by VEGF. Angiopoietin-2 is an antagonist to angiopoietin-1 that is found where vascular remodeling takes place.

However, VEGF and angiopoietins are not the only factors that potentially play a role in CNV formation, *basic fibroblast growth factor (bFGF2)* is detectable in the RPE cells in surgically excised CNV membranes [34, 35]. It is also overexpressed in RPE cells, choroidal vascular endothelial cells, and fibroblasts in laser-induced CNV [36]. It has been postulated that bFGF2 has an angiogenic action only in the setting of cellular injury [37].

Another important factor in angiogenesis is the *pigment epithelium-derived factor (PEDF)*. It is a neurotrophic growth factor for photoreceptors that has antiangiogenic action. Its reaction to oxygen is reciprocal to that of VEGF. In many animal models, it was shown that PEDF inhibits ischemia-induced retinopathy, VEGF-induced leakage as well as laser-induced CNV formation [38, 39]. Considering the antiangiogenetic activity, it seems that endogenous PEDF does not prevent the development of CNV. One reason might be the concentration of this factor. It has been shown that PEDF production decreases with age and that the vitreous concentration is decreased in patients with AMD [40] which is then overwhelmed by angiogenic factors.

Along with the pro-angiogenic and antiangiogenic factors, *extracellular matrix (ECM)* molecules also participate in several ways in the regulation of angiogenesis. Degradation of ECM releases and/or activates pro-angiogenic factors. Pro-angiogenic factors stimulate proteolytic activity, migration, proliferation, and tube formation in endothelial cells [41, 42].

Extracellular matrix molecules are able to directly inhibit or stimulate endothelial cell processes involved in angiogenesis by binding to integrins, which on its turn can upregulate and downregulate various intracellular signaling pathways. On the other hand, pro-angiogenic factors may act in part by altering the expression of integrins on endothelial cells [43–47]. This process is potentiated by the secretion of proteolytic enzymes. Two proteolytic systems have been implicated in the breakdown of ECM during angiogenesis, one involving urokinase type of plasminogen activator and one involving matrix metalloproteinases (MMPs) which are present in excised CNV specimens and increased in laser-induced CNV [48, 49].

Inflammation has also been proposed to play a role in the formation of CNV. Several histopathological studies have identified inflammatory reactions in autopsy eyes with CNV [50, 51]. It has been shown that the Bruch's membrane has thin areas around the breaks where CNV goes through to the subretinal space and that the choroid underneath those thinned areas is infiltrated with inflammation cells such as lymphocytes, macrophages, fibroblasts, and myofibroblasts [52]. Activated macrophages and other inflammatory cells secrete proteolytic enzymes such as collagenase and elastase that can degrade Bruch's membrane, and by releasing cytokines, inflammatory cells might foster CNV growth.

Another important point is the leucocytes-mediated angiogenesis and its role in the interaction of cellular adhesion molecules and VEGF. VEGF induces the expression of intracellular adhesion molecule-1 (ICAM-1) on tumor cells as well as vascular endothelial cells and regulates leukocyte adhesion to endothelial cells [53]. ICAM-1 blockade decreases VEGF-induced leukostasis in the retina [54]. These systems are intertwined: leukocytes, which possess receptors for and migrate in response to VEGF can also produce and release VEGF [55].

2.1 Choroidal Neovascularization in Other Diseases

The development of choroidal neovascularization is found in a heterogeneous group of diseases. In addition to choroidal neovascularization secondary to age-related macular degeneration, neovascular membranes are also found in patients with high myopia, pseudoxanthoma elasticum, after trauma, or after inflammatory diseases that affect the choroid.

2.2 What Do These Patients Have in Common?

Various diseases that are associated with an increased risk for the development of CNV have a disorder of the *Bruch's membrane* in common. In patients with high myopia or patients with Pseudoxanthoma elasticum who are known to have thinning of the Bruch's membrane, there is an increased risk of developing CNV [56]. Likewise, mechanical (i.e., trauma) or thermal (i.e., laser photocoagulation) damage to the Bruch's membrane leads to an increased risk for CNV. Another category of increased risk for CNV development is inflammatory diseases of the choroid such as multifocal choroiditis or ocular histoplasmosis. In Sorsby fundus dystrophy, an autosomal dominant disease, deposits on the

Bruch's membrane lead to CNV formation [57, 58]. Sorsby is caused by mutations in the tissue inhibitor of metalloproteinases 3 (TIMP-3) gene. The gene product is an inhibitor of metalloproteinases, which is involved in the regulation of ECM turnover [59]. Malattia Leventinese and Doyne honeycomb retinal dystrophy are two other autosomal dominant disorders with drusen formation and CNV, both caused by a mutation in the EFEMP1 gene that encodes a protein of extracellular matrix ("EGF-containing fibrillin-like extracellular matrix protein 1").

Therefore, these diseases and CNV secondary to AMD that exhibits abnormalities of the Bruch's membrane suggest that alteration of ECM of the RPE predisposes the development of CNV.

2.3 What Do We Know from Animal Models?

A central limitation in studies of CNV is the lack of adequate animal models that accurately reflect changes in AMD. In an established model, a rupture of the Bruch's membrane induced by laser burns results in CNV formation [60]. Although *laser-induced CNV* in animal models may not represent CNV secondary to AMD in humans, it gives us insights into important features of the human condition. Laser photocoagulation that disrupts the Bruch's membrane, especially in the macula, can induce CNV in humans [60, 61]. Other similar features are migration of choroidal vascular endothelial cells and newly formed vessels into the subretinal space through the disrupted Bruch's membrane, accumulation of subretinal fluid, presence of leucocytes adjacent to the neovascular membrane as well as fibrovascular scar formation [51, 62, 63].

Another animal model is the transgenic model. A transgenic mouse line with overexpression of VEGF in the photoreceptors showed new vessels originating from the deep retina capillary extending through the photoreceptors to the subretinal space. This model did not show choroidal neovascularization [64]. A sole overexpression of an angiogenic growth factor does not seem sufficient to induce CNV formation. The intact Bruch's membrane apparently forms a mechanical or biochemical barrier to VEGF from the retina into the choroid. Another transgenic mouse line with overexpression of VEGF in the RPE showed the development of intrachoroidal CNV that did not penetrate through the intact Bruch's membrane and RPE [65]. Viral models with a recombinant adenovirus vector encoding VEGF that was injected into the subretinal space showed the development of CNV that breached the Bruch's membrane and reached the subretinal space [66]. However, the localization into the subretinal space may be due to iatrogenic breaks in Bruch's membrane during the subretinal injection of the virus. Taking the abovementioned data together, it seems that the development of CNV requires different factors including the imbalance of the angiogenesis process as well as a defect in the Bruch's membrane.

Key Learning Points

- Choroidal neovascularization is one of the leading causes of vision impairment in developed countries.
- The pathogenesis of choroidal neovascularization is not completely clear.
- Using different image modalities impairment of choroidal blood flow has been shown to play a role in the development of choroidal neovascularization.
- Hemodynamic changes in the ocular vessels induced by accumulation of lipids leads to increased intravascular pressure and RPE detachment and CNV formation.
- Imbalance of the angiogenic process including different factors such as vascular endothelial growth factor, angiopoietins, basal fibroblast growth factor and pigment epithelium-derived factor as well as degradation of extracellular matrix are crucial for the development of CNV.
- Inflammation including infiltration of the choroid with inflammatory cells as well as leucocytes-mediated angiogenesis are part of CNV formation.

References

1. Bourne RR, Stevens GA, White RA, Smith JL, Flaxman SR, Price H, et al. Causes of vision loss worldwide, 1990–2010: a systematic analysis. Lancet Glob Health. 2013;1(6):e339–49.
2. Chang TS, Freund KB, de la Cruz Z, Yannuzzi LA, Green WR. Clinicopathologic correlation of choroidal neovascularization demonstrated by indocyanine green angiography in a patient with retention of good vision for almost four years. Retina. 1994;14(2):114–24.
3. Gass JD, Agarwal A, Lavina AM, Tawansy KA. Focal inner retinal hemorrhages in patients with drusen: an early sign of occult choroidal neovascularization and chorioretinal anastomosis. Retina. 2003;23(6):741–51.
4. Chong NH, Keonin J, Luthert PJ, Frennesson CI, Weingeist DM, Wolf RL, et al. Decreased thickness and integrity of the macular elastic layer of Bruch's membrane correspond to the distribution of lesions associated with age-related macular degeneration. Am J Pathol. 2005;166(1):241–51.
5. Ross RD, Barofsky JM, Cohen G, Baber WB, Palao SW, Gitter KA. Presumed macular choroidal watershed vascular filling, choroidal neovascularization, and systemic vascular disease in patients with age-related macular degeneration. Am J Ophthalmol. 1998;125(1):71–80.
6. Pauleikhoff D, Spital G, Radermacher M, Brumm GA, Lommatzsch A, Bird AC. A fluorescein and indocyanine green angiographic study of choriocapillaris in age-related macular disease. Arch Ophthalmol. 1999;117(10):1353–8.
7. Grunwald JE, Hariprasad SM, DuPont J. Effect of aging on foveolar choroidal circulation. Arch Ophthalmol. 1998;116(2):150–4.
8. Grunwald JE, Hariprasad SM, DuPont J, Maguire MG, Fine SL, Brucker AJ, et al. Foveolar choroidal blood flow in age-related macular degeneration. Invest Ophthalmol Vis Sci. 1998;39(2):385–90.
9. Moult EM, Alibhai AY, Rebhun C, Lee B, Ploner S, Schottenhamml J, et al. Spatial distribution of choriocapillaris impairment in eyes with choroidal neovascularization secondary to age-related macular degeneration: a quantitative OCT angiography study. Retina. 2020;40(3):428–45.
10. Friedman E. A hemodynamic model of the pathogenesis of age-related macular degeneration. Am J Ophthalmol. 1997;124(5):677–82.
11. Friedman E. The role of the atherosclerotic process in the pathogenesis of age-related macular degeneration. Am J Ophthalmol. 2000;130(5):658–63.
12. Mori F, Konno S, Hikichi T, Yamaguchi Y, Ishiko S, Yoshida A. Pulsatile ocular blood flow study: decreases in exudative age related macular degeneration. Br J Ophthalmol. 2001;85(5):531–3.
13. Remulla JF, Gaudio AR, Miller S, Sandberg MA. Foveal electroretinograms and choroidal perfusion characteristics in fellow eyes of patients with unilateral neovascular age-related macular degeneration. Br J Ophthalmol. 1995;79(6):558–61.
14. Senger DR, Galli SJ, Dvorak AM, Perruzzi CA, Harvey VS, Dvorak HF. Tumor cells secrete a vascular permeability factor that promotes accumulation of ascites fluid. Science. 1983;219(4587):983–5.
15. Keck PJ, Hauser SD, Krivi G, Sanzo K, Warren T, Feder J, et al. Vascular permeability factor, an endothelial cell mitogen related to PDGF. Science. 1989;246(4935):1309–12.
16. Leung DW, Cachianes G, Kuang WJ, Goeddel DV, Ferrara N. Vascular endothelial growth factor is a secreted angiogenic mitogen. Science. 1989;246(4935):1306–9.
17. Shweiki D, Itin A, Soffer D, Keshet E. Vascular endothelial growth factor induced by hypoxia may mediate hypoxia-initiated angiogenesis. Nature. 1992;359(6398):843–5.
18. Adamis AP, Miller JW, Bernal MT, D'Amico DJ, Folkman J, Yeo TK, et al. Increased vascular endothelial growth factor levels in the vitreous of eyes with proliferative diabetic retinopathy. Am J Ophthalmol. 1994;118(4):445–50.
19. Pe'er J, Shweiki D, Itin A, Hemo I, Gnessin H, Keshet E. Hypoxia-induced expression of vascular endothelial growth factor by retinal cells is a common factor in neovascularizing ocular diseases. Lab Investig. 1995;72(6):638–45.
20. Adamis AP, Shima DT, Tolentino MJ, Gragoudas ES, Ferrara N, Folkman J, et al. Inhibition of vascular endothelial growth factor prevents retinal ischemia-associated iris neovascularization in a nonhuman primate. Arch Ophthalmol. 1996;114(1):66–71.
21. Amano S, Rohan R, Kuroki M, Tolentino M, Adamis AP. Requirement for vascular endothelial growth factor in wound- and inflammation-related corneal neovascularization. Invest Ophthalmol Vis Sci. 1998;39(1):18–22.
22. Ferrara N, Henzel WJ. Pituitary follicular cells secrete a novel heparin-binding growth factor specific for vascular endothelial cells. Biochem Biophys Res Commun. 1989;161(2):851–8.
23. Miller JW, Adamis AP, Shima DT, D'Amore PA, Moulton RS, O'Reilly MS, et al. Vascular endothelial growth factor/vascular permeability factor is temporally and spatially correlated with ocular angiogenesis in a primate model. Am J Pathol. 1994;145(3):574–84.
24. Ashton N. Retinal vascularization in health and disease: proctor award lecture of the Association for Research in Ophthalmology. Am J Ophthalmol. 1957;44(4 Pt 2):7–17.
25. Shimizu K, Kobayashi Y, Muraoka K. Midperipheral fundus involvement in diabetic retinopathy. Ophthalmology. 1981;88(7):601–12.
26. Blaauwgeers HG, Holtkamp GM, Rutten H, Witmer AN, Koolwijk P, Partanen TA, et al. Polarized vascular endothelial growth factor secretion by human retinal pigment epithelium and localization of vascular endothelial growth factor receptors

on the inner choriocapillaris. Evidence for a trophic paracrine relation. Am J Pathol. 1999;155(2):421–8.
27. Roberts WG, Palade GE. Increased microvascular permeability and endothelial fenestration induced by vascular endothelial growth factor. J Cell Sci. 1995;108(Pt 6):2369–79.
28. Suri C, Jones PF, Patan S, Bartunkova S, Maisonpierre PC, Davis S, et al. Requisite role of angiopoietin-1, a ligand for the TIE2 receptor, during embryonic angiogenesis. Cell. 1996;87(7):1171–80.
29. Carmeliet P. Mechanisms of angiogenesis and arteriogenesis. Nat Med. 2000;6(4):389–95.
30. Potente M, Gerhardt H, Carmeliet P. Basic and therapeutic aspects of angiogenesis. Cell. 2011;146(6):873–87.
31. Suri C, McClain J, Thurston G, McDonald DM, Zhou H, Oldmixon EH, et al. Increased vascularization in mice overexpressing angiopoietin-1. Science. 1998;282(5388):468–71.
32. Thurston G, Suri C, Smith K, McClain J, Sato TN, Yancopoulos GD, et al. Leakage-resistant blood vessels in mice transgenically overexpressing angiopoietin-1. Science. 1999;286(5449):2511–4.
33. Witzenbichler B, Maisonpierre PC, Jones P, Yancopoulos GD, Isner JM. Chemotactic properties of angiopoietin-1 and -2, ligands for the endothelial-specific receptor tyrosine kinase Tie2. J Biol Chem. 1998;273(29):18514–21.
34. Amin R, Puklin JE, Frank RN. Growth factor localization in choroidal neovascular membranes of age-related macular degeneration. Invest Ophthalmol Vis Sci. 1994;35(8):3178–88.
35. Frank RN, Amin RH, Eliott D, Puklin JE, Abrams GW. Basic fibroblast growth factor and vascular endothelial growth factor are present in epiretinal and choroidal neovascular membranes. Am J Ophthalmol. 1996;122(3):393–403.
36. Ogata N, Matsushima M, Takada Y, Tobe T, Takahashi K, Yi X, et al. Expression of basic fibroblast growth factor mRNA in developing choroidal neovascularization. Curr Eye Res. 1996;15(10):1008–18.
37. Yamada H, Yamada E, Kwak N, Ando A, Suzuki A, Esumi N, et al. Cell injury unmasks a latent proangiogenic phenotype in mice with increased expression of FGF2 in the retina. J Cell Physiol. 2000;185(1):135–42.
38. Mori K, Gehlbach P, Yamamoto S, Duh E, Zack DJ, Li Q, et al. AAV-mediated gene transfer of pigment epithelium-derived factor inhibits choroidal neovascularization. Invest Ophthalmol Vis Sci. 2002;43(6):1994–2000.
39. Stellmach V, Crawford SE, Zhou W, Bouck N. Prevention of ischemia-induced retinopathy by the natural ocular antiangiogenic agent pigment epithelium-derived factor. Proc Natl Acad Sci USA. 2001;98(5):2593–7.
40. Holekamp NM, Bouck N, Volpert O. Pigment epithelium-derived factor is deficient in the vitreous of patients with choroidal neovascularization due to age-related macular degeneration. Am J Ophthalmol. 2002;134(2):220–7.
41. Gross JL, Moscatelli D, Rifkin DB. Increased capillary endothelial cell protease activity in response to angiogenic stimuli in vitro. Proc Natl Acad Sci USA. 1983;80(9):2623–7.
42. Sato Y, Rifkin DB. Autocrine activities of basic fibroblast growth factor: regulation of endothelial cell movement, plasminogen activator synthesis, and DNA synthesis. J Cell Biol. 1988;107(3):1199–205.
43. Asahara T, Chen D, Takahashi T, Fujikawa K, Kearney M, Magner M, et al. Tie2 receptor ligands, angiopoietin-1 and angiopoietin-2, modulate VEGF-induced postnatal neovascularization. Circ Res. 1998;83(3):233–40.
44. Campochiaro PA, Soloway P, Ryan SJ, Miller JW. The pathogenesis of choroidal neovascularization in patients with age-related macular degeneration. Mol Vis. 1999;5:34.
45. Murata T, He S, Hangai M, Ishibashi T, Xi XP, Kim S, et al. Peroxisome proliferator-activated receptor-gamma ligands inhibit choroidal neovascularization. Invest Ophthalmol Vis Sci. 2000;41(8):2309–17.
46. Seo MS, Kwak N, Ozaki H, Yamada H, Okamoto N, Yamada E, et al. Dramatic inhibition of retinal and choroidal neovascularization by oral administration of a kinase inhibitor. Am J Pathol. 1999;154(6):1743–53.
47. Miller JW, Stinson WG, Folkman J. Regression of experimental iris neovascularization with systemic alpha-interferon. Ophthalmology. 1993;100(1):9–14.
48. Cornelius LA, Nehring LC, Roby JD, Parks WC, Welgus HG. Human dermal microvascular endothelial cells produce matrix metalloproteinases in response to angiogenic factors and migration. J Invest Dermatol. 1995;105(2):170–6.
49. Pepper MS, Vassalli JD, Montesano R, Orci L. Urokinase-type plasminogen activator is induced in migrating capillary endothelial cells. J Cell Biol. 1987;105(6 Pt 1):2535–41.
50. Green WR, Key SN 3rd. Senile macular degeneration: a histopathologic study. Trans Am Ophthalmol Soc. 1977;75:180–254.
51. Penfold PL, Provis JM, Billson FA. Age-related macular degeneration: ultrastructural studies of the relationship of leucocytes to angiogenesis. Graefes Arch Clin Exp Ophthalmol. 1987;225(1):70–6.
52. van der Schaft TL, Mooy CM, de Bruijn WC, de Jong PT. Early stages of age-related macular degeneration: an immunofluorescence and electron microscopy study. Br J Ophthalmol. 1993;77(10):657–61.
53. Becker MD, Kruse FE, Azzam L, Nobiling R, Reichling J, Volcker HE. In vivo significance of ICAM-1—dependent leukocyte adhesion in early corneal angiogenesis. Invest Ophthalmol Vis Sci. 1999;40(3):612–8.
54. Miyamoto K, Khosrof S, Bursell SE, Moromizato Y, Aiello LP, Ogura Y, et al. Vascular endothelial growth factor (VEGF)-induced retinal vascular permeability is mediated by intercellular adhesion molecule-1 (ICAM-1). Am J Pathol. 2000;156(5):1733–9.

55. Harmey JH, Dimitriadis E, Kay E, Redmond HP, Bouchier-Hayes D. Regulation of macrophage production of vascular endothelial growth factor (VEGF) by hypoxia and transforming growth factor beta-1. Ann Surg Oncol. 1998;5(3):271–8.
56. Green WR, Wilson DJ. Choroidal neovascularization. Ophthalmology. 1986;93(9):1169–76.
57. Hoskin A, Sehmi K, Bird AC. Sorsby's pseudoinflammatory macular dystrophy. Br J Ophthalmol. 1981;65(12):859–65.
58. Sorsby A, Mason ME. A fundus dystrophy with unusual features. Br J Ophthalmol. 1949;33(2):67–97.
59. Weber BH, Vogt G, Pruett RC, Stohr H, Felbor U. Mutations in the tissue inhibitor of metalloproteinases-3 (TIMP3) in patients with Sorsby's fundus dystrophy. Nat Genet. 1994;8(4):352–6.
60. Ryan SJ. Subretinal neovascularization. Natural history of an experimental model. Arch Ophthalmol. 1982;100(11):1804–9.
61. Francois J, De Laey JJ, Cambie E, Hanssens M, Victoria-Troncoso V. Neovascularization after argon laser photocoagulation of macular lesions. Am J Ophthalmol. 1975;79(2):206–10.
62. Grossniklaus HE, Cingle KA, Yoon YD, Ketkar N, L'Hernault N, Brown S. Correlation of histologic 2-dimensional reconstruction and confocal scanning laser microscopic imaging of choroidal neovascularization in eyes with age-related maculopathy. Arch Ophthalmol. 2000;118(5):625–9.
63. Nishimura T, Goodnight R, Prendergast RA, Ryan SJ. Activated macrophages in experimental subretinal neovascularization. Ophthalmologica. 1990;200(1):39–44.
64. Okamoto N, Tobe T, Hackett SF, Ozaki H, Vinores MA, LaRochelle W, et al. Transgenic mice with increased expression of vascular endothelial growth factor in the retina: a new model of intraretinal and subretinal neovascularization. Am J Pathol. 1997;151(1):281–91.
65. Schwesinger C, Yee C, Rohan RM, Joussen AM, Fernandez A, Meyer TN, et al. Intrachoroidal neovascularization in transgenic mice overexpressing vascular endothelial growth factor in the retinal pigment epithelium. Am J Pathol. 2001;158(3):1161–72.
66. Baffi J, Byrnes G, Chan CC, Csaky KG. Choroidal neovascularization in the rat induced by adenovirus mediated expression of vascular endothelial growth factor. Invest Ophthalmol Vis Sci. 2000;41(11):3582–9.

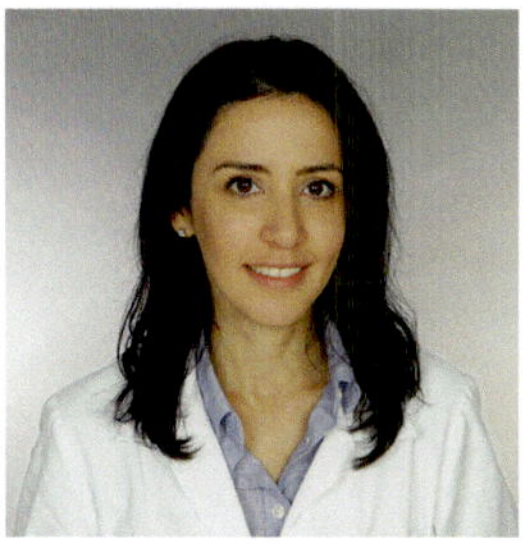

Dr. Mayss Al-Sheikh is a medical retina consultant at the University Hospital of Zurich, Switzerland. She achieved her medical degree at the University of Dusseldorf in Germany.

Dr. Mayss Al-Sheikh completed her residency at the University Hospital of Zurich, Switzerland, and an international fellowship in medical retina at the Doheny Eye Institute and Stein Eye Institute, University of California, Los Angeles, USA.

Dr. Mayss Al-Sheikh's main professional interest is multimodal and advanced imaging. She published more than 40 peer-reviewed articles and book chapters. She received her "venia legendi" in ophthalmology, in particular in retinal imaging from the University of Zurich in 2019. She is involved in training of medical students and residents in ophthalmology.

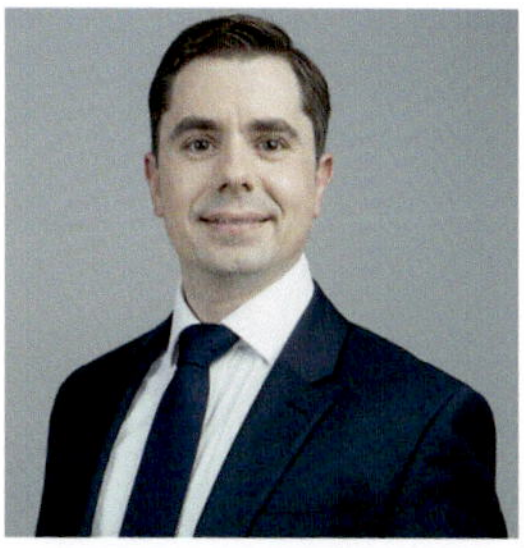

Daniel Barthelmes Director, Department of Ophthalmology, University Hospital Zurich and Chair of Ophthalmology, University of Zurich

Head, Clinical Neurosciences/Head and Neck Disease, University Hospital Zurich

Academic qualifications: MD, PhD, executive MBA, FEBO, FMH Ophthalmology and Ophthalmic Surgery.

After his specialty training in Switzerland, DB moved to Sydney (Australia). Besides his PhD in basic research on vascular stem cells at The University of Sydney, DB also did a clinical fellowship in vitreoretinal surgery and was closely involved in the Fight Retinal Blindness Project (FRB!). He was the first Swiss participant in the European Leadership Development Program, finished the executive MBA program at the University of Zurich in March 2018 and was appointed director of the Department of Ophthalmology at the University Hospital Zurich and chair of ophthalmology at the University of Zurich in August 2018.

DB's research topics for more than 12 years are age-related macular degeneration (AMD), hereditary retinal degeneration, and retinal vascular disease. Past and current research involves both clinical and basic research topics. He did his MD thesis on gene identification using a gene-trap approach and his PhD thesis on vascular stem cells. DB has coauthored more than 110 original manuscripts.

3 Histopathology of Choroidal Neovascularization

Evangelina Esposito, Julio A. Urrets-Zavalia, and Pablo Zoroquiain

3.1 General Histopathology of CNV

The globe is composed of three layers: fibrous sheet, vascular sheet, and nervous sheet. The first is composed of the cornea and the sclera, and provides the structure of the eye. The second, called the uveal tract, is composed of the iris, ciliary body, and the choroid. The third is composed of the retina. The choroid is a pigmented and highly vascularized component of the uveal tract in the eye, allowing for light absorption and providing oxygen and nutrients to the outer retina. Anatomically, the choroid extends from the ora serrata to the optic nerve head and is located at the posterior two-thirds of the eye between the sclera and retina. Anteriorly, it is followed by the ciliary body and the iris. Its thickness varies in humans from 0.1 mm anteriorly and 0.22 mm posteriorly (Fig. 3.1); however, it decreases by age 90 to about 80 μm [1]. The choroid is composed of vessels that are derived from the anastomosis of branches of the ophthalmic artery. These are the posterior ciliary arteries, and penetrate the sclera posteriorly, approximately 6 mm far from the optic nerve. The arteries then branch into terminal arterioles that feed the choriocapillaris. These subsequently drain into venules that merge to form the 4–5 vortex veins at the equator of the sclera [2].

The choroid and the retina are anatomically and functionally related, the retinal pigmentary epithelium (RPE), photoreceptors and the choriocapillaris are described as a functional unit [3]. Choroidal neovascularization is controlled by a dynamic balance between membrane-bound and diffusible substances with properties that either promote or inhibit blood vessel development [4].

Choroidal neovascularization is a major cause of blindness, and is characterized by the three patterns of growth of newly formed vessels from the choriocapillaris through Bruch's membrane, infiltrating sub-RPE space (type 1) (Fig. 3.2), between retina and RPE (type 2) or combined (type 3) [5]. The mechanism of this neovascularization is not well elucidated.

Any damage in the Bruch's membrane or RPE may lead to CNV, which represents an altered healing process secondary to a chorioretinal injury. In this scenario, no single cause for CNV

E. Esposito (✉)
Department of Ophthalmology, University Clinic Reina Fabiola, Universidad Catolica de Cordoba, Cordoba, Argentina

Department of Pathology, University Clinic Reina Fabiola, Universidad Catolica de Cordoba, Cordoba, Argentina

J. A. Urrets-Zavalia
Department of Ophthalmology, University Clinic Reina Fabiola, Universidad Catolica de Cordoba, Cordoba, Argentina

P. Zoroquiain
Department of Pathology, School of Medicine, Pontificia Universidad Católica de Chile, Santiago, Chile

J. Chhablani (ed.), *Choroidal Neovascularization*, https://doi.org/10.1007/978-981-15-2213-0_3

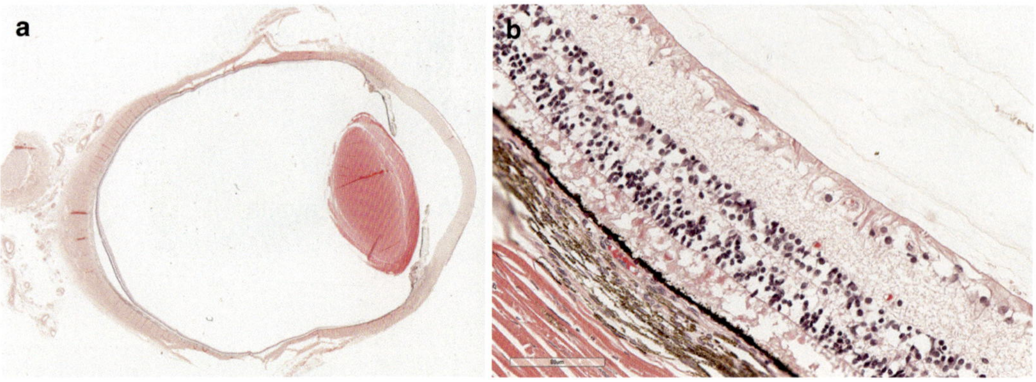

Fig. 3.1 Histology of the choroid. (**a**) The choroid is the posterior aspect of the uveal tract, located between the retina and the sclera (7×). (**b**) The sclera, choroid, and retina (400×)

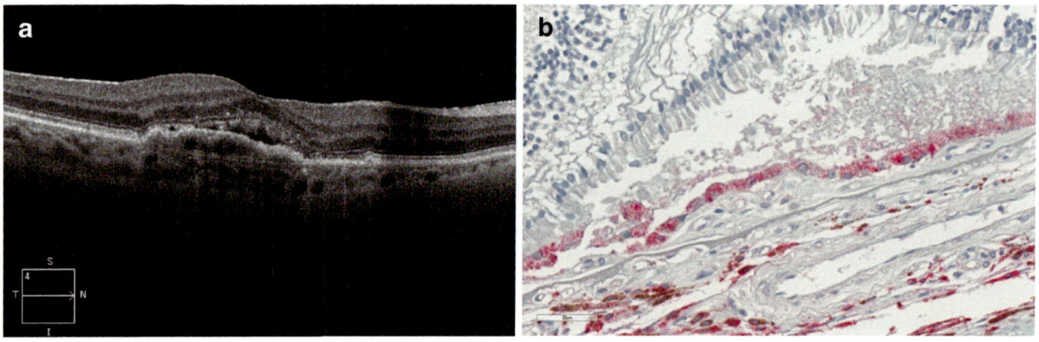

Fig. 3.2 Choroidal neovascularization. (**a**) SD-OCT image showing sub-RPE proliferation. (**b**) The histopathology of CNV, note the fibrovascular membrane located between Bruch's membrane and RPE. Bruch's membrane in this image is thickened and showed some external excrescences (400×)

is identifiable. Rather, it represents a broad spectrum of conditions arising from different etiologies. On light microscopy, different amounts and types of blood vessels, inflammatory exudate or infiltrate, fibrosis and scaring process are seen. A spectrum of findings can be found, with more "active" lesions, similar to any other granulation tissue or more "scarring" lesions on the other side. On electron microscopy, the most common cellular components are RPE, macrophages, erythrocytes, fibrocytes, and vascular endothelium. The most common extracellular components are 24-nm collagen and fibrin [6]. Clinically, this altered healing process is called CNV membranes. If this repair process is composed only by fibrous tissue without the proliferation of vessels above Bruch's membrane (or the blood vessels are fully regressed) the term scar is used.

In each disease, CNV may be accompanied by findings associated with the primary injury. In children and young adults, the development of CNV usually is secondary to choroidal osteoma, pathologic myopia, punctate inner choroidopathy, hereditary macular dystrophy, and angioid streaks but may also be idiopathic [7].

3.2 Inflammatory Associated CNV

Both infectious and noninfectious uveitic entities can lead to CNV [8]. Of the clinically evident inflammatory CNV, the vast majority are classic CNV on fluorescein angiography and type 2 CNV on optic coherence tomography imaging (OCT) [9, 10]. Inflammatory associations of

CNV are usually related to breaks in RPE or Bruch's membrane. Moreover, they are usually associated with granulomas, scars, or choroidal granulomas [11].

3.2.1 Non-granulomatous Inflammation

On histopathology, non-granulomatous processes can be defined as a predominantly exudative and distortive process. Contrary to this, proliferative changes are subtle (i.e., granulomas, lymphoid aggregates, exuberant granulation tissue). As a sequela of uveitis, the choroid may show focal or diffuse areas of atrophy or scarring. Retinochoroiditis or chorioretinitis may destroy Bruch's membrane and the retinal pigment epithelium. Due to the fact that the regenerative capabilities of these tissues are poor, most cases will develop CNV with the possibility of fibrosis and chorioretinal fusion [9].

3.2.1.1 Presumed Ocular Histoplasmosis Syndrome (POHS)

In focal disease processes, such as POHS, antigen deposition in the area of the Bruch's membrane leads to a focal inflammatory response, a break in the Bruch's membrane, and granulation tissue proliferation (CNV) into the subretinal space [5]. CNV may appear peripapillary (Fig. 3.3) or juxtafoveal, and is known to be a prominent feature in POHS [12, 13].

3.2.1.2 Punctate Inner Choroidopathy (PIC)

PIC is a multifocal choroiditis that affects young myopic women. It presents with blurred vision, photopsias, or paracentral scotomas. Multiple small, round, subretinal yellow-white lesions are observed in the posterior pole that heal and subsequently form small atrophic scars. Sometimes, a shallow neurosensory detachment may overlay the lesions. CNV may complicate PIC in more

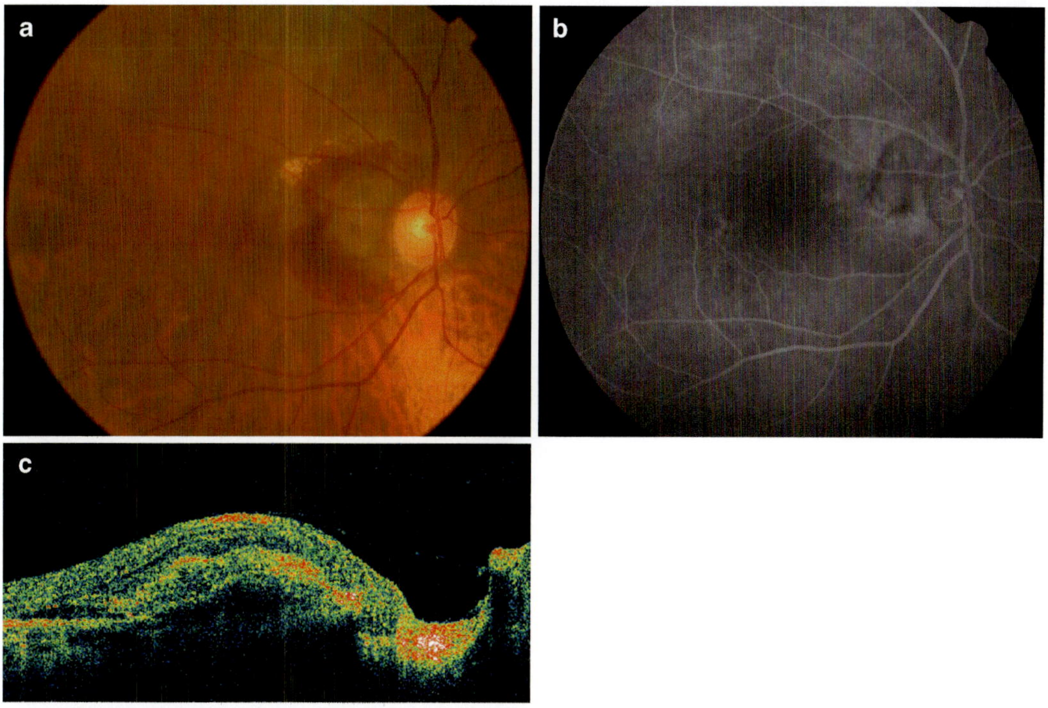

Fig. 3.3 Peripapillary CNV (**a**) Funduscopic image (**b**) Fluorescein angiography (**c**) OCT image

than 50% of cases, and they develop within 1 year of initial disease [9].

3.2.1.3 Serpiginous Choroiditis (SC)

Serpiginous choroiditis is a rare chronic, progressive, recurrent, bilateral asymmetric, posterior uveitis of unknown etiology. It is very important to differentiate between classic SC and serpiginous-like choroiditis before initiating aggressive immunomodulatory therapy, knowing the relationship of the latter with tuberculosis [14].

The disease extends centrifugally from the peripapillary region toward the posterior pole. Visual acuity may be severely compromised when the disease progresses through the macula, or when a submacular CNV membrane develops. CNV complicates serpiginous choroiditis in up to 35% of cases. As it occurs within an area of chorioretinal disturbance, it is sometimes difficult to detect clinically, and is more readily detected by fluorescein angiography and OCT.

3.2.1.4 Acute Posterior Multifocal Placoid Pigment Epitheliopathy (APMPPE)

APMPPE is a rare inflammatory bilateral intraocular disease that affects generally healthy young adults, characterized by sudden onset of paracentral scotomas, photopsia, and blurred vision, and the appearance of multifocal yellowish-white placoid lesions of different sizes in the posterior pole and mid-periphery. Visual symptoms recover after a course of a few weeks, and healing of fundus lesions leaves a mottled RPE or an irregularly pigmented and atrophic chorioretinal scar [15]. In the acute phase, on fluorescein angiography lesions show early hypofluorescence followed by late hyperfluorescence (Fig. 3.4). Very rarely, a CNV membrane may develop within an area of a healed lesion [16].

3.2.1.5 Behçet's Disease

Behçet's disease (syndrome) is characterized by retinal vasculitis, recurrent bilateral iridocyclitis with hypopyon, aphthous ulcers of the mouth and genitalia, dermatitis, arthralgia, thrombophlebitis, and neurologic disturbances. The disease is most common in men, especially between the ages of 20 and 30 years.

Pathological examination of the eyes diagnosed as Behçet's disease show a serohemorrhagic exudate containing polymorphonuclear leukocytes in the vitreous and in the anterior and posterior chambers. There are extensive areas of retinal necrosis. Depending on the stage of the disease, mononuclear and polymorphonuclear leukocytes can be found in the choroid. The choroidal infiltrate is predominantly composed of CD4 T lymphocytes, with some B lymphocytes and plasma cells (Fig. 3.5). If retinal necrosis affects Bruch's membrane it may develop CNV.

3.2.1.6 Pars Planitis

This disease usually affects children or young adults. The histopathologic features include detachment and collapse of the vitreous body with fibrous organization of the vitreous base, chronic inflammatory cells in the vitreous, edema of the optic nerve head and macula, retinal phlebitis and periphlebitis, preretinal membranes associated with breaks in the internal limiting membrane, anterior traction of the peripheral retina, and no significant choroiditis, cyclitis, or peripheral chorioretinal atrophy (Fig. 3.6) [17]. Choroidal neovascularization is a rare complication of intermediate uveitis, and pathophysiologic consideration suggests that chronic disc edema may be a risk factor for this condition [18].

3.2.2 Granulomatous Inflammation

Granulomatous inflammation is a type of chronic inflammation characterized by a cellular infiltrate of histiocytes. In addition, lymphocytes, plasma cells, and polymorphonuclear cells, such as eosinophils and neutrophils may be also observed [19, 20].

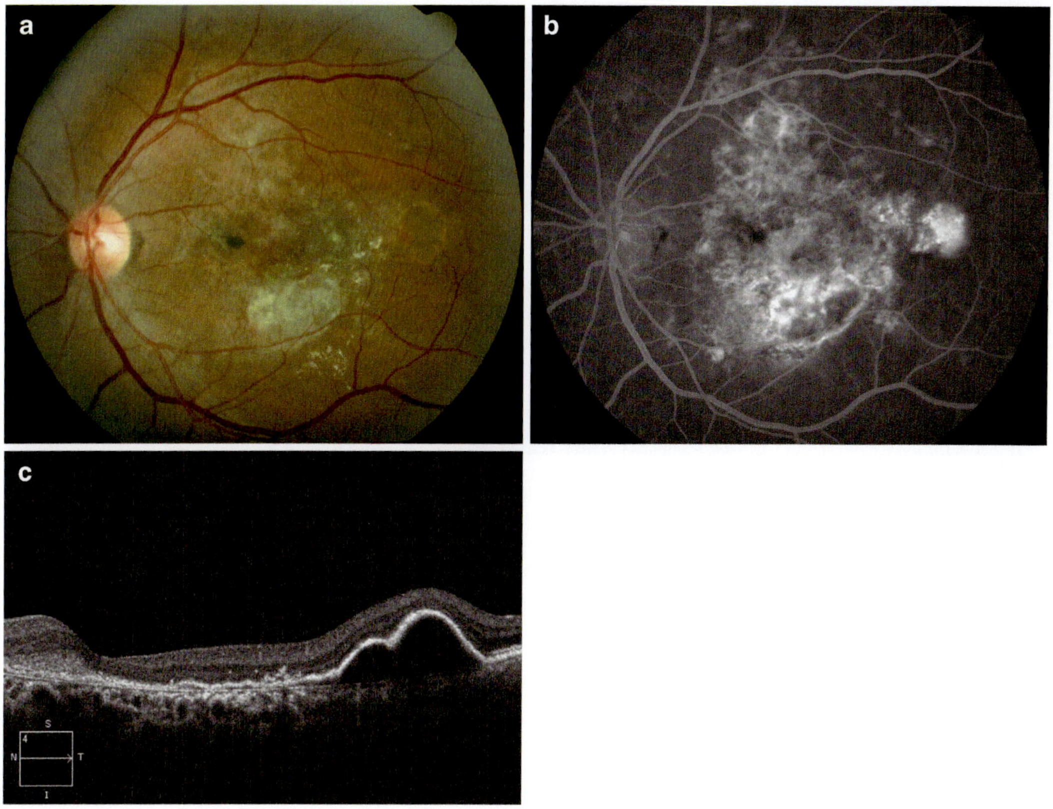

Fig. 3.4 Acute posterior multifocal placoid pigment epitheliopathy (**a**) Funduscopic image (**b**) Fluorescein angiography (**c**) SD-OCT image

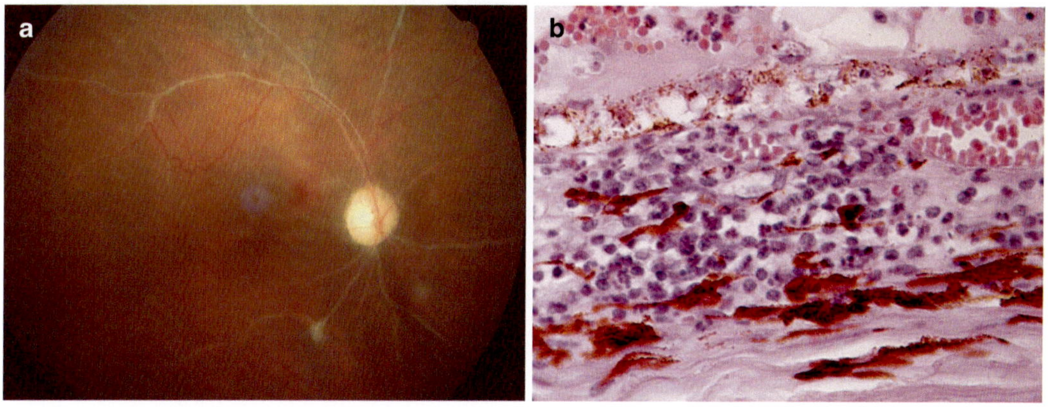

Fig. 3.5 Behçet's disease (**a**) Funduscopic image (**b**) Full thickness choroidal inflammatory infiltrate composed of lymphocytes, neutrophils, and plasma cells are seen. No vasculitis is present. Reprinted from Choroidal Disorders, 1st edition, Esposito, et al, Choroidal Histopathology, Pages No. 21-48, Copyright 2017, with permission from Elsevier

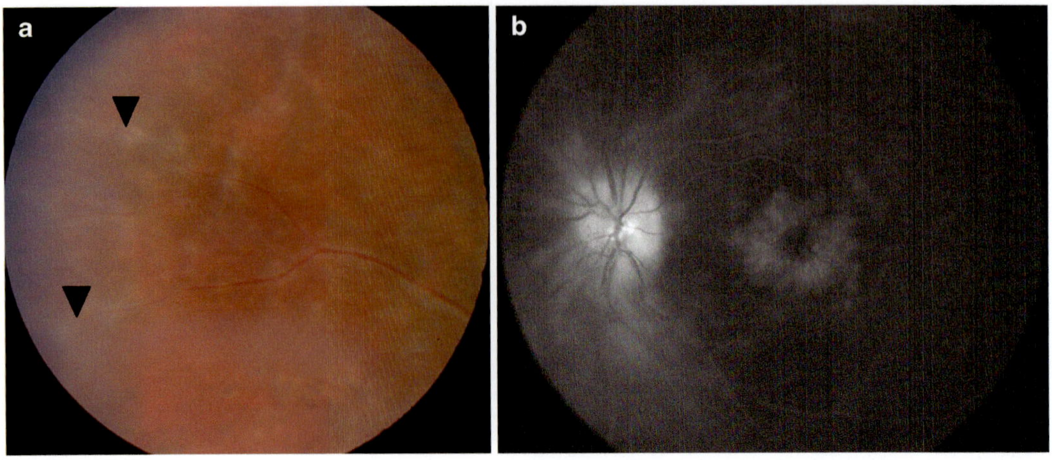

Fig. 3.6 Pars planitis (**a**) Funduscopic image showing peripheral vasculitis (arrowheads) (**b**) Fluorescein angiography showing macular edema

3.2.2.1 Toxoplasmosis

Ocular toxoplasmosis is a parasitic infection of the eye caused by the protozoan *Toxoplasma gondii*. Infections may be congenital or acquired through the ingestion of uncooked and infected meat, contaminated vegetables or water [21].

This disease typically affects the posterior pole of the eye and the lesions can be solitary or multiple and can further be subclassified as active or scaring. Active lesions are gray-white and accompanied by exudation, vasculitis, and choroiditis (Fig. 3.7).

The normally clear vitreous is compromised and becomes hazy due to the infiltration of inflammatory cells. The patient will generally not complain of pain, but rather of an increase in floaters and a possible decrease in vision in the affected eye [22]. The scarring begins from the periphery of the lesion, and progresses toward the center with variable pigmentation changes [23].

T. gondii primarily affects the retina and secondarily the choroid, although choroidal lesions do not occur in the absence of retinal infection.

Histopathological confirmation may be obtained by chorioretinal biopsies, and more rarely, enucleation. The toxoplasma cysts, bradyzoites, and tachyzoites can be identified with hematoxylin and eosin (H&E), immunohistochemistry, or by PCR [24]. However, the majority of the cases are diagnosed clinically and CNV complication is uncommon [25]. Although the parasite is confined to the retina, breaks in Bruch's membrane will permit the contact of the choroid with the infectious antigen, thereby causing an inflammatory response. This may lead to CNV that appears at the border of the scar and the healthy retina [25].

Ocular toxoplasmosis often presents as extensive granulomatous inflammatory infiltration of the choroid and areas of necrosis in Bruch's membrane. In immunocompromised patients, the inflammatory infiltrate may be minimal or absent. Therefore, the focal areas of necrosis are important clues to make the correct diagnosis of toxoplasmosis [24].

3.2.3 Tuberculosis

Tuberculosis is an infectious disease caused by the acid-fast bacilli *Mycobacterium tuberculosis* and is characterized pathologically by the formation of granulomas with a central area of caseous necrosis. The most frequent route that the bacilli reaches the eye is through the bloodstream [19].

In posterior uveitis caused by tuberculosis, the ocular changes can be divided into four groups: choroidal tubercles, choroidal tuberculoma, subretinal abscess, and serpiginous-like

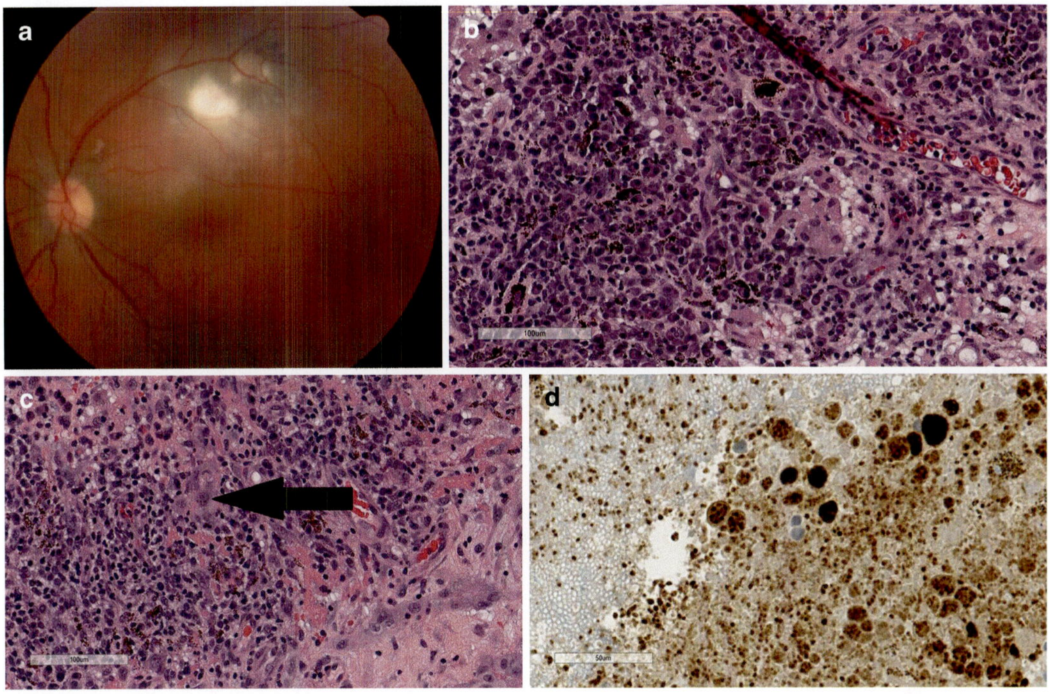

Fig. 3.7 Toxoplasmosis (**a**) Funduscopic image (**b**) The inflammation extends to the inner part of the choriocapillaris. Note the dense lymphocytic and plasmocytic reaction of the choroid and the multinucleated giant cell (arrow) H&E 200×. (**c**) Bradyzoites cyst (arrow) H&E 200×. (**d**) The microorganisms are highlighted with anti-toxoplasmosis immunohistochemistry (DAB 200×)

choroiditis (SLC) [26]. The exact mechanism of SLC in tuberculosis remains unknown. It may represent an immune-mediated hypersensitivity reaction (type IV) without the presence of acid-fast bacteria in the choroid or retinal pigment epithelium [26]. The lesions are usually multifocal, bilateral, noncontiguous to optic disc, and are commonly associated with mild vitreous inflammation. There are two distinct clinical patterns: discrete, multifocal choroiditis lesions that are initially noncontiguous but later progress to form diffuse lesions with an active edge, resembling serpiginous choroiditis; and less commonly, a solitary, plaque-like lesion. Neovascularization, when present, has been reported as Type 1 (sub-RPE) [27].

The disease is characterized pathologically by the formation of one or multiple granulomas [28]. The histology of the granuloma reveals central necrosis surrounded by histiocytes/epithelioid cells mixed with multinucleated giant cells, Langhans type, and a rim of small lymphocytes (Fig. 3.8).

These inflammatory phagocytes in turn are surrounded by lymphocytes. The necrotic area usually contains few bacteria, which can be visualized on Ziehl–Neelsen acid-fast stain as red rod-shaped organisms. However, several organisms can also be seen in the necrotic macrophages that line caseous necrosis. In some granulomas, the organisms can be seen in multinucleated giant cells (Fig. 3.3) or more frequently, they may not be detected by the histologic staining techniques [26]. Currently PCR-based diagnostic tools are highly sensitive and specific [29].

In the choroid, these tubercles/tuberculomas may involve all layers of the choroid. In the early stages, the overlying RPE remains normal but is disrupted during later stages as the tubercles increase in size. The surrounding choroid is essentially normal except for some lymphocytic infiltration [26, 30–33].

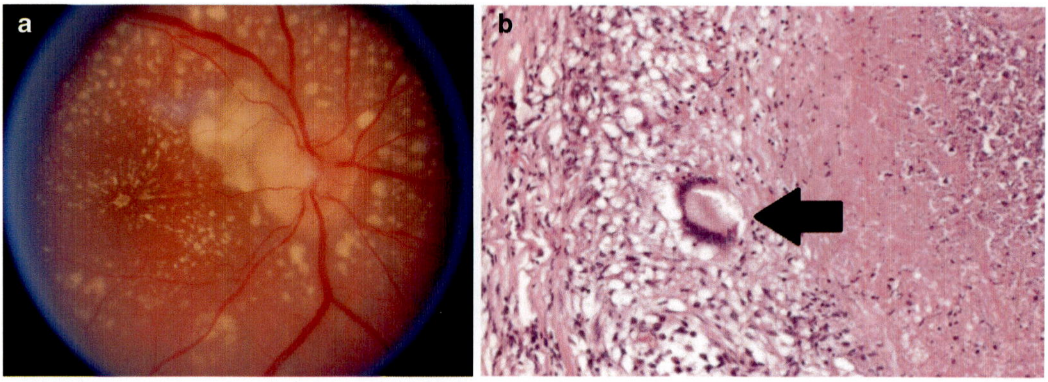

Fig. 3.8 (**a**) Fundus image of the left eye of a patient with tuberculosis (**b**) Chronic choroidal granulomatous inflammation with caseous necrosis and Langhans multinucleated giant cells (arrows). A rim of lymphocytes surrounding the granuloma is seen

3.2.4 Vogt–Koyanagi–Harada (VKH) Syndrome

Vogt–Koyanagi–Harada (VKH) syndrome is a bilateral granulomatous uveitis that is associated with integumentary, auditory, and central nervous manifestations [34].

The pathogenesis underlying VKH is thought to be autoimmune, with T cells mounting a response against melanocytes. There are acute and chronic stages of the disease, with the former responding well to corticosteroid treatment; chronic disease may have recurrent bouts of acute activity [35]. In the eye, VKH presents with posterior uveitis or diffuse granulomatous panuveitis, in association with serous exudative detachment and disc hyperemia, secondary to increased permeability and leakage of the choroidal vessels [34, 36]. Anterior segment inflammation can also occur concomitantly with subclinical posterior uveitis [37]. Chronic VKH can lead to the pathognomonic sunset glow fundus, corresponding to the degeneration of the retinal pigment epithelium [38].

Chronic VKH can also result in peripapillary atrophy [36] and subretinal fibrosis leading to neovascularization, which are poor prognostic factors [39]. Submacular choroidal neovascularization may be another cause of significant vision loss in VKH syndrome and may occur in up to 9% of cases [9, 40]. Type 2 accounts for all cases of CNV complicating these cases [9] and the macular and peripapillary areas seem to be the most frequently affected areas by this complication [41].

The histopathology of the choroid depends on the stage of the disease. In acute VKH, there is generalized granulomatous inflammation of the choroid with uveal thickening [42]. This is due to the infiltration with lymphocytes, macrophages, epithelioid cells [36], and plasma cells. The sensory retina may be detached from the pigment epithelium by a protein exudate with eosinophils [43]. Dalen-Fuchs nodules, which are clusters of macrophages and RPE cells located over Bruch's membrane, may also be observed (Fig. 3.9) [35]. In the early stages, the choriocapillaris is usually spared.

In contrast, the choroidal inflammation in chronic VKH is non-granulomatous [38]. Infiltrates are still primarily lymphocytic, and there is marked thinning of the uvea. There may be obliteration of the choriocapillaris. Dalen-Fuchs nodules are absent; instead, there is loss of the melanin granules in the retinal pigment epithelium. Nearby these are focal areas of hyperpigmentation, which are compensatory hyperproliferations of RPE; these tend to be arranged in papillary or tubular patterns [35]. Chronic recurrent VKH resembles acute VKH on histopathology, characterized by granulo-

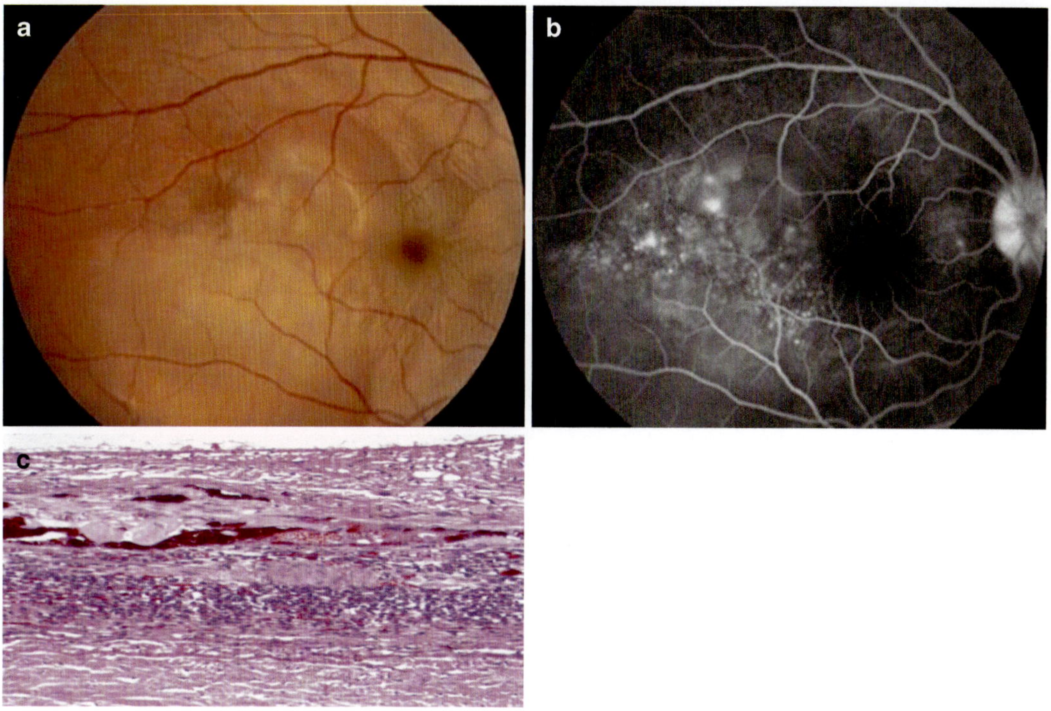

Fig. 3.9 Vogt–Koyanagi–Harada syndrome. (**a**) Funduscopic image (**b**) Fluorescein angiography (**c**) Dalen-Fuchs nodules are clusters of macrophages and RPE cells overlying Bruch's membrane. These are characteristic of acute VKH and chronic recurrent VKH. Note the dense choroidal lymphocytic infiltrate

matous inflammation and Dalen-Fuchs nodules but with less uveal thickening and loss of choroidal melanocytes [43].

3.2.5 Sarcoidosis

Sarcoidosis is a noninfectious inflammatory granulomatous disease that may involve a single or multiple systems. The lungs, lymph nodes, skin, the central nervous system, and the eye can be involved.

Posterior segment involvement is reported in 14–28% of patients [44], and these can present as posterior uveitis and sarcoid nodules of the optic nerve, retina, and choroid [45]; vitritis with or without inflammatory snowballs [46], retinal vasculitis, chorioretinitis, vascular occlusions, macular edema, papilledema [44] and retinal detachment [47]. The development of a CNV complex is not common, though when present, has been reported as type 2 CNV [10].

Sarcoid nodules or tubercles are pathognomonic of this disease. On histology, these are circumscribed noncaseating granulomas composed of primarily lymphocytes in association with Langerhans giant cells and macrophages [48]. Tubercles of the same size are usually seen in isolation, although these may sometimes coalesce. Clusters of the epithelioid and Langerhans cells are usually surrounded by lymphocytes or plasma cells and may either be separated by connective tissue or form conglomerates (Fig. 3.10) [49].

Also observed are perivascular exudates that correlate with "candle-wax drippings" on indirect ophthalmoscopy, perivascular lymphocytic and neutrophilic infiltration, and vascular sheathing [50]. Acid fast and Gomori methenamine silver stains for fungi and bacteria, respectively,

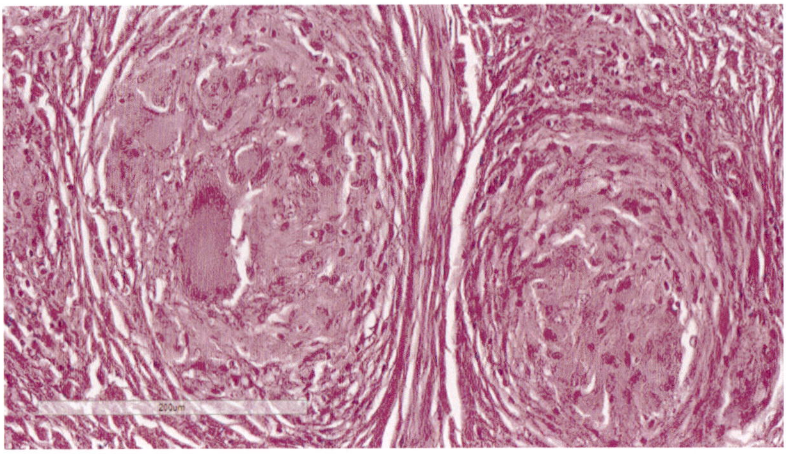

Fig. 3.10 Sarcoid nodules. Note the discrete, compact granulomas consisting of histiocytes, lymphocytes, and giant cells. The granulomas are separated by connective tissue. No necrosis is seen

should be negative, and there should be no signs of a foreign body inciting the reaction [51].

Sarcoidosis resembles other granulomatous diseases on histology, such as histoplasmosis, leprosy, and tuberculosis based on the discrete pattern in which cellular infiltration is arranged [49]; the infrequency of necrosis and the occasional distinctive asteroid and Schaumann bodies that can be seen on sarcoid nodules [52].

3.3 Degeneration Associated CNV

3.3.1 Neovascular Age-Related Macular Degeneration (AMD)

AMD classically presents in a person over 50 years old with sudden blurred central vision, metamorphopsia, and/or a central or paracentral relative scotoma.

Neovascular AMD, also known as wet or exudative AMD, affects 10–20% of all AMD patients, and is a leading cause of severe visual impairment among the elderly population living in high- or middle-income countries [53]. Inflammation can play a key role in the treatment and pathophysiology of this condition. It is considered that the primary event is the deposition of extracellular material (drusen). This material seems to be highly pro-inflammatory leading to the inflammatory state [54].

Almost always, choroidal submacular neovascularization occurs in the context of preexisting clinical manifestations of dry or non-exudative AMD, such as macular retinal pigment epithelium (RPE) irregularities, drusen, and/or patchy or geographic atrophy [55].

Biomicroscopy of the fundus shows a localized area of a shallow neurosensory detachment that may be exudative, hemorrhagic, or mixed. Also, an RPE detachment may be the initial clinical sign or accompany the neurosensory detachment, and is clinically observed as grayish or dark, well-delineated dome-shaped subretinal elevation.

CNV development among patients with AMD can be characterized as type 1 (subretinal), type 2 (outer retinal), or mixed based on clinical and examination (including imaging) findings Fig. 3.11 [56]. A majority of CNV are type 2 lesions with abnormal growth of vasculature into the outer retinal space. CNV seen in AMD are usually subfoveal and are associated with the presence of drusen and retinal pigment epithelial abnormalities due to the accumulation of lipofuscin material. On the other hand, the retinal pigment epithelium is often intact in individuals with CNV [57]. The proposed mechanism of development of CNV is the focal breach of the retinal pigment epithelium due to infection/inflammation leading to growth and entry.

Most of AMD CNV are type 2 (external sensory retinal) and are accompanied by drusen and

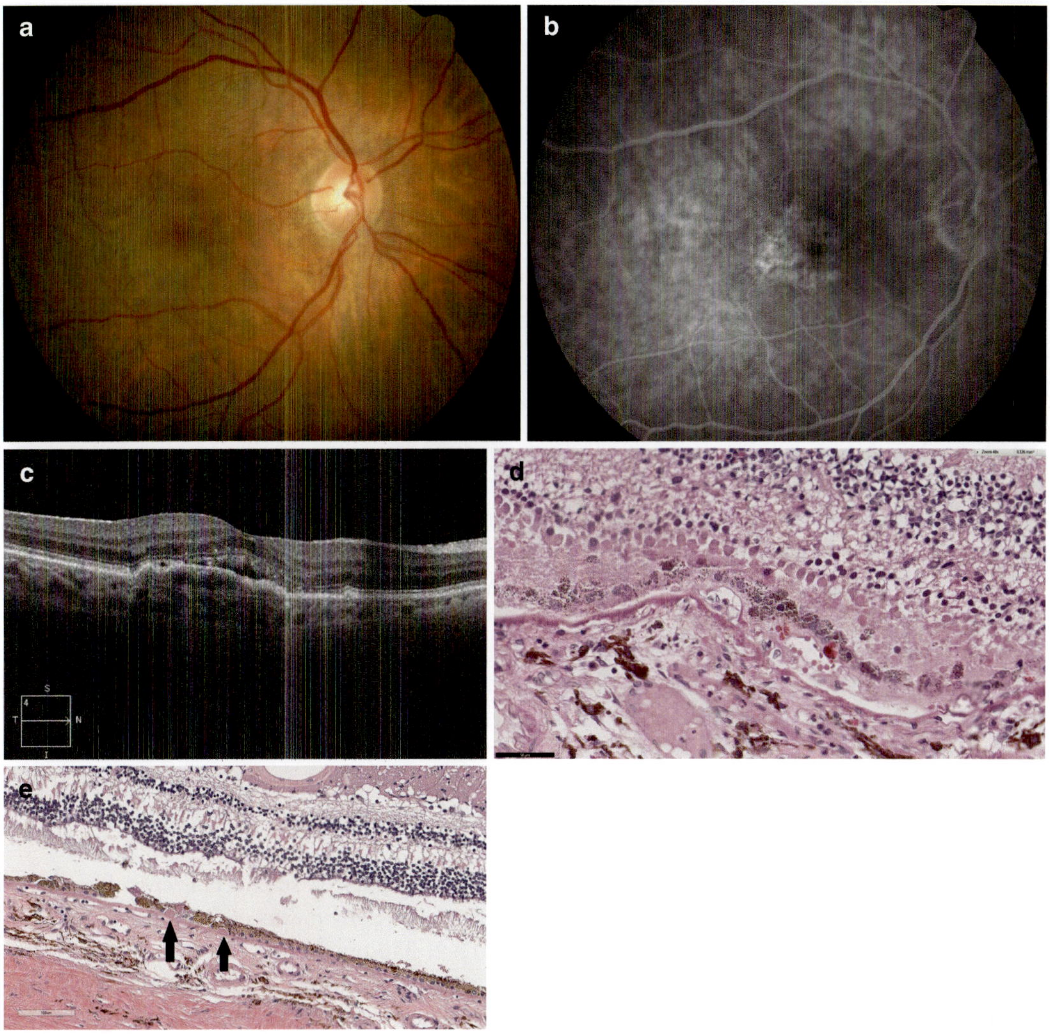

Fig. 3.11 Neovascular age-related macular degeneration type 1 (**a**) Funduscopic image (**b**) Fluorescein angiography (**c**) SD-OCT image (**d**) A thickened Bruch's membrane with diffuse drusen formation is seen. Note on the right two ghost vessels with red blood cells. (**e**) Dry AMD with drusen (arrows) and no CNV H&E (200×)

RPE abnormalities similar to those of Dry AMD such lipofuscin deposition [56] and is nicely delineated by fluorescein angiography [58].

Type 1 CNV can also be seen under the RPE, and presents clinically as an RPE detachment. Later, CNV membranes disrupt the RPE and invade the subretinal space (type 3). Type 2 gets through RPE directly into the sub-neurosensory space.

With optical coherence tomography (OCT), type 1 is observed as a well-delineated RPE detachment, or as an irregular elevation and later disruption of the submacular RPE, accompanied by subretinal hemorrhage or fluid, disruption of the outer neurosensory retina, and neurosensory cystoid edema. Type 2 CNV is easily identified between RPE and neurosensory retina, and also neurosensory detachment and edema are generally observed.

Progressively, in untreated or unresponsive-to-treatment cases, a disciform fibrotic scarring of the macula forms, surrounded by an area of chorioretinal atrophy [58].

3.3.2 Myopic Neovascular Maculopathy

Progressive elongation of the globe observed in high myopia produces a biomechanical stretching of the retina, RPE, and choroid [59] accompanied by a straightening and thinning of retinal vessels with reduction of retinal vascular flow, and a diminished density of the retinal capillary network and choriocapillaris [60–62]. These events appear to induce several degenerative processes of the macular region [63, 64]. In one study evaluating patients with unilateral myopia complicated with neovascular maculopathy by means of color Doppler imaging, higher resistivity index in posterior ciliary arteries were found when compared with the non-myopic fellow eye [65].

Myopic neovascular maculopathy is one of the most frequent and severe vision-threatening complications in highly myopic patients and is the most frequent cause of submacular choroidal neovascularization in persons under the age of 50 years [66]. It may be observed in up to 10% of patients with high myopia, being more frequent in women [67].

Although its pathogenesis is not well established, some predisposing risk factors have been found, such as degenerative changes in Bruch's membrane, thinning of choriocapillaris, and slowing of the choroidal circulation [68, 69].

Biomicroscopically, the subretinal choroidal neovascularization is generally observed as a round, flat, or minimally elevated brown or grayish spot, sometimes accompanied by a small hemorrhage in the surroundings. Although it may be observed in a highly myopic eye without evident myopic fundus changes at the posterior pole [66], it presents generally in an eye with diffuse macular atrophy, patchy atrophy in the macular area, and lacquer cracks [70]. Frequently, the subretinal neovascular membrane develops at the edges of a lacquer crack, atrophy plaque, or steep staphylomatous area [70].

About 35% of bilateral highly myopic patients with neovascular maculopathy in one eye may develop neovascular maculopathy in the contralateral eye within 8 years [70].

Choroidal neovascularization in high myopia is less aggressive and expansive than AMD and tends to regress and cicatrize spontaneously, leaving a subretinal scar area of irregular cicatricial hyperplasia of the RPE named Fuchs spot, surrounded by progressive chorioretinal atrophy [71].

Fluorescein angiography delineates quite well the generally small neovascular membrane. However, in cases with advanced macular patchy chorioretinal atrophy the lesion may become hardly identifiable.

In OCT, the acute neovascular membrane appears as a well-circumscribed non-homogenously hyper-reflective lesion in the subretinal space, with a subtle amount of subretinal exudation and intraretinal cystoid edema, not always present in the initial phase.

Long-term visual prognosis is poor for untreated or unresponsive-to-treatment lesions. At 10 years after onset 96% of cases will have a visual acuity of less than 20/200 [72].

3.3.3 Pachychoroid Related CNV

In normal subjects, submacular choroidal thickness measured by means of OCT ranges between 250 and 330 μm, and is thinner temporally and nasally. It may decrease with aging, in high axial length, and in certain diseases such as glaucoma, pseudoxanthoma elasticum, and birdshot chorioretinopathy [73]. A diffuse choroidal thickening may also be observed in normal eyes without any pathologic consequence.

Pachychoroid is a term to describe focal or diffuse choroidal thickening, dilated vessels in Haller's layer (pachyvessels) that may represent the full extent of choroidal thickness, and thinning of Sattler's layer and choriocapillaris [74, 75].

Another important feature of pachychoroid is choroidal vascular hyperpermeability, evidenced by indocyanine green (ICG) angiography [76].

Pachychoroid constitutes a clinical entity comprising a spectrum of diseases that includes central serous chorioretinopathy, pachychoroid pigment epitheliopathy, polypoidal choroidal vasculopathy, and pachychoroid neovasculopathy [74].

The latter consists in a choroidal neovascular complex that develops overlying the RPE (type 1 neovascularization) in a localized area of dilated choroidal vessels and choroidal thickening, diagnosed by means of OCT, and may progress to polypoidal choroidal vasculopathy [77].

Clinically, besides some focal RPE abnormalities, choroidal neovascularization occurs in the absence of age-related degenerative changes such as drusen and atrophy, or other types of degenerative disease [77]. Irregular and shallow RPE detachments are very characteristic of this entity. Under this area, a complex choroidal vein network may be visualized by OCT angiography [77, 78].

A variant of this syndrome is peripapillary pachychoroid, described recently by Phasukkijwatana et al., and is characterized by pachychoroid around the optic disc, choroidal folds, hyperopia, short axial length, nasal macular edema and/or detachment, and occasional optic disc edema [79].

The pathogenesis of pachychoroid and its associations remains unknown.

3.3.4 Polypoidal Choroidal Vasculopathy (PCV)

Polypoidal choroidal vasculopathy (PCV) is a variant of type 1 choroidal neovascularization, characterized by abnormal focal vascular branching network and terminal saccular dilatation resembling polyps that may bleed and exudate profusely under the neurosensory retina of the posterior pole in longstanding lesions. Polypoidal lesions may sometimes be identified as a subretinal orange bulging lesion principally located around the optic disc and the macular area, are frequently bilateral, and are less frequently observed with drusen than in AMD [80]. Risk factors include male gender, smoking, hyperlipidemia, obesity, and hypertension. ICGA is the gold standard for their diagnosis, but they can also be observed with fluorescein angiography as long as the anomalous network is not covered by a dense hemorrhage plaque [81].

3.3.5 Macular Telangiectasia

Macular telangiectasia comprises a variety of clinical pictures characterized by altered juxta- or parafoveolar retinal capillaries. It may be classified into two major forms. Type 1 is the congenital form, also known as mac tel type 1, and is usually unilateral. Type 2, also known as mac tel type 2, is presumably acquired, affecting both eyes of middle-aged and older individuals [82].

Intraretinal neovascularization is a frequent complication of mac tel type 2, and is more often observed temporal to the fovea, and may extend to the subretinal space and choriocapillaris. Intraretinal and subretinal lipid deposits, subretinal or retinal hemorrhage, and macular edema, and a right-angle retinal venule are reaching the center of the lesion are key clinical findings [83].

3.3.6 CNV Secondary to Angioid Streaks

Histopathology has shown that angioid streaks are caused by breaks within an abnormally thickened and often calcified Bruch's membrane [84]. The overlying RPE is atrophic but not necessarily discontinuous and the blood–retinal barrier is intact. CNV is represented by blood vessels that invade the break, breach the epithelium, and proliferate in the subretinal space [85].

3.3.7 Best Associated CNV

Usually the ganglion cell layer and inner and outer plexiform layers of the central retina are edematous, and the outer segments showed focal atrophy, lipofuscin-like material under the macular RPE. Bruch's membrane changes such as disruption or thickening were also observed along with CNV [86].

3.4 Traumatic Associated CNV

3.4.1 Post-trauma CNV

Ocular blunt trauma is a major cause of preventable visual loss secondary to posterior segment complications, such as vitreous hemorrhage, retinal detachment, macular hole, traumatic optic neuropathy, choroidal rupture, and CNV [87]. Choroidal rupture is a break in the choroid, Bruch's membrane, and RPE, and 5–10% of those eyes may develop a late CNV [88]. Choroidal ruptures located closer to the fovea, as well as longer ruptures, were at higher risk for developing CNV, 82% occurring within the first-year post trauma [88]. Clinically they present as a relatively small, flat, or slightly elevated hemorrhagic or grayish plaques that typically develop within or at the border of a chorioretinal traumatic scar.

3.4.2 LASER Induced CNV

Classically, immediately after laser treatment histopathology shows coagulative necrosis involving all retinal layers that in 3 weeks evolve to a marked retinal attenuation and chorioretinal scarring [89]. The irradiated cells show vacuolation damage to the inner retinal layers and some of them vacuolation in their inner segments, pyknotic nuclei, or degeneration in the fiber layer of Henle. Increase in output energy results in increasing trauma at damaged sites. According to the LASER power, a breakdown of the pigment epithelium and Bruch's membrane may be seen [90]. Neovascularization shares the common histopathological characteristics at the margin of the LASER scar.

3.5 Tumoral Associated CNV

3.5.1 Choroidal Osteoma

Choroidal osteoma is a benign ossifying tumor affecting more frequently young women that presents ophthalmoscopically as a white or pale well-defined flat or slightly elevated mass, found around the optic disc or in the macula. The high tissue density lesion is also evidenced by ultrasonography and CT of the orbit [91]. Vision may decrease slowly as the result of degenerative changes at the choriocapillaris and RPE over the years. However, sudden visual loss may occur as the consequence of serous or hemorrhagic macular detachment from choroidal neovascularization (CNV) [92].

The histopathological description of choroidal osteoma in the literature is limited. On histopathology, choroidal osteomas appear as mature bone with marrow spaces connected to each other and filled with connective tissue [93, 94]. The bony trabeculae contain osteoblasts, osteocytes, and occasionally osteoclasts [94]. Superficially, some of the marrow spaces will have feeder vessels that connect to choriocapillaris beneath Bruch's membrane. The lumen of the choriocapillaris can be obliterated by the tumor in most areas [94]. An atrophied and depigmented RPE layer is usually seen overlying the tumor [93, 94]. In addition, subretinal exudates and a degenerated photoreceptor layer above the tumor, with loss of nuclei, can be observed [93, 94].

3.5.2 Choroidal Nevus

Choroidal nevi are benign tumors, generally ophthalmoscopically observed as a dark-gray flat or minimally elevated lesion, and most frequently observed posterior to the equator and extrafoveolar. Patients with subfoveolar nevi are at certain risk of visual loss because of choriocapillaris disruption and subsequent disruption of photoreceptor outer segments. Also, a CNV complex may develop at the margins or over the choroidal nevus generating a serous neurosensory detachment [95]. In longstanding cases lipid deposition may precipitate in the subretinal space contouring the CNV lesion (Fig. 3.12).

Choroidal nevi arise from melanocytic cells derived from the neural crest [96, 97]. In general, the cells of a nevus cell are "plumper" than the normal melanocytes of the choroid and ciliary body. Morphologically, nevi are classified into

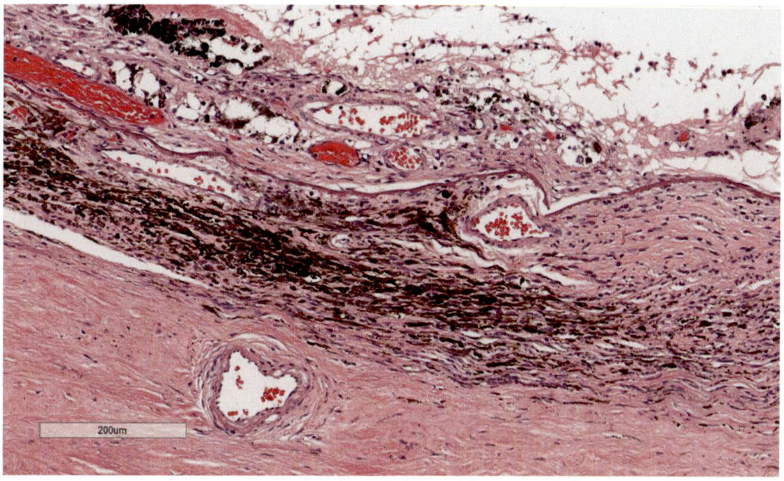

Fig. 3.12 Choroidal nevus. Note the CNV characterized by a vascularized fibrous membrane over Bruch's membrane. RPE and outer retinal segments are disrupted, H&E (100×)

four types: polyhedral, fusiform, spindle, and balloon cells [97].

1. Polyhedral nevus cells: This is the most common cell type found in nevi of the ciliary body and choroid. Its voluminous cytoplasm is densely packed with melanin, obscuring nuclear details. When sections are thoroughly bleached, a rather small, round, uniformly basophilic nucleus without a prominent nucleolus is seen. This cell accounts for over two-thirds of the mass in the majority of these nevi. It is indistinguishable from those cells that compose the melanocytomas of the optic disc and from those that diffusely thicken the choroid in congenital ocular melanocytosis.
2. Spindle nevus cells: This is considered the second most frequent cell type in benign pigmented tumors of the choroid. It is a small, spindle-shaped cell with a slender, intensely basophilic nucleus. Unlike polyhedral cells, these cells consistently contain little or no pigment and are often distributed in a striking manner in the outer portions of a nevus. Only rarely does this cell type make up the bulk of a nevus, which is then characteristically only lightly pigmented.
3. Fusiform and dendritic nevus cells: These cells are less intensely pigmented than the polyhedral cells and display a larger nucleus with a slightly loose chromatin pattern and occasionally even a small nucleolus. Furthermore, the cytoplasm is more abundant than in the spindle melanocytes.
4. Balloon cells: This subtype of cells is similar to cells found in cutaneous nevi. These are large cells with abundant foamy cytoplasm.

Histopathological alterations in the structures surrounding choroidal nevi include narrowing or dilatation of the choriocapillaris, atrophy and clumping of the retinal pigment epithelial (RPE), drusen formation, serous detachment of the neurosensory retina, subretinal neovascularization, and lipofuscin deposition [97–99].

3.6 Development Alterations or Malformations Associated CNV

3.6.1 Coloboma

Choroidal coloboma is a congenital malformation characterized by a failure during embryogenesis of the inner and outer layers to fuse along the optic fissure [100].

The simultaneous closure of the fissure and retinal differentiation, together with subsequent retinal growth, are vital with respect to the pathophysiology of the fissure in that only the inner neuroblastic layer of the retina, with its Müller cells, fuses across the fissure. The outer neuro-

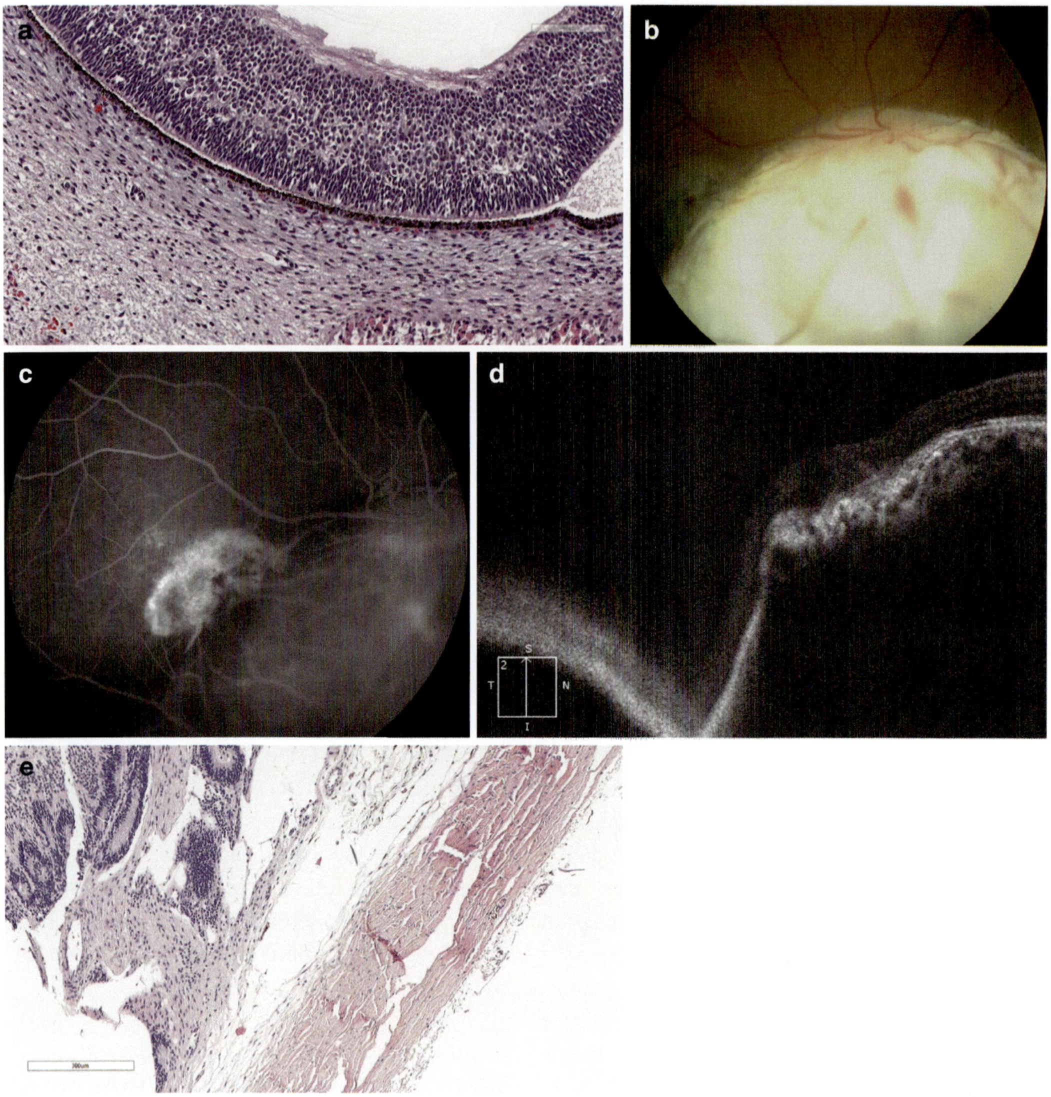

Fig. 3.13 Coloboma. (**a**) Histology of a normal developing eye in the 8th gestational week. Note the primitive two layers of the retina, immature choroid and sclera H&E 200× (**b**) Funduscopic image (**c**) Fluorescein angiography (**d**) SD-OCT image Histology of coloboma. The choroid is replaced only by a loose connective tissue. The retina in this image is dysplastic with rosette formation

blastic layer reverts and connects to the RPE (Fig. 3.13) [101].

As described by Schubert (2005), common histologic findings are [101]:

Pediatric coloboma is characterized by an intercalary membrane in direct contact with the sclera, central glial triangle, point of reversal and duplication of the photoreceptor layer, locus minoris resistentiae, and lateral displacement of the RPE. Also variable degrees of vascularization at the junction between the external limiting membrane and the RPE, the choroid ends together with the RPE and may be thickened and the sclera is thinned. Intrascleral rosettes may be present.

In adult coloboma marginal retinal vessels, marginal choroidal thickening and hyperplasia of the RPE are encountered together with vessels with intimal hyperplasia and absence of the glial triangle, point of reversal, duplication, and locus minoris resistentiae. The choroid is absent at the center and the sclera is thinned.

Choroidal neovascularization favors the margin of colobomas, with vessels tending to grow toward the intercalary membrane [102–104].

3.7 Unknown: Idiopathic CNV

The pathophysiological processes in idiopathic CNV remain unclear. Histopathology of this lesion may correspond to the general description of CNV [6].

Key Learning Points

CNV is a repair response during the healing process after injury due to the poor regenerative properties of the retina, Bruch's membrane, and choriocapillaris.

Choroidal neovascularization represents a nonspecific response to different etiologies.

In each disease, CNV may be accompanied by findings associated with the primary etiologic condition.

CNV may be localized in any part of the retina, but macular involvement is common.

References

1. Ramrattan RS, van der Schaft TL, Mooy CM, de Bruijn WC, Mulder PG, de Jong PT. Morphometric analysis of Bruch's membrane, the choriocapillaris, and the choroid in aging. Invest Ophthalmol Vis Sci. 1994;35(6):2857–64.
2. Kiel JW. The ocular circulation. In: Granger DN, Granger JP, editors. Integrated systems physiology: from molecule to function to disease. San Rafael, CA: Morgan & Claypool Life Sciences; 2010.
3. Strauss O. The retinal pigment epithelium in visual function. Physiol Rev. 2005;85(3):845–81.
4. Hanahan D, Folkman J. Patterns and emerging mechanisms of the angiogenic switch during tumorigenesis. Cell. 1996;86(3):353–64.
5. Grossniklaus HE, Green WR. Choroidal neovascularization. Am J Ophthalmol. 2004;137(3):496–503.
6. Grossniklaus HE, Miskala PH, Green WR, Bressler SB, Hawkins BS, Toth C, et al. Histopathologic and ultrastructural features of surgically excised subfoveal choroidal neovascular lesions: submacular surgery trials report no. 7. Arch Ophthalmol. 2005;123(7):914–21.
7. Barth T, Zeman F, Helbig H, Oberacher-Velten I. Etiology and treatment of choroidal neovascularization in pediatric patients. Eur J Ophthalmol. 2016;26(5):388–93.
8. Kuo IC, Cunningham ET Jr. Ocular neovascularization in patients with uveitis. Int Ophthalmol Clin. 2000;40(2):111–26.
9. Wu K, Zhang X, Su Y, Ji Y, Zuo C, Li M, et al. Clinical characteristics of inflammatory choroidal neovascularization in a Chinese population. Ocul Immunol Inflamm. 2016;24(3):261–7.
10. Querques L, Querques G, Miserocchi E, Modorati G, Bandello F. Intravitreal aflibercept for choroidal neovascularization in ocular sarcoidosis. Eur J Ophthalmol. 2016;26(5):e124–7.
11. Roy R, Saurabh K, Bansal A, Kumar A, Majumdar AK, Paul SS. Inflammatory choroidal neovascularization in Indian eyes: etiology, clinical features, and outcomes to anti-vascular endothelial growth factor. Indian J Ophthalmol. 2017;65(4):295–300.
12. Krill AE, Archer D. Choroidal neovascularization in multifocal (presumed histoplasmin) choroiditis. Arch Ophthalmol. 1970;84(5):595–604.
13. Macular Photocoagulation Study Group. Laser photocoagulation for neovascular lesions nasal to the fovea. Results from clinical trials for lesions secondary to ocular histoplasmosis or idiopathic causes. Arch Ophthalmol. 1995;113(1):56–61.
14. Dutta Majumder P, Biswas J, Gupta A. Enigma of serpiginous choroiditis. Indian J Ophthalmol. 2019;67(3):325–33.
15. Xerri O, Salah S, Monnet D, Brezin AP. Untreated acute posterior multifocal placoid pigment epitheliopathy (APMPPE): a case series. BMC Ophthalmol. 2018;18(1):76.
16. Bowie EM, Sletten KR, Kayser DL, Folk JC. Acute posterior multifocal placoid pigment epitheliopathy and choroidal neovascularization. Retina. 2005;25(3):362–4.
17. Pederson JE, Kenyon KR, Green WR, Maumenee AE. Pathology of pars planitis. Am J Ophthalmol. 1978;86(6):762–74.
18. Mehta S, Hariharan L, Ho AC, Kempen JH. Peripapillary choroidal neovascularization in pars planitis. J Ophthalmic Inflamm Infect. 2013;3(1):13.
19. Yanoff M, Sassani JW. Ocular pathology. 6th ed. Edinburgh: Mosby/Elsevier; 2009. p. x, 789.
20. Williams GT, Williams WJ. Granulomatous inflammation—a review. J Clin Pathol. 1983;36(7):723–33.
21. Silveira C, Belfort R Jr, Burnier M Jr, Nussenblatt R. Acquired toxoplasmic infection as the cause of toxoplasmic retinochoroiditis in families. Am J Ophthalmol. 1988;106(3):362–4.
22. Nussenblatt RB, Belfort R Jr. Ocular toxoplasmosis. An old disease revisited. JAMA. 1994;271(4):304–7.
23. Commodaro AG, Belfort RN, Rizzo LV, Muccioli C, Silveira C, Burnier MN Jr, et al. Ocular toxoplasmo-

sis: an update and review of the literature. Mem Inst Oswaldo Cruz. 2009;104(2):345–50.
24. Belfort RN, Rasmussen S, Kherani A, Lodha N, Williams G, Fernandes BF, et al. Bilateral progressive necrotizing retinochoroiditis in an immunocompromised patient: histopathological diagnosis. Acta Ophthalmol. 2010;88(5):614–5.
25. Benevento JD, Jager RD, Noble AG, Latkany P, Mieler WF, Sautter M, et al. Toxoplasmosis-associated neovascular lesions treated successfully with ranibizumab and antiparasitic therapy. Arch Ophthalmol. 2008;126(8):1152–6.
26. Gupta V, Gupta A, Rao NA. Intraocular tuberculosis—an update. Surv Ophthalmol. 2007;52(6):561–87.
27. Aggarwal K, Agarwal A, Sharma A, Sharma K, Gupta V, Group OS. Detection of type 1 choroidal neovascular membranes using optical coherence tomography angiography in tubercular posterior uveitis. Retina. 2019;39(8):1595–1606.
28. Centers for Disease Control and Prevention. Case definitions for infectious conditions under public health surveillance. MMWR Recomm Rep. 1997;46(RR-10):1–55.
29. Biswas J, Kazi MS, Agarwal VA, Alam MS, Therese KL. Polymerase chain reaction for Mycobacterium tuberculosis DNA detection from ocular fluids in patients with various types of choroiditis in a referral eye center in India. Indian J Ophthalmol. 2016;64(12):904–7.
30. Duke-Elder S, Perkin ES. System of ophthalmology: diseases of the uveal tract. St Louis: CV Mosby; 1966.
31. Lyon CE, Grimson BS, Peiffer RL Jr, Merritt JC. Clinicopathological correlation of a solitary choroidal tuberculoma. Ophthalmology. 1985;92(6):845–50.
32. Vrioni G, Levidiotou S, Matsiota-Bernard P, Marinis E. Molecular characterization of Mycobacterium tuberculosis isolates presenting various drug susceptibility from Greece using three DNA typing methods. J Infect. 2004;48(3):253–62.
33. Spencer WH. Ophthalmic pathology. 4rd ed. Philadelphia: W.B. Saunders; 1990.
34. Read RW, Rao NA. Utility of existing Vogt-Koyanagi-Harada syndrome diagnostic criteria at initial evaluation of the individual patient: a retrospective analysis. Ocul Immunol Inflamm. 2000;8(4):227–34.
35. Inomata H, Rao NA. Depigmented atrophic lesions in sunset glow fundi of Vogt-Koyanagi-Harada disease. Am J Ophthalmol. 2001;131(5):607–14.
36. Nakayama M, Keino H, Okada AA, Watanabe T, Taki W, Inoue M, et al. Enhanced depth imaging optical coherence tomography of the choroid in Vogt-Koyanagi-Harada disease. Retina. 2012;32(10):2061–9.
37. Bacsal K, Wen DS, Chee SP. Concomitant choroidal inflammation during anterior segment recurrence in Vogt-Koyanagi-Harada disease. Am J Ophthalmol. 2008;145(3):480–6.
38. Takahashi H, Takase H, Ishizuka A, Miyanaga M, Kawaguchi T, Ohno-Matsui K, et al. Choroidal thickness in convalescent Vogt-Koyanagi-Harada disease. Retina. 2014;34(4):775–80.
39. Lertsumitkul S, Whitcup SM, Nussenblatt RB, Chan CC. Subretinal fibrosis and choroidal neovascularization in Vogt-Koyanagi-Harada syndrome. Graefes Arch Clin Exp Ophthalmol. 1999;237(12):1039–45.
40. Rubsamen PE, Gass JD. Vogt-Koyanagi-Harada syndrome. Clinical course, therapy, and long-term visual outcome. Arch Ophthalmol. 1991;109(5):682–7.
41. Inomata H, Minei M, Taniguchi Y, Nishimura F. Choroidal neovascularization in long-standing case of Vogt-Koyanagi-Harada disease. Jpn J Ophthalmol. 1983;27(1):9–26.
42. Lubin JR, Ni C, Albert DM. Clinicopathological study of the Vogt-Koyanagi-Harada syndrome. Int Ophthalmol Clin. 1982;22(3):141–56.
43. Rao NA. Pathology of Vogt-Koyanagi-Harada disease. Int Ophthalmol. 2007;27(2–3):81–5.
44. Verma A, Biswas J. Choroidal granuloma as an initial manifestation of systemic sarcoidosis. Int Ophthalmol. 2010;30(5):603–6.
45. Cook BE Jr, Robertson DM. Confluent choroidal infiltrates with sarcoidosis. Retina. 2000;20(1):1–7.
46. Kawaguchi T, Hanada A, Horie S, Sugamoto Y, Sugita S, Mochizuki M. Evaluation of characteristic ocular signs and systemic investigations in ocular sarcoidosis patients. Jpn J Ophthalmol. 2007;51(2):121–6.
47. Olk RJ, Lipmann MJ, Cundiff HC, Daniels J. Solitary choroidal mass as the presenting sign in systemic sarcoidosis. Br J Ophthalmol. 1983;67(12):826–9.
48. Whitcup SM, Chan CC, Geiger GL. Diagnosis of corticosteroid resistant ocular sarcoidosis by chorioretinal biopsy. Br J Ophthalmol. 1999;83(4):504–5.
49. Hogan MJ, Zimmerman LE. Ophthalmic pathology, an atlas and textbook. 2nd ed. Philadelphia: W.B. Saunders; 1962. p. xiv, 797.
50. Gass JD, Olson CL. Sarcoidosis with optic nerve and retinal involvement. Arch Ophthalmol. 1976;94(6):945–50.
51. Frank KW, Weiss H. Unusual clinical and histopathological findings in ocular sarcoidosis. Br J Ophthalmol. 1983;67(1):8–16.
52. Spencer WH. Ophthalmic pathology: an atlas and textbook. 4th ed. Philadelphia: W.B. Saunders; 1996.
53. Mitchell P, Liew G, Gopinath B, Wong TY. Age-related macular degeneration. Lancet. 2018;392(10153):1147–59.
54. Anderson DH, Mullins RF, Hageman GS, et al. A role of for local inflammation in the formation of drusen in the aging eye. Am J Ophthalmol. 2002;134(3):411–31.
55. Kim JH, Chang YS, Kim JW, Kim CG, Lee DW. Age-related differences in the prevalence of subtypes of Neovascular age-related macular degeneration in the first diagnosed eye. Graefes Arch Clin Exp Ophthalmol. 2019;257(5):891–8.

56. Told R, Sacu S, Hecht A, Baratsits M, Eibenberger K, Kroh ME, et al. Comparison of SD-optical coherence tomography angiography and indocyanine green angiography in type 1 and 2 neovascular age-related macular degeneration. Invest Ophthalmol Vis Sci. 2018;59(6):2393–400.
57. D'Ambrosio E, Tortorella P, Iannetti L. Management of uveitis-related choroidal neovascularization: from the pathogenesis to the therapy. J Ophthalmol. 2014;2014:450428.
58. Yonekawa Y, Miller JW, Kim IK. Age-related macular degeneration: advances in management and diagnosis. J Clin Med. 2015;4(2):343–59.
59. Wu PC, Chen YJ, Chen CH, Chen YH, Shin SJ, Yang HJ, et al. Assessment of macular retinal thickness and volume in normal eyes and highly myopic eyes with third-generation optical coherence tomography. Eye. 2008;22(4):551–5.
60. Shimada N, Ohno-Matsui K, Harino S, Yoshida T, Yasuzumi K, Kojima A, et al. Reduction of retinal blood flow in high myopia. Graefes Arch Clin Exp Ophthalmol. 2004;242(4):284–8.
61. Shih YF, Fitzgerald ME, Norton TT, Gamlin PD, Hodos W, Reiner A. Reduction in choroidal blood flow occurs in chicks wearing goggles that induce eye growth toward myopia. Curr Eye Res. 1993;12(3):219–27.
62. Sayanagi K, Ikuno Y, Uematsu S, Nishida K. Features of the choriocapillaris in myopic maculopathy identified by optical coherence tomography angiography. Br J Ophthalmol. 2017;101(11):1524–9.
63. Steidl SM, Pruett RC. Macular complications associated with posterior staphyloma. Am J Ophthalmol. 1997;123(2):181–7.
64. Ohsugi H, Ikuno Y, Shoujou T, Oshima K, Ohsugi E, Tabuchi H. Axial length changes in highly myopic eyes and influence of myopic macular complications in Japanese adults. PLoS One. 2017;12(7):e0180851.
65. Dimitrova G, Tamaki Y, Kato S, Nagahara M. Retrobulbar circulation in myopic patients with or without myopic choroidal neovascularisation. Br J Ophthalmol. 2002;86(7):771–3.
66. Cohen SY, Laroche A, Leguen Y, Soubrane G, Coscas GJ. Etiology of choroidal neovascularization in young patients. Ophthalmology. 1996;103(8):1241–4.
67. Hotchkiss ML, Fine SL. Pathologic myopia and choroidal neovascularization. Am J Ophthalmol. 1981;91(2):177–83.
68. Fujiwara T, Imamura Y, Margolis R, Slakter JS, Spaide RF. Enhanced depth imaging optical coherence tomography of the choroid in highly myopic eyes. Am J Ophthalmol. 2009;148(3):445–50.
69. Ikuno Y, Jo Y, Hamasaki T, Tano Y. Ocular risk factors for choroidal neovascularization in pathologic myopia. Invest Ophthalmol Vis Sci. 2010;51(7):3721–5.
70. Ohno-Matsui K, Yoshida T, Futagami S, Yasuzumi K, Shimada N, Kojima A, et al. Patchy atrophy and lacquer cracks predispose to the development of choroidal neovascularisation in pathological myopia. Br J Ophthalmol. 2003;87(5):570–3.
71. Yokoi T, Ohno-Matsui K. Diagnosis and Treatment of Myopic Maculopathy. Asia Pac J Ophthalmol. 2018;7(6):415–21.
72. Yoshida T, Ohno-Matsui K, Yasuzumi K, Kojima A, Shimada N, Futagami S, et al. Myopic choroidal neovascularization: a 10-year follow-up. Ophthalmology. 2003;110(7):1297–305.
73. Nag TC, Kumari C. Electron microscopy of the human choroid. In: Chhablani J, Ruiz-Medrano J, editors. Choroidal disorders. London: Academic Press; 2017. p. 7–20.
74. Akkaya S. Spectrum of pachychoroid diseases. Int Ophthalmol. 2018;38(5):2239–46.
75. Cheung CMG, Lee WK, Koizumi H, Dansingani K, Lai TYY, Freund KB. Pachychoroid disease. Eye. 2019;33(1):14–33.
76. Ersoz MG, Arf S, Hocaoglu M, Sayman Muslubas I, Karacorlu M. Indocyanine green angiography of pachychoroid pigment epitheliopathy. Retina. 2018;38(9):1668–74.
77. Pang CE, Freund KB. Pachychoroid neovasculopathy. Retina. 2015;35(1):1–9.
78. Dansingani KK, Balaratnasingam C, Klufas MA, Sarraf D, Freund KB. Optical coherence tomography angiography of shallow irregular pigment epithelial detachments in pachychoroid spectrum disease. Am J Ophthalmol. 2015;160(6):1243–54.e2.
79. Phasukkijwatana N, Freund KB, Dolz-Marco R, Al-Sheikh M, Keane PA, Egan CA, et al. Peripapillary pachychoroid syndrome. Retina. 2018;38(9):1652–67.
80. Kumar A, Kumawat D, Sundar MD, Gagrani M, Gupta B, Roop P, et al. Polypoidal choroidal vasculopathy: a comprehensive clinical update. Ther Adv Ophthalmol. 2019;11:2515841419831152.
81. Goldhardt R, Rosen BS. Polypoidal choroidal vasculopathy. Curr Ophthalmol Rep. 2019;7(1):66–72.
82. Engelbert M, Chew EY, Yannuzzi LA. Macular telangiectasia. In: Ryan SJ, editor. Retina. 2. London: Elsevier; 2013. p. 1050–7.
83. Yannuzzi LA, Bardal AM, Freund KB, Chen KJ, Eandi CM, Blodi B. Idiopathic macular telangiectasia. Arch Ophthalmol. 2006;124(4):450–60.
84. Dreyer R, Green WR. The pathology of angioid streaks: a study of twenty-one cases. Trans Pa Acad Ophthalmol Otolaryngol. 1978;31(2):158–67.
85. Clarkson JG, Altman RD. Angioid streaks. Surv Ophthalmol. 1982;26(5):235–46.
86. Atmaca-Sonmez P, Heckenlively JR. Genetic disorders of the retina and optic nerve. In: Klintworth GK, Garner A, editors. Garner and Klintworth's pathobiology of ocular disease. 3rd ed. New York: Informa Healthcare; 2008. p. 753–94.
87. Venkatesh R, Bavaharan B, Yadav NK. Predictors for choroidal neovascular membrane formation and visual outcome following blunt ocular trauma. Ther Adv Ophthalmol. 2019;11:2515841419852011.

88. Ament CS, Zacks DN, Lane AM, Krzystolik M, D'Amico DJ, Mukai S, et al. Predictors of visual outcome and choroidal neovascular membrane formation after traumatic choroidal rupture. Arch Ophthalmol. 2006;124(7):957–66.
89. Smiddy WE, Hernandez E. Histopathologic characteristics of diode laser-induced chorioretinal adhesions for experimental retinal detachment in rabbit eyes. Arch Ophthalmol. 1992;110(11):1630–3.
90. Marshall J, Hamilton AM, Bird AC. Histopathology of ruby and argon laser lesions in monkey and human retina. A comparative study. Br J Ophthalmol. 1975;59(11):610–30.
91. Lehto KS, Tommila PV, Karma A. Choroidal osteoma: clues to diagnosis. Acta Ophthalmol Scand. 2007;85(2):218–20.
92. Shields CL, Sun H, Demirci H, Shields JA. Factors predictive of tumor growth, tumor decalcification, choroidal neovascularization, and visual outcome in 74 eyes with choroidal osteoma. Arch Ophthalmol. 2005;123(12):1658–66.
93. Gass JD, Guerry RK, Jack RL, Harris G. Choroidal osteoma. Arch Ophthalmol. 1978;96(3):428–35.
94. Williams AT, Font RL, Van Dyk HJ, Riekhof FT. Osseous choristoma of the choroid simulating a choroidal melanoma. Association with a positive 32P test. Arch Ophthalmol. 1978;96(10):1874–7.
95. Chien JL, Sioufi K, Surakiatchanukul T, Shields JA, Shields CL. Choroidal nevus: a review of prevalence, features, genetics, risks, and outcomes. Curr Opin Ophthalmol. 2017;28(3):228–37.
96. Jakobiec FA. Ocular anatomy, embryology, and teratology. Philadelphia: Harper & Row; 1982.
97. Naumann G, Yanoff M, Zimmerman LE. Histogenesis of malignant melanomas of the uvea. I. Histopathologic characteristics of nevi of the choroid and ciliary body. Arch Ophthalmol. 1966;76(6):784–96.
98. Naumann G, Zimmerman LE, Yanoff M. Visual field defect associated with choroidal nevus. Am J Ophthalmol. 1966;62(5):914–7.
99. Muscat S, Parks S, Kemp E, Keating D. Secondary retinal changes associated with choroidal naevi and melanomas documented by optical coherence tomography. Br J Ophthalmol. 2004;88(1):120–4.
100. Ammon V. Anatomische Untersuchung von Coloboma bulbi. Z Ophthalmol. 1830;1830:I.
101. Schubert HD. Structural organization of choroidal colobomas of young and adult patients and mechanism of retinal detachment. Trans Am Ophthalmol Soc. 2005;103:457–72.
102. Leff SR, Britton WA Jr, Brown GC, Lucier AC, Brown JF. Retinochoroidal coloboma associated with subretinal neovascularization. Retina. 1985;5(3):154–6.
103. Takenaka J, Yamane K, Minamoto A, Mishima HK, Hayashida H. Subretinal neovascularization associated with retinochoroidal coloboma. Eur J Ophthalmol. 2005;15(6):815–7.
104. Spitzer M, Grisanti S, Bartz-Schmidt KU, Gelisken F. Choroidal neovascularization in retinochoroidal coloboma: thermal laser treatment achieves long-term stabilization of visual acuity. Eye. 2006;20(8):969–72.

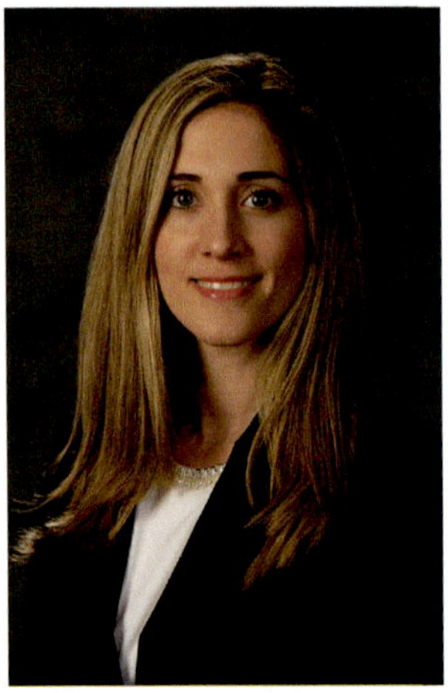

Evangelina Esposito, M.D., ChM., is an ophthalmologist from Argentina. Her fields are Ocular Pathology, Ocular Oncology, and Uveitis. She graduated as a physician in the National University of Córdoba, Argentina (2004–2009), and completed residency training in Ophthalmology at the Catholic University of Córdoba, Argentina (2011–2014). She finished an Ocular Pathology and Ocular Oncology fellowship at McGill University, Montreal, Canada (2015–2017). Dr. Esposito was awarded by the Argentinian Council of Ophthalmology (CAO) as a Distinguished Young Ophthalmologist in 2014 and by the McGill University Health Centre Foundation with the Leonard Ellen Ocular Pathology Fellowship in 2015. She also was awarded by the International Council of Ophthalmology (ICO) with The David E I Pyott Master of Surgery in Clinical Ophthalmology Scholarship (2017), and finished the second year of the ChM in Clinical Ophthalmology at the University of Edinburgh (2017–2019) with a distiction. She participates actively in teaching and research.

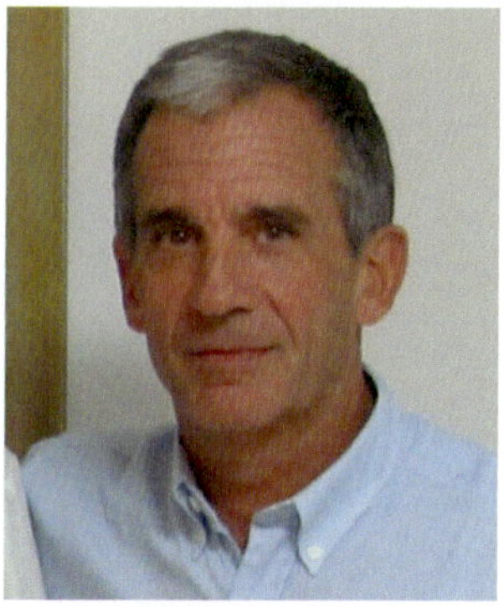

Julio A. Urrets-Zavalia, M.D., Ph.D., is a vitreo-retinal subspecialist and Chairman of the Department of Ophthalmology at the University Clinic Reina Fabiola, Catholic University of Cordoba, Argentina, since 1991.

He obtained his medical degree from the Faculty of Medical Sciences, National University of Cordoba, and his Ph.D. in Medicine from the Faculty of Health Sciences of the Catholic University of Cordoba, Argentina, and performed a fellowship in Retina at Department of Ophthalmology, Hôpital de la Croix-Rousse, Université Claude Bernard, Lyon, France.

Dr. Urrets-Zavalia is profesor and Chair of Ophthalmology Clinic, and director of the Postgraduate Degree in Ophthalmology at the Faculty of Health Sciences, Catholic University of Cordoba, Argentina.

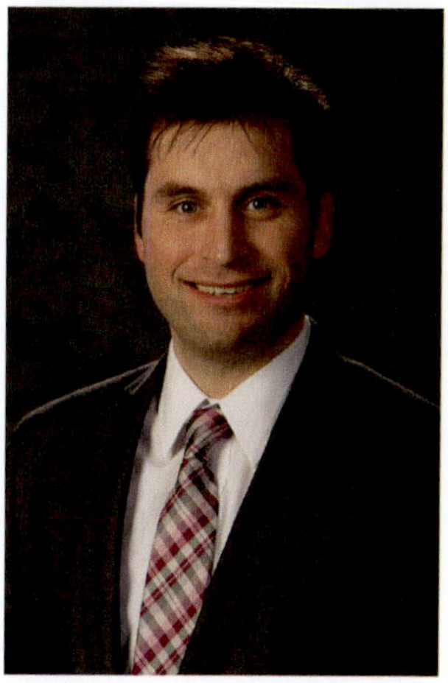

Pablo Zoroquiain is an Assistant Professor in the Department of Pathology and Ophthalmology, at Pontificia Universidad Católica de Chile, Santiago, Chile. He graduated from Universidad de los Andes, School of Medicine, and did a residency in Anatomical Pathology at Pontificia Universidad Católica de Chile, Santiago, Chile. He completed an Ocular Pathology Clinical and Research Fellowship at McGill University and a Doctorate in Ophthalmology and Visual Science at Universidad Federal de Sao Paulo (UNIFESP). Currently, he is an Ocular Pathologist, Cytopathologist, and the Director of the Cytopathology Laboratory at UC-Christus Health Center. He is author and co-author of over 80 publications including, 50 peer-reviewed papers, 32 peer-reviewed abstracts, and 2 book chapters. Dr. Zoroquiain is distinguished with several national and international awards. He has served as Guest Speaker at many conferences and symposia in the United States, England, Thailand, Brazil, Peru, and Chile.

4 Choroidal Neovascularization Animal Models

Takayuki Baba

4.1 Introduction

The wet type of age-related macular degeneration (AMD) is typically caused by choroidal neovascularization (CNV). The growing population of patients with wet AMD needs an effective modality of treatment. The treatment burden for patients and drug cost is still problematic although the extensive use of intravitreal anti-vascular endothelial growth factor (VEGF) injection enabled to treat wet AMD patients. To develop new drugs or treatment modality, an experimental model using animals is quite useful. Since the CNV grows only in vivo, there is no experimental model of CNV using cell or tissue culture. Therefore, the animal model which mimics human CNV is critical to test various molecules which have the potential to cure the CNV [1, 2]. The other pivotal role of an animal model is to investigate the mechanism of disease progression [3]. The exact cause of the development of CNV has not been determined yet although there were numerous studies conducted to elucidate the mechanism of disease. Since the tissues of active CNV are quite challenging to obtain, the investigation of an animal model is essential to understand the disease process.

T. Baba (✉)
Department of Ophthalmology and Visual Science, Chiba University Graduate School of Medicine, Chiba, Japan
e-mail: babatakayuki@nifty.com

The ideal animal model needs to have the following characteristics; (1) similarity to human CNV; (2) to clear ethical issues and to be justified for experimental use; and (3) the affordability for multiple purposes. Unfortunately, the perfect animal model which can duplicate human CNV is still not available. However, it is most important that the CNV should be very close to human CNV when the disease pathogenesisi is investigated. The ethical issue should be considered before starting experiments. For example, CNV in primate models is expected to have a similar response to the treatments as human CNV does. However, the advantage of using a primate model is limited to the ability to test the CNV located at macular. If the location of CNV does not matter for the experiment, the small animals such as mice or rats are good to be used. The use of small animals is also beneficial to reduce the cost of experiments. The price for animals themselves but also the expenses for maintaining animals are much less than keeping large animals and primates.

The history of an animal model of CNV started with the primate model of CNV created induced by laser [4]. They used Argon laser and found the subretinal neovascularization in 4 in 5 eyes after disruption of Bruch's membrane. Interestingly, the incidence of CNV formation is higher in eyes with laser-induced branch retinal vein occlusion in addition to the disruption of Bruch's membrane (9/11 eyes). It suggests the

J. Chhablani (ed.), *Choroidal Neovascularization*, https://doi.org/10.1007/978-981-15-2213-0_4

substantial effect of ischemia and inflammation which helps to grow CNV. The ischemic retina drives intraocular VEGF and seems to accelerate the development of CNV. At that point, this model is very reasonable.

Based on Ryan's CNV model, it has already suggested that the experimental CNV requires several factors to develop. First, the compensation of Bruch's membrane is always necessary. This can be explained by the fact that the increased level of angiogenic factors is not enough to cause the CNV [5, 6]. On the other hand, the CNV formation is confirmed simply after the disruption of Bruch's membrane using laser breaks or mechanical or chemical damage of Bruch's membrane [7]. For this instance, the size of CNV is relatively small suggesting the damage of Bruch's membrane is enough to grow CNV but not enough to extend to the large size. To create a large volume of CNV, the growth factors such as VEGF play an important role. The additional use of growth factor facilitates to obtain large and long-acting CNV [8]. The local inflammation and wound-healing process are also necessary to grow the large CNV. The inflammatory cytokines and growth factors can be increased in such occasions and result in helping the growth of the CNV.

The species mainly used for animal experiments are as follows: mice, rats, rabbits, pigs, and primates. The most commonly used are mice and rats. The size of the eyeball is small in mice but it is possible to create laser-induced CNV and subretinal injection with some difficulty. The availability of genetically engineered animals is an advantage of using mice models. On the other hand, the size of the rat's eyeball is larger than that of mice and enables subretinal injections more comfortable. The surgically induced CNV models with subretinal injection of various materials are available using rat. The low cost for maintaining those small rodents is another advantage when the cost is compared with those for large animals. The rabbit eye is much larger than the eyes of mice and rats and is more easily manipulated. The longitude of CNV is greater than the eyes of small rodents in the rabbit eyes. The disadvantage of rabbit eye is that they do not have macular and do have a different system of retinal vascular such as medullary ray from other animals including mice, rats, and primates. The size of the pig eye is similar to that of the human eye and surgical manipulation including vitrectomy is available. The disadvantages of using pig eyes are that the pig eye does not have macular and the expenses for obtaining and maintaining animals is high. The primate models have advantages such as the large size of the eyeball, the existence of macular, and close approximately to the human retina. The primate eyes also used for testing the drug delivery system and even used for clinical trials proceed to the human trial. The primate eye model is ideal for studying CNV but there is an ethical issue of using primate eyes when eyes of small rodents are already available as reliable models. The cost for animals itself and maintaining are also high.

4.2 Animal Models of CNV

4.2.1 Laser-Induced Model

The first laser-induced CNV model was reported by Ryan et al. in 1979 [4]. They used rhesus monkey and applied relatively strong Argon laser such as 200–900 mW with a duration of 0.1 s. The spot size was small about 50–100 micrometers and resulted in laser break of Bruch's membrane. The formation of CNV was confirmed in 4 of 5 eyes with laser break only and 9 of 11 eyes with a combination of laser break and retinal vein occlusion. Criswell et al. reported the characteristics of laser CNV in squirrel monkeys [9]. They used 532 nm and 664 nm diode laser mounted slit-lump and fundus was visualized using a Goldmann-type contact lens. Nine to twelve photocoagulations were placed as a grid pattern at the posterior fundus. Their laser setting was with laser power 104–650 mW, size with 70–75 micrometers, duration 0.01–1.0 s. They found 65% of lesions had CNV in squirrel monkey and 37% of lesions developed CNV in the macaque monkey. Histologically, the localized CNV tissue had the moderate to extensive thickening of choriocapillaris layer. Diffuse fibrovascular tissues expanded beyond laser spot and invaded into the retina in 76% of CNV in squirrel monkeys and 27% of macaque monkeys. They suggested that the CNVs have characteristics which are unique to spieces and squirrel monkey has more diffuse CNV allows studying neovascularization away from the trauma site.

The rat model of laser-induced CNV was first reported by Dobi et al. in 1989 [10]. They used 647 nm Krypton laser with a spot size of 100 micrometers, 50–160 mW, and duration of 0.1 s. The laser was mounted on the Zeiss-slit lump and the cover-slip was served as a contact lens. Long–Evans rats were used and the CNV was observed in 24–60% of eyes. One hundred and twenty megawatts of laser intensity was most reliable for inducing CNV in their settings. They also found the adequate power delivered shows the central bubble at the irradiated area and develops good CNV. If the laser is too weak or too strong, the CNV did not grow well. The excessively powerful laser made avascular scars without any CNV formation. The fluorescein angiography showed staining at 1 day corresponding to the acute injury and this hyperfluorescence disappeared at 1 week. The leakage of dye associated CNV was observed 2–6 weeks after the laser treatment. Sixty percent of the lesions presented the capillaries originating within the choroid extended through the disruption of Bruch's membrane into the subretinal space histologically. The overlying retina degenerated as well as pigment epithelium, outer nuclear layer, and outer plexiform layer. The disrupted area of Bruch's membrane had pigment-laden cells, fibroblasts, and collagen fibers.

The rabbit CNV model was reported in 1991 by El Dirini et al. [11] They used subretinal irradiation of laser using trans-vitreal glass pipette delivered into subretinal space. The argon laser power was 200–1100 mW and spot size was 100 micrometer with a duration of 0.05 s. They found no CNV formation in the eyes with low powers of 0.2–0.5 W but found CNV in 100% of lesions by histopathologically if the laser was applied with a high intensity such as 1000 mW. The fluorescein angiogram showed the hyperfluorescence at 1 and 3 days after the treatment but showed only faint tissue staining at 1–4 weeks postoperatively suggesting the proliferative retinal pigment epithelial cells ensheathed the CNV.

Tobe et al. used the mouse model of laser-induced CNV in 1998 [12]. The C57BL/6 J mice were used for the experiments. The laser was mounted on a slit-lump and a slide glass was used as a contact lens. They used Krypton laser with a spot size of 50 micrometers, 350–400 mW, and a duration of 0.05 s. They found CNV in 57% of treated eyes, and the central bubble formation which is the same as rat CNV is a good sign of initiating the CNV formation. Four weeks after the laser, the dye leakage was confirmed in 39% of the area by fluorescein angiography. Histological findings such as cellular tissue extending from choroid to subretinal space through the rupture of Bruch's membrane and pigment-laden macrophage-like cells and surrounding retinal pigment epithelial cells were observed at 3 days after the laser. One week after the laser, newly formed vessels with wide lumen from the choroid to subretinal space were found with pigment epithelial cells partly covering the new vessel.

A pig model was used by Saishin et al. for testing the effect of protein kinase inhibitors [13]. Four-week-old young Yorkshire pigs were treated by diode laser after the intubation and general anesthesia maintained with inhalation of 1–3% halothane, 2% O_2, and 1% NO_2. The Bruch's membrane rupture was made by laser with a power of 400 mW, size of 75 micrometers, and duration of 0.1 s. The minimal laser power was determined when the vaporization bubble was observed. They found CNV formation in 100% of eyes treated and it was confirmed by histologically. To test the ability to cease the formation of CNV via blocking VEGF, they measured the size of CNV by calculating the area of the GSA-lectin labeled vascular tissue in each slide through the laser spot.

Overall, the laser-induced model was strongly associated with the rupture of Bruch's membrane and if there is no damage to the Bruch's membrane, there was no CNV formation. At that point, this model is a wound-healing model and has a self-limited course. Although the mechanism of developing CNV is different from the human CNV, the advantage of the laser-induce CNV model should be evaluated. The simple technique of using the laser, the reproducibility of CNV if the proper setting of laser is used, the short time-course of CNV to develop are the merits of this model. Multiple lesions created in one eye enables the multiple evaluations of treatment modalities and contributes to increasing the efficacy of trials.

4.3 Surgically Induced Model

The formation is CNV can be obtained by injecting various materials into the subretinal space. For the technical reason, larger animals are preferred but there were numerous reports using mouse and rat for the background of this model. Subretinal injection is necessary to the process of this model; the mechanically induced CNV models are surgically induced models of CNV. The nature of these models varies based on the materials or drug injected subretinally.

VEGF is a major player to develop neovascularization. The induction of rat $VEGF_{164}$ cDNA using adenovirus vector which is injected in subretinal space of rat caused CNV in 86% of eyes [14]. The overexpression of mRNA of VEGF was observed in retinal pigment epithelial cells by 10–31 days postoperatively. The formation of CNV was confirmed by histologically at 80 days after the injection concomitant with the degeneration of overlying retina. The severity of CNV depended on the amount of vector. Baffi et al. used adenovirus vector coding $VEGF_{165}$ to promote CNV by subretinal injection [15]. They used Long–Evans rat and found the elevated expression of VEGF at retinal pigment epithelium 1 week after the injection. The formation of CNV was confirmed by fluorescein angiography, histology using flatmount choroid, and transmission electron microscope from 2 to 4 weeks post injection. Although their concentration of adenovirus coding $VEGF_{165}$ was much smaller than that used in Spilsbury's study, the mitogenic effect on vascular endothelial tissue was still significant. Julien and Kreppel et al. injected high-capacity adenoviral vector expressing VEGF-A_{165} into the subretinal space of Chinchilla bastard rabbits [8]. The leakage from CNV was observed by scanning laser ophthalmoscopy with fluorescein and indocyanine green at 2 and 4 weeks in 15 of 18 eyes (83%). Pathological subretinal vessel formation was confirmed with activated endothelial cells and macrophages. They demonstrated the elevation of basic fibrous growth factor as well as VEGF. Cui et al. used VEGF-impregnated gelatin microspheres injected intravitreally into the subretinal space of *Macaca mulatta* monkeys [16]. The CNV developed in 12 of 13 eyes (92%) and the leakage from CNV was confirmed by fluorescein angiography from 2 to 12 weeks after the injection. The immunohistochemical findings showed the CD31-positive new vessels at 1–8 weeks and glial fibrillary acidic protein at 6 weeks suggesting glial proliferation. Macrophages engaged early point at day 3 but not found on day 7 and after.

Schmack and Berglin et al. injected polystyrene microbeads and retinal epithelial cells into the subretinal space of C57BL6 mice [17]. The overall incidence of CNV was 94%. The CNV thickness became maximal at 7 days post injection of C57BL6-derived RPE cells and polystyrene microbeads simultaneously. The activated retinal pigment cells expressed not only VEGF but other chemotactic and inflammatory cytokines such as MCP-1, MMP-2, MMP-9 which lead to the development of CNV. The cell-2 deficient mouse showed smaller CNV after subretinal injection suggested the recruitment of macrophages in the process of CNV formation.

Matrigel, a basement membrane extract, is used for solidifying tissue and it can stimulate angiogenesis. Shen et al. used Matrigel to induce CNV by injecting subretinally [18]. They used wildtype and Ccl2-deficient mouse and found the CNV formation in 31% and 53% of eyes, respectively. Ccl2, a member of MCP of CC-chemokine is known to have a protective role against AMD. In their study, the CNV developed in 31% of eyes in wildtype and 53% of eyes in the Ccl2-deficient group suggesting the involvement of macrophages and chemotaxis in the formation of CNV. Qiu et al. used pigmented rabbit and injected Matrigel with or without a various concentration of VEGF [19]. They found CNV in 100% of eyes injected Matrigel and none of the eyes injected PBS. The CNV developed 2–4 weeks after injection and lasted at 9 weeks after that. The activity of CNV was confirmed by fluorescein angiography and the CNV was histologically confirmed. They also performed optical coherence tomography to reveal the subretinal fluid suggesting the leaky vessel within the lesion.

It resembles the laser rupture of Bruch's membrane that the perforation of Bruch's membrane by a needle developed CNV in rabbit eyes [7]. The subretinal neovascularization was observed arising from the site of the perforation of Bruch's membrane in the eyes of pigmented rabbits. The injury was made by a scalpel blade trans-sclerally. The degeneration of photoreceptors and proliferation of retinal pigment epithelium were also observed. The neovascularization extended beyond the scar of Bruch's membrane. Lassota et al. used 12-week-old domestic pigs and compared the techniques of perforating Bruch's membrane transvitreally with and without removal of the retinal pigment epithelium [20]. They found CNV formation with both techniques at 14 days after the injection but the CNV was more prominent in eyes with Bruch's rupture without retinal pigment epithelial removal. They suggested that the VEGF secreted by retinal pigment epithelium was reduced after the removal of cells and resulted in reduced stimuli to grow CNV. This model does not require any special agents or drugs to promote CNV growth. At that point, this is a good simple model but is eventually a wound-healing process and the lifetime of CNV is unknown.

Tamai et al. injected 12.5–25 micrograms of linoleic acid hydroperoxide (18:2/LHP) into the subretinal space of rabbits and found the CNV in 11 of 14 eyes (46%) histologically [21]. When they injected 150–200 micrograms of LHP, severe retinal and choroidal atrophy was observed, but no CNV developed. The fluorescein angiography showed no hyper fluorescence at 1 week but leakage was evident at 2 and 4 weeks postoperatively. After the injection of LHP, Armstrong et al. found that the level of VEGF, transforming growth factor-b, and platelet-derived growth factor peaked at 24 hours and sustained at the high level throughout the following 3 weeks in the postoperative period [22]. Those angiogenic cytokines play roles to develop CNV after the injection of LHP.

We used Sprague–Dawley rats to develop a lipid-induced CNV model [23]. 13(S)-Hydroperoxy-9Z,11E-octadecadienoic acid (HpODE) is one of several oxidized lipids, which exist under normal conditions in cell membranes of the human body [24]. We injected 13(S)-HPODE into the subretinal space using a glass needle and a pico-injector. The formation of CNV was confirmed by histology including JB-4 embedded thin sections, immunohistochemistry with a confocal microscope, and transmission electron microscope. The course of CNV development was observed by fluorescein angiography. Typically, some small hyperfluorescent spots were found at 1 week and more intense leakage was observed at 2 weeks and the leakage was most prominent at 3–4 weeks and decreased at 5 weeks suggesting the reduced or matured CNV (Fig. 4.1). We found the CNV in 6 of 7 eyes (85.7%) which were injected 30 microgram of HPODE in 2 microliters of borate buffer (Fig. 4.2). Lipids were confirmed at inside of CNV and surrounding retina, and ED1 (CD68) positive circulating monocyte and ED2 (CD163) positive resident macrophage were recruited in the CNV (Fig. 4.3). We suggested the 13(S) HPODE-stimulated inflammatory cells or retinal pigment epithelial cells degraded the Bruch's membrane by tissue protease and stimulated endothelial cells by secreting growth factors such as VEGF and eventually developed CNV. Since HPODE exists in Bruch's membrane naturally and was found more in the eyes of aged human and eyes with age-related macular degeneration [24], this model using subretinal HPODE is a good model that mimics human CNV with high reproducibility and ideal time course to evaluate therapeutic modalities.

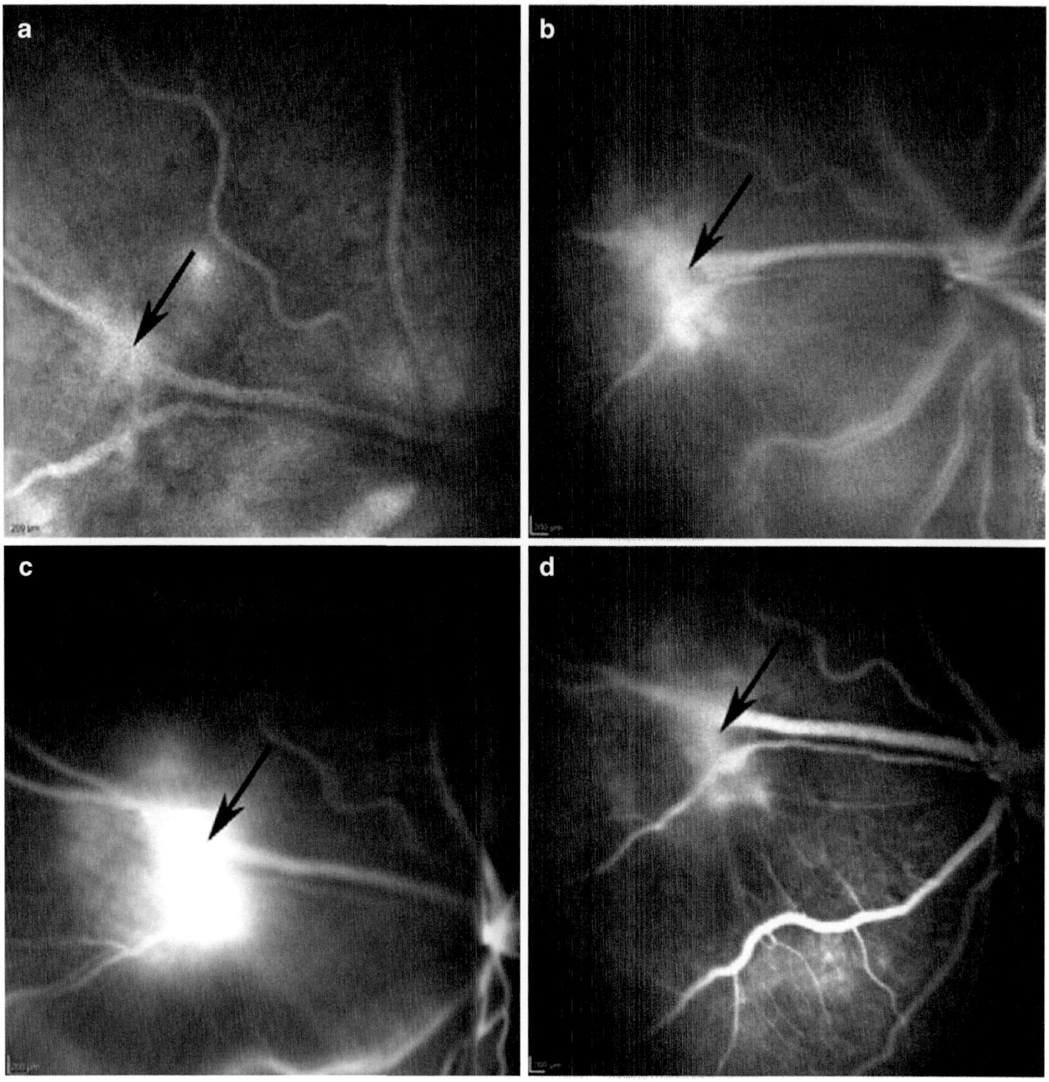

Fig. 4.1 Fluorescein angiographic image of the eye after subretinal injection of 30 micrograms of HpODE. The timing in each angiogram was about one and a half minutes after the injection of dye. (**a**) A small dye leakage was observed at 1 week (arrow). Greater leakage was observed at 2 weeks (**b**, arrow) and was greatest at 3 weeks (**c**, arrow). (**d**) The leakage area decreased at 5 weeks (arrow). (From Baba T et al., 2010 [23])

4.4 Genetically Engineered Model

The Ccr2/Ccl2 deficient mouse model was developed by Ambati et al. [25, 26]. Ccr2/Ccl2 deficient transgenic mouse fails to recruit macrophages to the area of the RPE and Bruch's membrane because those chemotactic cytokines and receptors control inflammatory cells. They found 25% of the eyes of their transgenic animals and the accumulation of C5a and IgG suggested the source of VEGF.

The Ccl2/Cx3cr1 deficient double knockout mouse was developed by Chan et al. [27] Their mouse had increased N-retinylidene-N-retinylethanolamine (A2E) and decreased DRp20 levels in the RPE. These mice had the changes of retinal pigment epithelium and drusen-like lesions if the mouse fed a diet low in omega-3 polyunsaturated fatty acids (PUFAs). Ccl2 is

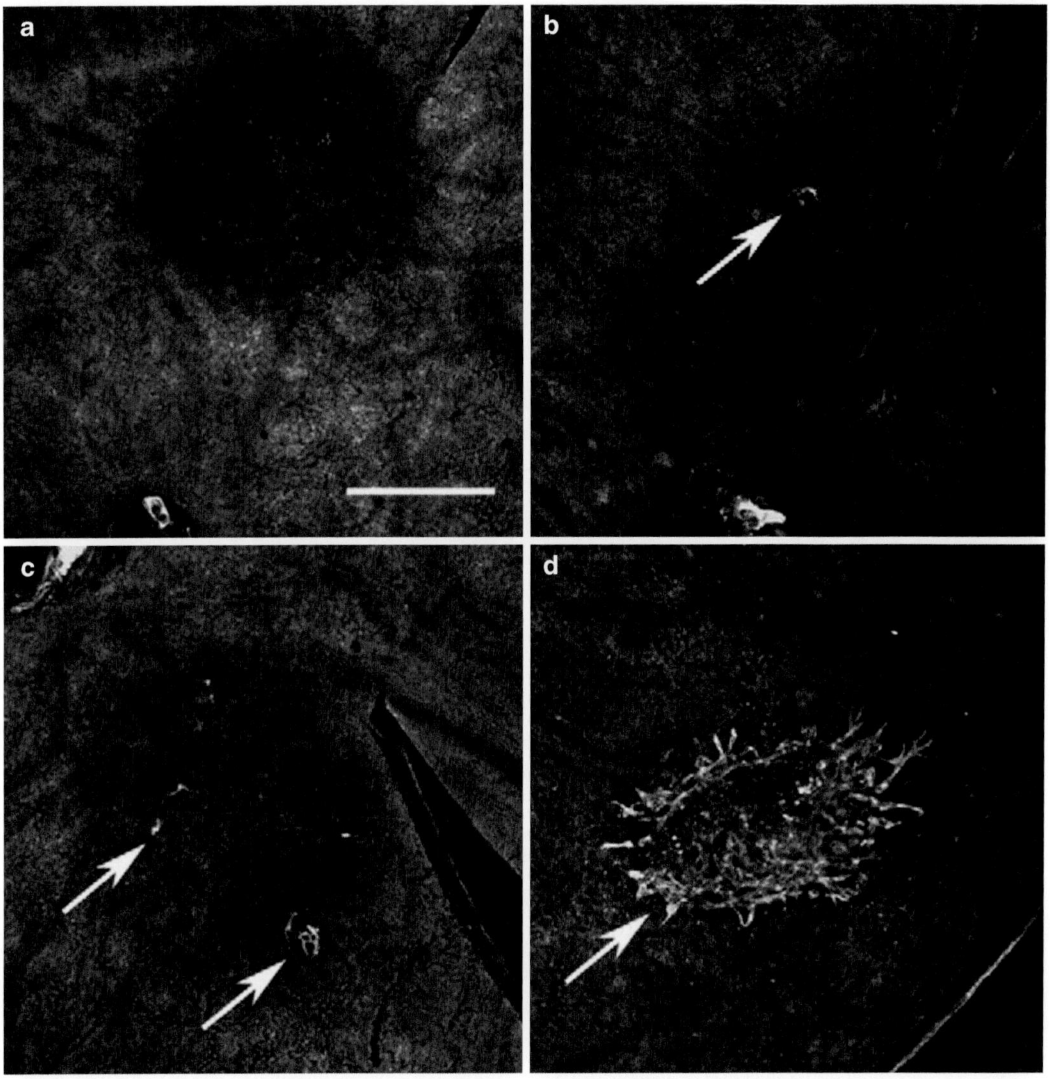

Fig. 4.2 Images of HpODE-induced CNV. GSA-lectin visualized the neovascularization in flatmount choroid at 3 weeks after injection. (**a**) No CNV was observed after one microgram of HpODE injection. (**b** and **c**) Five micrograms (**b**) and 15 micrograms (**c**) of HpODE caused CNV (arrows); Relatively small CNV was observed. (**d**) Thirty micrograms of HpODE caused significantly large CNV (arrow). Scale bar: 500 micrometers. (From Baba T et al., [23])

necessary to recruit monocyte and CX3CR1 moves circulating monocytes to tissues and makes them into resident macrophages and dendritic cells [28]. In these mice, CNV was found histologically in 15% of animals in 6 weeks.

The Cu, Zn-superoxide dismutase (SOD1) deficient mice had funduscopically and histologically evident CNV in 8.3% and 10% of animals [29]. One of the antioxidative systems in the eye is Cu, Zn-SOD1 in the cytosol and the most major scavenger of oxidative stress. In 3 of 30 animals (10%) which is older than 10 months, they found the CNV histologically. In the animals that had a CNV formation, the fibrovascular tissue extended through the rupture of Bruch's membrane. The drusen formation and thickened Bruch's membrane were commonly observed in the older mice. Therefore, the senecient SOD1−/− mice had characteristics of dry and wet human AMD.

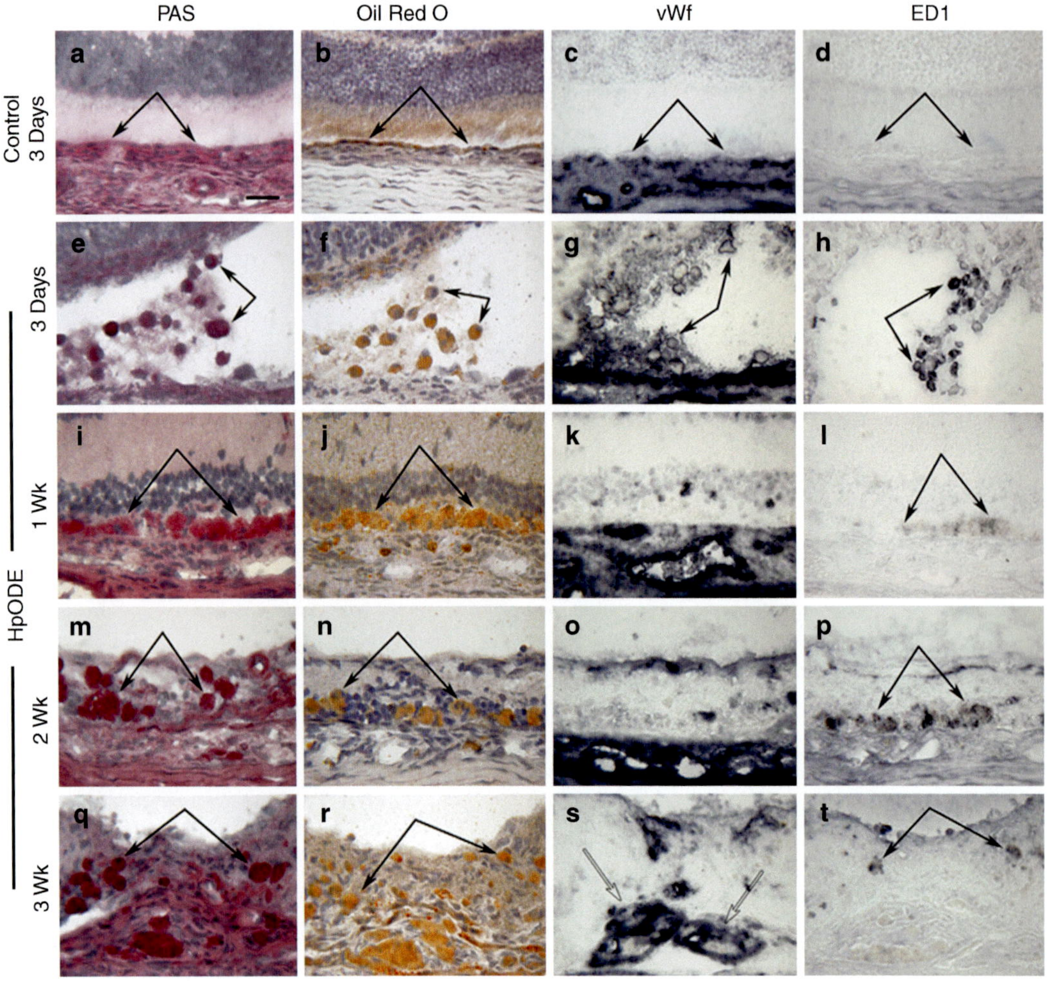

Fig. 4.3 Histological images after buffer (A–D) or HpODE (E–T) injection. PAS-positive RPE cells were observed at 3 days after buffer injection (**a**, paired arrows). The RPE cells contained no lipids (**b**, paired arrows). There was no labelling by vWF (**c**, paired arrows) or ED1 of the cells (**d**, paired arrows) in the subretinal space. (**e**) At 3 days after the HpODE injection, PAS-positive cells were abundant (paired arrows) in the space between retina and RPE. (**f**) These cells contained lipids (paired arrows) and soluble vWF (**g**, paired arrows) was observed around the ED1-positive cells (**h**, paired arrows). One week after the injection of HpODE there were PAS-positive cells on Bruch's membrane (**i**, paired arrows) with lipids (**j**, paired arrows). There were ED1-positive cells among them (L, paired arrows). (**k**) Some vWF structures suggesting retinal capillaries are observed in the inner nuclear layer. (**m**) At 2 weeks after the injection of HpODE, the degenerated photoreceptors were observed. (**m** and **n**) In the subretinal space, PAS-positive, lipid-laden cells were observed (paired arrows). (**o**) There is a vWF structure suggesting a deep retinal capillary in the inner nuclear layer. (**p**) There were some subretinal ED1-positive cells (paired arrows). (**s**) By 3 weeks, a subretinal CNV formation was clearly labeled with vWF (open arrows). PAS-positive material and cells are observed in subretinal space (**q**, paired arrows), lipids (**r**, paired arrows), and some ED1-labeled cells (**t**, paired arrows) above the CNV. Scale bar 30 micrometers. (From Baba T et al., [23])

The nuclear factor erythroid-2 related factor 2 (Nrf2) is important for cell response to oxidative stress and toxification. The Nrf2 deficient mouse had an age-dependent degenerative change of retinal pigment epithelium and drusen-like deposition and accumulation of lipofuscin, deposition of sub pigment epithelial inflammatory protein [30]. The CNV was confirmed using histology in 3 of 17 eyes (18%) of animals with age 11–17 months. The eyes with CNV also presented subretinal hemorrhage and exudate which are typical findings of human CNV.

4.5 Conclusion

Excellent quality of experimental models needs the comparability to human disease and reproducibility for repeating experiments. Also, the affordability of animal is vital for continuing the project and clearing ethical problems is also necessary to justify the use of animals for research for a human being. Therefore, the perfect animal model is desirable, but it is quite challenging to obtain. In terms of the CNV model for wet AMD, there is a variety of experimental models. Three major approaches to develop CNV are laser, surgery, and genetic manipulation. Each option can be used to small to large animals except for genetic engineering is mainly for mice. It is important to use the proper model suitable for what to see through the experiments. Because the response to drug is different from human CNV, e.g., less response of rodent CNV to bevacizumab and ranibizumab, great caution should be paid to test the treatment modalities [31].

Key Learning Messages

- There are three major types of experimental CNV models.
- A laser-induced CNV model is reproducible but the mechanism is a wound-healing process which has a relatively short time course.
- A surgically induced CNV model is more physiological but technically challenging in some models using small rodents.
- Some of the genetically engineered models mimic human disease very well but it takes a relatively long time to develop CNV.
- Models using small rodents are affordable and reproducible but do not have macular.
- Models using large animals including primates have high comparability to human CNV but have ethical and financial issues.
- The selection of models varies based on the purpose of investigation or trial for treatment modalities.

References

1. Grossniklaus HE, Kang SJ, Berglin L. Animal models of choroidal and retinal neovascularization. Prog Retin Eye Res. 2010;29:500–19.
2. Pennesi ME, Neuringer M, Courtney RJ. Animal models of age related macular degeneration. Mol Asp Med. 2012;33:487–509.
3. Campochiaro PA. Molecular pathogenesis of retinal and choroidal vascular diseases. Prog Retin Eye Res. 2015;49:67–81.
4. Ryan SJ. The development of an experimental model of subretinal neovascularization in disciform macular degeneration. Trans Am Ophthalmol Soc. 1979;77:707–45.
5. Ohno-Matsui K, Hirose A, Yamamoto S, et al. Inducible expression of vascular endothelial growth factor in adult mice causes severe proliferative retinopathy and retinal detachment. Am J Pathol. 2002;160:711–9.
6. Oshima Y, Oshima S, Nambu H, et al. Increased expression of VEGF in retinal pigmented epithelial cells is not sufficient to cause choroidal neovascularization. J Cell Physiol. 2004;201:393–400.
7. Hsu HT, Goodnight R, Ryan SJ. Subretinal choroidal neovascularization as a response to penetrating retinal injury in the pigmented rabbit. Jpn J Ophthalmol. 1989;33:358–66.
8. Julien S, Kreppel F, Beck S, et al. A reproducible and quantifiable model of choroidal neovascularization induced by VEGF A165 after subretinal adenoviral gene transfer in the rabbit. Mol Vis. 2008;14:1358–72.
9. Criswell MH, Ciulla TA, Hill TE, et al. The squirrel monkey: characterization of a new-world primate model of experimental Choroidal neovascularization and comparison with the macaque. Invest Ophthalmol Vis Sci. 2004;45:625–34.
10. Dobi ET, Puliafito CA, Destro M. A new model of experimental choroidal neovascularization in the rat. Arch Ophthalmol. 1989;107:264–9.
11. elDirini AA, Ogden TE, Ryan SJ. Subretinal endophotocoagulation. A new model of subretinal neovascularization in the rabbit. Retina. 1991;11:244–9.
12. Tobe T, Ortega S, Luna JD, et al. Targeted disruption of the FGF2 gene does not prevent choroidal neovascularization in a murine model. Am J Pathol. 1998;153:1641–6.
13. Saishin Y, Silva RL, Saishin Y, et al. Periocular injection of microspheres containing PKC412 inhibits Choroidal neovascularization in a porcine model. Invest Ophthalmol Vis Sci. 2003;44:4989–93.
14. Spilsbury K, Garrett KL, Shen WY, et al. Overexpression of vascular endothelial growth factor (VEGF) in the retinal pigment epithelium leads to the development of choroidal neovascularization. Am J Pathol. 2000;157:135–44.
15. Baffi J, Byrnes G, Chan CC, Csaky KG. Choroidal neovascularization in the rat induced by adenovirus

mediated expression of vascular endothelial growth factor. Invest Ophthalmol Vis Sci. 2000;41:3582–9.
16. Cui JZ, Kimura H, Spee C, et al. Natural history of choroidal neovascularization induced by vascular endothelial growth factor in the primate. Graefes Arch Clin Exp Ophthalmol. 2000;238:326–33.
17. Schmack I, Berglin L, Nie X, et al. Modulation of choroidal neovascularization by subretinal injection of retinal pigment epithelium and polystyrene microbeads. Mol Vis. 2009;15:146–61.
18. Shen D, Wen R, Tuo J, et al. Exacerbation of retinal degeneration and choroidal neovascularization induced by subretinal injection of Matrigel in CCL2/MCP-1-deficient mice. Ophthalmic Res. 2006;38:71–3.
19. Qiu G, Stewart JM, Sadda S, et al. A new model of experimental subretinal neovascularization in the rabbit. Exp Eye Res. 2006;83:141–52.
20. Lassota N, Kiilgaard JF, Prause JU, et al. Surgical induction of choroidal neovascularization in a porcine model. Graefes Arch Clin Exp Ophthalmol. 2007;245:1189–98.
21. Tamai K, Spaide RF, Ellis EA, et al. Lipid hydroperoxide stimulates subretinal choroidal neovascularization in the rabbit. Exp Eye Res. 2002;74:301–8.
22. Armstrong D, Ueda T, Ueda T, et al. Lipid hydroperoxide stimulates retinal neovascularization in rabbit retina through expression of tumor necrosis factor-alpha, vascular endothelial growth factor and platelet-derived growth factor. Angiogenesis. 1998;2:93–104.
23. Baba T, Bhutto IA, Merges C, et al. A rat model for choroidal neovascularization using subretinal lipid hydroperoxide injection. Am J Pathol. 2010;176:3085–97.
24. Spaide RF, Ho-Spaide WC, Browne RW, Armstrong D. Characterization of peroxidized lipids in Bruch's membrane. Retina. 1999;19:141–7.
25. Ambati J, Anand A, Fernandez S, et al. An animal model of age-related macular degeneration in senescent Ccl-2- or Ccr-2-deficient mice. Nat Med. 2003;9:1390–7.
26. Takeda A, Baffi JZ, Kleinman ME, et al. CCR3 is a target for age-related macular degeneration diagnosis and therapy. Nature. 2009;460:225–30.
27. Chan CC, Ross RJ, Shen D, et al. Ccl2/Cx3cr1-deficient mice: an animal model for age-related macular degeneration. Ophthalmic Res. 2008;40:124–8.
28. Geissmann F, Jung S, Littman DR. Blood monocytes consist of two principal subsets with distinct migratory properties. Immunity. 2003;19:71–82.
29. Imamura Y, Noda S, Hashizume K, et al. Drusen, choroidal neovascularization, and retinal pigment epithelium dysfunction in SOD1-deficient mice: a model of age-related macular degeneration. Proc Natl Acad Sci U S A. 2006;103:11282–7.
30. Zhao Z, Chen Y, Wang J, et al. Age-related retinopathy in NRF2-deficient mice. PLoS One. 2011;6:e19456.
31. Lu F, Adelman RA. Are intravitreal bevacizumab and ranibizumab effective in a rat model of choroidal neovascularization? Graefes Arch Clin Exp Ophthalmol. 2009;247:171–7.

Electron Microscopy of the Choroidal Neovascularization

5

Tapas C. Nag and Sneha Gupta

5.1 Introduction

Age-related macular degeneration is a serious ocular problem of the elderly (>50 years), especially those living in the advanced countries. In this disease, the capillary layer of the choroid, called the choriocapillaris [1–3] is critically affected, along with Bruch's membrane, a collagenous layer that separates the retina from it [4], and the outer retina comprising the retinal pigment epithelium and photoreceptor cells [5–9]. Aging is considered a risk factor that initiates the development of age-related macular degeneration. There are gradual alterations in the contents of retinal pigment epithelium, Bruch's membrane (BM), and the choriocapillaris with progressive aging, resulting in the death of capillaries. Due to some unknown situations, these changes culminate in the disease manifestations, wherein excessive tissue changes and capillary loss result in the diminished supply of oxygen and vital nutrients to the retinal pigment epithelium. As a result, the retinal pigment epithelium becomes hypofunctional, and gradually photoreceptor cells die from the macula. The latter is ultimately responsible for vision loss, affecting the regular activities and lifestyle patterns in the elderly.

The initial course of the disease, called dry age-related macular degeneration (accounting for 90% of all cases), begins with the formation and deposition of some yellowish materials, called drusen, in the macula with aging. Electron microscopy has confirmed these materials as degenerative tissue remnants that most likely arise from degenerated retinal pigment epithelium, besides other undefined sources. There is a limitation in visual capabilities (e.g., difficulty in reading) in the affected individuals, though it is not severe at this early stage with dry age-related macular degeneration. The situation progresses slowly in untreated cases (and if the diet lacks carotenoids and vitamins) and over a period of years, there is substantial death of macular photoreceptors and retinal pigment epithelium. The loss of the retinal pigment epithelium may be extensive in another clinical condition, called geographic atrophy [7, 9, 10]. In rather unfavorable situations in about 10% of the total victims, the dry age-related macular degeneration may take a sight threatening form, called wet or exudative age-related macular degeneration. Choroidal neovascularization (CNV) is clinically a devastating event in wet age-related macular degeneration. This chapter deals with the electron microscope data of CNV reported in affected individuals secondary to age-related macular degeneration.

T. C. Nag (✉) · S. Gupta
Neurobiology Laboratory, Department of Anatomy, All India Institute of Medical Sciences, New Delhi, India

J. Chhablani (ed.), *Choroidal Neovascularization*, https://doi.org/10.1007/978-981-15-2213-0_5

5.1.1 Choroidal Neovascularization

Figure 5.1 demonstrates the capillary layer of the choriocapillaris in a normal, aged human donor. In wet age-related macular degeneration, CNV results in abnormal development of vessels from the choriocapillaris. It has two well-recognized categories: (1) occult CNV, when the growth of vessels is not marked, and there is minimal leakage from those vessels, and (2) classical CNV, when the growth of vessels is prominent beneath the retina, which leads to more leakage of blood and severe loss of central vision. Depending on the site and spreading of new vessels, CNV can be categorized into three types: (1) type 1, when CNV is limited predominantly between BM and retinal pigment epithelium (subretinal pigment epithelium pattern; Figs. 5.2 and 5.3); (2) type 2, when vessel growth is reached between the retinal pigment epithelium and retina (subretinal pattern); and (3) the combined pattern, when subretinal pigment epithelium new vessels extend into the subretinal space [11–13].

5.2 Risk Factors for CNV

In wet age-related macular degeneration, the abnormal development of new vessels is linked with certain altered histophysiological alterations of the BM and retinal pigment epithelium. These changes are likely to be the risk factors

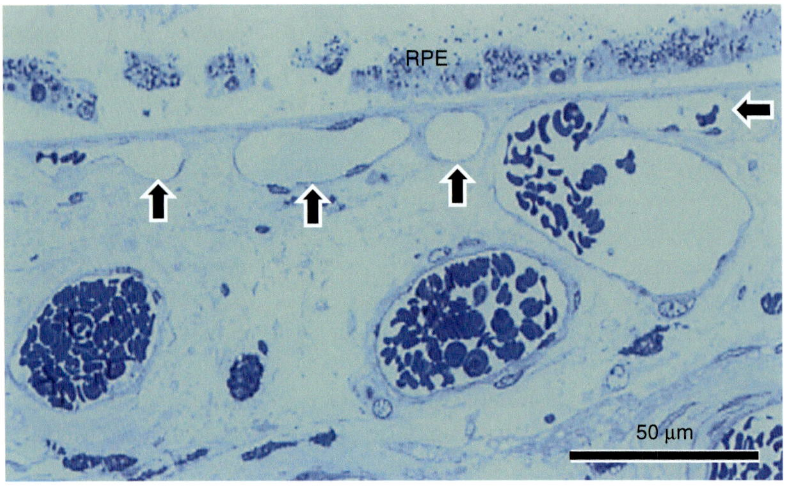

Fig. 5.1 Light micrograph of toluidine blue-stained choroid from a normal 64-year-old donor, showing capillaries (arrows) of the choriocapillaris layer, from which pathological neovascularization begins in wet AMD

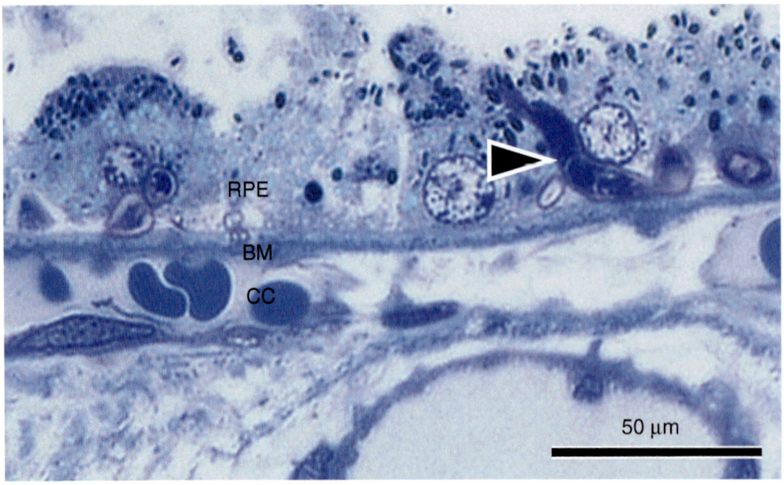

Fig. 5.2 Light micrograph showing a capillary lying in the RPE layer (arrowhead) of 89-year-old donor retina. Bruch's membrane (BM) and choriocapillaris (CC) are indicated

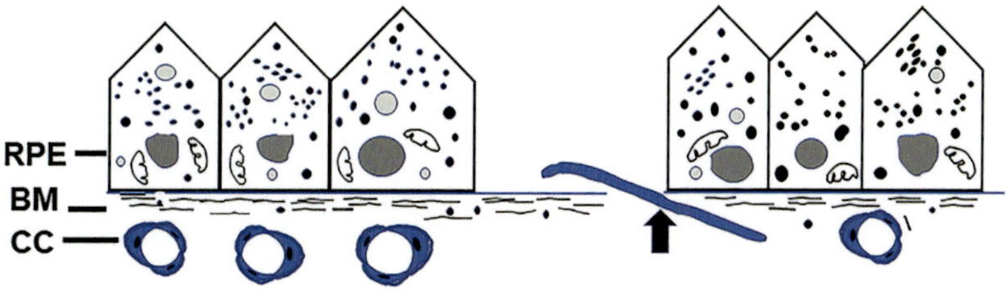

Fig. 5.3 Diagram showing the formation of a new vessel (arrow) between Bruch's membrane (BM) and RPE (sub-RPE pattern). The vessel originates from the choriocapillaris (CC)

for CNV. Currently, the identified major risk factors are:

1. Drusen characteristics
2. Calcification and disintegration of BM
3. Focal hyperpigmentation of the macular RPE
4. Accumulation of polar phospholipids in BM
5. Choriocapillaris loss

The significance of these individual factors predisposing CNV is analyzed below from the published work in this field.

5.2.1 Role of Drusen and Basal Deposits in CNV

The unusual build-up of drusen in the macula is a characteristic feature for age-related macular degeneration [14–18]. Drusen occupy two favored sites: (1) in spaces created between the retinal pigment epithelium basal and plasma membrane, and (2) in BM, especially between the retinal pigment epithelium basal membrane and inner collagenous layer. The histological and histochemical characteristics of drusen are to specific forms of age-related macular degeneration and CNV pathogenesis. Soft, diffuse, large, and hyperfluorescent drusen, which originate from the degeneration of the retinal pigment epithelium, are considered a major risk factor for the progress of CNV [7, 17, 19–27]. Besides drusen, other amorphous and fibrillar deposits are associated with CNV (frank as well as occult) secondary to the pathogenesis of age-related macular degeneration [8, 24, 25, 28–33]. The slow, diffuse thickening of BM and progressive accumulation of basal linear deposits in this layer create a diffusion barrier for the retinal pigment epithelium [16, 34], thereby depriving it from receiving oxygen and water-soluble substances from the choroidal circulation.

5.2.2 Focal Macular Hyperpigmentation of the Retinal Pigment Epithelium

The reports of Bressler et al. [14], Abdelsalam et al. [19], Wang et al. [18], and CAPT Research Group [35] asserted that focal macular hyperpigmentation is linked with an increased risk of emergent CNV.

5.3 Calcification of Bruch's Membrane

Histological examination of eyes with different stages of age-related macular degeneration [36] revealed high grade of calcification and disintegration of BM in exudative age-related macular degeneration, unlike in nonexudative cases. These changes imply that calcification as well as fragmentation of BM may be involved in CNV, especially by helping ingrowth of choroidal neovascular membranes [33, 36–38].

5.3.1 Role of Phospholipids in CNV Growth

The soft, large, and diffuse drusen of the macula contain predominantly polar phospholipids and are found to be associated with the development of CNV [23, 24]. Lommatzsch et al. [31] showed by electron microscopy the presence of vesicles and droplets in basal deposits that stained intensely for phospholipids. The phospholipid content most likely undergoes oxidative damage and the lipid deposition in association with changes in BM are believed to induce inflammatory reactions, resulting in the ingrowth of choroidal new vessels beneath the retinal pigment epithelium [23]. Experimentally, in rodent models, subretinal injection of oxidized lipids can induce CNV [39, 40] by inducing increased expressions of genes involved in inflammatory cascade [26]. The latter can be inhibited by blocking monocyte chemoattractant protein-1, a potent molecule involved in inflammation [40]. Finally, the chemical modification of BM likely generates a furrow between the inner collagenous layer and the basal lamina of the retinal pigment epithelium through which new vessels can grow.

5.4 Choriocapillaris Loss

There is clear evidence for CNV development in response to choriocapillaris loss. Histological studies revealed degenerative capillaries to be frequent in cases with exudative age-related macular degeneration and loss of capillaries was attended by neovascularization [41–43]. The retinal pigment epithelium then suffers from hypoxia, a condition that favors the release of vascular endothelial growth factor by retinal pigment epithelium, stimulating neovascularization from preexisting choriocapillaris.

5.4.1 The Process of CNV in General

The early features of CNV in wet age-related macular degeneration were described by examining tissues from patients with an advanced form of the disease. Neovascularization appears to proceed from preexisting choroidal capillaries and venules [24, 44–46]. This is also evident in experimental studies using laser photocoagulation in monkeys [47] and in newly formed subretinal vessels after photocoagulation, demonstrating features that are essentially present in choroidal capillaries [48]. In CNV, initially there is budding and sprouting of endothelial cells (Fig. 5.4) and enlargement of pericytes, the latter appear to surround endothelial cell sprouts in neovascular development [45]. These vessels enter the inner collagenous layer of BM and extend into BM and basal laminar deposits, spreading over the subretinal pigment epithelial zone [8]. Killingsworth [45] described two phases of neovascular growth: (1) the initial phase, being restricted within the choroid, is low in turnover of vessels and these vessels penetrate BM. This is followed by a "high-turnover" phase, showing extensive proliferation of endothelial cells and migration and invasion of new vessels

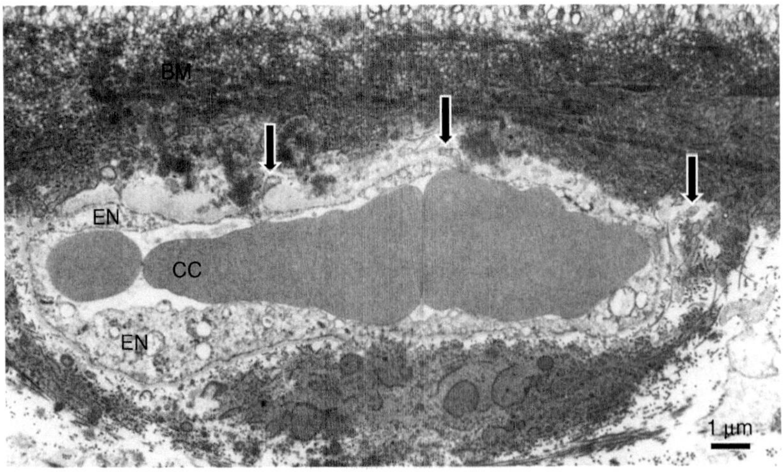

Fig. 5.4 A capillary of the choriocapillaris (CC), showing slender, endothelial sprouts (arrows), passing through the basal lamina into the perivascular matrix. BM, Bruch's membrane; EN, endothelial cell. Reprinted from Killingsworth (Graefe's Arch Clin Exp Ophthalmol 1995; 233: 313–323), with permission from Springer-Verlag

in the subretinal pigment epithelial zone. Hemorrhage and lipid exudates in the subretinal or subretinal pigment epithelial zones are considered to be the earliest sign of CNV symptoms. The new vessels are leaky, and clinically this can be identified from hyperfluorescence in fluorescein angiography, indicating leakage of fluorescein from the new vessels [24, 48]. Excessive leakage of serum fluid can lead to the formation of disciform scars that trigger photoreceptor cell death.

5.4.2 Role of Macrophages and Leukocytes in CNV

The spatiotemporal distribution of macrophages and leukocytes in areas of neovascularization (Figs. 5.5 and 5.6) led several authors to imply the involvement of these cells in the development of neovascular age-related macular degeneration [46, 49–51]. These cells, upon activation, can liberate vasoproliferative agents as part of inflammatory response, thereby inducing neovascularization [46, 51]. The new vessels of the choriocapillaris can penetrate BM in the absence of a prior break [52], or the activated leukocytes and macrophages may cause focal thinning and break the integrity of BM [50, 53], favoring neovascular growth in age-related macular degeneration [54]. This is evident from the appearance of macrophages and lymphocytes near the region of breaks of BM (Fig. 5.5), suggesting their involvement in the growth of new vessels. Matrix metalloproteinases, collagenase, and elastase released by them disrupts the integrity of BM, allowing the incursion of new vessels into the subretinal pigment epithelial to subretinal space [55–57]. Nishimura et al. [58] reported the presence of activated macrophages in experimental subretinal neovascularization, implying them to play a potential angiogenic role [59]. Other cellular phenotypes, namely fibrocytes, mast cells, monocytes, lymphocytes, and collagen and fibrin as extracellular materials have been found in and around the new vessels [13, 29, 32, 46, 49, 53, 60, 61]. The cellular elements noted are possibly involved in the formation of

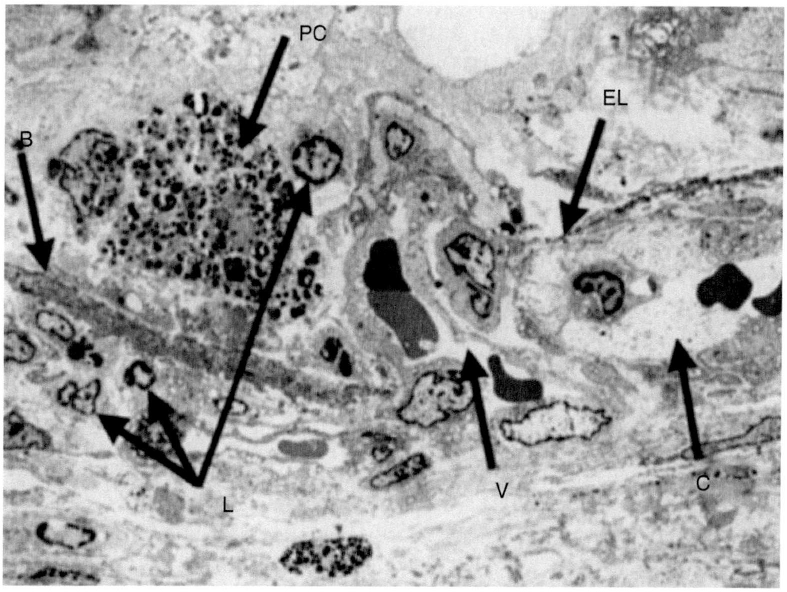

Fig. 5.5 Electron micrograph showing a capillary (C) and a venule (V) ingress the sub-RPE area via a break in Bruch's membrane (B). Leukocytes (L) lie closely adhered to Bruch's membrane and on the retinal side of Bruch's membrane. A pigment clump (PC) is seen immediately above Bruch's membrane. EL, elastic layer of Bruch's membrane. Final magnification x1,226.4. Reprinted from Penfold et al. (Graefe's Arch Clin Exp Ophthalmol 1987; 225:70–76), with permission from Springer-Verlag

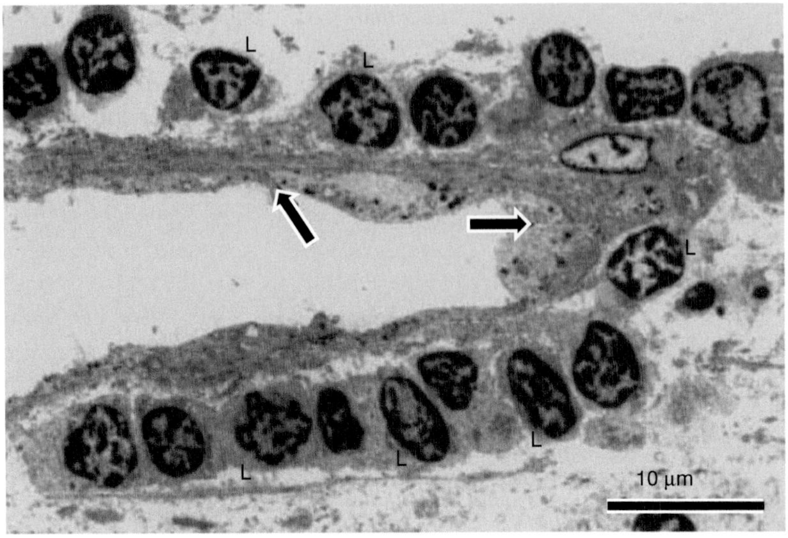

Fig. 5.6 Electron micrograph depicting the accumulation of lymphocytes (L) adherent to the abluminal surface of a subretinal vessel. Arrows denote tight junctions between apposing endothelial cells that lack fenestrae. Reprinted from Penfold et al. (Prog Ret Eye Res 2001; 20:385–414, with permission from Elsevier)

breaks in BM in age-related macular degeneration [46, 53], favoring CNV growth and progression [62, 63], while fibrin is suggested to act as a scaffold for the growth of new vessels [49]. There is evidence for the dissolution of elastic lamina of BM in CNV, allowing new vessels to grow toward the retinal pigment epithelium. Also, experimental studies hint to the possible involvement of abnormal elastin metabolism in the formation of neovascular membrane in age-related macular degeneration [64]. In addition, leukocytes are implicated in the formation as well as exudation from new vessels [46]. Thus, it is likely that inflammation plays a critical role in CNV pathogenesis in age-related macular degeneration [31, 54, 65].

5.4.3 Role of RPE in CNV

The retinal pigment epithelium is vital for the regular maintenance of the choriocapillaris [66] via the release of trophic substances. However, it plays a role in CNV by releasing an excess of certain angiogenic cytokines [56], e.g., VEGF [42, 43, 49, 67]. The presence of VEGF immunoreactivity in the neovascular membrane has been shown [32, 68, 69]. Other factors, e.g., fibroblast growth factors, released by injured RPE could also be involved in this process [70]. There are also antiangiogenic molecules like pigment epithelial-derived factor from retinal pigment epithelium [71] that can arrest CNV progression [72]. A balance between the secretory levels of vascular endothelial growth factor and pigment epithelial-derived factor therefore determines the course of CNV pathogenesis [73].

5.5 Conclusions

Although extensive research has been carried out in the last two decades, the pathological basis of CNV development in wet age-related macular degeneration remains poorly understood. Therapeutic measures to combat CNV can be useful only when we have an unambiguous understanding of the process. Earlier, the Eye Disease Case–Control Study Group [74] in its preliminary report pointed out that carotenoid-based antioxidant supplementation could retard neovascular growth in age-related macular degeneration, an approach that needs additional studies for evaluation. Second, because numerous reports have linked the presence of inflammatory cells with CNV pathogenesis, experimental studies to decipher their precise contributory role (friends or foe? [75]) in this disease and therapeutic interventions to suppress/modulate the activities of local inflammatory cells can be considered. Further, inhibition of angiogenesis proper, in a strict sense, seems a promising plan for the management of CNV. For example, inhibitors of metalloproteinases, e.g., TIMP-3 [76], have been shown to offer good protection. The precise regulation of secretion of pigment epithelial-derived factor in CNV is not clear; it is known that its loss could be a problem for ischemia-induced neovascularization [77]. Paradoxically, its high level is reported to increase CNV development [78], a fact that just repeats that much remains to be known about this factor. Considering that it is a potent antiangiogenic factor [77], its use can be manipulated to have benefit over CNV growth. Intraocular or subretinal injection of adeno-associated viral vector with PEDF gene is reported to partially inhibit laser-induced neovascularization in murine models [79], raising the hope that sustained release of pigment epithelial-derived factor may cause regression even in established neovascularization.

References

1. Krebs W, Krebs I. Fine structure of the choroid. In: Primate retina and choroid. New York, NY: Springer; 1991.
2. Nag TC, Kumari C. Electron microscopy of the human choroid. In: Chhablani J, Ruiz-Medrano J, editors. Choroidal disorders. London: Academic Press; 2017. p. 7–20.
3. Nickla DL, Wallman J. The multifunctional choroid. Prog Ret Eye Res. 2010;29:144–68.
4. Nag TC, Wadhwa S. Ultrastructure of human retina in aging and various pathological states. Micron. 2012;43:859–71.
5. Ambati J, Ambati BK, Yoo SH, Ianchulev S, Adamis AP. Age-related macular degeneration: etiology, pathogenesis, and therapeutic strategies. Surv Ophthalmol. 2003;48:257–93.
6. Bhutto I, Lutty G. Understanding age-related macular degeneration (AMD): relationships between the photoreceptor/retinal pigment epithelium/Bruch's membrane/choriocapillaris complex. Mol Asp Med. 2012;33:295–317.
7. Green WR. Histopathology of age-related macular degeneration. Mol Vis. 1999;5:27.
8. Green WR, Enger C. Age-related macular degeneration histopathologic studies: the 1992 Lorenz E. Zimmerman Lecture. Ophthalmology. 1993;100:1519–35.
9. Zarbin MA. Current concepts in the pathogenesis of age related macular degeneration. Arch Ophthalmol. 2004;122:598–614.
10. McLeod DS, Taomoto M, Otsuji T, Green WR, Sunness JS, Lutty GA. Quantifying changes in RPE and choroidal vasculature in eyes with age-related macular degeneration. Invest Ophthalmol Vis Sci. 2002;43:1986–93.
11. Gass JD. Biomicroscopic and histopathologic considerations regarding the feasibility of surgical excision of subfoveal neovascular membranes. Am J Ophthalmol. 1994;118:285–98.
12. Grossniklaus HE, Gass JDM. Clinicopathologic correlations of surgically excised type 1 and type 2 submacular choroidal neovascular membranes. Am J Ophthalmol. 1998;126:59–69.
13. Grossniklaus HE, Green WR. Choroidal neovascularization. Am J Ophthalmol. 2004;137:496–503.
14. Bressler NM, Bressler SB, Seddon JM, Gragoudas ES, Jacobson LP. Drusen characteristics in patients with exudative versus non-exudative age-related macular degeneration. Retina. 1998;8:109–14.
15. Mullins RF, Johnson MN, Faidley EA, Skeie JM, Huang J. Choriocapillaris vascular dropout related to density of drusen in human eyes with early age-related macular degeneration. Invest Ophthalmol Vis Sci. 2011;52:1606–12.
16. Pauleikhoff D, Chen J, Chisholm I, Bird A. Choroidal perfusion abnormality with age-related Bruch's membrane change. Am J Ophthalmol. 1990;109:211–7.
17. Sarks SH. Council lecture: drusen and their relationship to senile macular degeneration. Aust J Ophthalmol. 1980;8:117–30.
18. Wang JJ, Foran S, Smith W, Mitchell P. Risk of age-related macular degeneration in eyes with macular drusen or hyperpigmentation: the Blue Mountains eye study cohort. Arch Ophthalmol. 2003;121:658–63.
19. Abdelsalam A, Del Priore L, Zarbin MA. Drusen in age-related macular degeneration: pathogenesis, natural course, and laser photocoagulation-induced regression. Surv Ophthalmol. 1999;44:1–29.
20. Bressler SB, Maguire MG, Bressler NM, Fine SL. Relationship of drusen and abnormalities of the retinal pigment epithelium to the prognosis of neovascular macular degeneration. The macular photocoagulation study group. Arch Ophthalmol. 1990;108:1442–7.
21. Bressler NM, Silva JC, Bressler SB, Fine SL, Green WR. Clinicopathologic correlation of drusen and retinal pigment epithelial abnormalities in age-related macular degeneration. Retina. 1994;14:130–42.
22. Fine SL, Berger JW, Maguire MG, Ho AC. Age-related macular degeneration. New Eng J Med. 2000;342:483–92.
23. Pauleikhoff D. Drusen in Bruch's membrane. Their significance for the pathogenesis and therapy of age-associated macular degeneration. Ophthalmologe. 1992;89:363–86. [Article in German]

24. Sarks SH, Van Driel D, Maxwell L, Killingsworth M. Softening of drusen and subretinal neovascularization. Trans Ophthalmol Soc UK. 1980;100:414–22.
25. Sarks JP, Sarks SH, Killingsworth MC. Evolution of soft drusen in age-related macular degeneration. Eye. 1994;8:269–83.
26. Shaw PX, Zhang L, Zhang M, Du H, Zhao L, Lee C, Grob S, Lim SL, Hughes G, Lee J, Bedell M, Nelson MH, Lu F, Krupa M, Luo J, Ouyang H, Tu Z, Su Z, Zhu J, Wei X, Feng Z, Duan Y, Yang Z, Ferreyra H, Bartsch DU, Kozak I, Zhang L, Lin F, Sun H, Feng H, Zhang K. Complement factor H genotypes impact risk of age-related macular degeneration by interaction with oxidized phospholipids. Proc Natl Acad Sci U S A. 2012;109:13757–62.
27. Sarks S, Cherepanoff S, Killingsworth M, Sarks J. Relationship of basal laminar deposit and membranous debris to the clinical presentation of early age-related macular degeneration. Invest Ophthalmol Vis Sci. 2007;48:968–77.
28. Chang TS, Freund KB, de la Cruz Z, Yannuzzi LA, Green WR. Clinicopathologic correlation of choroidal neovascularization demonstrated by indocyanine green angiography in a patient with retention of good vision for almost four years. Retina. 1994;14:114–24.
29. Grossniklaus HE, Green WR. Histopathologic and ultrastructural findings of surgically excised choroidal neovascularization. Submacular surgery trials research group. Arch Opthalmol. 1998;116:745–9.
30. Hermans P, Lommatzsch A, Bornfeld N, Pauleikhoff D. Angiographic-histological correlation of late exudative age-related macular degeneration. Ophthalmologe. 2003;100:378–83.
31. Lommatzsch A, Hermans P, Müller KD, Bornfeld N, Bird AC, Pauleikhoff D. Are low inflammatory reactions involved in exudative age-related macular degeneration? Morphological and immunhistochemical analysis of AMD associated with basal deposits. Graefes Arch Clin Exp Ophthalmol. 2008;246:803–10.
32. Lopez PF, Grossniklaus HE, Lambert HM, Aaberg TM, Capone A Jr, Sternberg P Jr, L'Hernault N. Pathologic features of surgically excised subretinal neovascular membranes in age-related macular degeneration. Am J Ophthalmol. 1991;112:647–56.
33. Spraul CW, Lang GE, Grossniklaus HE, Lang GK. Histologic and morphometric analysis of the choroid, Bruch's membrane, and retinal pigment epithelium in postmortem eyes with age-related macular degeneration and histologic examination of surgically excised choroidal neovascular membranes. Surv Ophthalmol. 1999;44(Suppl 1):S10–32.
34. Moore DJ, Hussain AA, Marshall J. Age-related variation in the hydraulic conductivity of Bruch's membrane. Invest Ophthalmol Vis Sci. 1995;36:1290–7.
35. Complications of Age-related Macular Degeneration Prevention Trial (CAPT) Research Group. Risk factors for choroidal neovascularization and geographic atrophy in the complications of age-related macular degeneration prevention trial. Ophthalmology. 2008;115:1474–9.
36. Spraul CW, Grossniklaus HE. Characteristics of Drusen and Bruch's membrane in postmortem eyes with age-related macular degeneration. Arch Ophthalmol. 1997;115:267–73.
37. Friedman E. The pathogenesis of age-related macular degeneration. Am J Ophthalmol. 2008;146:348–9.
38. Spraul CW, Lang GE, Grossniklaus HE, Lang GK. Characteristics of drusen and changes in Bruch's membrane in eyes with age-related macular degeneration. Histological study. Ophthalmologe. 1998;95:73–9. [Article in German]
39. Lu Z, Lin V, May A, Che B, Xiao X, Shaw DH, Su F, Wang Z, Du H, Shaw PX. HTRA1 synergizes with oxidized phospholipids in promoting inflammation and macrophage infiltration essential for ocular VEGF expression. PLoS One. 2019;14:e0216808.
40. Suzuki M, Tsujikawa M, Itabe H, Du ZJ, Xie P, Matsumura N, Fu X, Zhang R, Sonoda KH, Egashira K, Hazen SL, Kamei M. Chronic photo-oxidative stress and subsequent MCP-1 activation as causative factors for age-related macular degeneration. J Cell Sci. 2012;125:2407–15.
41. Biesemeier A, Taubitz T, Julien S, Yoeruek E, Schraermeyer U. Choriocapillaris breakdown precedes retinal degeneration in age-related macular degeneration. Neurobiol Aging. 2014;35:2562–73.
42. McLeod DS, Grebe R, Bhutto I, Merges C, Baba T, Lutty GA. Relationship between RPE and choriocapillaris in age-related macular degeneration. Invest Ophthalmol Vis Sci. 2009;50:4982–91.
43. Seddon JM, McLeod DS, Bhutto IA, Villalonga MB, Silver RE, Wenick AS, Edwards MM, Lutty GA. Histopathological insights into choroidal vascular loss in clinically documented cases of age-related macular degeneration. JAMA Ophthalmol. 2016;134:1272–80.
44. Green WR, Key SN 3rd. Senile macular degeneration: a histopathologic study. Trans Am Ophthalmol Soc. 1977;75:180–254.
45. Killingsworth MC. Angiogenesis in early choroidal neovascularization secondary to age-related macular degeneration. Graefes Arch Clin Exp Ophthalmol. 1995;233:313–23.
46. Penfold PL, Provis JM, Billson FA. Age-related macular degeneration: ultrastructural studies of the relationship of leucocytes to angiogenesis. Graefes Arch Clin Exp Ophthalmol. 1987;225:70–6.
47. Archer DB, Gardiner TA. Electron microscopic features of experimental choroidal neovascularization. Am J Ophthalmol. 1981;91:433–57.
48. Miller H, Miller B, Ryan SJ. Newly-formed subretinal vessels. Fine structure and fluorescein leakage. Invest Ophthalmol Vis Sci. 1986;27:204–13.
49. Grossniklaus HE, Ling JX, Wallace TM, Dithmar S, Lawson DH, Cohen C, Elner VM, Elner SG,

Sternberg P Jr. Macrophage and retinal pigment epithelium expression of angiogenic cytokines in choroidal neovascularization. Mol Vis. 2002;8: 119–26.
50. Killingsworth MC, Sarks JP, Sarks SH. Macrophages related to Bruch's membrane in age-related macular degeneration. Eye. 1990;4:613–21.
51. Ryan SJ. Subretinal neovascularization after laser coagulation. Graefes Arch Clin Exp Ophthalmol. 1980;215:29–42.
52. Heriot WJ, Henkind P, Bellhorn DVN, Burns MS. Choroidal neovascularisation can digest Bruch's membrane: a prior break is not essential. Ophthalmology. 1984;91:1603–8.
53. Penfold P, Killingsworth M, Sarks S. An ultrastructural study of the role of leucocytes and fibroblasts in the breakdown of Bruch's membrane. Aust NZ J Ophthalmol. 1984;12:23–31.
54. Penfold PL, Killingsworth MC, Sarks SH. Senile macular degeneration: the involvement of immunocompetent cells. Graefes Arch Clin Exp Ophthalmol. 1985;223:69–76.
55. Kadonosono K, Yazama F, Itoh N, et al. Expression of matrix metalloproteinase-7 in choroidal neovascular membranes in age-related macular degeneration. Am J Ophthalmol. 1999;128:382–4.
56. Lambert V, Munaut C, Jost M, Noël A, Werb Z, Foidart JM, Rakic JM. Matrix metalloproteinase-9 contributes to choroidal neovascularization. Am J Pathol. 2002;161:1247–53.
57. van der Schaft TL, Mooy CM, de Bruijn WC, de Jong PT. Early stages of age-related macular degeneration: an immunofluorescence and electron microscopy study. Br J Ophthalmol. 1993;77:657–61.
58. Nishimura T, Goodnight R, Prendergast RA, Ryan SJ. Activated macrophages in experimental subretinal neovascularization. Ophthalmologica. 1990;200:39–44.
59. Oh H, Takagi H, Takagi C, et al. The potential angiogenic role of macrophages in the formation of choroidal neovascular membranes. Invest Ophthalmol Vis Sci. 1999;40:1891–8.
60. Grossniklaus HE, Miskala PH, Green WR, Bressler SB, Hawkins BS, Toth C, Wilson DJ, Bressler NM. Histopathologic and ultrastructural features of surgically excised subfoveal choroidal neovascular lesions: submacular surgery trials report no. 7. Arch Ophthalmol. 2005;123:914–21.
61. Lafaut BA, Aisenbrey S, Vanden Broecke C, Di Tizio F, Bartz-Schmidt KU. Clinicopathological correlation in exudative age-related macular degeneration: recurrent choroidal neovascularization. Graefes Arch Clin Exp Ophthalmol. 2001;239:5–11.
62. Gehrs KM, Heriot WJ, de Juan E Jr. Transmission electron microscopic study of a subretinal choroidal neovascular membrane due to age-related macular degeneration. Arch Ophthalmol. 1992;110:833–7.
63. Grossniklaus HE, Cingle KA, Yoon YD, Ketkar N, L'Hernault N, Brown S. Correlation of histologic 2-dimensional reconstruction and confocal scanning laser microscopic imaging of choroidal neovascularization in eyes with age-related maculopathy. Arch Ophthalmol. 2000;118:625–9.
64. Skeie JM, Mullins RF. Elastin-mediated choroidal endothelial cell migration: possible role in age-related macular degeneration. Invest Ophthalmol Vis Sci. 2008;49:5574–80.
65. Penfold PL, Madigan MC, Gillies MC, Provis JM. Immunological and aetiological aspects of macular degeneration. Prog Ret Eye Res. 2001;20:385–414.
66. Korte GE, Repucci V, Henkind P. RPE destruction causes choriocapillary atrophy. Invest Ophthalmol Vis Sci. 1984;25:1135–45.
67. Spilsbury K, Garrett KL, Shen WY, Constable IJ, Rakoczy PE. Overexpression of vascular endothelial growth factor (VEGF) in the retinal pigment epithelium leads to the development of choroidal neovascularization. Am J Pathol. 2000;157:135–44.
68. Frank RN, Amin RH, Eliott D, Puklin JE, Abrams GW. Basic fibroblast growth factor and vascular endothelial growth factor are present in epiretinal and choroidal neovascular membranes. Am J Ophthalmol. 1996;122:393–403.
69. Kvanta A, Algvere PV, Berglin L, Seregard S. Subfoveal fibrovascular membranes in age-related macular degeneration express vascular endothelial growth factor. Invest Ophthalmol Vis Sci. 1996;37:1929–34.
70. Amin R, Puklin JE, Frank RN. Growth factor localization in choroidal neovascular membranes of age-related macular degeneration. Invest Ophthalmol Vis Sci. 1994;35:3178–88.
71. Campochiaro PA, Sugg R, Grotendorst G, Hjelmeland LM. Retinal pigment epithelial cells produce PDGF-like proteins and secrete them into their media. Exp Eye Res. 1989;49:217–27.
72. Mori K, Duh E, Gehlbach P, Ando A, Takahashi K, Pearlman J, Mori K, Yang HS, Zack DJ, Ettyreddy D, Brough DE, Wei LL, Campochiaro PA. Pigment epithelium derived factor inhibits retinal and choroidal neovascularization. J Cell Physiol. 2001;188: 253–63.
73. Bhutto IA, McLeod DS, Hasegawa T, Kim SY, Merges C, Tong P, Lutty GA. Pigment epithelium-derived factor (PEDF) and vascular endothelial growth factor (VEGF) in aged human choroid and eyes with age-related macular degeneration. Exp Eye Res. 2006;82:99–110.
74. Eye Disease Case Control Study Group. Antioxidant status and neovascular age-related macular degeneration. Arch Ophthalmol. 1993;111:104–9.
75. Skeie JM, Mullins RF. Macrophages in neovascular age-related macular degeneration: friends or foes? Eye (Lond). 2009;23:747–55.

76. Anand-Apte B, Pepper MS, Voest E, Montesano R, Olsen B, Murphy G, Apte SS, Zetter B. Inhibition of angiogenesis by tissue inhibitor of metalloproteinase-3. Invest Ophthalmol Vis Sci. 1997;38:817–23.
77. Dawson DW, Volpert OV, Gillis P, Crawford SE, Xu H, Benedict W, Bouck NP. Pigment epithelium derived factor: a potent inhibitor of angiogenesis. Science. 1999;285:245–8.
78. Ferguson TA. Kaplan H, Tezel T, et al: augmentation of choroidal neovascularization in a laser induced mouse model by PEDF. ARVO Annual Meeting, Abstract. 2002;2756
79. Mori K, Gehlbach P, Yamamoto S, et al. AAV-mediated gene transfer of pigment epithelium-derived factor inhibits choroidal neovascularization. Invest Ophthalmol Vis Sci. 2002;43:1994–2000.

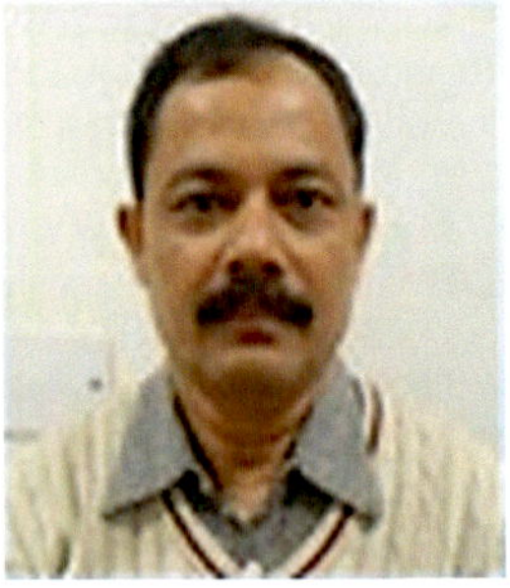

Dr. TC Nag is a professor in the Department of Anatomy, All India Institute of Medical Sciences, New Delhi, India. His main research interest is to see age-related changes in the human retina and choroid, to find a basis/link that triggers for the pathogenesis of age-related macular degeneration.

He has published about 142 papers in peer-reviewed journals and 7 invited chapters in books published by Elsevier and Springer-Verlag.

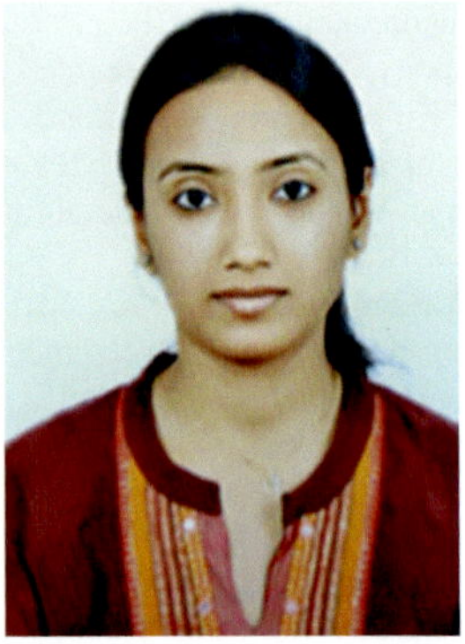

Dr. Sneha Gupta is currently in her final year of residency (MD) in the Department of Anatomy, All India Institute of Medical Sciences, New Delhi, India. Her research interest includes light-induced retinal changes in rodent models, especially to understand the role of continuous exposure to light on the pathophysiology of age-related macular degeneration.

6 Genomics in Choroidal Neovascularization

Kenji Yamashiro

6.1 Genes Associated with Age-Related Macular Degeneration

Age-related macular degeneration (AMD) is a multifactorial disease, and its development is affected by both genetic and environmental factors. Aging and smoking are the major environmental factors for AMD, and genes affecting AMD development are called susceptibility genes.

Since the discovery of associations between the *CFH* gene and AMD development in 2005 [1], many genome-wide association studies (GWASs) have investigated AMD pathogenesis. The first GWAS successfully discovered an association between *CFH* and AMD by comparing 116,204 genetic variations between 96 cases and 50 controls [1]. In 2006, GWASs comparing 97,824 genetic variations between 130 cases and 96 controls discovered the second AMD susceptibility locus, *ARMS2/HTRA1* [2]. After these discoveries, several candidate-gene approach studies confirmed significant associations between AMD and complement pathway genes, such as *C2/CFB*, *C3*, and *CFI,* using 1287–2172 samples [3–6]. In 2010, two GWASs using 2688 and 3307 samples found further AMD susceptibility genes of *LIPC* and *TIMP3*, respectively [7, 8]. The first GWAS from Japan discovered a significant association between *TNFRSF10A* and AMD using 827 cases and 3323 controls [9], and the first GWAS combining East Asian samples of 2119 cases and 5691 controls discovered genome-wide significance of *CETP* with AMD [10].

In 2013, a large-scale GWAS comparing 2,442,884 genetic variations between 7650 cases and 51,844 controls discovered seven new loci associated with AMD [11]. This study group further performed a large-scale GWAS comparing 12,023,830 genetic variations between 16,144 cases and 17,832 controls and discovered 34 AMD-susceptibility loci in 2016 (Table 6.1) [12]. Since GWAS can sometimes provide false positive results, the results should be carefully understood by referring to reports from other groups.

6.2 Genes Associated with Neovascular AMD

To date, the mechanisms by which susceptibility genes affect AMD development have not been thoroughly elucidated. Some AMD susceptibility genes might promote drusen accumulation, vulnerability of the Bruch's membrane or retinal pigment epithelium, CNV development, or geographic atrophy (GA) development. Since most previous

K. Yamashiro (✉)
Department of Ophthalmology, Otsu Red Cross Hospital, Otsu, Japan

Department of Ophthalmology and Visual Sciences, Kyoto University Graduate School of Medicine, Kyoto, Japan
e-mail: yamashro@kuhp.kyoto-u.ac.jp

J. Chhablani (ed.), *Choroidal Neovascularization*, https://doi.org/10.1007/978-981-15-2213-0_6

GWASs on AMD have included both neovascular AMD and atrophic AMD in case samples, it is unclear whether susceptibility genes for CNV development and GA development are similar. However, one study reported that *MMP9* was significantly associated only with neovascular AMD, and it was not significantly associated with GA [12]. To confirm the reproducibility of these findings, associations between *MMP9* and CNV or GA should be further evaluated in the future.

Table 6.1 Susceptibility genes for age-related macular degeneration

Chromosome	Locus
1	*CFH*
2	*COL4A3*
3	*ADAMTS9-AS*
3	*COL8A1*
4	*CFI*
5	*SPEF2*
5	*C9*
6	*C2/CFB-SKIV2L*
6	*VEGFA*
7	*KMT2E-SRPK2*
7	*PILRB-PILRA*
8	*TNFRSF10A*
9	*TRPM3*
9	*MIR6130-RORB*
9	*TGFBR1*
9	*ABCA1*
10	*ARHGAP21*
10	*ARMS2-HTRA1*
12	*RDH5-CD63*
12	*ACAD10*
13	*B2GALTL*
14	*RAD51B*
15	*LIPC*
16	*CETP*
16	*CTRB2-CTRB1*
17	*TMEM97-VTN*
17	*NPLOC4-TSPAN10*
19	*CNN2*
19	*C3*
19	*APOE*
20	*MMP9*
20	*C20orf85*
22	*SYN3-TIMP3*
22	*SLC16A8*

6.3 Genes Associated with CNV Subtypes

Neovascular AMD is usually divided into three subtypes: typical AMD, polypoidal choroidal vasculopathy (PCV), and retinal angiomatous proliferation (RAP). Typical AMD develops as type 1 or type 2 CNV, PCV develops as type 1 CNV with polypoidal lesions at its edge, and RAP develops as type 3 CNV. Among previously reported susceptibility genes for AMD, *ARMS2/HTRA1* has demonstrated different associations to these three subtypes [13–16]. Its association is weaker for PCV and stronger for RAP (Table 6.2). *ARMS2/HTRA1* might determine the type of CNV in eyes with AMD.

Although most susceptibility genes are significantly associated with all AMD subtypes, *FGD6* might be associated only with PCV. One study from East Asia reported that a rare variant of *FGD6* was significantly associated with PCV, but not with typical AMD [17]. Therefore, associations between *FGD6* and PCV or typical AMD should be evaluated in Caucasian populations. Further investigation of *FGD6* might determine whether it is a true susceptibility gene of PCV only.

6.4 Genes Associated with Natural Course of PCV

In addition to its potential roles in the divergence of AMD into typical AMD, PCV, or RAP, *ARMS2/HTRA1* might be useful to predict PCV

Table 6.2 Genetic associations to polypoidal choroidal vasculopathy

Genes	Association to			Ref
	PCV	tAMD	RAP	
ARMS2/HTRA1	Association (+) (weak)	Association (+)	Association (+) (strong)	13–16
FGD6	Association (+)	Association (−)		17

PCV polypoidal choroidal vasculopathy, *tAMD* typical age-related macular degeneration, *RAP* retinal angiomatous proliferation, *Ref* references prognosis. One Japanese group reported that the T allele in *ARMS2/HTRA1* rs10490924 was a risk allele for vitreous hemorrhage, retinal hemorrhage, hemorrhagic pigment epithelial detachment (PED), and serous PED in eyes with PCV [18, 19]. Since hemorrhagic complications significantly worsen visual prognosis of eyes with PCV, *ARMS2/HTRA1* would determine the natural prognosis of PCV. In contrast to *ARMS2/HTRA1*, *CFH* has not shown clear associations to the natural course of PCV in previous studies.

6.5 Genes Associated with CNV Size in AMD

Since CNV size determines scotoma size in patients with AMD, genes associated with CNV size are clinically important. In a GWAS from Japan, *ARMS2/HTRA1* and *MMP20* were discovered as significantly associated with CNV size in AMD [20]. The association between *ARMS2/HTRA1* and CNV size in AMD has been reported in previous studies on *ARMS2/HTRA1* association to AMD [21–23]. Therefore, *ARMS2/HTRA1* would be a key gene to determine CNV size in AMD. As for *MMP20*, its association with CNV size should be confirmed using other cohorts, due to the potential of false-positive results from GWAS. Similar to genetic associations in PCV prognosis, *CFH* does not show a clear association to CNV size in AMD.

6.6 Genes Associated with AMD Bilaterality

Early genetic studies for AMD reported that associations between *ARMS2/HTRA1* and AMD were stronger for patients with bilateral AMD than patients with unilateral AMD [24, 25]. Later studies confirmed significant genotype distribution differences in *ARMS2/HTRA1* between patients with bilateral AMD and patients with unilateral AMD [19, 26–28]. In 2017, a GWAS from Japan confirmed a genome-wide level significant association between *ARMS2/HTRA1* and AMD bilaterality. Although the CATT study did not show associations between *ARMS2/HTRA1* and AMD bilaterality [29], many previous studies reported positive associations between *ARMS2/HTRA1* and AMD bilaterality. Additionally, one study reported further genome-wide level associations. Genotype data of *ARMS2/HTRA1* could be useful to predict future development of AMD in the unaffected eye of patients with unilateral AMD.

In a study on 207 patients with unilateral AMD, the rate of AMD development in the unaffected eye at 10 years was reportedly about 10%, 50%, and 70% in patients with GG, GT, and TT genotype in *ARMS2/HTRA1* rs10490924, respectively [30].

6.7 Genes Associated with Treatment Outcomes for CNV in AMD

After approval of anti-VEGF drugs for AMD, anti-VEGF treatment has become the first-line treatment for AMD. As such, photodynamic therapy (PDT) is rarely used to treat AMD. However, recent studies suggest that PDT would be a better treatment for some eyes with PCV [31, 32]. Although outcomes of PDT treatment for AMD are not always favorable, the genetic information of *ARMS2/HTRA1* might be useful to predict the response to PDT in AMD. Three studies from Japan reported that patients with risk alleles for AMD in *ARMS2/HTRA1* showed worse visual outcomes after PDT for typical AMD and PCV. Genotype information of *ARMS2/HTRA1* might enable prediction of PDT treatment outcomes for typical AMD and PCV. In Caucasian populations, however, two reports did not find associations between *ARMS2/HTRA1* and PDT outcomes for AMD [33, 34]. Since PDT is rarely used for typical AMD, yet PDT can be a suitable treatment for some PCV, associations between *ARMS2/HTRA1* and PDT outcomes should be further confirmed in eyes with PCV to enable precision/personalized medicine with PDT for PCV.

In addition to *ARMS2/HTRA1*, several genes have been reported to be associated with treatment outcomes after PDT for AMD, including

VEGFA [35, 36], *PEDF* [37], *CRP* [38], and coagulation balance genes [39, 40]. Therefore, use of genetic information might be able to improve the prediction accuracy of treatment outcomes for AMD. However, limited evidence is available for the associations between these genes and treatment outcomes. Further studies are warranted to use these genes for precision/personalized medicine in AMD.

In contrast to genes associated with PDT outcomes, genes associated with treatment outcomes after anti-VEGF treatment have not been clearly elucidated. In candidate gene approach studies, various genes have been evaluated for their associations to anti-VEGF treatment outcomes, such as *ARMS2/HTRA1*, *CFH*, *VEGFA*, *C2/CFB*, *C3*, *CFI*, *APOE*, *IL8*, and *PEDF*. Although some studies reported significant associations of these genes with treatment outcomes after anti-VEGF treatment for AMD, many other studies did not find associations (Tables 6.3, 6.4, 6.5, and 6.6).

Table 6.3 Associations of *CFH* gene with treatment outcome after anti-VEGF treatment for AMD

	N	Association to treatment outcome
McKibbin, et al. [41]	104	Significant association
Menghini, et al. [42]	204	Significant association
Tian, et al. [43]	144	Significant association
Kloeckener-Gruissem, et al. [44]	122	Significant association
Brantley, et al. [45]	86	Significant association
Dikmetas, et al. [46]	193	Significant association
Smailhodzic, et al. [47]	420	Significant association
Lee, et al. [48]	156	Significant association
Nischler, et al. [49]	197	Significant association
Imai, et al. [50]	83	Significant association
Yamashiro, et al. [51]	75	No association
Orlin, et al. [52]	150	No association
Hata, et al. [53]	105	No association
Hagstrom, et al. [54]	834	No association
Abedi, et al. [55]	224	No association
Teper, et al. [56]	90	No association
Kang, et al. [57]	75	No association
Kitchens, et al. [58]	101	No association
Yuan, et al. [59]	168	No association
Chang, et al. [60]	102	No association
Habibi, et al. [61]	70	No association
Park et al. [62]	273	No association

Although GWASs on associations for AMD treatment outcomes are rare, one GWAS from Japan reported that *ARMS2/HTRA1* might be useful to predict the number of anti-VEGF drug injections

Table 6.4 Associations of *ARMS2/HTRA1* gene with treatment outcome after anti-VEGF treatment for AMD

	N	Association to treatment outcome
Kang, et al. [57]	75	Significant association
McKibbin, et al. [41]	104	Significant association
Abedi, et al. [55]	224	Significant association
Tian, et al. [43]	144	Significant association
Teper, et al. [56]	90	Significant association
Yuan, et al. [59]	168	Significant association
Kitchens, et al. [58]	101	Significant association
Smailhodzic, et al. [47]	420	No association
Van Asten, et al. [63]	391	No association
Orlin, et al. [52]	150	No association
Hagstrom, et al. [54]	834	No association
Hata, et al. [53]	105	No association
Kloeckener-Gruissem, et al. [44]	122	No association
Yamashiro, et al. [51]	75	No association
Brantley, et al. [45]	86	No association
Chang, et al. [60]	102	No association
Park et al. [62]	273	No association
Imai, et al. [50]	83	No association

Table 6.5 Associations of *VEGFA* gene with treatment outcome after anti-VEGF treatment for AMD

	N	Association to treatment outcome
Abedi, et al. [64]	201	Significant association
Nakata, et al. [36]	94	Significant association
Kitchens, et al. [58]	101	Significant association
Park et al. [62]	273	Significant association
Imai, et al. [50]	83	Significant association
Lazzeri, et al. [65]	64	Significant association
McKibbin, et al. [41]	104	No association
Smailhodzic, et al. [47]	420	No association
van Asten, et al. [63]	391	No association
Hagstrom, et al. [54]	834	No association
Wang, et al. [66]	106	No association
Boltz, et al. [67]	141	No association
Yuan, et al. [59]	168	No association
Chang, et al. [60]	102	No association

Table 6.6 Associations of other genes with treatment outcome after anti-VEGF treatment for AMD

	Loci	N	Association to treatment outcome
Kloeckener-Gruissem, et al. [44]	*C2/CFB*	122	No association
Abedi, et al. [55]	*C2/CFB*	224	No association
Park, et al. [62]	*C2/CFB*	273	No association
Abedi, et al. [55]	*C3*	224	No association
Hagstrom, et al. [54]	*C3*	834	No association
Park, et al. [62]	*CFI*	273	No association
Park, et al. [62]	*APOE*	273	No association
Wickremasinghe, et al. [68]	*APOE*	192	Significant association
Hautamaki, et al. [69]	*IL8*	96	Significant association
Hautamaki, et al. [70]	*IL8*	50	Significant association
Park, et al. [62]	*PEDF*	273	No association
Imai, et al. [50]	*PEDF*	83	Significant association

required to maintain dry macula after initial treatment [71]. In AMD, *ARMS2/HTRA1* would be the most attractive gene for precision/personalized medicine with anti-VEGF treatment.

Most previous genetic association studies on treatment outcomes after anti-VEGF treatment for AMD analyzed samples treated with a pro re nata (PRN) regimen. Eyes with AMD treated with the PRN regimen receive an initial treatment of anti-VEGF injections to inactivate CNV and then were followed up monthly to determine recurrence of retinal exudative changes. Although additional treatment is required immediately following the detection of retinal exudative change recurrence with the PRN regimen, many patients do not follow-up monthly and receive immediate treatment partly due to patient decisions in the real world. As a result, insufficient treatment can lead to false results in genetic association studies on treatment outcomes.

Recently, the treat and extend (TAE) regimen has become popular to treat AMD with anti-VEGF drugs. In this regimen, patients continue to receive treatment at every visit, and the interval between visits is extended or shortened to adjust to each patient's needs. TAE regimen can theoretically prevent undertreatment for AMD, and many studies have reported favorable treatment results [72, 73]. Therefore, genetic association studies analyzing samples treated with the TAE regimen could reveal usefulness of genetic information for precision/personalized medicine in AMD.

6.8 Genes Associated with Pachychoroid Diseases

Although late AMD has been thought to develop from early AMD with drusen and retinal pigmentary abnormalities, some eyes with late AMD do not have drusen or pigmentary abnormalities. In 2012, it was proposed that some eyes with previously diagnosed neovascular AMD should be diagnosed as having CNV secondary to central serous chorioretinopathy (CSC) rather than AMD [74]. Before this proposal, it had been demonstrated that eyes with CSC had thicker choroid [75]. To mention the thick choroid status, a new term "pachychoroid" was coined in 2013, and the CNV secondary to CSC was termed as "pachychoroid neovasculopathy" that develops in association with choroidal thickening [76]. Detailed clinical phenotypes of pachychoroid neovasculopathy were described in 2015 [77], and the genetic characteristics of pachychoroid neovasculopathy were reported in 2016 [78].

In Japanese populations, about 20% of previously diagnosed AMD cases were reportedly pachychoroid neovasculopathy [79]. To date, clinically significant differences have not been reported on treatment outcomes between neovascular AMD and pachychoroid neovasculopathy. However, a recent genetic study confirmed the significance of differentiating pachychoroid neovasculopathy from AMD. Risk alleles for AMD in *CFH* were determined to function as protective alleles for pachychoroid, while risk alleles for pachychoroid were protective alleles for AMD, suggesting that AMD and pachychoroid are genetically distinct relative to *CFH* [80].

Thus far, genetic studies on pachychoroid diseases have been limited. Previously reported fre-

Table 6.7 Frequencies of risk alleles for age-related macular degeneration in Caucasians

Loci	SNP	Risk allele	Risk allele frequencies				Ref
			Pachychoroid	Control	Pachychoroid neovasculopathy	AMD	
CFH	Y402H	C	0.24	0.31	0.46	0.63	48
ARMS2/HTRA1	A69S	T	0.15	0.22	0.41	0.44	

Table 6.8 Frequencies of risk alleles for age-related macular degeneration in Japanese

Loci	SNP	Risk allele	Risk allele frequencies			Ref
			Control	Pachychoroid neovasculopathy	AMD	
CFH	I62V	G	0.59	0.59	0.75	49
ARMS2/HTRA1	A69S	T	0.39	0.51	0.65	

quencies of risk alleles for AMD in *CFH* and *ARMS2/HTRA1* are summarized in Tables 6.7 and 6.8. The C allele frequencies of *CFH* Y402H were found to be 0.24 in pachychoroid subjects and 0.31 in controls among Caucasians, suggesting that the AMD risk allele in *CFH*, C, has protective roles against pachychoroid development in Caucasians. The higher frequency of C allele (0.46) in pachychoroid neovasculopathy patients suggests that the C allele is a risk allele for progression of pachychoroid to pachychoroid neovasculopathy after CNV development. The risk allele of *CFH* for AMD would be a risk allele for CNV development in pachychoroid neovasculopathy in Caucasian subjects.

Although the risk allele frequency of *CFH* in pachychoroid subjects has not been reported in Japanese populations, recent GWAS has discovered that the risk allele of *CFH* for AMD has a protective effect against pachychoroid [80]. The risk allele frequency in pachychoroid must be lower than the control. Taken together with the risk allele frequency of 0.59 in controls, the risk allele frequency of 0.59 in pachychoroid neovascularization suggests that the *CFH* risk allele in AMD contributes to development of pachychoroid neovasculopathy. *CFH* should have similar effects on CNV development in pachychoroid neovasculopathy, as it affects CNV development in AMD both in Caucasian and Japanese populations. As for *ARMS2/HTRA1*, it might also contribute to CNV development both in pachychoroid neovasculopathy and AMD. However, further studies are warranted to confirm the association between *ARMS2/HTRA1* and CNV development in pachychoroid neovasculopathy.

Elucidation of genetic background for pachychoroid diseases might enable highly accurate precision/personalized medicine for AMD. Previous genetic studies on AMD treatment outcomes have included pachychoroid neovasculopathy as AMD. However, AMD and pachychoroid disease are genetically opposite diseases from the viewpoint of *CFH*. Genetic studies on treatment outcomes for pachychoroid neovascularization and AMD will lead to highly accurate precision/personalized medicine for pachychoroid neovasculopathy and AMD.

6.9 Genes Associated with Myopia

Myopia is also a multifactorial disease, and its heritability has long been widely known. The first established susceptibility gene for myopia, *GJD2*, was discovered in 2010 through GWAS [81]. Its association with high myopia was also confirmed [82]. Since the effect of each susceptibility gene is weak for myopia, large-scale GWAS is required to discover susceptibility genes for myopia. In 2018, the CREAM Consortium conducted a meta-analysis of GWASs using 160,420 samples and discovered 161 genetic regions associated with myopia [83].

Table 6.9 Susceptibility genes for myopia 1

Cornea	Lens	Retina (cell type not specified)		Vascular endothelium (Choroid)	Extracellular matrix (Sclera)
CHD7	*BMP4*	*ACP2*	*MYO1D*	*BMP2*	*ANTXR2*
CLU	*CLU*	*AKAP6*	*MYO5B*	*BMP4*	*COL10A1*
COL6A1	*KCNA4*	*API5*	*NCOA2*	*CD34*	*EFEMP1*
CYP26A1	*MAF*	*ARID2*	*NDUFBI*	*CD55*	*LAMA2*
EFEMP1	*SIX3*	*C14orf39*	*PCAT4*	*FLT1*	*SNTB1*
FBN1	*ST8SIA1*	*C2CD5*	*PDE11A*	*MED1*	*TCF7L2*
FLT1		*CD55*	*PDE3A*	*TGFBR1*	*TGFBR1*
PBX1		*CHD7*	*PNPT1*	*TMEM98*	*TMEM98*
RASGRF1		*CLU*	*PTPRR*	*TNFSF12*	*VIPR2*
SETMAR		*CYP26A1*	*RALY*		*ZIC2*
TCF7L2		*DNAJB12*	*RASGRFI*		
TGFBR1		*DRD1*	*RPP14*		
VIPR2		*GRIK1*	*SH3GL2*		
		KCNA4	*SIX3*		
		KCNMA1	*SNTB1*		
		KIRREL	*SYN3*		
		LINC00461	*TFAP2D*		
		LYPLAL1	*THEM184A*		
		MYCN			

Many myopia susceptibility genes were expressed in the retina (Tables 6.9 and 6.10), and it is now thought that the retina plays important roles to promote myopia development.

When myopia progression is severe, it develops into high myopia. High myopia is usually defined as eyes with refractive error greater than −6.0D or axial length more than 26.0 mm. Although similarities between backgrounds of myopia and high myopia development have not been cleared, most myopia susceptibility genes are suspected to susceptibility genes for high myopia. In addition to myopia susceptibility genes, GWASs on high myopia have reported possible susceptibility genes for high myopia (Table 6.11). Interestingly, most susceptibility genes for high myopia have not been included as myopia susceptibility genes discovered through a recent large-scale myopia GWAS. There might be background that is associated only with high myopia development, but not myopia.

6.10 Genes Associated with Myopic CNV

Established susceptibility genes for CNV development secondary to high myopia have not been discovered. Some susceptibility genes for AMD, myopia, and high myopia have been evaluated for their associations to myopic CNV development [20, 82, 91–95]. However, associations were not found for most genes and myopic CNV.

A recent GWAS from Japan discovered that *CCDC102B* was associated with fundus pathologic change secondary to high myopia, but not with myopia development [96]. Therefore, *CCDC102B* might contribute to the development of pathologic changes in high myopia. *CCDC102B* might be associated with myopic CNV development, and elucidation of *CCDC102B* mechanisms contributing to pathologic change development could lead to preventive treatments for myopic CNV in highly myopic eyes.

Table 6.10 Susceptibility genes for myopia 2

Retina									
Ganglion cell	Amacrine cell	Rod bipolar cell	Cone ON bipolar cell	Cone OFF bipolar cell	Mueller cell	Horizontal cell	Cone	Rod	Retinal pigment epithelium
BMP4	*FRMPD2*	*GRM3*	*GJD2*	*LRIT2*	*CA8*	*DLG2*	*CABP4*	*CABP4*	*ANO2*
GRIA4	*GJD2*	*KCNA4*	*GNB3*		*EDN2*	*TFAP2B*	*CACNA1D*	*CACNA1D*	*BMP2*
GRM3	*GRM3*	*KCNMA1*	*GRIA4*		*KCNJ2*	*ZEB2*	*EDN2*	*DYNLRB2*	*BMP4*
KCNJ2	*KCNA4*	*RORB*	*TJP2*		*PRSS56*		*GJD2*	*EDN2*	*C8orf84*
MED1	*KCNMA1*				*RGR*		*GNB3*	*FRMPD2*	*CLU*
NMT	*POU6F2*						*KCNQ5*	*GJD2*	*EFEMP1*
POU6F2	*SEMA3D*						*LRITI1*	*KCNQ5*	*IL4*
ZIC2	*TJP2*						*MED1*	*KCNA4*	*KCNJ5*
	TFAP2B						*RP1L1*	*LRIT1*	*KCNQ5*
	ZEB2						*THRB*	*LRIT2*	*MED1*
							TSPAN10	*MAF*	*RDH5*
							TTC8	*MED1*	*RGR*
								RORB	*TGFBR1*
								RP1L1	*TMEM98*
								TSPAN10	*TTC8*
								TTC8	*TRAF1*

Table 6.11 Previously reported possible susceptibility genes for high myopia

Nakanishi et al. [84]	*11q24.1*
Li et al. [85]	*CTNND2*
Li et al. [86]	*4q25*
Shi et al. [87]	*13q12.12*
Fan et al. [88]	*1q41*
Shi et al. [89]	*VIPR2*
Shi et al. [89]	*SNTB1*
Khor et al. [90]	*ZFHX1B*

Key Learning Points: 5–7 Key Messages

1. Major susceptibility genes for AMD are *CFH* and *ARMS2/HTRA1*.
2. *MMP9* might be a susceptibility gene for neovascular AMD but not for dry AMD.
3. *FGD6* might be a susceptibility gene for PCV but not for typical AMD.
4. *ARMS2/HTRA1* might be useful for precision/personalized medicine for AMD.
5. Pachychoroid disease and AMD are genetically distinct diseases, as related to *CFH*.
6. *GJD2* is a major susceptibility gene for myopia.
7. *CCDC102B* is a major susceptibility gene for pathologic myopia.

References

1. Klein RJ, Zeiss C, Chew EY, et al. Complement factor H polymorphism in age-related macular degeneration. Science. 2005;308(5720):385–9.
2. Dewan A, Liu M, Hartman S, et al. HTRA1 promoter polymorphism in wet age-related macular degeneration. Science. 2006;314(5801):989–92.
3. Gold B, Merriam JE, Zernant J, et al. Variation in factor B (BF) and complement component 2 (C2) genes is associated with age-related macular degeneration. Nat Genet. 2006;38(4):458–62.
4. Maller JB, Fagerness JA, Reynolds RC, Neale BM, Daly MJ, Seddon JM. Variation in complement factor 3 is associated with risk of age-related macular degeneration. Nat Genet. 2007;39(10):1200–1.
5. Yates JR, Sepp T, Matharu BK, et al. Complement C3 variant and the risk of age-related macular degeneration. N Engl J Med. 2007;357(6):553–61.
6. Fagerness JA, Maller JB, Neale BM, Reynolds RC, Daly MJ, Seddon JM. Variation near complement factor I is associated with risk of advanced AMD. Eur J Hum Genet. 2009;17(1):100–4.
7. Chen W, Stambolian D, Edwards AO, et al. Genetic variants near TIMP3 and high-density lipoprotein-associated loci influence susceptibility to age-related macular degeneration. Proc Natl Acad Sci U S A. 2010;107(16):7401–6.
8. Neale BM, Fagerness J, Reynolds R, et al. Genome-wide association study of advanced age-related macular degeneration identifies a role of the hepatic lipase gene (LIPC). Proc Natl Acad Sci U S A. 2010;107(16):7395–400.
9. Arakawa S, Takahashi A, Ashikawa K, et al. Genome-wide association study identifies two susceptibility loci for exudative age-related macular degeneration in the Japanese population. Nat Genet. 2011;43(10):1001–4.
10. Cheng CY, Yamashiro K, Chen LJ, et al. New loci and coding variants confer risk for age-related macular degeneration in east Asians. Nat Commun. 2015;6:6063.
11. Fritsche LG, Chen W, Schu M, et al. Seven new loci associated with age-related macular degeneration. Nat Genet. 2013;45(4):433–9. 439e431-432
12. Fritsche LG, Igl W, Bailey JN, et al. A large genome-wide association study of age-related macular degeneration highlights contributions of rare and common variants. Nat Genet. 2016;48(2):134–43.
13. Hayashi H, Yamashiro K, Gotoh N, et al. CFH and ARMS2 variations in age-related macular degeneration, polypoidal choroidal vasculopathy, and retinal angiomatous proliferation. Invest Ophthalmol Vis Sci. 2010;51(11):5914–9.
14. Tanaka K, Nakayama T, Yuzawa M, et al. Analysis of candidate genes for age-related macular degeneration subtypes in the Japanese population. Mol Vis. 2011;17:2751–8.
15. Liang XY, Lai TY, Liu DT, et al. Differentiation of exudative age-related macular degeneration and polypoidal choroidal vasculopathy in the ARMS2/HTRA1 locus. Invest Ophthalmol Vis Sci. 2012;53(6):3175–82.
16. Yuan D, Yuan D, Yuan S, Liu Q. The age-related maculopathy susceptibility 2 polymorphism and polypoidal choroidal vasculopathy in Asian populations: a meta-analysis. Ophthalmology. 2013;120(10):2051–7.
17. Huang L, Zhang H, Cheng CY, et al. A missense variant in FGD6 confers increased risk of polypoidal choroidal vasculopathy. Nat Genet. 2016;48(6):640–7.
18. Sakurada Y, Kubota T, Mabuchi F, Imasawa M, Tanabe N, Iijima H. Association of LOC387715 A69S with vitreous hemorrhage in polypoidal choroidal vasculopathy. Am J Ophthalmol. 2008;145(6):1058–62.
19. Sakurada Y, Kubota T, Imasawa M, et al. Role of complement factor H I62V and age-related maculopathy susceptibility 2 A69S variants in the clinical expression of polypoidal choroidal vasculopathy. Ophthalmology. 2011;118(7):1402–7.
20. Akagi-Kurashige Y, Yamashiro K, Gotoh N, et al. MMP20 and ARMS2/HTRA1 are associated with Neovascular lesion size in age-related macular degeneration. Ophthalmology. 2015;122(11):2295–302. e2292

21. Gotoh N, Yamada R, Nakanishi H, et al. Correlation between CFH Y402H and HTRA1 rs11200638 genotype to typical exudative age-related macular degeneration and polypoidal choroidal vasculopathy phenotype in the Japanese population. Clin Exp Ophthalmol. 2008;36(5):437–42.
22. Andreoli MT, Morrison MA, Kim BJ, et al. Comprehensive analysis of complement factor H and LOC387715/ARMS2/HTRA1 variants with respect to phenotype in advanced age-related macular degeneration. Am J Ophthalmol. 2009;148(6):869–74.
23. Bessho H, Honda S, Kondo N, Negi A. The association of age-related maculopathy susceptibility 2 polymorphisms with phenotype in typical neovascular age-related macular degeneration and polypoidal choroidal vasculopathy. Mol Vis. 2011;17:977–82.
24. Seddon JM, Francis PJ, George S, Schultz DW, Rosner B, Klein ML. Association of CFH Y402H and LOC387715 A69S with progression of age-related macular degeneration. JAMA. 2007;297(16):1793–800.
25. Seddon JM, Reynolds R, Maller J, Fagerness JA, Daly MJ, Rosner B. Prediction model for prevalence and incidence of advanced age-related macular degeneration based on genetic, demographic, and environmental variables. Invest Ophthalmol Vis Sci. 2009;50(5):2044–53.
26. Chen H, Yang Z, Gibbs D, et al. Association of HTRA1 polymorphism and bilaterality in advanced age-related macular degeneration. Vis Res. 2008;48(5):690–4.
27. Chen Y, Zeng J, Zhao C, et al. Assessing susceptibility to age-related macular degeneration with genetic markers and environmental factors. Arch Ophthalmol. 2011;129(3):344–51.
28. Schwartz SG, Agarwal A, Kovach JL, et al. The ARMS2 A69S variant and bilateral advanced age-related macular degeneration. Retina. 2012;32(8):1486–91.
29. Maguire MG, Daniel E, Shah AR, et al. Incidence of choroidal neovascularization in the fellow eye in the comparison of age-related macular degeneration treatments trials. Ophthalmology. 2013;120(10):2035–41.
30. Tamura H, Tsujikawa A, Yamashiro K, et al. Association of ARMS2 genotype with bilateral involvement of exudative age-related macular degeneration. Am J Ophthalmol. 2012;154(3):542–8. e541
31. Koh A, Lee WK, Chen LJ, et al. EVEREST study: efficacy and safety of verteporfin photodynamic therapy in combination with ranibizumab or alone versus ranibizumab monotherapy in patients with symptomatic macular polypoidal choroidal vasculopathy. Retina. 2012;32(8):1453–64.
32. Koh A, Lai TYY, Takahashi K, et al. Efficacy and safety of Ranibizumab with or without Verteporfin photodynamic therapy for Polypoidal Choroidal vasculopathy: a randomized clinical trial. JAMA Ophthalmol. 2017;135(11):1206–13.
33. Chowers I, Meir T, Lederman M, et al. Sequence variants in HTRA1 and LOC387715/ARMS2 and phenotype and response to photodynamic therapy in neovascular age-related macular degeneration in populations from Israel. Mol Vis. 2008;14:2263–71.
34. Brantley MA Jr, Edelstein SL, King JM, et al. Association of complement factor H and LOC387715 genotypes with response of exudative age-related macular degeneration to photodynamic therapy. Eye (Lond). 2009;23(3):626–31.
35. Immonen I, Seitsonen S, Tommila P, et al. Vascular endothelial growth factor gene variation and the response to photodynamic therapy in age-related macular degeneration. Ophthalmology. 2010;117(1):103–8.
36. Nakata I, Yamashiro K, Nakanishi H, Tsujikawa A, Otani A, Yoshimura N. VEGF gene polymorphism and response to intravitreal bevacizumab and triple therapy in age-related macular degeneration. Jpn J Ophthalmol. 2011;55(5):435–43.
37. Nakata I, Yamashiro K, Yamada R, et al. Genetic variants in pigment epithelium-derived factor influence response of polypoidal choroidal vasculopathy to photodynamic therapy. Ophthalmology. 2011;118(7):1408–15.
38. Feng X, Xiao J, Longville B, et al. Complement factor H Y402H and C-reactive protein polymorphism and photodynamic therapy response in age-related macular degeneration. Ophthalmology. 2009;116(10):1908–12. e1901
39. Parmeggiani F, Costagliola C, Gemmati D, et al. Predictive role of coagulation-balance gene polymorphisms in the efficacy of photodynamic therapy with verteporfin for classic choroidal neovascularization secondary to age-related macular degeneration. Pharmacogenet Genomics. 2007;17(12):1039–46.
40. Parmeggiani F, Costagliola C, Gemmati D, et al. Coagulation gene predictors of photodynamic therapy for occult choroidal neovascularization in age-related macular degeneration. Invest Ophthalmol Vis Sci. 2008;49(7):3100–6.
41. McKibbin M, Ali M, Bansal S, et al. CFH, VEGF and HTRA1 promoter genotype may influence the response to intravitreal ranibizumab therapy for neovascular age-related macular degeneration. Br J Ophthalmol. 2012;96(2):208–12.
42. Menghini M, Kloeckener-Gruissem B, Fleischhauer J, et al. Impact of loading phase, initial response and CFH genotype on the long-term outcome of treatment for neovascular age-related macular degeneration. PLoS One. 2012;7(7):e42014.
43. Tian J, Qin X, Fang K, et al. Association of genetic polymorphisms with response to bevacizumab for neovascular age-related macular degeneration in the Chinese population. Pharmacogenomics. 2012;13(7):779–87.
44. Kloeckener-Gruissem B, Barthelmes D, Labs S, et al. Genetic association with response to intravitreal ranibizumab in patients with neovascular AMD. Invest Ophthalmol Vis Sci. 2011;52(7):4694–702.
45. Brantley MA Jr, Fang AM, King JM, Tewari A, Kymes SM, Shiels A. Association of complement factor H and LOC387715 genotypes with response of exudative

age-related macular degeneration to intravitreal bevacizumab. Ophthalmology. 2007;114(12):2168–73.
46. Dikmetas O, Kadayifcilar S, Eldem B. The effect of CFH polymorphisms on the response to the treatment of age-related macular degeneration (AMD) with intravitreal ranibizumab. Mol Vis. 2013;19:2571–8.
47. Smailhodzic D, Muether PS, Chen J, et al. Cumulative effect of risk alleles in CFH, ARMS2, and VEGFA on the response to ranibizumab treatment in age-related macular degeneration. Ophthalmology. 2012;119(11):2304–11.
48. Lee AY, Raya AK, Kymes SM, Shiels A, Brantley MA Jr. Pharmacogenetics of complement factor H (Y402H) and treatment of exudative age-related macular degeneration with ranibizumab. Br J Ophthalmol. 2009;93(5):610–3.
49. Nischler C, Oberkofler H, Ortner C, et al. Complement factor H Y402H gene polymorphism and response to intravitreal bevacizumab in exudative age-related macular degeneration. Acta Ophthalmol. 2011;89(4):e344–9.
50. Imai D, Mori K, Horie-Inoue K, et al. CFH, VEGF, and PEDF genotypes and the response to intravitreous injection of bevacizumab for the treatment of age-related macular degeneration. J Ocul Biol Dis Infor. 2010;3(2):53–9.
51. Yamashiro K, Tomita K, Tsujikawa A, et al. Factors associated with the response of age-related macular degeneration to intravitreal ranibizumab treatment. Am J Ophthalmol. 2012;154(1):125–36.
52. Orlin A, Hadley D, Chang W, et al. Association between high-risk disease loci and response to anti-vascular endothelial growth factor treatment for wet age-related macular degeneration. Retina. 2012;32(1):4–9.
53. Hata M, Tsujikawa A, Miyake M, et al. Two-year visual outcome of ranibizumab in typical neovascular age-related macular degeneration and polypoidal choroidal vasculopathy. Graefes Arch Clin Exp Ophthalmol. 2015;253(2):221–7.
54. Hagstrom SA, Ying GS, Pauer GJT, et al. Pharmacogenetics for genes associated with age-related macular degeneration in the comparison of AMD treatments trials (CATT). Ophthalmology. 2013;120(3):593–9.
55. Abedi F, Wickremasinghe S, Richardson AJ, Islam AF, Guymer RH, Baird PN. Genetic influences on the outcome of anti-vascular endothelial growth factor treatment in neovascular age-related macular degeneration. Ophthalmology. 2013;120(8):1641–8.
56. Teper SJ, Nowinska A, Pilat J, Palucha A, Wylegala E. Involvement of genetic factors in the response to a variable-dosing ranibizumab treatment regimen for age-related macular degeneration. Mol Vis. 2010;16:2598–604.
57. Kang HK, Yoon MH, Lee DH, Chin HS. Pharmacogenetic influence of LOC387715/HTRA1 on the efficacy of bevacizumab treatment for age-related macular degeneration in a Korean population. Korean J Ophthalmol. 2012;26(6):414–22.
58. Kitchens JW, Kassem N, Wood W, et al. A pharmacogenetics study to predict outcome in patients receiving anti-VEGF therapy in age related macular degeneration. Clin Ophthalmol. 2013;7:1987–93.
59. Yuan D, Yuan D, Liu X, Yuan S, Xie P, Liu Q. Genetic association with response to intravitreal ranibizumab for neovascular age-related macular degeneration in the Han Chinese population. Ophthalmologica. 2013;230(4):227–32.
60. Chang W, Noh DH, Sagong M, Kim IT. Pharmacogenetic association with early response to intravitreal ranibizumab for age-related macular degeneration in a Korean population. Mol Vis. 2013;19:702–9.
61. Habibi I, Sfar I, Kort F, et al. Y402H polymorphism in complement factor H and age-related macular degeneration in the Tunisian population. Ophthalmic Res. 2013;49(4):177–84.
62. Park UC, Shin JY, Kim SJ, et al. Genetic factors associated with response to intravitreal ranibizumab in Korean patients with neovascular age-related macular degeneration. Retina. 2014;34(2):288–97.
63. van Asten F, Rovers MM, Lechanteur YT, et al. Predicting non-response to ranibizumab in patients with neovascular age-related macular degeneration. Ophthalmic Epidemiol. 2014;21(6):347–55.
64. Abedi F, Wickremasinghe S, Richardson AJ, et al. Variants in the VEGFA gene and treatment outcome after anti-VEGF treatment for neovascular age-related macular degeneration. Ophthalmology. 2013;120(1):115–21.
65. Lazzeri S, Figus M, Orlandi P, et al. VEGF-A polymorphisms predict short-term functional response to intravitreal ranibizumab in exudative age-related macular degeneration. Pharmacogenomics. 2013;14(6):623–30.
66. Wang JJ, Rochtchina E, Smith W, et al. Combined effects of complement factor H genotypes, fish consumption, and inflammatory markers on long-term risk for age-related macular degeneration in a cohort. Am J Epidemiol. 2009;169(5):633–41.
67. Boltz A, Ruiss M, Jonas JB, et al. Role of vascular endothelial growth factor polymorphisms in the treatment success in patients with wet age-related macular degeneration. Ophthalmology. 2012;119(8):1615–20.
68. Wickremasinghe SS, Xie J, Lim J, et al. Variants in the APOE gene are associated with improved outcome after anti-VEGF treatment for neovascular AMD. Invest Ophthalmol Vis Sci. 2011;52(7):4072–9.
69. Hautamaki A, Kivioja J, Vavuli S, et al. Interleukin 8 promoter polymorphism predicts the initial response to bevacizumab treatment for exudative age-related macular degeneration. Retina. 2013;33(9):1815–27.
70. Hautamaki A, Kivioja J, Seitsonen S, et al. The IL-8, VEGF, and CFH polymorphisms and bevacizumab in age-related macular degeneration. Ophthalmology. 2014;121(4):973–973.e971.
71. Yamashiro K, Mori K, Honda S, et al. A prospective multicenter study on genome wide associations to

ranibizumab treatment outcome for age-related macular degeneration. Sci Rep. 2017;7(1):9196.
72. Okada M, Kandasamy R, Chong EW, McGuiness M, Guymer RH. The treat-and-extend injection regimen versus alternate dosing strategies in age-related macular degeneration: a systematic review and meta-analysis. Am J Ophthalmol. 2018;192:184–97.
73. Silva R, Berta A, Larsen M, et al. Treat-and-extend versus monthly regimen in Neovascular age-related macular degeneration: results with Ranibizumab from the TREND study. Ophthalmology. 2018;125(1):57–65.
74. Fung AT, Yannuzzi LA, Freund KB. Type 1 (sub-retinal pigment epithelial) neovascularization in central serous chorioretinopathy masquerading as neovascular age-related macular degeneration. Retina. 2012;32(9):1829–37.
75. Imamura Y, Iida T, Maruko I, Zweifel SA, Spaide RF. Enhanced depth imaging optical coherence tomography of the sclera in dome-shaped macula. Am J Ophthalmol. 2011;151(2):297–302.
76. Warrow DJ, Hoang QV, Freund KB. Pachychoroid pigment epitheliopathy. Retina. 2013;33(8):1659–72.
77. Pang CE, Freund KB. Pachychoroid neovasculopathy. Retina. 2015;35(1):1–9.
78. Dansingani KK, Perlee LT, Hamon S, et al. Risk alleles associated with neovascularization in a Pachychoroid phenotype. Ophthalmology. 2016;123(12):2628–30.
79. Miyake M, Ooto S, Yamashiro K, et al. Pachychoroid neovasculopathy and age-related macular degeneration. Sci Rep. 2015;5:16204.
80. Hosoda Y, Yoshikawa M, Miyake M, et al. CFH and VIPR2 as susceptibility loci in choroidal thickness and pachychoroid disease central serous chorioretinopathy. Proc Natl Acad Sci U S A. 2018;115(24):6261–6.
81. Solouki AM, Verhoeven VJ, van Duijn CM, et al. A genome-wide association study identifies a susceptibility locus for refractive errors and myopia at 15q14. Nat Genet. 2010;42(10):897–901.
82. Hayashi H, Yamashiro K, Nakanishi H, et al. Association of 15q14 and 15q25 with high myopia in Japanese. Invest Ophthalmol Vis Sci. 2011;52(7):4853–8.
83. Tedja MS, Wojciechowski R, Hysi PG, et al. Genome-wide association meta-analysis highlights light-induced signaling as a driver for refractive error. Nat Genet. 2018;50(6):834–48.
84. Nakanishi H, Yamada R, Gotoh N, et al. A genome-wide association analysis identified a novel susceptible locus for pathological myopia at 11q24.1. PLoS Genet. 2009;5(9):e1000660.
85. Li YJ, Goh L, Khor CC, et al. Genome-wide association studies reveal genetic variants in CTNND2 for high myopia in Singapore Chinese. Ophthalmology. 2011;118(2):368–75.
86. Li Z, Qu J, Xu X, et al. A genome-wide association study reveals association between common variants in an intergenic region of 4q25 and high-grade myopia in the Chinese Han population. Hum Mol Genet. 2011;20(14):2861–8.
87. Shi Y, Qu J, Zhang D, et al. Genetic variants at 13q12.12 are associated with high myopia in the Han Chinese population. Am J Hum Genet. 2011;88(6):805–13.
88. Fan Q, Barathi VA, Cheng CY, et al. Genetic variants on chromosome 1q41 influence ocular axial length and high myopia. PLoS Genet. 2012;8(6):e1002753.
89. Shi Y, Gong B, Chen L, et al. A genome-wide meta-analysis identifies two novel loci associated with high myopia in the Han Chinese population. Hum Mol Genet. 2013;22(11):2325–33.
90. Khor CC, Miyake M, Chen LJ, et al. Genome-wide association study identifies ZFHX1B as a susceptibility locus for severe myopia. Hum Mol Genet. 2013;22(25):5288–94.
91. Fernandez-Robredo P, Maestre SR, Zarranz-Ventura J, Mulero HH, Salinas-Alaman A, Garcia-Layana A. Myopic choroidal neovascularization genetics. Ophthalmology. 2008;115(9):1632. 1632 e1631
92. Nakanishi H, Gotoh N, Yamada R, et al. ARMS2/HTRA1 and CFH polymorphisms are not associated with choroidal neovascularization in highly myopic eyes of the elderly Japanese population. Eye (Lond). 2010;24(6):1078–84.
93. Leveziel N, Yu Y, Reynolds R, et al. Genetic factors for choroidal neovascularization associated with high myopia. Invest Ophthalmol Vis Sci. 2012;53(8):5004–9.
94. Miyake M, Yamashiro K, Nakanishi H, et al. Evaluation of pigment epithelium-derived factor and complement factor I polymorphisms as a cause of choroidal neovascularization in highly myopic eyes. Invest Ophthalmol Vis Sci. 2013;54(6):4208–12.
95. Oishi M, Yamashiro K, Miyake M, et al. Association between ZIC2, RASGRF1, and SHISA6 genes and high myopia in Japanese subjects. Invest Ophthalmol Vis Sci. 2013;54(12):7492–7.
96. Hosoda Y, Yoshikawa M, Miyake M, et al. CCDC102B confers risk of low vision and blindness in high myopia. Nat Commun. 2018;9(1):1782.

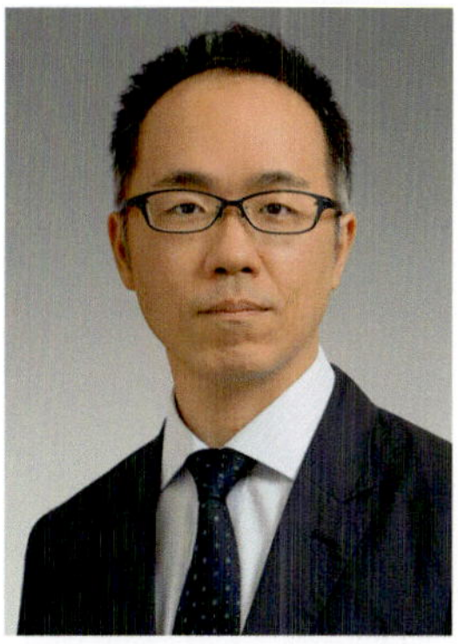

Kenji Yamashiro received MD from Kyoto University Medical School in1995 and PhD from Kyoto University Graduate School of Medicine in 2002 after joining Angiogenesis lab in Massachusetts Eye and Ear Infirmary at Harvard Medical School. Dr. Yamashiro is an author on over 180 scientific publications (impact factor: over 850) and currently a Director of Ophthalmology at Otsu Red Cross Hospital and a Clinical Professor of Ophthalmology at the Kyoto University Graduate School of Medicine, Japan. His recent interest is in improving medical and surgical treatment for retinal diseases.

Part II

Clinical Entities

7 Neovascular AMD: Clinical Features and Imaging

Cláudia Farinha and Rufino Silva

7.1 Introduction

Age-related macular degeneration (AMD) is the leading cause of irreversible visual impairment and blindness in the elderly in developed countries [1, 2]. It is well recognized that global population aging is expected in the next decades, and therefore, the number of patients affected by AMD is expected to increase significantly. Recent estimates point to a projected number of people with AMD in 2020 of 196 million, and 288 million in 2040 [3, 4]. Importantly, approximately 10% of AMD patients manifest the neovascular form of the disease, which if left untreated leads to severe irreversible visual loss. Neovascular AMD (nAMD) is, in fact, responsible for approximately 80% of cases of severe vision loss due to AMD [2]. Therefore, a worldwide increase in the burden of nAMD and associated risk of blindness seems to be certain in the near future [5, 6].

Neovascular AMD reports to the development of choroidal neovascularization (CNV) and the presence of its associated features, such as retinal pigment epithelial detachment (PED), retinal and subretinal hemorrhage and fluid, fibrovascular disciform scarring and retinal pigment epithelial tear [6]. This designation also includes specific neovascular phenotypes such as retinal angiomatous proliferation (RAP), or type 3 neovascularization, and polypoidal choroidal vasculopathy (PCV) [7–9].

Histologically, a CNV is a neovascular proliferation that grows through breaks in the Bruch's membrane and progresses laterally between the RPE and Bruch's. Grossniklaus and Gass described two different histologic types of neovascular growth: type 1 (confined beneath the retinal pigmented epithelium (RPE)) and type 2 (when the neovascularization grows between the neurosensory retina and the RPE) [10, 11]. However, the two types can often coexist in AMD (mixed CNV). In 1996, Hartnett et al. [12] described a new distinct

C. Farinha
Ophthalmology Department, Coimbra Hospital and Universitary Centre (CHUC), Coimbra, Portugal

Association for Innovation and Biomedical Research on Light and Image (AIBILI), Coimbra, Portugal

Faculty of Medicine, University of Coimbra (FMUC), Coimbra, Portugal

R. Silva (✉)
Ophthalmology Department, Coimbra Hospital and Universitary Centre (CHUC), Coimbra, Portugal

Association for Innovation and Biomedical Research on Light and Image (AIBILI), Coimbra, Portugal

Faculty of Medicine, Coimbra Institute for Clinical and Biomedical Research. University of Coimbra (iCBR- FMUC), Coimbra, Portugal

Coimbra Medical Space, Coimbra, Portugal
e-mail: rufino.silva@oftalmologia.co.pt

J. Chhablani (ed.), *Choroidal Neovascularization*, https://doi.org/10.1007/978-981-15-2213-0_7

phenotype of neovascularization, which originates from the deeper retina and eventually extends posteriorly toward the choroid, this was later denominated by Yannuzzi and colleagues as RAP, and more recently as type 3 neovascularization [7, 13]. The diagnosis of different neovascular histologic subtypes in AMD is nowadays regarded as non-crucial in deciding treatment, as all neovascular AMD can be treated with anti-vascular endothelial growth factors (VEGF). However, it may be important for predicting therapeutic response and prognosis and for consideration of adjunctive photodynamic therapy in PCV cases [14].

7.2 Clinical Presentation of Neovascular AMD

Neovascular AMD presents clinically by typical signs and symptoms, usually in the elder patient. Blurred or decreased vision and distortion in the image (metamorphopsia), especially when reading, are the main complaints. Micropsia and central scotoma can be referred, but sometimes there may be no complaints at all. The patient can be truly asymptomatic, or the visual changes are too subtle in the early stages for the patient to notice them.

In fundoscopy, there are several features that can be appreciated. The CNV may appear as a gray lesion located deep to the retina, elevating it, and often with associated presence of blood (intra and/or subretinal), hard exudates, and intraretinal edema with or without a neurosensorial detachment (Fig. 7.1). This gray color of the CNV is not always seen, and the presence of the remaining features in an older patient with AMD and vision loss indicates the presence of the membrane. Associated serous or hemorrhagic PED is also typical, with the latter being more frequent in the context of PCV. In other cases, the only presenting sign is a small neurosensory detachment, and a careful analysis of the fundus together with a high clinical suspicion and imagiological ancillary tests is fundamental to the correct diagnosis and timely treatment [6].

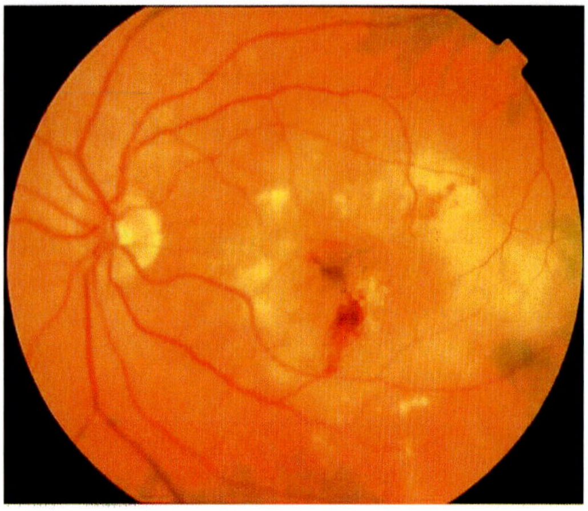

Fig. 7.1 Clinical presentation of nAMD. Retinal edema and elevation associated with retinal hemorrhages, hard exudates, and subretinal fibrosis are typical signs of late exudative AMD

7.2.1 Pigment Epithelial Detachment

A PED refers to the anatomical separation of the RPE from the underlying Bruch's membrane. In neovascular AMD they can be serous, fibrovascular (type 1 CNV), mixed (with both serous and fibrovascular components), and might also be hemorrhagic as a complication of the associated CNV [15, 16]. In eyes with nAMD, it is not uncommon to see more than one type of PED.

On funduscopic examination, a serous PED is seen as a sharply demarcated circular or ovoid dome-shaped elevation of the RPE with a clear or yellowish–orange color. When chronic there may be pigment migration and deposition in a reticular or radial pattern over the PED [6]. The serous PED is usually related to CNV in nAMD and an associated notched appearance is considered typical. However, avascular PEDs may also be seen without evidence of CNV. Of patients with neovascular AMD only 1% present with a pure serous PED, whereas 31% present with a vascularized serous PED [15]. The natural history of a serous PED is relatively more favorable, compared to vascularized PEDs associated with type 1 (sub-RPE) neovascularization, which have a high risk for vision loss. Subfoveal avascular serous PEDs can, in fact, remain unchanged over significant periods of time and visual acuity may stabilize without treatment [15].

A hemorrhagic PED, this is blood within a PED, implies a diagnosis of CNV. It appears as an elevated, dark-red-greenish mound. The hemorrhage can dissect through the RPE into the subretinal space or into the retina. Rarely, it may pass through the retina into the vitreous cavity, causing hemovitreous [6].

In some cases, a pure fibrovascular PED (fvPED) can present with a homogeneous dark red color in fundoscopy. This feature can be misinterpreted as blood in the sub-RPE space; however, it corresponds only to an engorged neovascular complex with large-caliber vessels. These vessels may be more mature and possibly contain stagnated blood that appears dark red. One should be aware of this variant of fibrovascular PEDs because these large neovascular vessels may bleed and necessitate aggressive treatment [15].

7.2.2 Retinal Pigment Epithelial Tear

Tears of the RPE were first described in 1981 by Hoskin and colleagues [17]. A retinal pigment epithelial tear usually occurs in an eye with a serous or fibrovascular PED, and can occur in up to 27% of eyes, depending on the study population. The spontaneous tear rate in the natural history of fvPEDs in nAMD has been reported to be between 10% and 12.5%. There are conflicting reports on the incidence of RPE tears after anti-VEGF therapies, but it is estimated to affect 15% to 20%, especially when the PED is 600 μm or greater in height. Visual acuity usually drops suddenly with the event if the tear involves the foveal center; however, it is often stabilized if anti-VEGF therapy is continued [16, 17].

A RPE tear probably results from growing tension in the junction of the attached and detached areas of the RPE, from increasing fluid beneath it and/or from contraction of an associated CNV when an RPE-adherent fibrovascular component is present in the PED [6]. The edge of the elevated RPE curls in the direction of the CNV, leaving bare Bruch's membrane and choroid in the area exposed, which gives rise to a sharply depigmented area, usually with a crescent-shaped configuration. The curled and rolled RPE is seen adjacent to this hypopigmented area as an area of increased brownish pigmentation [15]. Sometimes concentric tears may develop and only an island of scrolled RPE remains at the center of the tear. Diagnosing small tears is easier with fundus autofluorescence imaging, as the tear crescent area shows profound hypoautofluorescence, with a slight increase in autofluorescence in the area of the torn and retracted RPE [17].

7.2.3 Disciform Scar

A CNV is a fibrovascular tissue since the neovessels are accompanied by fibrous tissue. With time, and despite treatment, the fibrotic turnover might progress, and the plane of the RPE is destroyed, making the CNV classification by type no longer discernible. When the fibrous tissue becomes clinically visible, the CNV and fibrous tissue complex are called a disciform scar.

Clinically, disciform lesions vary in color from white to yellow. Hyperpigmented areas may be present depending on the degree of RPE hyperplasia within the scar tissue. Disciform scars may continue to grow, with new areas of neovascularization proliferating along their edge. Reading vision is severely compromised at this point and rarely is better than 20/200 [6].

7.3 Imaging in Neovascular AMD

Imaging is essential in the diagnosis and treatment of nAMD. Fluorescein angiography (FA) is traditionally considered the *gold standard* for the diagnosis, because it can provide useful information concerning lesion subtype and activity through the dynamic visualization of dye leakage [18]. In the last years, however, Spectral Domain Optical Coherence Tomography (SD-OCT) has become an indispensable tool in the diagnosis and follow-up of nAMD, as it allows for noninvasive high-resolution visualization of the CNV and associated features related to angiographic leakage, such as intraretinal and subretinal fluid [19]. In the clinical setting, other ancillary exams used in nAMD management include indocyanine green angiography (ICGA) and more recently OCT Angiography (OCT-A).

OCT Angiography is a new technology that is rapidly growing and gaining popularity in the daily practice of AMD clinics because it allows to noninvasively detect the neovascular network, giving information on flow and vessel density, while simultaneously providing all the structural B-scan information of a conventional OCT device.

7.3.1 Fluorescein Angiography

As stated above, FA is still considered today the *gold standard* for the diagnosis and management of nAMD in clinical practice. In the era of OCT, FA remains important in CNV diagnosis because it reduces the possibility of error or misdiagnosis. In fact, multimodal imaging including FA and OCT is currently the state of the art in the assessment of nAMD. Fluorescein angiography is also used to this day in major nAMD clinical trials and the imaging features analyzed are recognized as valid and reliable endpoints [20].

The study of a CNV lesion with FA allows the clinic to determine patterns of fluorescence such as classic and occult, and the relative composition (predominantly classic, minimally classic, and occult CNV). There is an assumed relationship between the histopathologic types 1 and 2 and the occult and classic CNV patterns, respectively, however, there is little evidence to support the universality of this correlation. FA also allows to analyze on the boundaries of the lesion as "well defined" or "poorly defined" and the location of the CNV in respect to the fovea (subfoveal, juxtafoveal if the border is within 199 μm of the center, and extrafoveal if the margin is at least 200 μm from the foveal center) [6]. Fluorescein angiography is particularly useful in assessing CNV activity through the dynamic visualization of dye leakage. Other features of an active CNV such as neurosensorial detachment and serous PED are easily assessed by FA, as dye pools in these potential spaces, with increased fluorescence through the angiogram [18].

The nomenclature of classic vs occult CNV provided by FA is, however, becoming less used in the clinical setting because of the relatively uniform treatment given to these patients with anti-VEGFs, and because of the major role attributed to SD-OCT in the diagnosis and follow-up of nAMD. Despite this, the knowledge is still essential because response to treatment may be different on different lesion subtypes, and because most clinical trials still rely on these angiographic features for the inclusion of patients.

7.3.1.1 Classic CNV

A classic CNV is seen in the early phases of the angiogram as a hyperfluorescent area, with well-defined borders, sometimes surrounded by a hypofluorescent halo. The individual vessels in the CNV may be seen, often with a "wagon wheel" appearance composed by the feeding central vessels and the centripetally oriented neovessels that radiate from them. The hyperfluorescence associated with the classic CNV typically increases as the angiogram progresses, with marked leakage extending beyond the borders of the CNV in the late frames (Fig. 7.2) [6, 21–23].

7.3.1.2 Occult CNV

The term occult CNV reports to two patterns in angiography: *fibrovascular PED* and *late leakage of undetermined source* (LLUS).

A fvPED is best appreciated at 1–2 min in the angiogram, as an irregular elevated area of stippled or pinpoint-like hyperfluorescence, with or without leakage or with staining in the late frames. The hyperfluorescence, in this case, is much weaker compared to classic CNVs, and the borders of the detachment are often indistinct (Fig. 7.3). Fibrovascular PEDs must be distinguished from purely serous PEDs, but it is not uncommon to visualize a serous PED contiguous with a fvPED.

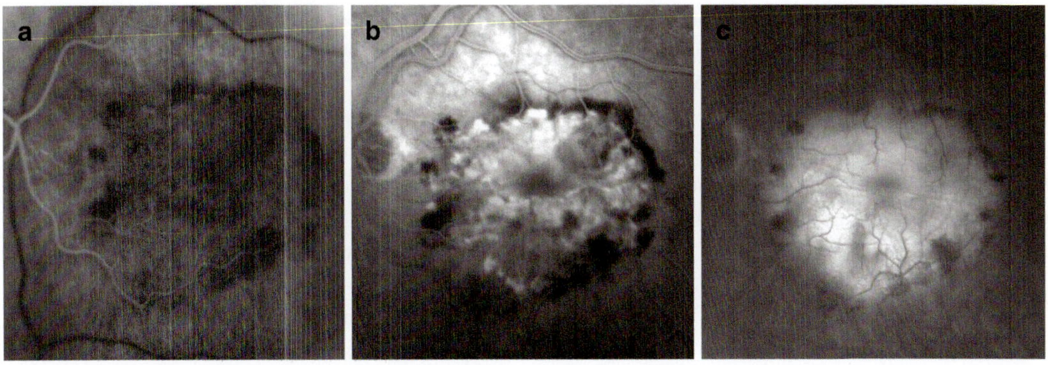

Fig. 7.2 Classic CNV in FA. (**a**) The classic lesion presents with well-defined limits in early phase and the neovascular network is seen with great detail; (**b**) in intermediate phase it increases significantly in brightness further enhancing the visualization of the neovessels; (**c**) in late phase there is intense leakage obscuring the CNV borders and neovascular network details

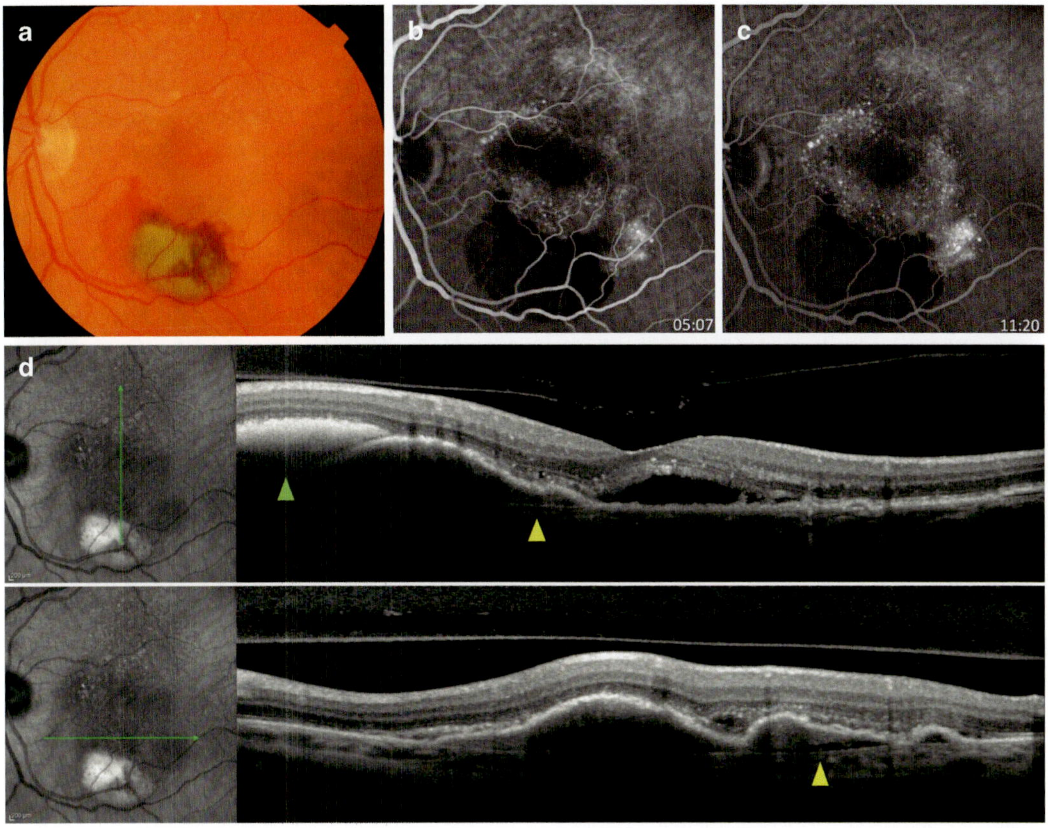

Fig. 7.3 Multimodal imaging of occult CNV/type 1 CNV. (**a**) CFP image shows the presence of a PED in the central macula with soft drusen and subretinal fluid, and an inferior subretinal hemorrhage with dehemoglobinized blood; (**b**, **c**) FA shows occult CNV with fibrovascular PED pattern as an irregular area of stippled hyperfluorescence in intermediate transit phase, with persistent staining and discrete leakage in late phase; there is also blocked fluorescence of the choroid from the subretinal blood; (**d**) SD-OCT scans show the presence of the fvPED corresponding to type 1 CNV, seen as irregularly elevated RPE with underlying heterogenous laminar tissue, separating it from the Bruch's membrane; there is a fluid cleft beneath the fibrovascular tissue (triple layer sign) (yellow arrows). Subretinal fluid involving the foveal center and subretinal hemorrhage, hyperreflective, and blocking the RPE and choroidal details, are also seen (green arrow)

The LLUS term is used when there is late choroidal-based leakage with no clearly corresponding identifiable classic CNV or fvPED in the early or mid-phase of the angiogram. It appears as speckled hyperfluorescence, often with overlying subretinal pooling of dye, and the CNV boundaries cannot be determined precisely [6, 15, 21–23].

7.3.2 Indocyanine Green Angiography

Indocyanine green is a dye that is more protein-bound than sodium fluorescein and fluoresces in the near-infrared wavelength, which enhances its transmission through the RPE, but also through blood and exudative material, thus providing a more detailed visualization of the choroidal vasculature and its pathology [23, 24].

ICGA is very useful in the context of nAMD for accurate detection of occult CNV, especially in cases that otherwise would be difficult to discern using only FA [25], for example, when occult CNV does not fluoresce enough to be clearly seen in FA or when a serous or hemorrhagic PED mask the underlying membrane. ICGA is also of great interest in diagnosing specific neovascular phenotypes such as RAP lesions, especially in the early stages, and PCV [20]. ICGA is the *gold standard* for the diagnosis of the latter because it allows the clear detection of polyps or aneurysmatic dilatations, as more recently described.

ICGA Patterns in nAMD:

- **Plaque**: The most common pattern, is a hyperfluorescent area larger than one disk area, usually well defined, that shows relatively late in the angiogram. The plaques may exhibit progressive growth.
- **Hot spot or focal CNV**: When lesions appear as occult CNV on FA but demonstrate hyperfluorescence in ICGA of less than one disk area. They usually show by the mid-phase of the angiogram and often correspond to elements of RAP or PCV [23].

  Area of ill-defined fluorescence.

7.3.3 Optical Coherence Tomography

Optical coherence tomography has become an indispensable tool in the assessment of retinal pathology, and by extension in the diagnosis and follow-up of patients with nAMD. Compared to dye-based FA and ICGA, OCT is a noninvasive and less-time consuming exam that gives precious information on the morphologic microstructural characteristics of a CNV and associated features, and their response to treatment. Currently, two OCT technologies are in wide-spread use: the spectral-domain OCT (SD-OCT), that operates at scanning rates of approximately 27,000–70,000 A-scans/second; and the swept source OCT (SS-OCT). The latter has faster scanning speeds (100,000–400,000 A-scans/second) and operates at a longer wavelength, increasing the visualization of structures beneath the RPE [26, 27].

In nAMD, the use of OCT combined with FA and ICGA provided a better understanding on how to correlate the abundant information from multimodal imaging with the previous histologic findings described by Grossniklaus and Gass on types 1 and 2 neovascular membranes [10, 11]. This multimodal approach is superior to FA alone to determine the presence, location and size of CNV, and these are factors that may be predictive of prognosis and treatment response.

Thus, a new imagiological CNV classification emerged based on this OCT-driven multimodal approach: **type 1**, **type 2** and **type 3** neovascularization [23]. Type 1 and type 3 neovascular membranes are the most prevalent subtypes of neovascular AMD, when using FA and OCT combined, and are estimated to represent 40% and 34% of cases, respectively. Pure type 2 lesions account for only 9% and mixed membranes are seen in 17% of cases, as reported by Jung et al. [28].

Type 1 and 2 lesions characteristics in OCT are presented below. Type 3 neovascular membrane or RAP and PCV, as a variant of type 1, will be discussed separately.

7.3.3.1 Type 1 Neovascular Membrane

Corresponds to a CNV that occurs and grows beneath the RPE, creating a separation between the RPE and the Bruch's membrane. A type 1 CNV corresponds to a vascularized PED and is the most common in nAMD.

On OCT it appears as moderate to high reflective material located between the RPE and the Bruch, clearly separating them. Some authors have called this the "*double layer sign*" when it is relatively thin [29]. This fibrovascular tissue is seen with various degrees of thickness and volume, usually with a fusiform or nodular shape. Its inner reflectivity varies according to the composition, typically having a heterogeneous multilaminar structure with moderate to high reflectivity, that adheres to the elevated RPE (Fig. 7.3). Spaide et al. [30] proposed that the CNV vessels adhere to the basal surface of the RPE when the RPE becomes elevated by sub-RPE exudation. Hyporeflective oval spaces and channels may be seen within the fibrovascular tissue and are thought to correspond to the neovessels' vascular lumen.

Fluid clefts are also observed as optically empty spaces within or beneath the fibrovascular tissue. Khan et al. [31] described the "*triple layer sign*" when a hyporeflective space or cleft appears immediately underneath the fibrovascular multilayered PED. The "*onion sign*" was described by Mukkamala et al. [32], and corresponds to a pattern of layered hyperreflective bands beneath the RPE line and within the fvPED that correlates clinically with areas of yellow exudates. They hypothesized that these hyperreflective bands correspond to exudation of lipid in the sub-RPE space from the CNV.

A type 1 CNV may be associated with larger serous components, and the CNV may be seen adjacent to the borders of the serous detachment and/or as hyperreflective material that lines along the back surface of the elevated PED. The appearance of vascularized and serous PEDs may be similar in OCT and FA/ICGA is essential to identify the associated CNV.

Type 1 CNVs may be non-exudative, slowly enlarging over years, with the patient remaining asymptomatic. This silent growth can be noninvasively monitored by OCT, and more recently by OCT-A. Grossniklaus and Green hypothesized that the type 1 CNV may be a compensatory response supporting an ischemic outer retina, and theoretically that could protect against the advent or progression of geographic atrophy [33].

Eyes become symptomatic when subretinal or intraretinal exudation develops and this is seen in OCT as subretinal (SRF) or intraretinal fluid (IRF). IRF occurs either diffusely, with increased retinal thickness and reduced retinal reflectivity, or localized in nonreflective cysts (cystic macular edema). Subretinal fluid is the predominant form of exudation in type 1 CNV. OCT is thus of great value in assessing the CNV activity during follow-up [15]. Although the clinical course is variable, a type 1 CNV tends to behave less aggressively than types 2 and 3, as these cause more active exudation and more rapid vision loss [15].

A type 1 CNV corresponds usually to an occult CNV in FA (both fvPED and LLUS), and to a plaque pattern in ICGA.

7.3.3.2 Type 2 Neovascular Membrane

Corresponds to a CNV that has penetrated the RPE/Bruch's membrane complex and proliferates in the subretinal space. Pure type 2 CNV is rare in nAMD and Naysan and colleagues [34] reported that type 2 CNV occurs almost exclusively in AMD patients with pure subretinal drusenoid deposits (reticular pseudodrusen) phenotype and thin choroids. In fact, in AMD a type 2 CNV is usually seen in association with a type 1 that has grown vertically to penetrate the RPE and is now proliferating in the subretinal space, this is, a mixed CNV (Fig. 7.4) [23, 28].

In OCT type 2 neovessels are seen above the RPE band and beneath the photoreceptor outer segments. The CNV is seen as moderately to hyperreflective material that may appear more laminar in structure or with a more amorphous appearance with fuzzy borders. This depends on the size, degree of exudation, and associated features such as fibrin deposition or presence of subretinal hemorrhage. Usually, there is disorganization of the photoreceptors' layers with disruption of the ellipsoid zone and external limiting membrane. In this context, intraretinal cystic edema is common and predominates over subretinal fluid [23].

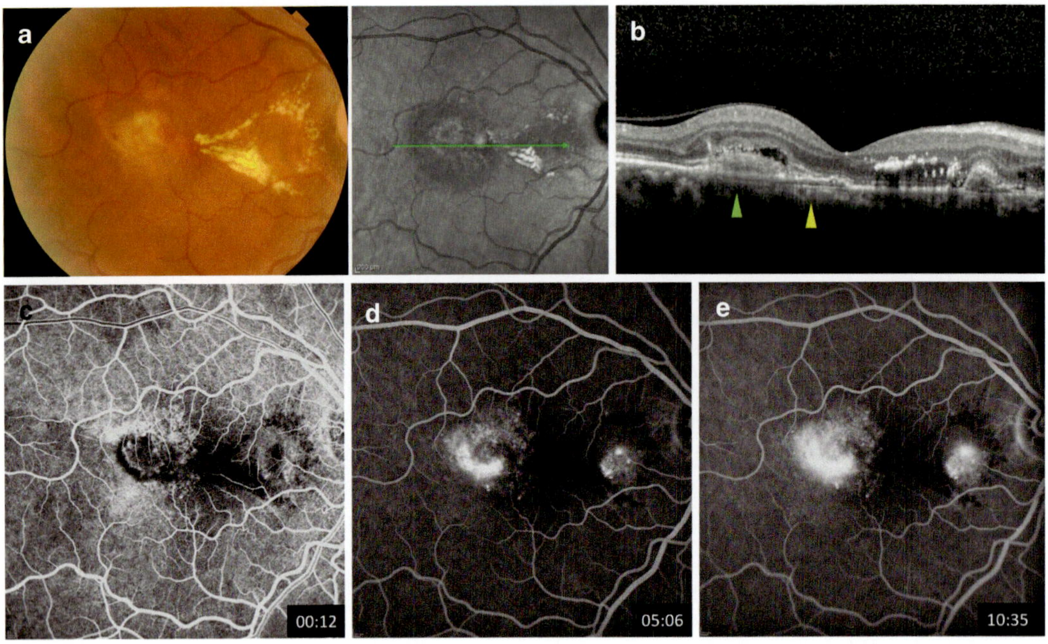

Fig. 7.4 Multimodal imaging of mixed type 1 and 2 CNV. (**a**) CFP image shows the presence hard exudates in the macula and some degree of subretinal fibrosis temporal to the fovea; (**b**) SD-OCT scan shows the presence of a fvPED corresponding to type 1 CNV, in a double layer configuration (yellow arrow), with overlying subretinal type 2 CNV (green arrow) and subretinal fluid; (**c**) FA shows a classic CNV in the early phase corresponding to the type 2 lesion, with well-defined limits and a surrounding hypofluorescent halo; (**d**, **e**) in intermediate and late FA phases occult CNV (type 1) is seen as irregular, stippled hyperfluorescence adjacent to the classic CNV and in the nasal fovea, with leakage in late phases less intense compared to the classic component

As the CNV matures, progression to subretinal fibrosis may ensue and appear on OCT as a hyperreflective band overlying the RPE with substantial disorganization and thinning of the outer retina.

A type 2 CNV corresponds usually to a classic CNV in FA. In ICGA, the vascular networks are seen but can be difficult to detect overlying the intense hyperfluorescence of the background choroidal circulation. A hypofluorescent outer border can surround the CNV [21].

7.3.4 Other Features of nAMD in Multimodal Imaging

7.3.4.1 Pigment Epithelial Detachments

The FA pattern through the angiogram together with OCT and, whenever necessary, ICGA, allows the differentiation between the different PED types that can be present in AMD. These include *drusenoid PED* not associated with CNV, *fibrovascular PED* or type 1 CNV, *serous PED* (vascularized or avascular), and *hemorrhagic PED* [6, 15]:

- ***Drusenoid PEDs*** are not a feature of nAMD but they will be referred as it is important to accurately differentiate them from fvPEDs. They are seen as an extensive area of large confluent soft drusen, often with overlying reticulated pigment clumping and a scalloped border. They fluoresce faintly during the angiogram and become less fluorescent in the late phase. They do not progress to bright hyperfluorescence like a serous PED, neither present with stippled hyperfluorescence, differentiating them from fvPED. Focal hypofluorescent areas correspond to the blocking effect of overlying pigment hyperplasia [35].

- In ICGA using a confocal scanning laser ophthalmoscope (SLO) system, the PED will appear as a homogeneous hypofluorescent area during the transit, because the drusen-like content will block the fluorescence from the choroidal vasculature. With ICGA using a traditional fundus camera-based system the drusenoid PED can appear isofluorescent or slightly hypofluorescent.
- On OCT the PED will appear as a smooth elevation of the RPE band with or without undulation, with material underneath that typically has a dense homogeneous appearance with moderate or high reflectivity. Sub-RPE fluid pockets above the deposited material may be present. Hyperreflective foci with posterior shadowing are commonly seen immediately above the PED and correspond to pigment clumping from RPE in histologic examination [36]. Subretinal or intraretinal fluid is not typical and should raise suspicion of CNV. However, there may be a small pocket of benign subretinal fluid or an acquired vitelliform lesion. This must be differentiated from an active CNV as treatment is not indicated.
- A ***serous PED*** appears in FA as a uniform bright hyperfluorescent area in the early phase with smooth borders, increasing in intensity toward the late phase, with little or no leakage along its borders. A serous PED might obscure any CNV contained in its area. However, a typical fluorescein pattern of the vascularized serous PED is when a serous PED has a *notch* or *hot spot* corresponding to CNV. The FA shows early intense hyperfluorescence and late homogeneous pooling of the serous component while the notch has stippled hyperfluorescence indicating the associated occult membrane.
- In ICGA, the serous PED is hypofluorescent in both the early and the late phases when using a confocal SLO system, because fluid blocks the normal fluorescence of the choroid. If there is early hyperfluorescence and late staining adjacent to the serous PED or within, this corresponds to associated occult CNV.
- On OCT a serous PED appears as a smooth, sharply demarcated dome-shaped elevation of the RPE, overlying a homogeneously hyporeflective space, with a clearly visible Bruch's membrane beneath it, seen as a thin hyperreflective line [37].
- A ***hemorrhagic PED*** presents in FA as a dark area through the angiogram, as the blood beneath the RPE will block choroidal fluorescence. In ICGA, a focal or plaque-like area of hyperfluorescence corresponding to the CNV may be seen through the blood or at its border. The OCT shows a dome-shaped elevation of the RPE with the blood beneath appearing hyperreflective. Because of this, there is substantial attenuation of the signal from deeper structures and the sub-RPE CNV, as well as the Bruch's membrane and the choroid, are not easily discerned or not seen at all.

7.3.4.2 RPE Tear

In FA, the areas where the RPE is missing cause a window defect showing the early choroidal fluorescence, with staining till the late frames, but generally there is no leakage from the stripped area. The area with the retracted and curled RPE blocks the background fluorescence, thus being hypofluorescent through all angiographic examinations. There may be leakage from this area later from an underlying CNV.

Sarraf et al. [38] published a grading system for RPE tears that is based on the greatest linear diameter of the tear measured with FA: grade 1 are those <200 μm, grade 2 when between 200 μm and 1 disk diameter, grade 3 if >1 disk diameter, and grade 4 if they are >1 disk diameter and involve the center of the fovea. This grading system was shown to have prognostic significance in the response to treatment with anti-VEGF and functional outcome.

In ICGA, the bare choroid is hypofluorescent or isofluorescent, and the rolled RPE is moderately hypofluorescent [17].

The OCT shows disruption of the RPE monolayer in the PED, varying from a microscopic defect to a large discontinuity. The retracted RPE is seen with an irregular shape, often with the free edge curled under the PED, showing dense hyperreflectivity from duplication of the RPE, and a shadowing effect beneath it. The bare choroid area shows hyperreflectivity as a result of deeper penetration due to the absence of the RPE. The retina overlying this zone remains intact with or without associated subretinal fluid. OCT is the preferred method for definite diagnosis of RPE tear (Fig. 7.5) [17, 37].

7.3.4.3 Disciform Scarring

Usually the disciform scar is hyperfluorescent from both fluorescein dye leakage and staining. The fluorescence may fade away in the late frames or increase, if there is still exudation with fluid. Hypofluorescent areas may be seen when RPE pigmentary reaction blocks fluorescence. In ICGA anastomoses between the retina and the choroid are often observed [21].

On OCT the scar corresponds to a highly reflective outer retinal or subretinal lesion. There is extensive damage to the photoreceptors inner and outer segments with disruption of the ellipsoid zone and external limiting membrane and thinning of the outer nuclear layer [37]. At this point, *outer-retinal tubulations (ORTs)* may appear over the scar and in associated areas of outer retina and RPE atrophy (Fig. 7.6). ORTs should be differentiated from intraretinal fluid from exudation. They were first described histologically as interconnecting tubes containing degenerate photoreceptors and enveloping Müller cells in AMD patients. In OCT ORTs appear as round or oval lesions with hyporeflective lumen and hyperreflective borders located in the outer nuclear layer, overlying an RPE that is either disrupted or absent. They may form branching networks of channels best appreciated in *en face* OCT [39, 40]. *Degenerative cysts,* usually small

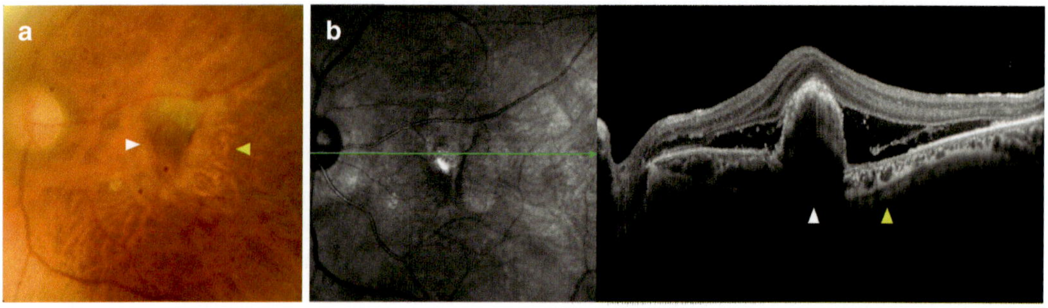

Fig. 7.5 RPE tear. (**a**) CFP shows the ruptured and retracted RPE as an area of increased pigmentation (white arrow) and an associated geographic area of depigmentation from denuded choroid (yellow arrow); fibrosis and retinal hemorrhages are also seen; (**b**) the corresponding SD-OCT B-scan shows the elevated fibrovascular PED with RPE retraction and shadowing effect over the underlying choroid from the folded RPE (white arrow) and the area of bare choroid, where the RPE is absent, with increased reflectivity (yellow arrow)

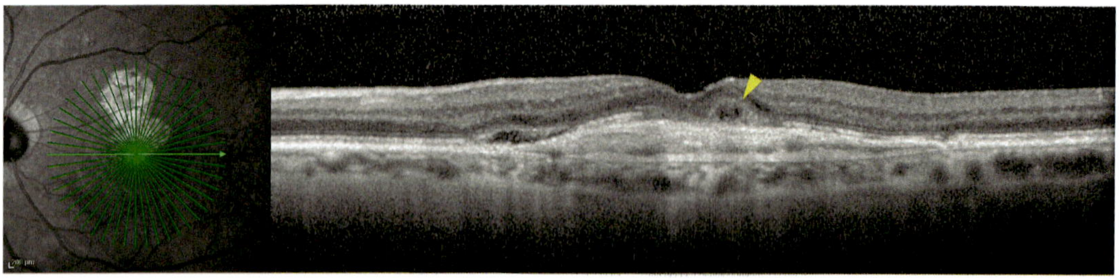

Fig. 7.6 Disciform scar in OCT. The scar is seen as a highly reflective subretinal lesion with disruption of the overlying ellipsoid zone and external limiting membrane and thinning of the outer nuclear layer. Outer-retinal tubulations with hyperreflective borders are seen over the fibrotic lesion (yellow arrow)

and more quadrangular in shape, may also appear overlying the scar and/or atrophy and are thought to be related to a degenerative process, perhaps Müller cell degeneration, rather than to exudation. In accordance with this, leakage is usually absent in FA [41]. Both ORTs and degenerative cysts detected in OCT are important for the clinician to recognize because they can interfere with treatment decisions.

7.4 Specific Neovascular Phenotypes in AMD

7.4.1 Retinal Angiomatous Proliferation (Type 3 Neovascularization)

First described by Hartnett et al. [12] as intraretinal vascular proliferation without any choroidal vascular involvement or "deep retinal anomalous complexes," this type of neovascularization was later denominated by Yannuzzi and colleagues as retinal angiomatous proliferation or RAP [13]. There was, however, doubt on the primary origin of the lesion: the retina or the choroid, the latter being proposed by Gass [42]. Studies with SD-OCT imaging concluded that the neovascular process could originate from either the retina or choroid, but histopathologic studies suggest that neovascularization is in the retina [7, 43, 44]. Following the intraretinal origin, a RAP staging system was proposed by Yannuzi et al. [13]: *Stage 1*—intraretinal neovascularization; *Stage 2*—subretinal neovascularization with retinal–retinal anastomosis; and *Stage 3*—neovascularization with a vascularized pigment epithelial detachment and a retinal–choroidal anastomosis.

Despite this, RAP was more recently proposed to be designated as type 3 neovascularization, following the logic of type 1 and 2 neovascularization classification [7, 13, 23, 43].

RAP is estimated to represent about 10% to 15% of new nAMD cases. Another important notion is that a patient with RAP in one eye has a high chance of developing another RAP lesion in the fellow eye. This is estimated to be 80% after 1 year, and increases to 100% at 3 years [45]. The presence of reticular pseudodrusen and thinner choroid also seems to be associated with RAP development [8].

Clinically, RAP lesions are usually seen in the parafoveal region presenting with retinal edema, hard exudates, and preretinal, intraretinal, and subretinal small spot hemorrhages. Sometimes it is possible to see the deepening of the dilated anastomotic vessel at 90° orientation, typically over a PED. Retinal–retinal anastomosis is also seen in RAP. When a larger fibrovascular PED develops in later stages other features of nAMD may appear making the diagnosis of this distinct phenotype more difficult based only in fundoscopy [13, 15, 46].

On fluorescein angiography, a RAP lesion in the initial stage typically presents as a focal area of hyperfuorescence in the early phase located outside the foveal avascular zone. This focal area progressively increases in brightness during the angiogram with leakage in the late frames. A retinal-retinal or retinal–choroidal anastomosis may be seen. If a fvPED develops from progression of the type 3 membrane, signs of occult CNV will appear and diagnosis of RAP becomes difficult with FA only. Both intraretinal leakage with pooling in cystoid spaces and subretinal leakage may be seen.

ICG angiography is very useful in identifying the intraretinal neovascular complex as a characteristic "hot spot." Another typical feature is the intraretinal leakage in the late phase of the ICGA into the cystoid macular edema (CME) spaces, presumably because of the presence of fibrin in these and the affinity of the ICG molecule to fibrin [7, 8, 13].

Findings in OCT also depend on the stage of the RAP lesion. An incipient RAP lesion can be seen as a punctate or focal intraretinal hyperreflective lesion located in the outer retina above the external limiting membrane (ELM), overlying an area of outer nuclear layer thinning and photoreceptors loss, or overlying a PED. There can be associated CME at this point (Fig. 7.7) [37]. In more advanced stages, the most common appearance is that of a serous PED (or sometimes a fvPED) with overlying CME. It is possible to observe a focal break in the RPE band of the PED through which a continuous hyperreflective band connects the intraretinal component to the sub-RPE component. A distinctive feature is the disruption of the external limiting membrane that accompanies the CME above the PED as opposed to a Type 2 CNV that is usually associated with a neurosensory detachment and an intact ELM. Even in highly active lesions with extensive sub-RPE fluid and CME, the latter can extend greatly along the outer plexiform layer without significant subretinal fluid [8, 15, 47].

Recently OCT-A proved to be useful not only in the diagnosis but also in the study of RAP pathophysiology. Characteristic findings of RAP in OCT-A will be discussed further below.

7.4.2 Polypoidal Choroidal Vasculopathy/Aneurysmal Type 1 Neovascularization

Polypoidal choroidal vasculopathy is currently considered a subtype of type 1 neovasculariza-

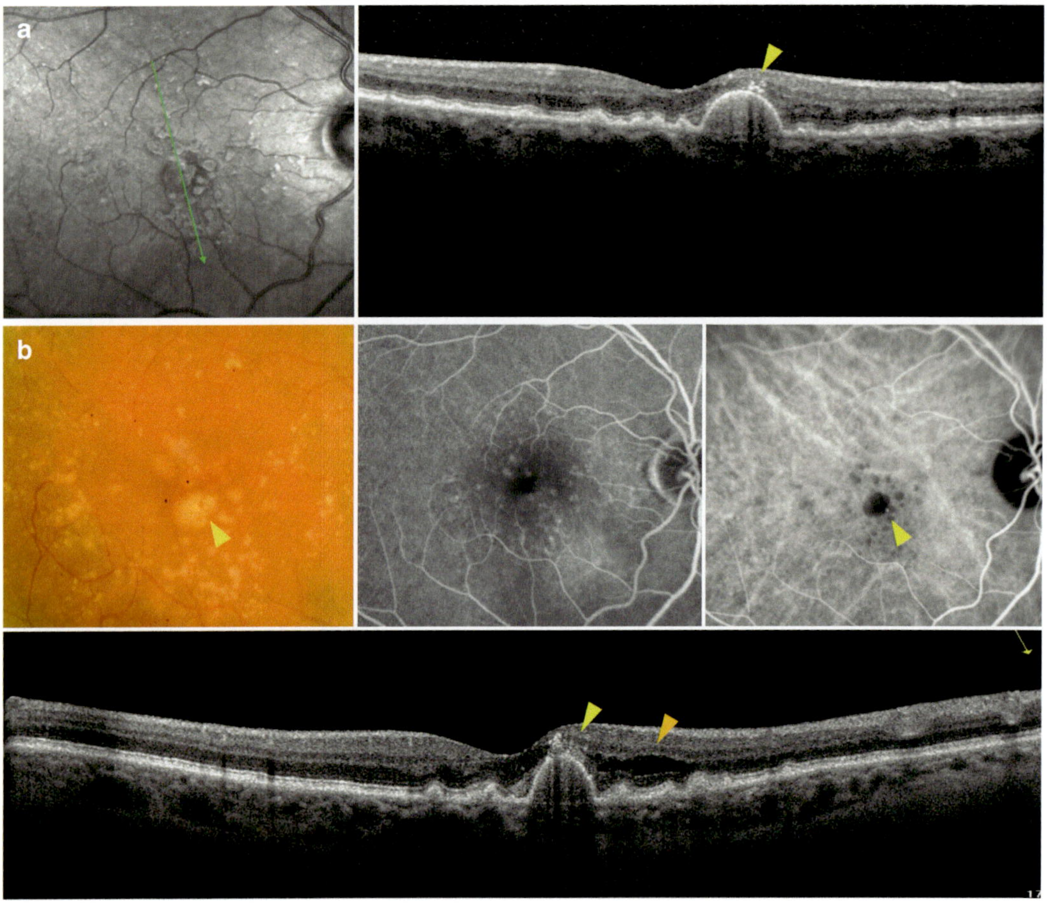

Fig. 7.7 Multimodal imaging of stage 1 RAP lesion progression over 2 months. (**a**) At baseline, SD-OCT scan shows drusenoid-like PED with relatively homogenous content and hyperreflective foci overlying the RPE (yellow arrow). (**b**) after 2 months, one can see in the same orientation SD-OCT scan the disruption of the RPE below the hyperreflective foci, with an ill-defined band of increased reflectivity extending to the RPE, accompanied by the development of cystoid spaces corresponding to cystoid macular edema (orange arrow); CFP shows only increased pigmentation in the area above the soft drusen and ICGA (top, right) shows a small hot spot representing the incipient RAP lesion (yellow arrow)

tion in which polypoidal or aneurysmal vascular dilations develop, usually in the fringe of the neovascular network or "branch vascular network" (BVN).

This entity was first coined by Yannuzi and colleagues as Idiopathic Polypoidal Choroidal Vasculopathy in 1982, as it presented in a group of patients with distinct demographic characteristics—younger middle-aged women of black American background—and had better prognosis compared to "conventional" nAMD [48, 49]. Subsequent reports extended the superior prevalence to the Asian population and recent studies have shown that a greater proportion of these patients may be white and older.

Controversy persists if PCV is a subset of nAMD or a separate entity as polypoidal lesions can be seen in the context of other clinical entities, such as in the pachychoroid spectrum [50]. Besides, PCV was shown in multimodal imaging studies to represent a neovasculopathy, rather than a distinct abnormality of the inner choroidal vasculature as initially proposed. This led to the notion that PCV should not be seen as a single disease, but as a common manifestation of many. In this regard, PCV is seen today as a variant of type 1 CNV predominantly affecting eyes with longstanding neovascularization, and the designation of Aneurysmal Type 1 Neovascularization was introduced [31, 51]. Being a type 1 CNV, both the BVN and the polyps or aneurysms are located in the sub-RPE space, but rarely the polyps can erode through the RPE and are seen as a type 2 lesion [15, 31].

Clinically the PCV patient presents with multiple, recurrent, sero-hemorrhagic pigment epithelial and neurosensorial detachments, sometimes with intraretinal lipid deposition, around the optic nerve or in the central macula. Orange nodules are sometimes seen in the borders of the lesion, or within the top of the PED, and correspond to polyps in ICGA. Vitreous hemorrhage is possible when subretinal hemorrhage is significant. PCV often follows a remitting-relapsing course and bilateral involvement is common (up to 86%) [52, 53].

The use of fluorescein angiography in PCV diagnosis is limited because it does not allow to clearly image the polypoidal lesion. FA usually shows only occult CNV patterns with intermediate or late leakage from undetermined source. But it can be useful to analyze the lesion's activity, as leakage is better imaged in FA compared to ICGA [9, 52].

ICGA is still considered the *gold standard* in PCV diagnosis as it allows to image both the BVN and the aneurysmal dilatations or polyps. Single or multiple polyps organized in grape-like clusters are better seen in the early phase of ICGA and make the diagnosis [37]. The area surrounding the vascular network is hypofluorescent in early phases but in the late phases there is often a reversal of the pattern with hyperfluorescence around the polypoidal lesion and hypofluorescence in the center. In very late phases ICGA shows *washout* in non-active lesions.

The EVEREST study group defined in the grading protocol PCV as the presence of early subretinal ICGA hyperfluorescence (appearing within the first 5–6 minutes of dye injection) and at least one of the following criteria: (1) nodular appearance of the polyp on stereoscopic viewing; (2) hypofluorescent halo around the nodule; (3) abnormal vascular channel(s) supplying the polyps, this is, the BVN; (4) pulsatile filling of polyps in dynamic ICGA; (5) orange subretinal nodules in the fundus corresponding to the hyperfluorescent nodular areas in ICGA; and (6) massive submacular hemorrhage. Nodular hyperfluorescence on stereoscopic ICGA was seen in the EVEREST study in 91.8% of cases, a hypofluorescent halo in 68.9%, and pulsatile polyps in only 6.6%. Byeon et al. described pulsatile polyps as more prone to rupture and causing severe hemorrhage [54, 55].

OCT findings are highly reliable in suggesting a PCV phenotype: an isolated highly protruded RPE with underlying moderate reflectivity, sometimes round shaped with hyperreflective borders and hyporeflective lumen; a notched PED; nodular structures adhering to the elevated back surface of the RPE like "pearls on a string"—all these features corresponding to the polyps; and the *double-layer sign,* composed by the hyperreflective lines formed by the separation of the RPE and Bruch's membrane, with an intervening layer of moderate to high reflectivity that corresponds to the BVN/type 1 CNV [31]. De Salvo and colleagues reported that with a combination of OCT-based signs: multiple PEDs, sharp PED peak, PED notch, and rounded sub-RPE hyporeflective lesions, the sensitivity and specificity of PCV diagnosis with SD-OCT alone was of 94.6% and 92.9%, respectively [56]. Therefore, the OCT can be very helpful as a screening tool for PCV suspected cases that should undergo ICGA procedure for confirmation, as ICGA is not routinely performed in the majority of clinics worldwide (Fig. 7.8).

OCT is also very useful to detect associated intraretinal, subretinal, and sub-RPE fluid, thus inferring on lesion activity. In PCV different components of the lesion may be active or inactive. The predominant active component can be determined by co-localization of fluid in OCT with the polyps, the BVN, or both in ICGA. This multimodal analysis of the lesion activity is important as it may impact on the choice of treatment (anti-VEGF, photodynamic therapy, or both) [9, 23].

7.5 Optical Coherence Tomography Angiography in nAMD

OCT angiography is a new imaging modality that uses the OCT principles to detect blood flow within the vascular structures of the eye without the need to intravenously administer fluorescent dyes. Currently, available OCT-A devices provide detailed 3-dimensional volumes of the retinal and choroidal vasculatures that can be analyzed layer-by-layer in both *en-face* or cross-sectional display, simultaneously co-localizing blood flow with microstructural changes in conventional OCT B-scans.

Technically, OCT-A refers to a group of OCT imaging methods that allow the visualization of moving particles, such as erythrocytes in biological tissues. These methods ignore the quantitative measurement of blood flow and use motion as a contrast mechanism to visualize the location of the moving cells [57]. These methods detect differences in amplitude, intensity or

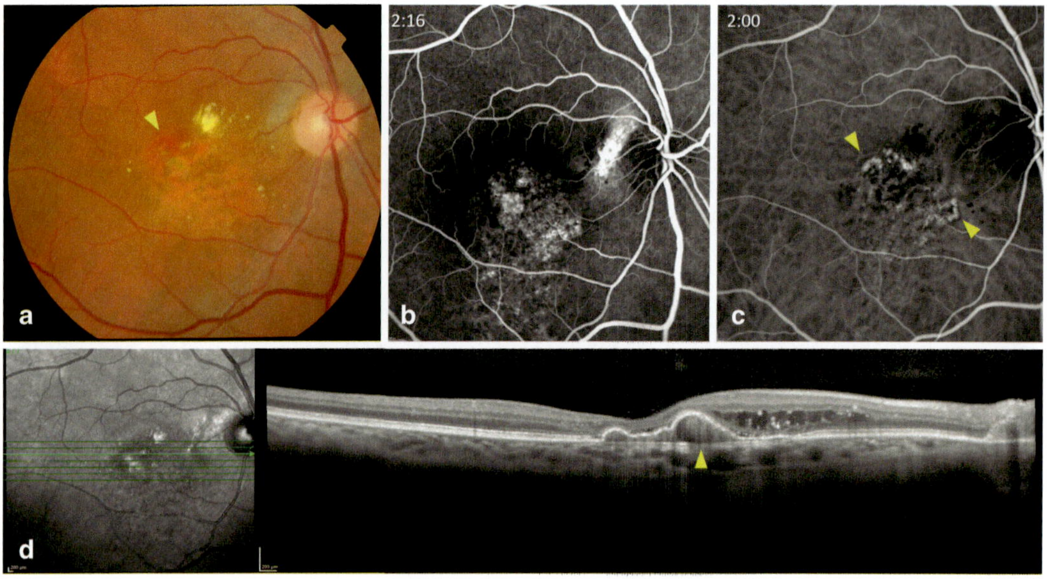

Fig. 7.8 Multimodal imaging of PCV lesion. (**a**) CFP shows typical orange round lesions (yellow arrow) with hard exudates in the macula. (**b**) FA only shows occult CNV pattern and it is with ICGA (**c**) that the clusters of polyps are identified (yellow arrow), surrounded by a hypofluorescent halo and located in the fringes of the BVN. (**d**) The SD-OCT scan shows round structures adhering to the back surface of the elevated RPE, with a hypo-reflective lumen and hyperreflective borders, corresponding to the polyps, along with the double-layer sign corresponding to the BVN located between the RPE and the Bruch's membrane

phase variance in a series of sequential B-scans taken at the same location, with high-frequency and dense volumetric scanning, from which proprietary algorithms such as the split-spectrum amplitude-decorrelation angiography (SSADA), the optical microangiography (OMAG), and the OCT angiography ratio analysis (OCTARA), are used to reconstruct the blood flow network in the acquired volume. In general, OCT-A systems can be divided into SD-OCT or SS-OCT-based systems. Some platforms already give automated, objective, quantitative data of flow (angio-analytics), but these features are not yet fully developed and must be validated prior to widespread use in clinics and clinical trials [58, 59]. Compared to conventional angiography the primary limitation is the absence of dynamic information such as filling speed and leakage, however, OCT-A can show collections of fluid in structural analysis, suggesting that leakage is present. Motion and retinal vascular projections are additional limitations, but these tend to be corrected as technology improves [20].

In nAMD, CNVs can be visualized as a network of abnormal, dilated, tortuous neovessels in the normally avascular outer retina or under the RPE, with several reports published detailing the OCT-A characteristics of type 1 and 2 neovascular membranes [60]. Appropriate segmentation of the layer containing the CNV is necessary to good visualization, with some platforms allowing for customized layer segmentation.

Neovascular membranes in AMD may present as well-circumscribed high-flow networks with larger feeder vessel trunks, fine arborizing vessels in the periphery and anastomotic loops or arcades at vessel termini, producing patterns described as "lacy wheel," "sea-fan," or "medusa-head" (Fig. 7.9); or poorly circumscribed, irregular vascular networks, said as "filamentous," "tangled," or "dead tree" CNVs (Fig. 7.10) [14]. Coscas et al. suggested different patterns and features for differentiating active from inactive CNVs in OCT-A: (1) shape, a well-defined (lacy-wheel or sea-fan shaped) CNV lesion in contrast to one with long filamentous linear vessels; (2) branching, numerous tiny capillaries, in contrast to rare large mature vessels; (3) the presence of anastomoses and loops; (4) morphology of the vessel termini, assessing the presence of a peripheral arcade in contrast to a "dead tree" appearance; and (5) pres-

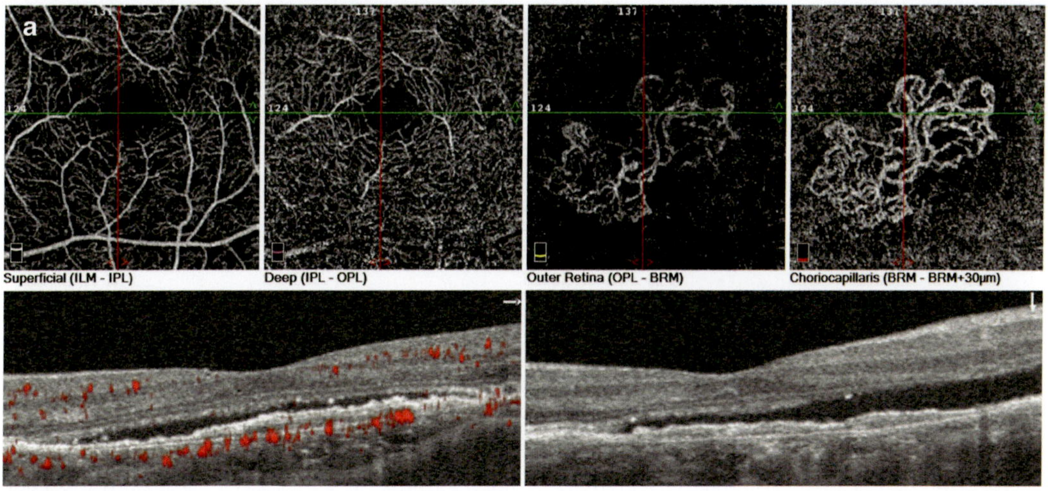

Fig. 7.9 OCT-A 3x3 mm *en face* and B-scans with superimposed flow (in red) of two cases presenting with type 1 neovascularization (**a**, **b**). In both cases the *en face* reconstruction shows more clearly the neovascular network in the choriocapillaris slab segmented bellow the RPE; the simultaneous B-scan allows for identification of the double-layer sign, corresponding to the CNV and of subretinal fluid, a marker of lesion activity. *En face* images show the CNV typical lacy pattern with peripheral arcades and loops, and surrounding hyposignal halo, correlating to activity status

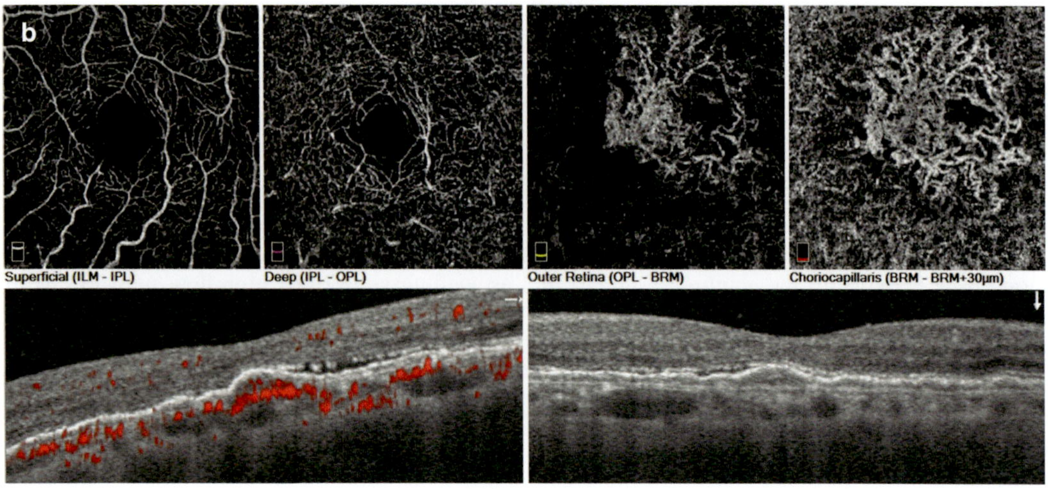

Fig. 7.9 (continued)

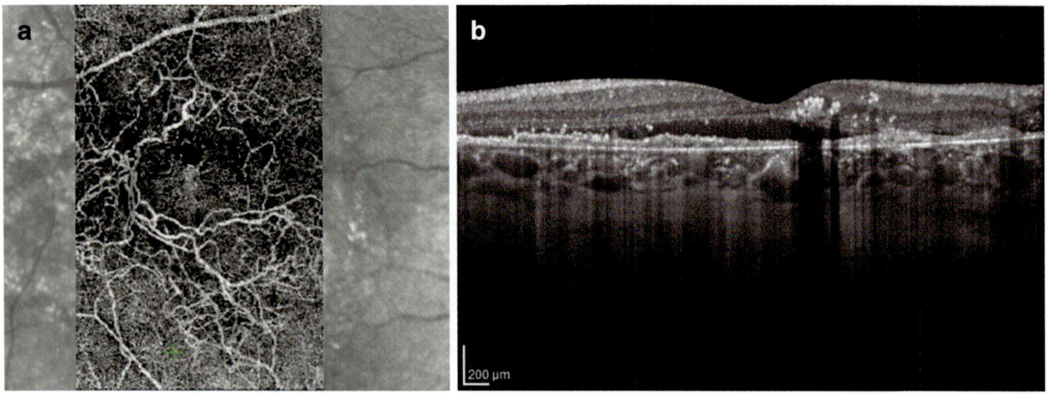

Fig. 7.10 "Dead tree" CNV pattern in OCT-A. (**a**) A poorly circumscribed, irregular vascular network is observed after treatment with anti-VEGF. Larger mature vessels predominate, and no loops, peripheral arcade, or perilesional hyposignal halo is seen. The "filamentous," "tangled," or "dead tree" patterns are associated with inactive or chronic CNVs; (**b**) the CNV corresponds to a shallow PED in SD-OCT (double-layer sign), and subretinal fluid is seen indicating lesion activity

ence of a perilesional hypointense halo, considered as regions of choriocapillaris alteration, either corresponding to flow impairment, steal or localized atrophy [61]. However, despite the attempts in establishing criteria for activity status in OCT-A, these are not validated, and the clinician must complement information with structural OCT showing indirect signs of leakage, such as subretinal or intraretinal fluid.

OCT-A also improves the detection of CNV in nAMD before it develops exudation, this is, quiescent CNV (qCNV) (Fig. 7.11). Rates of qCNV are reported to vary from 6% to 27% [37, 62]. The importance of the recognition of these lesions is the associated risk of exudation. De Oliveira Dias and colleagues reported an incidence at 1-year of 21% in exudation when qCNV was present at baseline compared to 4% when it was not, which translated to superior a risk of exudation of 15.2 times. Although no treatment for qCNVs is recommended at the present time, closer monitoring is warranted in order to detect exudation as early as possible and start appropriate treatment [62, 63].

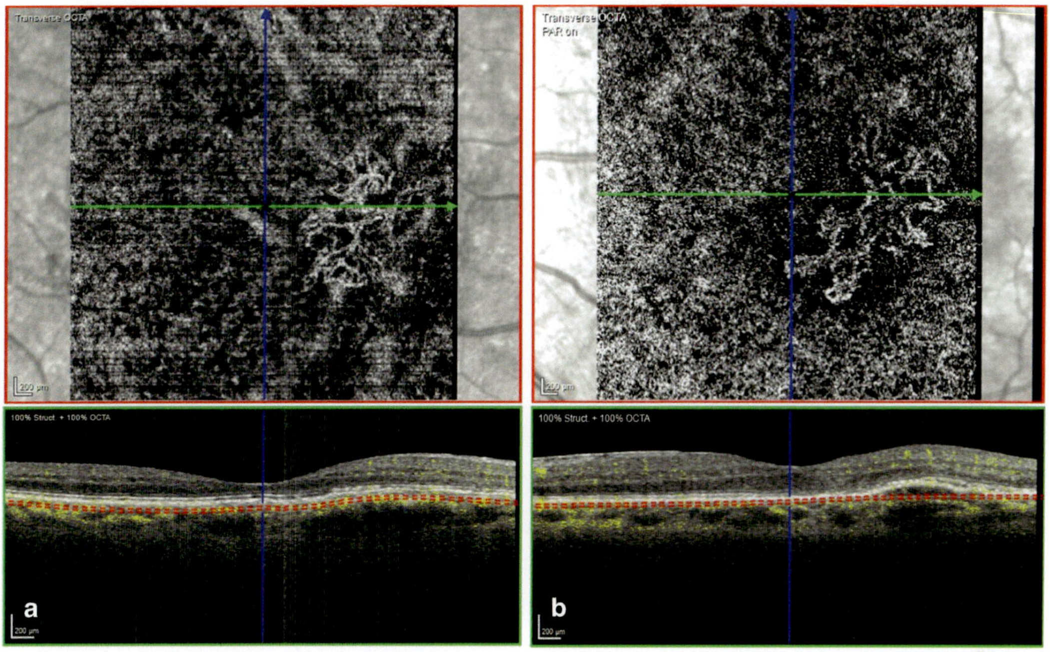

Fig. 7.11 Two exemplifying cases with quiescent type 1 CNV detected in OCT-A (**a**, **b**). Structural OCT scans show RPE irregularity and elevation (**a**) and a small PED (**b**), without associated intraretinal or subretinal fluid, and preserved retinal architecture. *En face* OCT-A clearly shows the CNV presence in the corresponding B-scan areas, with typical lacy pattern in the choriocapillaris slab

OCT-A combined with structural OCT thus emerges as a noninvasive tool with high potential for both the diagnosis and follow-up of the nAMD patient, and in the evaluation of the response to treatment over time. Treatment-naive CNV shows numerous fine, arborizing vessels, but during treatment with anti-VEGF there is a regression of the most fine vessels, while central, perhaps more mature trunks containing pericyte protected endothelial cells, seem to prevail [60, 64]. The area of CNV can also be measured by OCT-A, and its change with treatment is reported (Fig. 7.12) [37, 65, 66]. Other parameters, such as fractal dimension analysis, are being used to measure the branching pattern complexity of the CNV. Studies reported on reduced fractal dimension after treatment, suggesting less complexity due to the attenuation and pruning of small-caliber vessels [60]. OCT-A-based studies further revealed that CNV re-proliferation with the reopening of neovessels is observed from week 2 to week 4 post-treatment [64]. The revascularized CNV progressively changes to a more mature and less active phenotype over time, with larger vessel diameters, less network branching, and capillary rarefaction [62].

Altogether, the advantages of OCT-A in nAMD could lead to decreasing necessity of conventional invasive angiography in the clinical setting. Several studies compared the sensitivity and specificity of OCT-A alone or in combination with structural OCT to the *gold standard* FA (and/or ICGA) [67]. These reports vary between 50% and 87% in sensitivity and 91% to 98% in specificity for nAMD diagnosis with OCT-A. Lower sensitivities for CNV are usually associated with the presence of hemorrhage and large PEDs [62]. Perrott-Reynolds and colleagues conducted a review on the diagnostic accuracy of OCT-A for nAMD compared to FA/ICGA, and found only moderate consistency of sensitivity and specificity among the different studies analyzed. The majority had small sample sizes and none reported confidence intervals, limiting their results [68]. Compared to ICGA, measurements of CNV area in nAMD were significantly smaller

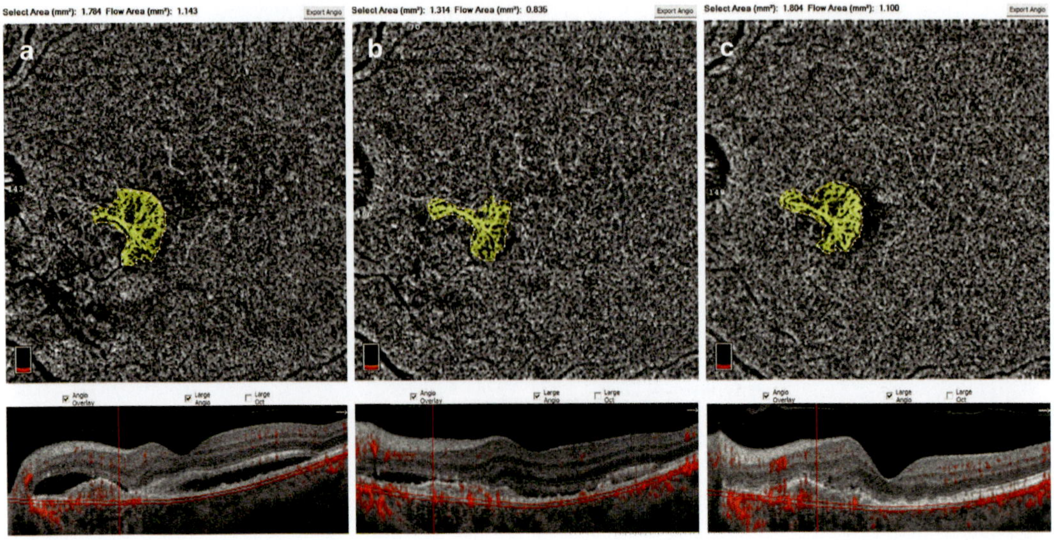

Fig. 7.12 CNV change with anti-VEGF therapy in OCT-A. (**a**) CNV lesion area is marked in yellow in *en face* image, B-scan shows type 1 CNV with subretinal fluid; (**b**) after treatment the CNV area decreases, with persistence of the central trunk and disappearance of flow in the more peripheral capillaries; (**c**) after the initial response there is repermeabilization of the peripheral capillaries with visualization of loops, peripheral arcades, and surrounding hyposignal halo, indicating that CNV activity is likely increasing

in OCT-A in both type 1 and type 2 membranes, despite the good correlation between measurements [14, 69].

Because of this inconsistent data, and despite the clear utility of OCT-A in nAMD diagnosis and follow-up, FA and ICGA are still considered the *gold standard* for a comprehensive evaluation of lesion location and morphology, and OCT-A stands for now as an auxiliary imaging method. Others propose, however, a new algorithm in that OCT and OCT-A are to be performed first and if the diagnosis is certain one should proceed to treatment, however, if the result is negative or there is doubt, dye-based examinations should always be performed [70].

7.5.1 RAP and PCV Phenotypes in OCT-A

OCT-A features of RAP lesions are now well documented. RAP lesions present in the earliest stages as small intraretinal neovascular complexes seen as tufts-shaped lesions in the outer retinal layers, descending from the deep capillary plexus to the RPE (Fig. 7.13). Feeder vessels in the deep capillary plexus dragging toward the outer retinal layers can be observed. In some cases, a clew-like flow signal in the choriocapillaris is also seen underneath the tuft-shaped lesion and corresponds to proliferation in the sub-RPE space. Careful assessment combined with structural OCT with superimposed flow signal is needed, as the RAP connections may be missed if only the *en face* image is examined [14, 71, 72]. OCT-A was shown to detect growth and morphologic changes in the incipient RAP lesion before the exudation develops and also enables the distinction from avascular hyperreflective foci from pigment migration seen in structural OCT [73].

OCT-A is also useful in documenting the response of type 3 lesions to treatment, as studies showed that the microvascular structure of RAP is highly responsive to anti-VEGF therapy, with a clear decrease in size [74].

At present, the role of OCT-A in PCV is less clear compared to other types of CNV. The BVN is visualized in OCT-A as any type 1 CNV, but polyps are not very well detected, at least using only automated segmentation. The detection rates of polyps using OCT-A are in fact much

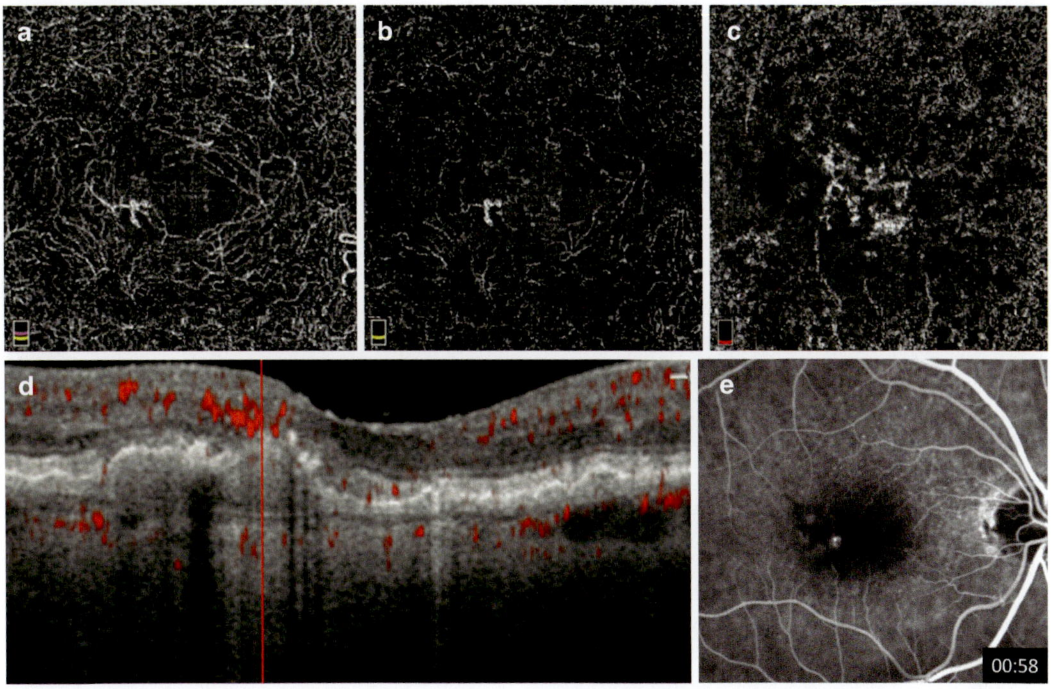

Fig. 7.13 RAP lesion in OCT-A. (**a**, **b**) A high-flow tuft-shaped abnormal neovascular network is seen mainly in deep retinal plexus and outer retina slabs; (**c**, **d**) there is a connection of the neovascular process to the subretinal space; this is best appreciated in the B-scan with superimposed blood flow (in red) where the flow is seen deepening and merging with the PED, with focal disruption of the RPE layer; (**e**) correspondent FA showing a hot spot from RAP lesion

lower compared with ICGA, which is the *gold standard* in PCV diagnosis. The hypothesis is that turbulent or very slow flow inside the polyp is below the threshold of motion detection by the device [14, 75].

Analyzing the B-scans obtained with OCT-A, the blood flow in polyps was shown to be just below the top of the PED, or focally located in the upper part of the peak caused by the polyp [76]. Because of this, it may be necessary to analyze the automated outer retina slab or to change manually the segmentation to above the choriocapillaris slab (where the BVN is seen), to detect the flow in the polyps in *en face* images.

According to level of segmentation and flow characteristics within the polyps, they are seen as a hyposignal round structure, a hypersignal ring of flow devoid of flow inside, or they can present in hypersignal patterns such as nodular, dot, or cluster (Figs. 7.14 and 7.15). The BVN is very well seen between the RPE and the Bruch's membrane and in patterns similar to other type 1 CNVs, including *seafan*, *medusa,* and *tangle* [76, 77].

One group using a novel OCT-A algorithm termed variable interscan time analysis (VISTA), that allows to visualize variations in relative blood flow, in conjunction with a prototype high-speed swept-source OCT, showed heterogeneous blood flow speeds within the polyps. Some had faster blood flow in the periphery and slower blood flow in the center, perhaps from turbulence within. The BVNs showed relatively faster flow in the larger trunk vessels and slower flow speeds in the smaller vessels [78, 79].

When there is a severe distortion of the retinal architecture from large serosanguineous PEDs, visualization of the BVN and polyps may not be possible or is very poor. This is another limitation of OCT-A in PCV where this type of complication is common. Therefore, OCT-A is currently

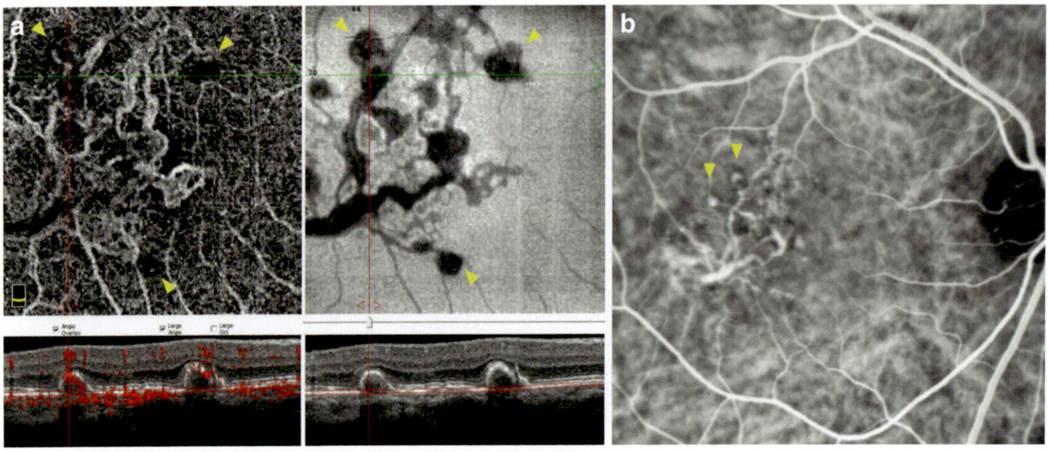

Fig. 7.14 Macular PCV lesion in OCT-A (**a**) and ICGA (**b**). OCT-A *en face* image in the left (**a**) shows the BVN with more detail compared to ICGA (**b**), however, the polyps are devoid of flow in the choriocapillaris slab where the BVN is best seen, and appear as round hyposignal structures (yellow arrows); in the B-scan image with superimposed flow (**a**, below, in the left) one can appreciate the presence of flow (in red) in the top of the peaked RPE elevations corresponding to polyps in ICGA (**b**). *En face* structural OCT (**a**, above, in the right) shows very nicely the BVN and polyps of the PCV lesion in close correspondence with the PCV lesion observed in ICGA (**b**)

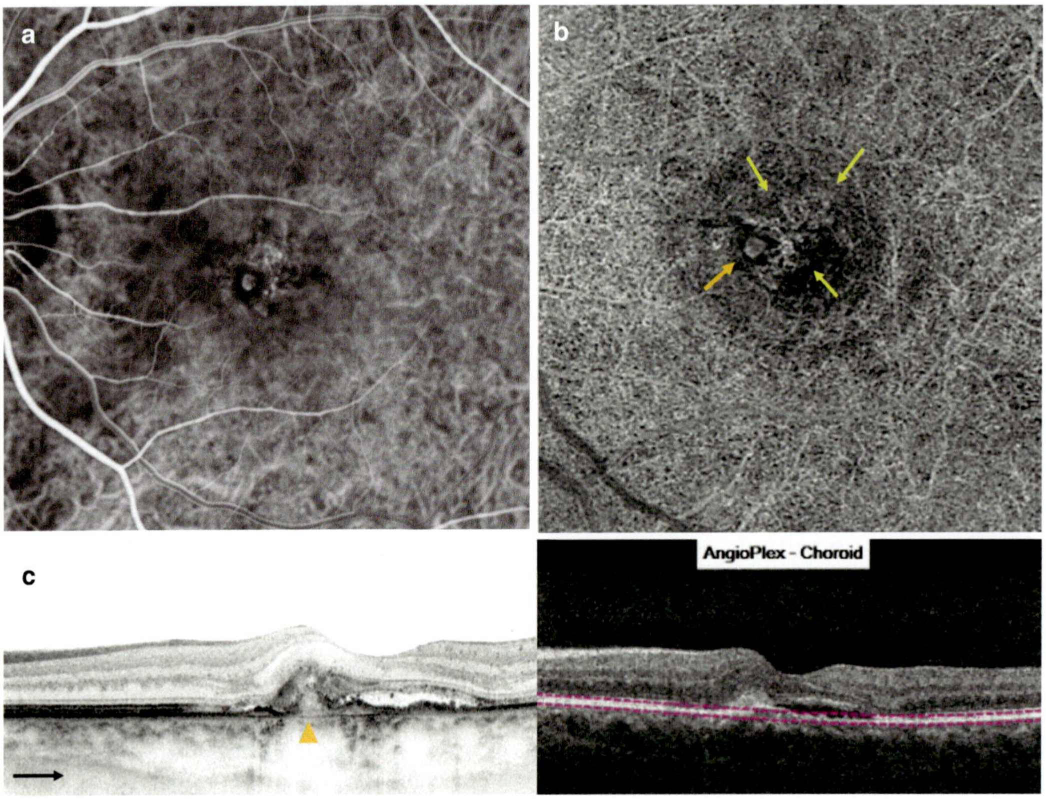

Fig. 7.15 PCV lesion in OCT-A (**a**), ICGA (**b**), and SD-OCT (**c**). In this case, the polyp component is seen in both ICGA and OCT-A as a round hypersignal structure with flow, surrounded by a hyposignal halo (orange arrow). The BVN is best appreciated in *en face* OCT-A (yellow arrows). (**c**) SD-OCT shows the peaked RPE elevation (orange arrow) typical for the underlying presence of polyps and the double layer sign in both sides representing the BVN, along with subretinal fluid

unable to replace ICGA in the assessment of PCV but can provide important supplementary information [9, 77]. In the future, further improvements in OCT-A will allow this technology to play a greater role in PCV diagnosis and management.

7.6 Concluding Remarks

Neovascular AMD is an entity extensively characterized by the clinical and imagiological perspectives. First with dye-based examinations, which for years served as the cornerstone for systematic clinical classification and treatment guidance, and afterward with the historical introduction of OCT. The latter, in constant improvement, lead to refinement in CNV classification in the last decade. A conciliation was finally achieved between the earliest histopathologic studies conducted by Gass and colleagues and the new imaging findings at the microstructural level that OCT provided complemented with FA and ICGA.

Today with the introduction of OCT-A we are again on the verge of exciting changes in both how nAMD is diagnosed and how patients will be managed during treatment. New algorithms and ultra-high-speed OCT systems are being developed and improved. Noninvasive, fast, and reliable new technologies will not only allow to detect CNVs' flow and vessel density, correlating them to microstructural analysis at the histological level, but they will enable flow velocity measurements, with distinction of regions of high and low flow that were not seen before. Progression to quantitative absolute measurements of flow in the future might be of great value, especially in analyzing for CNV activity and response to treatment.

Multimodal imaging is the future in nAMD assessment, and the future is promising.

Key Learning Points

1. Neovascular AMD must be promptly recognized, as treatments must be implemented early in the natural history of the disease to prevent severe visual loss.
2. Clinical and imagiological characteristics of nAMD are subject to constant study and development, as new technologies provide new means to accurately diagnose and to evaluate the response to treatment.
3. Currently, there is a transition in the way nAMD is classified. The classification in occult/classic CNV patterns diagnosed with the *gold standard* fluorescein angiography changed to a multimodal-based classification mainly guided by SD-OCT and closer to the histology of different nAMD phenotypes.
4. Neovascularization type 1 (bellow the RPE), type 2 (above the RPE), and type 3 (RAP lesion) classifications are now preferred. PCV is considered more as a variant of type 1 neovascularization in which polypoidal or aneurysmal vascular dilations develop.
5. Neovascular AMD phenotype distinction might not be as important as in the past in treatment decision, but might be important for prognosis, possible involvement of fellow eye and in considering adjuvant therapies such as PDT.
6. Multimodal-imaging with FA and SD-OCT (and ICGA when necessary) is the *gold standard* for nAMD diagnosis and follow-up. However, OCT-A is a breakthrough technology recently introduced in clinical practice that might change this paradigm. Neovascular AMD diagnosis and decision to treat might soon change to a purely non-invasive imaging approach.

Acknowledgments We are grateful to Ana Rita Santos for her help in assembling the figures.

References

1. Tomany SC, Wang JJ, Van Leeuwen R, et al. Risk factors for incident age-related macular degeneration: pooled findings from 3 continents. Ophthalmology. 2004;111(7):1280–7.
2. Shao J, Choudhary MM, Schachat AP. Neovascular age-related macular degeneration. Dev Ophthalmol. 2016;55:125–36.
3. Wong WL, Su X, Li X, et al. Global prevalence of age-related macular degeneration and disease burden projection for 2020 and 2040: a systematic

review and meta-analysis. Lancet Glob Health. 2014;2(2):e106–16.
4. Buch H, Nielsen NV, Vinding T, Jensen GB, Prause JU, La cour M. 14-year incidence, progression, and visual morbidity of age-related maculopathy: the Copenhagen City eye study. Ophthalmology. 2005;112(5):787–98.
5. Ferris FL, Fine SL, Hyman L. Age-related macular degeneration and blindness due to neovascular maculopathy. Arch Ophthalmol. 1984;102(11): 1640–2.
6. Bressler NM, Bressler SB. Neovascular (exudative or "wet") age-related macular degeneration. 6th ed. Retina Fifth Edition. Elsevier Inc; 2012. p. 1345–1372.
7. Yannuzzi LA, Freund KB, Takahashi BS. Review of retinal angiomatous proliferation or type 3 neovascularization. Retina. 2008;28(3):375–84.
8. Tsai ASH, Cheung N, Gan ATL, et al. Retinal angiomatous proliferation. Surv Ophthalmol. 2017;62(4):462–92.
9. Cheung CMG, Lai TYY, Ruamviboonsuk P, et al. Polypoidal Choroidal vasculopathy: definition, pathogenesis, diagnosis, and management. Ophthalmology. 2018;125(5):708–24.
10. Gass JD. Biomicroscopic and histopathologic considerations regarding the feasibility of surgical excision of subfoveal neovascular membranes. Am J Ophthalmol. 1994;118(3):285–98.
11. Grossniklaus HE, Gass JD. Clinicopathologic correlations of surgically excised type 1 and type 2 submacular choroidal neovascular membranes. Am J Ophthalmol. 1998;126(1):59–69.
12. Hartnett ME, Weiter JJ, Staurenghi G, Elsner AE. Deep retinal vascular anomalous complexes in advanced age-related macular degeneration. Ophthalmology. 1996;103(12):2042–53.
13. Yannuzzi LA, Negrão S, Iida T, et al. Retinal Angiomatous proliferation in age-related macular degeneration. Retina. 2001;21:416–34.
14. Talks SJ, Aftab AM, Ashfaq I, Soomro T. The role of new imaging methods in managing age-related macular degeneration. Asia Pac J Ophthalmol (Phila). 2017;6(6):498–507.
15. Mrejen S, Sarraf D, Mukkamala SK, Freund KB. Multimodal imaging of pigment epithelial detachment: a guide to evaluation. Retina (Philadelphia, Pa). 2013;33(9):1735–62.
16. Khanani AM, Eichenbaum D, Schlottmann PG, Tuomi L, Sarraf D. Optimal Management of Pigment Epithelial Detachments in eyes with Neovascular age-related macular degeneration. Retina (Philadelphia, Pa). 2018;38(11):2103–17.
17. Ersoz MG, Karacorlu M, Arf S. Sayman muslubas I, Hocaoglu M. retinal pigment epithelium tears: classification, pathogenesis, predictors, and management. Surv Ophthalmol. 2017;62(4):493–505.
18. Ravera V, Giani A, Pellegrini M, et al. Comparison among different diagnostic methods in the study of type and activity of Choroidal Neovascular membranes in age-related macular degeneration. Retina (Philadelphia, Pa). 2019;39(2):281–7.
19. Giani A, Luiselli C, Esmaili DD, et al. Spectral-domain optical coherence tomography as an indicator of fluorescein angiography leakage from choroidal neovascularization. Invest Ophthalmol Vis Sci. 2011;52(8):5579–86.
20. Holz FG, Sadda SR, Staurenghi G, et al. Imaging protocols in clinical studies in advanced age-related macular degeneration: recommendations from classification of atrophy consensus meetings. Ophthalmology. 2017;124(4):464–78.
21. Ditthmar F, Holz FG. Fluorescein angiography in ophthalmology. Heidelberg: Springer; 2007. p. 56–88. https://www.springer.com/gp/book/9783540783596.
22. Subfoveal neovascular lesions in age-related macular degeneration. Guidelines for evaluation and treatment in the macular photocoagulation study. Macular photocoagulation study group. Arch Ophthalmol. 1991;109(9):1242–57.
23. Freund KB, Zweifel SA, Engelbert M. Do we need a new classification for choroidal neovascularization in age-related macular degeneration? Retina (Philadelphia, Pa). 2010;30(9):1333–49.
24. Yannuzzi LA, Slakter JS, Sorenson JA, Guyer DR, Orlock DA. Digital Indocyanine Green Videoangiography and Choroidal neovascularization. Retina. 1992;12:191–223.
25. Regillo CD, Benson WE, Maguire JI, Annesley WH Jr. Indocyanine Green angiography and occult Choroidal neovascularization. Ophthalmology. 1994;101(2):280–8.
26. Gabriele ML, Wollstein G, Ishikawa H, et al. Optical coherence tomography: history, current status, and laboratory work. Invest Ophthalmol Vis Sci. 2011;52(5):2425–36.
27. Potsaid B, Baumann B, Huang D, et al. Ultrahigh speed 1050nm swept source/Fourier domain OCT retinal and anterior segment imaging at 100,000 to 400,000 axial scans per second. Opt Express. 2010;18(19):20029–48.
28. Jung JJ, Chen CY, Mrejen S, et al. The incidence of neovascular subtypes in newly diagnosed neovascular age-related macular degeneration. Am J Ophthalmol. 2014;158(4):769–79. e2
29. Sato T, Kishi S, Watanabe G, Matsumoto H, Mukai R. Tomographic features of branching vascular networks in polypoidal choroidal vasculopathy. Retina (Philadelphia, Pa). 2007;27(5):589–94.
30. Spaide RF. Enhanced depth imaging optical coherence tomography of retinal pigment epithelial detachment in age-related macular degeneration. Am J Ophthalmol. 2009;147(4):644–52.
31. Khan S, Engelbert M, Imamura Y, Freund KB. Polypoidal choroidal vasculopathy: simultaneous indocyanine green angiography and eye-tracked spectral domain optical coherence tomography findings. Retina (Philadelphia, Pa). 2012;32(6):1057–68.
32. Mukkamala SK, Costa RA, Fung A, Sarraf D, Gallego-pinazo R, Freund KB. Optical coherence

tomographic imaging of sub-retinal pigment epithelium lipid. Arch Ophthalmol. 2012;130(12):1547–53.
33. Grossniklaus HE, Green WR. Choroidal neovascularization. Am J Ophthalmol. 2004;137(3):496–503.
34. Naysan J, Jung JJ, Dansingani KK, Balaratnasingam C, Freund KB. Type 2 (subretinal) neovascularization in age-related macular degeneration associated with pure reticular pseudodrusen phenotype. Retina (Philadelphia, Pa). 2016;36(3):449–57.
35. Roquet W, Roudot-Thoraval F, Coscas G, Soubrane G. Clinical features of drusenoid pigment epithelial detachment in age related macular degeneration. Br J Ophthalmol. 2004;88(5):638–42.
36. Balaratnasingam C, Messinger JD, Sloan KR, Yannuzzi LA, Freund KB, Curcio CA. Histologic and optical coherence tomographic correlates in Drusenoid pigment epithelium detachment in age-related macular degeneration. Ophthalmology. 2017;124(5):644–56.
37. Waheed NK, Kashani AH, Alexandre C, Garcia DA, Duker JS, Rosenfeld PJ. Optical coherence tomography. 6th ed. Ryan's Retina. Elsevier Inc; 2019. p. 77–119.
38. Sarraf D, Reddy S, Chiang A, Yu F, Jain A. A new grading system for retinal pigment epithelial tears. Retina (Philadelphia, Pa). 2010;30(7):1039–45.
39. Schaal KB, Freund KB, Litts KM, Zhang Y, Messinger JD, Curcio CA. Outer retinal Tubulation in advanced age-related macular degeneration: optical coherence tomographic findings correspond to histology. Retina (Philadelphia, Pa). 2015;35(7):1339–50.
40. Preti RC, Govetto A, Filho RGA, et al. Optical coherence tomography analysis of outer retinal Tubulations, sequential evolution and pathophysiological insights. Retina (Philadelphia, Pa). 2018;38(8):1518–25.
41. Cohen SY, Dubois L, Nghiem-buffet S, et al. Retinal pseudocysts in age-related geographic atrophy. Am J Ophthalmol. 2010;150(2):211–7. e1
42. Gass JD, Agarwal A, Lavina AM, Tawansy KA. Focal inner retinal hemorrhages in patients with drusen: an early sign of occult choroidal neovascularization and chorioretinal anastomosis. Retina (Philadelphia, Pa). 2003;23(6):741–51.
43. Freund KB, Ho IV, Barbazetto IA, et al. Type 3 neovascularization: the expanded spectrum of retinal angiomatous proliferation. Retina (Philadelphia, Pa). 2008;28(2):201–11.
44. Monson DM, Smith JR, Klein ML, Wilson DJ. Clinicopathologic correlation of retinal Angiomatous proliferation. Arch Ophthalmol. 2008;37(8):1664–8.
45. Gross NE, Aizman A, Brucker A, Klancnik JM, Yannuzzi LA. Nature and risk of neovascularization in the fellow eye of patients with unilateral retinal angiomatous proliferation. Retina (Philadelphia, Pa). 2005;25(6):713–8.
46. Silva R. Neovascular phenotypes: retinal Angiomatous proliferation (RAP) or type 3 neovascularization. In: Age-related macular degeneration. 1st ed; 2010. p. 117–27.
47. Nagiel A, Sarraf D, Sadda SR, et al. Type 3 neovascularization: evolution, association with pigment epithelial detachment, and treatment response as revealed by spectral domain optical coherence tomography. Retina (Philadelphia, Pa). 2015;35(4):638–47.
48. Yannuzzi LA, Sorenson J, Spaide RF, Lipson B. Idiopathic polypoidal choroidal vasculopathy (IPCV). Retina. 1990;10:1–8.
49. Yannuzzi LA, Wong DW, Sforzolini BS, et al. Polypoidal choroidal vasculopathy and neovascularized age-related macular degeneration. Arch Ophthalmol. 1999;117(11):1503–10.
50. Dansingani KK, Balaratnasingam C, Naysan J, Freund KB. En face imaging of Pachychoroid Spectrum disorders with swept-source optical coherence tomography. Retina (Philadelphia, Pa). 2016;36(3):499–516.
51. Dansingani KK, Gal-or O, Sadda SR, Yannuzzi LA, Freund KB. Understanding aneurysmal type 1 neovascularization (polypoidal choroidal vasculopathy): a lesson in the taxonomy of 'expanded spectra'–a review. Clin Exp Ophthalmol. 2018;46(2):189–200.
52. Silva R. Neovascular phenotypes: Polypoidal Choroidal vasculopathy. In: Age-related macular degeneration. 1st ed; 2010. p. 129–39.
53. Li X. 74–Polypoidal Choroidal vasculopathy. 6th ed. Ryan's Retina. Elsevier Inc; 2019. p. 1458–1464.
54. Tan CS, Ngo WK, Chen JP, Tan NW, Lim TH. EVEREST study report 2: imaging and grading protocol, and baseline characteristics of a randomised controlled trial of polypoidal choroidal vasculopathy. Br J Ophthalmol. 2015;99(5):624–8.
55. Byeon SH, Lew YJ, Lee SC, Kwon OW. Clinical features and follow-up results of pulsating polypoidal choroidal vasculopathy treated with photodynamic therapy. Acta Ophthalmol. 2010;88(6):660–8.
56. De Salvo G, Vaz-Pereira S, Keane PA, Tufail A, Liew G. Sensitivity and specificity of spectral-domain optical coherence tomography in detecting idiopathic polypoidal choroidal vasculopathy. Am J Ophthalmol. 2014;158(6):1228–38.
57. Gorczynska I, Migacz JV, Zawadzki RJ, Capps AG, Werner JS. Comparison of amplitude-decorrelation, speckle-variance and phase-variance OCT angiography methods for imaging the human retina and choroid. Biomed Opt Express. 2016;7(3):911–42.
58. Tan ACS, Tan GS, Denniston AK, et al. An overview of the clinical applications of optical coherence tomography angiography. Eye (Lond). 2018;32(2):262–86.
59. De carlo TE, Romano A, Waheed NK, Duker JS. A review of optical coherence tomography angiography (OCTA). Int J Retina Vitreous. 2015;1:5.
60. Al-Sheikh M, Iafe NA, Phasukkijwatana N, Sadda SR, Sarraf D. Biomarkers of Neovascular activity in age-related macular degeneration using optical coherence tomography angiography. Retina (Philadelphia, Pa). 2018;38(2):220–30.
61. Coscas GJ, Lupidi M, Coscas F, Cagini C, Souied EH. Optical coherence tomography angiography versus traditional multimodal imaging in assessing the

activity of exudative age-related macular degeneration: a new diagnostic challenge. Retina (Philadelphia, Pa). 2015;35(11):2219–28.
62. Schneider EW, Fowler SC. Optical coherence tomography angiography in the management of age-related macular degeneration. Curr Opin Ophthalmol. 2018;29(3):217–25.
63. De Oliveira dias JR, Zhang Q, JMB G, et al. Natural history of subclinical neovascularization in non-exudative age-related macular degeneration using swept-source OCT angiography. Ophthalmology. 2018;125(2):255–66.
64. Mar ques JP, Costa JF, Marques M, Cachulo ML, Figueira J, Silva R. Sequential morphological changes in the CNV net after Intravitreal anti-VEGF evaluated with OCT angiography. Ophthalmic Res. 2016;55(3):145–51.
65. Coscas G, Lupidi M, Coscas F, Français C, Cagini C, Souied EH. Optical coherence tomography angiography during follow-up: qualitative and quantitative analysis of mixed type I and II choroidal neovascularization after vascular endothelial growth factor trap therapy. Ophthalmic Res. 2015;54(2):57–63.
66. Pilotto E, Frizziero L, Daniele AR, et al. Early OCT angiography changes of type 1 CNV in exudative AMD treated with anti-VEGF. Br J Ophthalmol. 2019;103(1):67–71.
67. De Carlo TE, Bonini filho MA, Chin AT, et al. Spectral-domain optical coherence tomography angiography of choroidal neovascularization. Ophthalmology. 2015;122(6):1228–38.
68. Perrott-reynolds R, Cann R, Cronbach N, et al. The diagnostic accuracy of OCT angiography in naive and treated neovascular age-related macular degeneration: a review. Eye (Lond). 2019;33(2):274–82.
69. Told R, Sacu S, Hecht A, Baratsits M, Eibenberger K, et al. Comparison of SD-optical coherence tomography angiography and Indocyanine Green angiography in type. Investig Opthalmology Vis Sci. 2018;59:2393–400.
70. Imaging of exudative age-related macular degeneration: toward a shift in the diagnostic paradigm? Retina (Philadelphia, Pa). 2017;38(Suppl 1):1–12.
71. Miere A, Querques G, Semoun O, et al. Optical coherence tomography angiography changes in early type 3 neovascularization after anti-VEGF treatment. Retina (Philadelphia, Pa). 2017;37(10):1873–9.
72. Querques G, Miere A, Souied EH. Optical coherence tomography angiography features of type 3 neovascularization in age-related macular degeneration. Dev Ophthalmol. 2016;56:57–61.
73. Tan ACS, Dansingani KK, Yannuzzi LA, Sarraf D, Freund KB. Type 3 neovascularization imaged with cross-sectional and en face optical coherence tomography angiography. Retina (Philadelphia, Pa). 2017;37(2):234–46.
74. Phasukkijwatana N, Tan ACS, Chen X, Freund KB, Sarraf D. Optical coherence tomography angiography of type 3 neovascularisation in age-related macular degeneration after antiangiogenic therapy. Br J Ophthalmol. 2017;101(5):597–602.
75. Tomiyasu T, Nozaki M, Yoshida M, Ogura Y. Characteristics of Polypoidal Choroidal vasculopathy evaluated by optical coherence tomography angiography. Invest Ophthalmol Vis Sci. 2016;57(9):OCT324–30.
76. Wang M, Zhou Y, Gao SS, et al. Evaluating Polypoidal Choroidal vasculopathy with optical coherence tomography angiography. Invest Ophthalmol Vis Sci. 2016;57(9):OCT526–32.
77. Inoue M, Balaratnasingam C, Freund KB. Optical coherence tomography angiography of polypoidal choroidal vasculopathy and polypoidal choroidal neovascularization. Retina (Philadelphia, Pa). 2015;35(11):2265–74.
78. Arya M, Rashad R, Sorour O, Moult EM, Fujimoto JG, Waheed NK. Optical coherence tomography angiography (OCTA) flow speed mapping technology for retinal diseases. Expert Rev Med Devices. 2018;21:1–8.
79. Rebhun CB, Moult EM, Novais EA, et al. Polypoidal Choroidal vasculopathy on swept-source optical coherence tomography angiography with variable Interscan time analysis. Transl Vis Sci Technol. 2017;6(6):4.

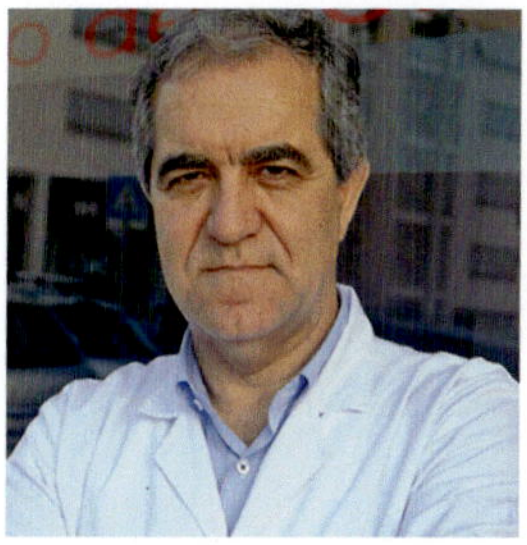

Rufino Silva MD, PhD, FEBO is an Assistant Professor of Ophthalmology at the Faculty of Medicine, University of Coimbra, Portugal (FMUC). He is also the Head of Medical Retina Unit at the Ophthalmology Department, Centro Hospitalar e Universitário de Coimbra, Portugal (CHUC) and an investigator at the Association for Innovation and Biomedical Research on Light and Image (AIBILI), Coimbra, Portugal.

Prof. Rufino Silva is an ophthalmologist with more than 25 years of experience, primarily committed to the study and treatment of retinal diseases, mainly focused on AMD, diabetic retinopathy, retinal vein occlusion (RVO), and pathologic myopia. His research is mainly focused on AMD: epidemiology, diet and lifestyle, imaging biomarkers, metabolomics, and genetics. He is author and co-author of more than 140 articles, chapters, and books.

Orcid: https://orcid.org/0000-0001-8676-0833

Management Strategies for Neovascular AMD

8

Irmela Mantel

8.1 The Story of Anti-VEGF Treatment: Molecules and Regimens

The current treatment of neovascular age-related macular degeneration (nAMD) is mainly based on the inhibition of the vascular endothelial growth factor (VEGF) in the retinal tissue by intravitreal injection of anti-VEGF agents. This approach allowed for the first time in history, a mean visual improvement from treatment start (baseline) [1–3], whereas preceding treatment options such as laser photocoagulation or photodynamic therapy (PDT) with verteporfin were only able to reduce the degree of visual loss. Although both laser and PDT are still occasionally used, these treatment options are reserved for exceptional cases.

VEGF was identified in the 1990s as a key factor in the development of neovascular membranes [4, 5]. VEGF was not only sufficient to promote a neovascular response [5] but also required; when VEGF was blocked in a nonhuman primate, no vasoproliferation was detected [4]. Subsequent studies have well established the central role of VEGF in neovascular disorders. The first commercially available anti-VEGF molecule was *pegaptanib* (brand name Macugen), licensed in 2000. It showed in a phase 3 clinical study an efficacy for nAMD which was yet limited to a reduction in visual loss compared to sham [6], similar to the efficacy of PDT with verteporfin [7]. Pegaptanib is a molecule that competitively binds to the VEGF isoform 165, which was considered the main pathogenic isoform. However, later studies showed that this approach neglected other VEGF isoforms with significant pathogenic potential that need to be targeted as well. *Ranibizumab* (brand name Lucentis), a specific affinity-mature fragment of a recombinant humanized IgG1 monoclonal antibody that neutralizes all active VEGF-A isoforms of the human VEGF protein, was licensed in 2006. With its arrival, a true efficacy revolution was started: Using monthly intravitreal injections, a mean visual acuity improvement was obtained after 1 and after 2 years of treatment, ranging between a mean gain of 5.4 ETDRS letters and 11.3 letters according to the study [1, 2, 8].

These pivotal trials did set the reference for the best visual outcomes under currently available treatment options. This astounding improvement in the prognosis of nAMD was achieved on the basis of *fixed monthly injections*. The high treatment frequency placed a heavy burden on the management of patients with chronic nAMD, thereby requiring many clinical and therapeutic interventions over the course of a patient's lifespan due to the repetitive treatment scheme.

I. Mantel (✉)
Department of Ophthalmology, University of Lausanne, Jules Gonin Eye Hospital, Fondation Asile des Aveugles, CP, Lausanne, Switzerland
e-mail: irmela.mantel@fa2.ch

J. Chhablani (ed.), *Choroidal Neovascularization*, https://doi.org/10.1007/978-981-15-2213-0_8

Therefore, many attempts were made to reduce the burden, both on the level of the total number of injections (cost factor) as well as on the level of the number of monitoring visits (human and technical resource factor). Quarterly fixed ranibizumab injections resulted in a loss of the initial VA improvement and were shown to be significantly inferior to monthly injections, although a subset of patients did well on this regimen [9–11]. A small study with the first *pro re nata (PRN) dosing* showed the feasibility and efficiency of a re-treatment strategy based on monthly assessments of visual acuity, fundus examination, and most importantly optical coherence tomography (OCT), allowing for a reduction in the mean number of injections [12, 13]. However, the inter-individual range of treatment needs varied widely, between monthly injections and no re-treatment after the loading dose. A later study showed that the mean treatment interval in a PRN regimen is approximately 2 months for ranibizumab [14]. The PRN regimen was the first approach to be widely adopted in clinical practice. It was validated as a valuable treatment option with a non-inferior outcome as compared to a fixed monthly re-treatment [15]. Both ranibizumab and the entire antibody *bevacizumab* were shown to be adequate treatment options [15]. However, some differences were found favoring ranibizumab: Pathological fluid was less frequently present when using ranibizumab, and the functional outcome of ranibizumab in the fixed monthly treatment was significantly better than bevacizumab in a PRN regimen [15]. In addition, bevacizumab is not licensed for intravitreal use but for intravenous use in oncology. In conclusion, bevacizumab is a less expensive second-choice off-label anti-VEGF drug, which has shown close to optimal efficacy for intravitreal use in nAMD.

Aflibercept is a recombinant fusion protein consisting of VEGF-binding portions from the extracellular domains of the human VEGF receptors 1 and 2 that are fused to the Fc portion of the human IgG1 immunoglobulin. Aflibercept was first labeled in 2011 for an intravitreal use in nAMD. The pivotal phase 3 clinical trial used in the first year a fixed injection regimen every 2 months for aflibercept (as compared to monthly injections with ranibizumab) and a PRN regimen in the second year. In both study periods, the efficacy of aflibercept was equivalent to that of ranibizumab. Thus, aflibercept was labeled for intravitreal injection in nAMD, and the recommended regimen was a fixed injection every 2 months. Although this is a valid approach, concerns were raised due to a subset of patients with significant monthly recurrences, leading to a zigzag curve of structural OCT outcomes when treating every other month [15]. It is unclear whether these patients would have had a better functional outcome with a monthly instead of the bimonthly aflibercept treatment.

Very recently, the new anti-VEGF agent *brolucizumab*, a very small single-chain antibody fragment allowing a high drug concentration, has shown its efficacy in a phase 3 study. The non-inferiority in comparison to aflibercept was shown for visual acuity and structural results, although the regimen was based on fixed injections every 3 months. Apparently, this new molecule might have a long-lasting activity, possibly related to the higher molecular dose. However, roughly half of the patients showed some disease activity when treated at 3-month intervals, and their regimen was changed to an injection every 2 months. Brolucizumab has recently become available on the market.

While fixed regimens have the major advantage of the ability to plan ahead with little necessity for monitoring visits, they result inevitably in overtreatment of some patients and/or undertreatment of others due to the large variability in treatment needs. In addition, economic concerns, limited resources, and considerations regarding possible side effects of the intravitreal injection procedure (endophthalmitis) lead to an inclination to reduce the number of injections. Individually adjusted variable dosing regimens have the potential to respond adequately to these requirements. Variable dosing regimens aiming for an individualized treatment, use the minimum number of injections needed for the best possible outcome. Independent of the choice of the anti-VEGF agent, variable dosing regimens rely on best practice in terms of *visit intervals and re-treatment criteria.* Major efficacy losses arise if the follow-up is neglected or unsuitable re-treatment criteria are used. Real-life results of PRN regimens have shown that visit interval longer than a month are unsuitable to achieve the best outcome. This is not surprising, as not only the treatment needs are extremely variable among patients, but longer monitoring intervals in a PRN regimen lead in many patients also to protracted recurrence periods. Thus, re-treatment may come too late in order to prevent progressive retinal damage due to recurrence. In other words, PRN with anti-VEGF antibodies is only a valuable strategy if monthly monitoring visits and prompt re-treatment in case of a recurrence can be guaranteed. The re-treatment criteria are discussed in a separate paragraph below.

The need for strict monthly monitoring visits in a PRN regimen with anti-VEGF drugs has rapidly revealed the capacity limits of healthcare providers. The high incidence of new cases and the required treatment chronicity have led to an overwhelming number of patients to be cared for. Moreover, PRN has the major disadvantage that planning is impossible, which is a logistic challenge to the institution and a psychological burden for the patient. Thus, alternative regimens have been developed, based on the idea that the past experience with a given eye may allow anticipating the future need for injections.

The *treat-and-extend regimen* applies this idea. After a loading dose of one to three monthly injections, the treatment interval is progressively extended by 2 weeks as long as no signs of activity (the criteria are discussed below) are detected. Monitoring is performed immediately before an injection, and its result determines the length of the next interval, without modifying the planned imminent injection. As soon as a monitoring visit reveals any signs of activity, the interval is shortened by 2 weeks. The interval between visits combining monitoring with treatment should usually not exceed approximately 3 months (12–16 weeks). If the macula of a treated eye remains dry at this three-month interval, a choice between the default treatment every 3 months or a change to monitoring visits without injections every 2 months is suggested. The outcomes with this strategy are comparable to those with a PRN regimen and statistically non-inferior to monthly re-treatment [16]. The treat-and-extend regimen needs a significantly lower number of monitoring visits (the mean value is approximately eight per year), and planning is clearly facilitated as nearly each monitoring visit goes along with an injection. Thus, this strategy has been widely adopted as the first-choice regimen for anti-VEGF treatment in nAMD.

The *observe-and-plan regimen* also applies the idea to schedule treatment intervals, however, to a series of injections instead of single injection intervals. Based on the regularity of individual treatment needs [17], the observe-and-plan regimen evaluates after the loading doses the time to the first recurrence signs using monthly monitoring visits ("observe"), thereafter applying this interval slightly shortened by 2 weeks in a series of planned injections with a fixed interval (up to three injections, interval between 1 and 3 months, treatment plan up to 6 months) [18, 19]. The monitoring visits after a series of fixed injections are therefore less frequent (the mean being approximately four per year) than in the treat-and-extend regimen, and the ability to plan ahead is excellent. However, the longest treatment interval without a monitoring visit should not exceed 3 months. This regimen has the potential for excellent patient care with limited ressources.

8.2 Re-Treatment Criteria for Variable Dosing Regimen

Sensitive re-treatment criteria are the cornerstone of any variable dosing regimen with anti-VEGF drugs. Most studies consider primarily OCT criteria, combined with fundus examination and visual acuity loss.

- *Visual acuity*: Visual loss relative to any preceding monitoring visit (typically 5 ETDRS letters or 1 line) is a clinically meaningful but unreliable criterion for re-treatment with anti-VEGF drugs. This re-treatment criterion was used due to its ease of examination. However, pathological changes are usually first detectable by OCT and manifest as a decline in visual acuity later. In addition, vision loss may be caused by many other conditions than exudative recurrence, and they may be completely unresponsive to anti-VEGF treatment, such as progressive macular atrophy or cataract. Therefore, it cannot be a stand alone criterion. In addition, retreatment should not wait for visual loss to happen, if other signs of activity are present. For best functional results it is important to treat before irreversible damage occurs to the photoreceptors.

- *OCT criteria*: With the arrival of high-precision spectral-domain OCT (SD-OCT) allowing a precise examination of the entire 6 × 6 mm macular cube, OCT has become the cornerstone of re-treatment strategies. Any pathological retinal fluid is easily detected by scanning through all acquired B-scans. However, a single line would be insufficient for decision making, as not only the fovea but also extrafoveal areas are relevant, needing treatment to prevent further neovascuar growth. Intra- or subretinal fluid is commonly considered a solid re-treatment criterion because it is usually a sign of active exudation from the neovascular membrane, requiring anti-VEGF re-treatment. However, fluid under the retinal pigment epithelium is only by some studies considered a re-treatment criterion [15]. This type of fluid is - after an initial improvement - insufficiently responsive to anti-VEGF treatment and appears to be not relevant for re-treatment. Considering this type of fluid a re-treatment criterion does not change the visual prognosis. However, cases of high retinal pigment epithelium detachment generally require anyway a high number of injections as intra- or subretinal fluid is frequently present and poorly responsive.
- *Retinal hemorrhage*: The fundus examination is the most useful investigation technique to identify retinal hemorrhage. New retinal hemorrhage may be a sign of nAMD activity requiring anti-VEGF re-treatment. Most variable dosing regimens consider a new hemorrhage to be a re-treatment criterion. However, hemorrhage might occur independently of VEGF levels and may not necessarily represent nAMD activity. For instance, large neovascular feeder vessels in combination with systemic hypertensive peaks or sustained Valsalva pressure might be the cause. Thus, hemorrhage might occur even under monthly anti-VEGF treatments and a complete VEGF suppression.

In summary, SD-OCT is the most important investigation for variable dosing regimens with anti-VEGF drugs. The general strategy is to apply the minimal number of injections in order to nearly completely suppress VEGF activity. Re-treatment is indicated at the earliest signs of exudative recurrence such as the presence of intra- or subretinal fluids, in particular foveal fluids. However, even extrafoveal fluids represent a threat to visual acuity due to underlying reactivation of neovascular processes. Any such reactivation might ultimately lead to further growth of the neovascular complex. As this could result in further loss of vision, any identification of relevant fluids is considered a criterion for re-treatment in order to prevent a disease progression.

Recent studies revealed a difference in the functional and prognostic relevance of intra- versus subretinal fluids. It has been shown that intraretinal fluids are associated with a worse visual outcome, whereas subretinal fluids appear to be well tolerated [20, 21]. Another recent study revealed that subretinal fluids up to 200 μm can be tolerated even under the fovea without a visual disadvantage, and the authors found non-inferiority versus no fluid tolerance [22]. Thus, the re-treatment criteria in variable dosing regimens with anti-VEGF drugs for nAMD might undergo some changes in the near future, differentiating the roles of subretinal from those of intraretinal fluids.

Some open questions still need to be addressed:

- *Degenerative* fluid accumulation due to a loss of retinal substance might simulate exudative fluids. However, reliable criteria to differentiate between them are missing. The best indicators of degenerative fluids might be so far: non-responsiveness to anti-VEGF drugs, overlying atrophy or fibrosis, no retinal thickness increase, and small intraretinal spaces.
- A subset of eyes presents *refractory fluids despite monthly treatments* with anti-VEGF medication. The causes of such a refractory fluid are variable and often difficult to identify.

Some patients might just have high intraretinal VEGF levels and an early recurrence, requiring ongoing monthly re-treatment with anti-VEGF drugs, while others might have a pathological exudation of an origin other than VEGF, being completely non-responsive to anti-VEGF treatment and, thus, not requiring monthly anti-VEGF injections. A non-responsive fluid might be linked to inflammation, degenerative changes, central serous chorioretinopathy, polypoidal choroidal vasculopathy, or other disorders. Obviously, adjuvant or alternative treatment strategies could be considered according to the cause of the refractory fluid. Steroids will be most useful in cases involving inflammatory components, while PDT with verteporfin would be an interesting treatment adjuvant for polypoidal choroidal vasculopathy (recently termed aneurysmal type 1 neovascularization). A triple therapy combining anti-VEGF medication with both intravitreal steroids and PDT has also been suggested.

- The role of switching from one anti-VEGF molecule to another has been largely discussed in the literature, however, without a convincing conclusion. It seems that refractory cases might sometimes benefit from changing the anti-VEGF agent, and drug tolerance may play a role [23]. However, clear clinical indicators are missing.
- The degree of structural and functional damage to the retina is currently poorly taken into account in the treatment regimen. Progressive fibrosis and atrophy are the main reasons for progressive visual loss despite careful re-treatments with anti-VEGF drugs [24]. Anti-VEGF treatment only addresses the exudative part of the disorder. However, if visual loss becomes severe (<0.1) due to irreversible fibrosis or atrophy, the usefulness of continued intravitreal injections is very limited. At some point, the anti-VEGF treatment does not make sense anymore. In the absence of a clearly defined limit, most clinicians will abandon the treatment when the vision is reduced to counting fingers.
- The topographic correlation between exudation and structural–functional retinal damage is another point that has so far been poorly addressed by variable dosing regimens with anti-VEGF drugs. While there is an agreement that exudative fluid should be treated independently of its location with respect to the fovea, it might well be that a location within a nonfunctional atrophic or fibrotic area is not a good re-treatment criterion: As long as functional regions of the retina are not threatened by exudation or neovascular membrane growth, it might not be needed to insist on VEGF suppression. However, the available evidence is insufficient to give recommendations on this point.

8.3 Screening and Early Discovery

Anti-VEGF treatment has introduced a new era in the treatment of nAMD improving its prognosis. Its efficacy with strong control over exudation and vasoproliferation allows for good visual acuity improvements as compared to the treatment baseline. The relative improvement is particularly good in eyes with poorer baseline vision [25]. However, the resulting vision level is the most relevant outcome for patients. Even if a lower baseline vision gains statistically more with anti-VEGF drugs, the resulting visual acuity remains lower than that of an early treated nAMD. A long-standing untreated nAMD will show more fibrosis and irreversible retinal damage, limiting the potential functional gain of any treatment. Thus, it is well recognized that the *early discovery of a neovascular complication in AMD* is extremely important for the final visual outcome.

A variety of screening approaches are available for the clinician and the patient. Clinical visits with visual acuity and SD-OCT are sensitive, but they cannot be performed frequently enough for efficient screening. The cornerstone of screening is the *home monitoring* of well-educated patients. The oldest method goes back to Prof. *Amsler*, who developed a simple *grid* with a central fixation point, printed on paper, to identify *metamorphopsia* (monocular examination reading correction and reading illumination). The appearance of new metamorphopsia is an early sign of retinal deformation, usually in the context of macular edema. In a patient with known early signs of AMD such as drusen and pigmentary changes, there is a high probability that new metamorphopsia indicates early exudative changes of nAMD. Such a patient needs to be seen by an ophthalmologist as soon as possible within 2 weeks.

Recently, a specially designed home monitoring device (ForseeHome™) has been tested for its sensitivity and specificity in the screening of neovascular complications in AMD [26]. It uses preferential *hyperacuity perimetry*. The use of this device led to the earlier recognition of neovascular complications and a better visual outcome than regular office visits (in combination with the Amsler grid at the discretion of the investigator). It is the first commercially available device for this use and approved by the US Food and Drug Administration (FDA).

In recent years, many *electronic applications* have emerged, proposing nAMD screening based on both Amsler grid analysis and hyperacuity perimetry. There are many minor and major variations available, and it is impossible to give clear recommendations for one or the other application. However, a minimum of scientific evaluation should be required in order to guarantee the quality of size, contrast, color setting, etc. Approval by the FDA is available for some of the applications.

8.4 Safety of Anti-VEGF Treatment

Anti-VEGF treatment for nAMD is applied using intravitreal injections. Both ocular and systemic safety concerns of the drug and the injection procedure need to be considered.

Safety issues of systemic treatments, including arterial hypertension and thromboembolic events, are not applicable in the same way as the eye globe is a relatively closed system. However, small quantities of anti-VEGF antibodies are absorbed into the systemic circulation, and in some patients, the systemic VEGF levels were critically reduced by 50%. However, the reported rates of systemic adverse events are low in all studies. No study showed a significant difference between anti-VEGF and comparison arms. However, minor nonsignificant differences with slightly more cardiovascular events in the anti-VEGF arms have initiated meta-analysis studies. In a meta-analysis including 21 studies with 9557 patients, anti-VEGF treatment did not significantly increase overall mortality or cardiovascular mortality [27]. The occurrence of serious systemic adverse events was comparable across anti-VEGF-treated groups and control groups.

Ocular inflammation and increased intraocular pressure after intravitreal injection were the most frequently reported serious ocular adverse events [28]. Endophthalmitis was reported in fewer than 1% of anti-VEGF-treated participants; no cases were reported in control groups. The transient increase in intraocular pressure after intravitreal injection of 0.05 ml of the anti-VEGF drug might need special consideration in advanced glaucoma patients with low target pressure.

8.5 Combination Treatment and Alternative Treatment Options

Anti-VEGF monotherapy is currently the best available treatment strategy for nAMD. Its strong control over exudation and vasoproliferation results in a high level of disease control. No alternative or adjuvant treatment has been able to improve this excellent outcome further. However, nAMD is a complex, multifactorial disorder. Therefore, it appears attractive to add a second line of action by an adjuvant treatment, potentially complementary to the anti-VEGF action. So far, no combination treatment was able to improve the visual results. Recently, the promising approach of combining anti-VEGF antibodies with pegpleranib E10030 (Fovista), an anti-platelet-derived growth factor antibody, failed to reach superiority to anti-VEGF monotherapy (ClinicalTrials.gov Identifier: NCT01940900), although its pathophysiological basis was highly attractive (acting on pericytes in semi-mature neovessels in order to increase the anti-VEGF sensitivity).

However, several other combination therapies are able to reduce the number of anti-VEGF injections. This appears to be particularly attractive for the so-called "anti-VEGF-refractory nAMD." However, little is known about possible unwanted effects on visual acuity in these cases. This would be important to avoid unnecessary additional risks of unwanted effects due to adjuvant treatments.

PDT with verteporfin was the standard treatment for subfoveal nAMD before the arrival of anti-VEGF drugs. Although it improves the final outcome compared to sham to some extent, a loss in the mean visual acuity was still a reality and the efficacy, therefore, not satisfactory [29]. However, in cases of a contraindication of the anti-VEGF treatment for whatever reason, PDT might be an alternative to reduce visual loss, but patients need to be informed about its inferiority compared to anti-VEGF therapy.

The *combination of anti-VEGF drugs with PDT* has been investigated in numerous studies. A recent meta-analysis included 16 randomized controlled trials comparing anti-VEGF monotherapy and the combination treatment of anti-VEGF antibodies with PDT (standard or reduced fluence) [30]. This meta-analysis confirmed that they only differed in the number of anti-VEGF injections needed, whereas visual acuity and central retinal thickness changes did not differ [30]. Interestingly, a subgroup analysis of adjuvant full-fluence PDT did reveal a lower central retinal thickness. This could be a warning sign, as full-fluence PDT has the potential to damage the choriocapillaris and the pigment epithelium.

Particular interest has been given to the role of PDT in *polypoidal choroidal vasculopathy (PCV)*, a special subtype of nAMD. Before the arrival of anti-VEGF therapy, PDT showed some promising results in PCV [31], while being relatively poorly efficient in other types of nAMD. Since the arrival of the anti-VEGF treatment, an improved visual benefit was found not only for nAMD in general but also for PCV. However, several studies have shown in PCV an interesting potential of anti-VEGF drugs with adjuvant PDT [32]. Their results are moderately variable; some of them suggesting a superior visual outcome and a higher rate of polyp closure along with a decreased number of anti-VEGF injections in the combination therapy [33], whereas others found a very high rate of disease control in anti-VEGF monotherapy with no added benefit from additional PDT treatment [34]. Thus, both options are currently considered valuable treatment approaches. In a setting with readily available anti-VEGF medication, PCV patients will undergo anti-VEGF monotherapy as a first-line treatment and change to a combination with PDT in case of persisting exudative signs. However, in cases with a priority for reduced numbers of injections and appointments, the first-line combination of anti-VEGF drugs and PDT might be an interesting option. However, this approach requires indocyanine green angiography for diagnosis and treatment guidance.

A broad combination treatment with *anti-VEGF antibodies, PDT, and intraocular steroid injections* (triamcinolone) has also been proposed as the so-called triple therapy [35]. The rationale combines the anti-VEGF and anti-inflammatory effects to act on both the neovascular processes and the PDT-related unwanted effects, increasing the benefits of adjuvant PDT on vascular occlusion. Although this treatment has been reported to be beneficial, there is no controlled clinical trial available. Therefore, no clear recommendation can be made. This treatment option might be of interest in some highly exudative, anti-VEGF-refractory cases.

The combination of anti-VEGF medication with *stereotactic radiotherapy* has been investigated in nAMD eyes with high anti-VEGF demand. The INTREPID trial found a reduced number of anti-VEGF injections over 2 years following a single stereotactic radiotherapy session [36]. However, some radiation-related unwanted effects were also described but considered non-significant for visual outcomes. Currently, a larger clinical trial is underway (ClinicalTrials.gov Identifier: NCT02243878), and first results might be expected for 2024.

Large submacular hemorrhage is a particular challenge in the management of nAMD. Dramatic visual loss occurs if the hemorrhage is central, and photoreceptors rapidly suffer from irreversible damage when in direct contact with a thick layer of blood (subretinal hemorrhage). In such cases, a combination of vitrectomy, subretinal tissue plasminogen activator, and intravitreal gas might be considered, if the bleeding is very recent. Outcomes vary widely, and systematic trials are lacking [37].

Very recently, the mineralocorticoid receptor pathway has been suggested to be implicated in the pathogenesis of choroidal neovascularization, based on animal models [38]. The clinical application has only been tested in a clinical pilot study [38] but may potentially become an interesting future option.

8.6 Future Challenges

Despite the breakthrough in the nAMD prognosis due to anti-VEGF treatment options, there are many unmet needs in nAMD. The underlying degenerative process frequently leads to macular atrophy and profound visual loss despite "successful" control of the neovascular process. Fibrosis is not inhibited by anti-VEGF treatment, a major problem particularly in type 2 neovascularization (classic neovascular membrane), and responsible for irreversible visual losses. Massive macular hemorrhage may occur in nAMD despite maximal monthly re-treatment with anti-VEGF medication, causing a profound acute loss in visual acuity. The chronicity of the exudative disorder requiring repetitive intravitreal injections is a major problem for patients and healthcare providers. More durable and less expensive solutions would be beneficial. Long-term delivery systems or small interfering RNAs are promising future possibilities. Artificial intelligence might become a useful tool to monitor and manage large numbers of patients. Finally, it could become a reality to recover lost vision with stem cell techniques or artificial retinal implants. Obviously, the best solution would be to find an efficient prophylactic treatment to prevent that AMD compromises the vision.

Key Learning Points

- The clinical management of nAMD requires careful monitoring and sensitive re-treatment criteria for anti-VEGF treatment. SD-OCT plays a key role in follow-up and decision-making.
- A variety of treatment regimens are available to the clinician. The key to functional success is not the choice of the regimen but the careful application of its rules, including monitoring intervals and re-treatment criteria.
- Undertreatment threatens the vision more than overtreatment.
- Most importantly, early discovery is crucial for good final visual results. Screening methods and patient education are most helpful.
- Some cases do not entirely respond to anti-VEGF treatment. Their best management is not well established. Combination treatment with other modalities may be considered.

References

1. Brown DM, Kaiser PK, Michels M, et al. Ranibizumab versus verteporfin for neovascular age-related macular degeneration. N Engl J Med. 2006;355:1432–44.
2. Rosenfeld PJ, Brown DM, Heier JS, et al. Ranibizumab for neovascular age-related macular degeneration. N Engl J Med. 2006;355:1419–31.
3. Heier JS, Brown DM, Chong V, et al. Intravitreal aflibercept (VEGF trap-eye) in wet age-related macular degeneration. Ophthalmology. 2012;119:2537–48.
4. Adamis AP, Shima DT, Tolentino MJ, et al. Inhibition of vascular endothelial growth factor prevents retinal ischemia-associated iris neovascularization in a nonhuman primate. Arch Ophthalmol. 1996;114:66–71.
5. Tolentino MJ, Miller JW, Gragoudas ES, Chatzistefanou K, Ferrara N, Adamis AP. Vascular endothelial growth factor is sufficient to produce iris neovascularization and neovascular glaucoma in a nonhuman primate. Arch Ophthalmol. 1996;114:964–70.
6. Gragoudas ES, Adamis AP, Cunningham ET Jr, Feinsod M, Guyer DR. Group VISiONCT. Pegaptanib for neovascular age-related macular degeneration. N Engl J Med. 2004;351:2805–16.
7. Bressler NM, Bressler SB. Photodynamic therapy with verteporfin (Visudyne): impact on ophthalmology and visual sciences. Invest Ophthalmol Vis Sci. 2000;41:624–8.
8. Brown DM, Michels M, Kaiser PK, Heier JS, Sy JP, Ianchulev T. Ranibizumab versus verteporfin photodynamic therapy for neovascular age-related macular degeneration: two-year results of the ANCHOR study. Ophthalmology. 2009;116:57–65.

9. Abraham P, Yue H, Wilson L. Randomized, double-masked, sham-controlled trial of ranibizumab for neovascular age-related macular degeneration: PIER study year 2. Am J Ophthalmol. 2010;150:315–24.
10. Schmidt-Erfurth U, Eldem B, Guymer R, et al. Efficacy and safety of monthly versus quarterly ranibizumab treatment in neovascular age-related macular degeneration: the EXCITE study. Ophthalmology. 2011;118:831–9.
11. Regillo CD, Brown DM, Abraham P, et al. Randomized, double-masked, sham-controlled trial of ranibizumab for neovascular age-related macular degeneration: PIER study year 1. Am J Ophthalmol. 2008;145:239–48.
12. Fung AE, Lalwani GA, Rosenfeld PJ, et al. An optical coherence tomography-guided, variable dosing regimen with intravitreal ranibizumab (Lucentis) for neovascular age-related macular degeneration. Am J Ophthalmol. 2007;143:566–83.
13. Lalwani GA, Rosenfeld PJ, Fung AE, et al. A variable-dosing regimen with intravitreal ranibizumab for neovascular age-related macular degeneration: year 2 of the PrONTO study. Am J Ophthalmol. 2009;148:43–58.
14. Busbee BG, Ho AC, Brown DM, et al. Twelve-month efficacy and safety of 0.5 mg or 2.0 mg ranibizumab in patients with subfoveal neovascular age-related macular degeneration. Ophthalmology. 2013;120:1046–56.
15. Martin DF, Maguire MG, Ying GS, Grunwald JE, Fine SL, Jaffe GJ. Ranibizumab and bevacizumab for neovascular age-related macular degeneration. N Engl J Med. 2011;364:1897–908.
16. Silva R, Berta A, Larsen M, et al. Treat-and-extend versus monthly regimen in Neovascular age-related macular degeneration: results with Ranibizumab from the TREND study. Ophthalmology. 2018;125:57–65.
17. Mantel I, Deli A, Iglesias K, Ambresin A. Prospective study evaluating the predictability of need for retreatment with intravitreal ranibizumab for age-related macular degeneration. Graefe's Arch Clin Exp Ophthalmol. 2013;251:697–704.
18. Gianniou C, Dirani A, Ferrini W, et al. Two-year outcome of an observe-and-plan regimen for neovascular age-related macular degeneration: how to alleviate the clinical burden with maintained functional results. Eye (London). 2015;29:342–9.
19. Mantel I, Niderprim SA, Gianniou C, Deli A, Ambresin A. Reducing the clinical burden of ranibizumab treatment for neovascular age-related macular degeneration using an individually planned regimen. Br J Ophthalmol. 2014;98:1192–6.
20. Jaffe GJ, Martin DF, Toth CA, et al. Macular morphology and visual acuity in the comparison of age-related macular degeneration treatments trials. Ophthalmology. 2013;120:1860–70.
21. Sharma S, Toth CA, Daniel E, et al. Macular morphology and visual acuity in the second year of the comparison of age-related macular degeneration treatments trials. Ophthalmology. 2016;123:865–75.
22. Guymer RH, Markey CM, McAllister IL, Gillies MC, Hunyor AP, Arnold JJ. Tolerating subretinal fluid in neovascular age-related macular degeneration treated with ranibizumab using a treat-and-extend regimen: FLUID study 24-month results. Ophthalmology. 2019;126:723–34.
23. Mantel I, Gillies MC, Souied EH. Switching between ranibizumab and aflibercept for the treatment of neovascular age-related macular degeneration. Surv Ophthalmol. 2018;63:638–45.
24. Rosenfeld PJ, Shapiro H, Tuomi L, et al. Characteristics of patients losing vision after 2 years of monthly dosing in the phase III ranibizumab clinical trials. Ophthalmology. 2011;118:523–30.
25. Kaiser PK, Brown DM, Zhang K, et al. Ranibizumab for predominantly classic neovascular age-related macular degeneration: subgroup analysis of first-year ANCHOR results. AmJ Ophthalmol. 2007;144:850–7.
26. Group AHSR, Chew EY, Clemons TE, et al. Randomized trial of a home monitoring system for early detection of choroidal neovascularization home monitoring of the eye (HOME) study. Ophthalmology. 2014;121:535–44.
27. Thulliez M, Angoulvant D, Le Lez ML, et al. Cardiovascular events and bleeding risk associated with intravitreal antivascular endothelial growth factor monoclonal antibodies: systematic review and meta-analysis. JAMA Ophthalmol. 2014;132:1317–26.
28. Solomon SD, Lindsley K, Vedula SS, Krzystolik MG, Hawkins BS. Anti-vascular endothelial growth factor for neovascular age-related macular degeneration. Cochrane Database Syst Rev. 2014;8(8):CD005139.
29. Bressler NM, Treatment of Age-Related Macular Degeneration with Photodynamic Therapy Study G. Photodynamic therapy of subfoveal choroidal neovascularization in age-related macular degeneration with verteporfin: two-year results of 2 randomized clinical trials-tap report 2. Arch Ophthalmol. 2001;119:198–207.
30. Gao Y, Yu T, Zhang Y, Dang G. Anti-VEGF Monotherapy versus photodynamic therapy and anti-VEGF combination treatment for Neovascular age-related macular degeneration: a meta-analysis. Invest Ophthalmol Vis Sci. 2018;59:4307–17.
31. Nowak-Sliwinska P, van den Bergh H, Sickenberg M, Koh AH. Photodynamic therapy for polypoidal choroidal vasculopathy. Prog Retin Eye Res. 2013;37:182–99.
32. Teo KYC, Gillies M, Fraser-Bell S. The use of vascular endothelial growth factor inhibitors and complementary treatment options in Polypoidal Choroidal vasculopathy: a subtype of Neovascular age-related macular degeneration. Int J Mol Sci. 2018;19(9):2611.
33. Koh A, Lai TYY, Takahashi K, et al. Efficacy and safety of Ranibizumab with or without Verteporfin photodynamic therapy for Polypoidal Choroidal vasculopathy: a randomized clinical trial. JAMA Ophthalmol. 2017;135:1206–13.
34. Lee WK, Iida T, Ogura Y, et al. Efficacy and safety of Intravitreal Aflibercept for Polypoidal Choroidal

vasculopathy in the PLANET study: a randomized clinical trial. JAMA Ophthalmol. 2018;136:786–93.
35. Augustin AJ, Puls S, Offermann I. Triple therapy for choroidal neovascularization due to age-related macular degeneration: verteporfin PDT, bevacizumab, and dexamethasone. Retina. 2007;27:133–40.
36. Jackson TL, Chakravarthy U, Slakter JS, et al. Stereotactic radiotherapy for neovascular age-related macular degeneration: year 2 results of the INTREPID study. Ophthalmology. 2015;122:138–45.
37. Stanescu-Segall D, Balta F, Jackson TL. Submacular hemorrhage in neovascular age-related macular degeneration: a synthesis of the literature. Surv Ophthalmol. 2016;61:18–32.
38. Zhao M, Mantel I, Gelize E, et al. Mineralocorticoid receptor antagonism limits experimental choroidal neovascularization and structural changes associated with neovascular age-related macular degeneration. Nat Commun. 2019;10:369.

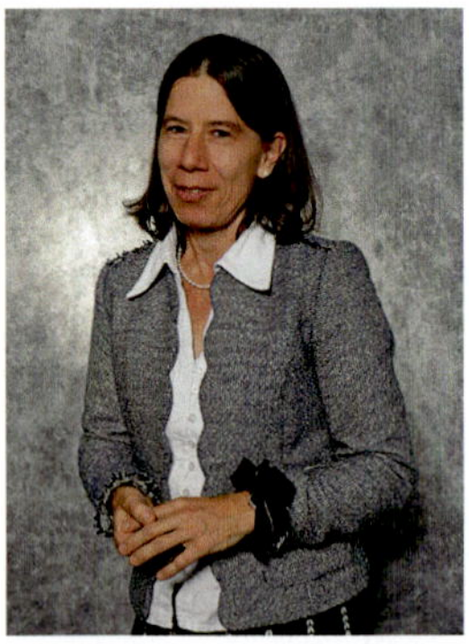

Irmela Mantel, MD is currently a medical retina lead consultant at the Jules Gonin Eye Hospital in Lausanne, Switzerland. She is actively involved in a number of research projects investigating retinal degenerative disorders and in particular age-related macular degeneration. Dr. Mantel received her medical degree from the University of Zurich, Switzerland. She has been a medical retina fellow to Professor Alan Bird at Moorfields Eye Hospital in London, England.

9 Myopic Choroidal Neovascularization

Seung-Young Yu and Kiyoung Kim

9.1 Incidence and Related Lesions

Pathologic myopia, termed "myopic macular degeneration," "myopic maculopathy," or "degenerative myopia," is a consequence of myopia progression, particularly in eyes with high myopia (typically defined as spherical equivalent less than −6.0 diopters). One of the most serious complications of pathologic myopia is myopic choroidal neovascularization (CNV), which frequently leads to a sudden but progressive loss of central vision.

Myopic CNV occurs in 5–11% of pathologic myopia, and the second common lesion in macular CNV followed by age-related macular degeneration (AMD). The prevalence and incidence of myopic CNV may differ between each geographic area and maybe underestimated or inaccurate because of insufficient screening. Since 1991, Fuchs named fibrovascular tissue elevated with dome-shaped retinal pigment epithelium (RPE) as Foester–Fuch's spot in high myopia, Gass defined that acute hemorrhage detachment primary occurs after the formation of neovascular membrane from Fuch's spot, secondly, organized sub-RPE hemorrhage accompanied with RPE proliferation remains as a blackish brown spot in the macula. Through slit examination, gray circular or oval-shaped pigmentation is observed in the border of macular lesions, and lesions can be confined in the macular or elsewhere. Fuch's spot is regarded as evidence of myopic CNV, which as Curtin and Karlin detected Fuch's spot in 5.2% of myopic eyes longer than 26.5 mm, and Hotchkiss and Fine found neovascularization in 40.7% of high myopia. Incidence of bilateral Fuch's spot has been reported between 12 and 41% by different authors. Particularly, 62% of total myopic CNV has developed in younger aged than 50, and when CNV occurs in one eye, the possibility of development in the fellow eye is estimated to be higher than 30% within 8 years.

9.2 Clinical Manifestation

Although, vision progressively decreases from the 40s in general pathologic myopia, a rapid vision decreases and metamorphopsia cab be caused by marginal exudation and hemorrhage in myopic CNV. Focal retinal detachment and hemorrhage can develop around CNV, but hard exudates are rarely detected [1].

Neovascular tissue is usually located underneath fovea. 58–74% of subretinal CNV involve fovea and size is less than half of optic disc. The other CNVs also exist within 100–300 μm of fovea. These foveal CNV is one of the specific clinical characteristics of myopic CNV [2].

S.-Y. Yu (✉) · K. Kim
Department of Ophthalmology, Kyung Hee University Hospital, Seoul, South Korea
e-mail: syyu@khu.ac.kr

J. Chhablani (ed.), *Choroidal Neovascularization*, https://doi.org/10.1007/978-981-15-2213-0_9

9.3 Fluorescein Angiography and Indocyanine Green Angiography

Early hyperfluorescence and late leakage of foveal CNV were observed in Fluorescein angiography (FA). However, leakage is not severely increased as CNV of AMD, and confined to the border of neovascular membrane. If a relatively large amount of leakage is present in old myopic patients, AMD should be considered as a main cause.

Avila et al. [3] reported that 91% of myopic eyes with severe choroidal degeneration did not present fluorescein leakage in CNV and 80% of myopic eyes with mild choroidal degeneration presented fluorescein leakage. This result supports that choroidal change of pathologic myopia is related to neovascularization which comes from the choroid. Choroidal blood flow decreases and choriocapillaris circulation are severely impaired in pathologic myopia. Furthermore, extensive choroidal atrophy causes loss of choroidal stroma and partial occlusion of the vessel, which consequently induces the formation of a relatively small size of CNV. In the early phase of indocyanine green angiography (ICGA), CNV appears as a hyperfluorescent lesion of similar intensity with choroidal background. ICGA can be used in addition to FA, because it can provide more informative data on the choroidal circulation, along with the presence and extent of lacquer cracks. CVN is delineated with hypofluorescent border and hyperfluorescent CNV continuously increases with choroidal arterial filling and maintains during choroidal venous phase. Neovascular membrane can remain as relatively hypofluorescent spot in late phase, but leakage does not occur. Although, it can be difficult to identify the exact margin and range of neovascular membrane, ICGA is a useful method to investigate the relationship between CNV and lacquer crack and detect hidden CNV which cannot be discovered with FA in myopic CNV patients with subretinal hemorrhage.

9.4 Optical Coherence Tomography (OCT) Findings

High-resolution OCT is a rapid, noninvasive technique that has been used efficiently to determine disease activity of myopic CNV. Several studies have successfully demonstrated the effectiveness of SD-OCT in assessing the activity and stage of the disease [1]. Compared with FA, myopic CNV presents as a hyper-reflective material above the RPE band (type 2 CNV) on SD-OCT, with a variable amount of subretinal fluid. Especially, it is helpful to evaluate the effectiveness of treatment by measuring subretinal fluid from CNV. If CNV locates above RPE layer and enough space is available around the lesion, it can be an indication for surgical removal of CNV.

9.5 Optical Coherence Tomography Angiography (OCTA)

The recent development of OCTA has allowed accurate delineation of structural and blood flow information from different retina and choroid layers. OCTA has been investigated to the study of several retinal disorders, and it also has proven particularly useful for the diagnosis of CNV in pathologic myopia. In OCTA, CNV appears as a large hyperintense vascular anastomotic network (Fig. 9.1). The use of OCTA may further clarify the role of choroidal blood flow and retinal function.

A recently developed swept-source OCTA (SS-OCTA) uses longer wavelength of approximately 1050 nm compared with spectral-domain OCTA (SD-OCTA: 840–880 nm). The main advantages of SS-OCTA over SD-OCTA is the higher scanning speed, which allows for denser A-scan and B-scans and larger scan areas for a same acquisition time. Additional advantages of SS-OCTA technology are enhanced light penetration through the RPE, as well as better detection of signals from the deeper retinal layers. This potentially allows for more detailed visualization, enhanced penetration through exudative

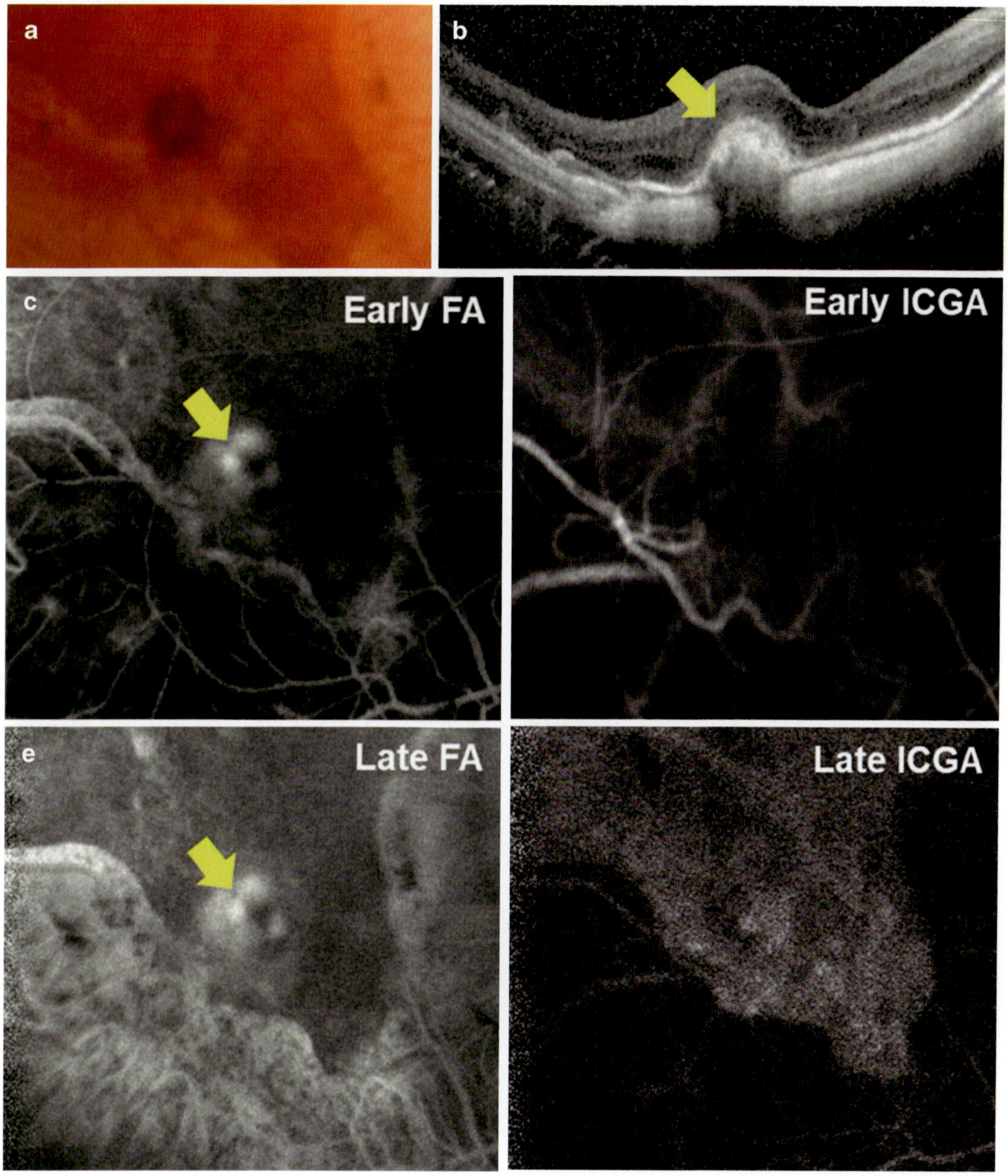

Fig. 9.1 Multimodal imaging of a 56-year-old female patient presenting myopic choroidal neovascularization (CNV). (**a**) Fundus color photo, (**b**) Optical coherence tomography (OCT), (**c–d**) Early and late fluorescein angiography (FA), (**e–f**) early and late indocyanine green angiography (**g–i**) Comparisons of three different OCT angiography (OCTA) devices in myopic CNV. Both spectral-domain and swept-source OCTA shows a clear vascular network in myopic CNV (yellow circle). (**g**) AngioPlex (spectral-domain OCTA): Carl Zeiss Meditec, Inc., Dublin, CA, USA; (**h**) Spectralis (Spectral-domain OCTA): Heidelberg Engineering, Heidelberg, Germany; (**i**) Swept-source OCTA: PLEX Elite 9000; Carl Zeiss Meditec, Inc., Dublin, CA, USA

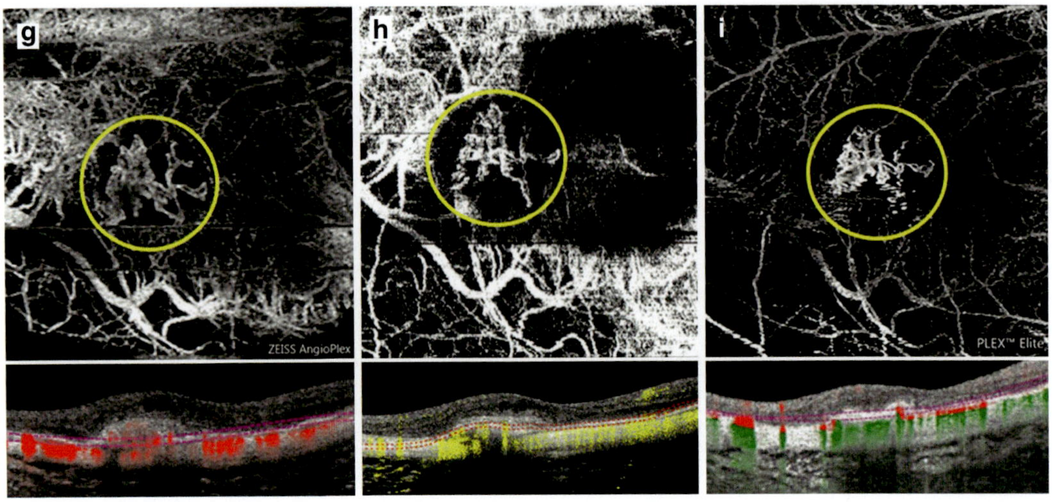

Fig. 9.1 (continued)

material or subretinal fluid, and better detection of neovascular complex compared with SD-OCTA. SS-OCTA can also provide better visualization of the choroid and choriocapillaris layer, which can detect neovascularization or abnormal choriocapillaris circulation. Novais et al. [4] showed that SS-OCTA is more accurately able to demarcate the full lesions of CNV vasculature compared with SD-OCTA.

Although OCTA may delineate the total area of neovascularization, there are still clinical limitations owing to its diagnostic sensitivity and specificity. OCTA is not able to reflect the level of activity and reveals new vessels with blood flow even in the scar or atrophic phase of myopic CNV. Secondly, the presence of macular hemorrhage may result in the masking of CNV signals. In these cases, OCTA may not detect any blood flow signal, while FA presents leakage in corresponding lesions.

9.6 Clinical Course

Yoshida et al. [5]. reported natural course of myopic CNV for 10 years. At baseline, the percentage of patients with visual acuity better than 20/40 was 22.2%, lower than 20/200 was 29.6%. However, at 10 years of final visit, only one eye remains with visual acuity over 20/40, and 96.3% of patients presented decreased visual acuity lower than 20/200. Hemorrhage associated with CNV is absorbed after an average 7.6 months, and rebleeding is rare. All neovascularization generally totally regresses and flattens after 5–10 years of occurrence, and is even difficult to identify in some cases. CNV activity shows generally weaker than AMD and spontaneous remission. However, regressed neovascular membrane itself and surrounding atrophy progress and expands. This enlargement of atrophy can cause progressive central visual loss.

According to the long-term retrospective observational study, the visual prognosis of myopic CNV is determined by age at onset, with patients aged >40 years having a worse prognosis compared to early-onset disease. Therefore, patient age at which an individual develops disease should be considered when evaluating the therapeutic management and course. Kojima et al. [6] reported that areas of chorioretinal atrophy are the most significant factors of poor long-term visual prognosis, and older age and larger CNV area were also associated factors for the onset of atrophy.

9.7 Treatment

9.7.1 Laser

Krypton red laser photocoagulation has been developed to prevent visual loss in extra-foveal myopic CNV. Krypton red laser was used to treat myopic eyes with less macular pigment because red laser light of a krypton laser is preferentially absorbed in melanin of choroid and occlude choroid derived neovascularization. At 2 years follow-up, there was a significant difference in treatment and control group in regard to far and near vision, but no significant difference at 5-year follow-up. Central visual acuity decreased as recurrence of CNV and enlargement of laser scar after photocoagulation. Recurrence rate is 31–71% and usually occurs with laser scars. With other wavelength lasers, treatment scar progressively expands in 92–100%. As photocoagulation scar and atrophic lesion are progressively enlarged and cause final visual loss, photocoagulation treatment is not recommended; otherwise, lesion locates far away from the fovea.

9.7.2 Photodynamic Therapy (PDT)

VIP (verteporfin in photodynamic therapy) study group attempted PDT in myopic CNV occurring in the fovea. Percentage of subjects with best-corrected visual acuity (BCVA) increasing over eight letters was 72%, higher than the control group (44%) at 1 year, but there was no significant difference between the two groups at 2-year follow-up. VIP group suggested that even results based on increase of BCVA over eight letters did not show a significant difference; overall BCVA distribution is better in the treatment group than the control group, which can be an evidence of superiority for PDT in myopic CNV.

9.7.3 Surgery

Surgical method was tried to remove CNV or macular translocation. Uemura and Thomas reported results of 23 eyes with surgical removal of CNV: visual increase in 39%, stable visual acuity in 26%, and visual decrease in 35%. However, Ruiz-Moreno et al. reported no significant visual increase in 22 eyes. Recurrence rate was reported between 18 and 57%.

Macular translocation is a surgical method that relocates the fovea away from CNV. There are two surgical methods which are vitrectomy, posterior vitreous detachment, relocating foveal with air–fluid exchange, and moving macula enough by 360 degree peripheral retinotomy. Tano et al. reported outcomes of macular translocation in 28 eyes, in which 75% showed BCVA improvement over 2 lines, 11% showed stable BCVA, and 14% exhibited BCVA decreases. However, this method is recently rarely performed due to postoperative complications such as retinal detachment, rotational diplopia, and difficulty of surgical procedure.

9.7.4 Anti-vascular Endothelial Growth Factor (Anti-VEGF) Treatment

Since 2005, Nguyen et al. reported visual increase after bevacizumab injection in two myopic CNV, anti-VEGF treatment including intravitreal ranibizumab injection has been widely used as myopic CNV. A total of four intravitreal anti-VEGF drugs have been clinically studied for the treatment of myopic CNV. Of these, only Ranibizumab and Aflibercept are currently approved for the use of myopic CNV [7–9]. Twenty-four months' comparison study between PDT and intravitreal bevacizumab injection showed that PDT can regress CNV and decrease central retinal thickness while being less effective in BCVA improvement [10]. Intravitreal bevacizumab treatment was reported to maintain stable visual acuity until 24 months [11]. A systematic review and meta-analysis of anti-VEGF therapy for myopic CNV has concluded that intravitreal anti-VEGF injection should be considered as a first-line treatment [12, 13].

9.7.5 Prognostic Factors Associated with Anti-VEGF Treatment Outcomes

Yang et al. [14] reported that baseline CNV lesion size was significantly associated with recurrence, and recurrence rate during follow-up was 23%. Ahn et al. [15] found that a thinner baseline choroid thickness was associated with incomplete regression of myopic CNV after a single anti-VEGF injection and with higher 1-year recurrence of myopic CNV. Baseline BCVA and location of neovascularization have been significantly correlated with visual outcome at the end of follow-up and associated with the need for re-treatment. A systematic review of intravitreal bevacizumab studies identified a lower rate of development of chorioretinal atrophy, younger age, and smaller myopic CNV size as the factors most consistently associated with BCVA improvement [16, 17]. Other factors identified as less frequently correlated with visual outcome included spherical equivalent, chorioretinal atrophy enlargement, choroidal thickness, presence of lacquer crack extending to the fovea, and size of peripapillary chorioretinal atrophy [18].

9.7.6 First-Line Therapy

The first-line treatment for myopic CNV recently has become anti-VEGF therapy [19]. If myopic CNV activity is confirmed using FA with OCT, prompt treatment with intravitreal anti-VEGF therapy should be administered. Beneficial evidences of pro re nata (PRN) dosing regimen is supported by the results of the REPAIR (Ranibizumabfor trEatment of CNV secondary to Pathological myopia: An Individualized Regimen) and RADIANCE (Ranibizumab And PDT evAluation iN myopic Choroidal nEovascularization) studies, in which patients were treated with a single injection of ranibizumab followed by PRN dosing based on the disease activity present at each follow-up visit (Fig. 9.2). The results 1 or 3 number of initial dosing schedules of intravitreal injection have been compared, resulting that similar visual outcome was reported in both injection strategies [20].

9.8 Follow-Up

After anti-VEGF treatment, SD-OCT should be performed monthly to identify the presence or absence of CNV activity and the need for additional treatment. Disease activity is determined by decreased visual acuity, new or persistent visual symptoms or signs of myopic CNV disease activity on FA and on SD-OCT. OCTA might be also helpful to confirm the presence of newly developed CNV. FA is recommended to determine CNV activity when considering re-treatment. For the recurrent CNV, intravitreal anti-VEGF should be promptly re-administered.

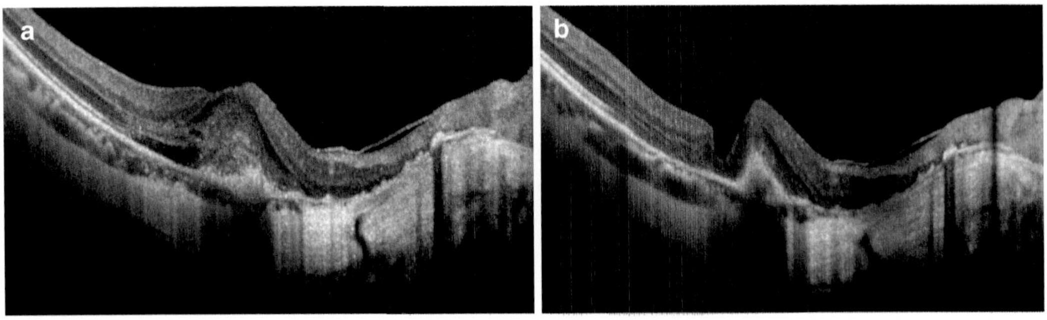

Fig. 9.2 Changes of SD-OCT after intravitreal anti-VEGF injection in myopic CNV. (**a**) The baseline spectral-domain-optical coherence tomography (SD-OCT) scan shows subretinal hyper-reflective material with fuzzy margin and the absence of the inner segment/outer segment junction (**b**) Six months after 3 times anti-VEGF injection, SD-OCT scan shows the disappearance of the subretinal fluid with a reduced size of the subretinal hyper-reflective material

Annual retinal screening and examination should be conducted with an increased risk of developing myopic CNV without any visual symptoms. Bilateral myopic CNV can occur in up to one-third of patients. So, the fellow eye is also required to be examined for the development of CNV. In a view of a stable period over 1 year without recurrence, the major concern is the development of chorioretinal atrophy which progressively involves central fovea. The most challenging problem of long-term therapy for myopic CNV is decreased visual acuity due to CNV-related macular atrophy even after successful CNV remission. Therefore, regular check-up should include fundus autofluorescence imaging to detect early changes of macular atrophy.

References

1. Liang IC, Shimada N, Tanaka Y, Nagaoka N, Moriyama M, Yoshida T, Ohno-Matsui K. Comparison of clinical features in highly myopic eyes with and without a dome-shaped macula. Ophthalmology. 2015;122:1591–600.
2. Ohno-Matsui K, Yoshida T. Myopic choroidal neovascularization: natural course and treatment. Curr Opin Ophthalmol. 2004;15:197–202.
3. Avila MP, Weiter JJ, Jalkh AE, Trempe CL, Pruett RC, Schepens CL. Natural history of choroidal neovascularization in degenerative myopia. Ophthalmology. 1984;91:1573–81.
4. Novais EA, Adhi M, Moult EM, Louzada RN, Cole ED, Husvogt L, Lee B, Dang S, Regatieri CV, Witkin AJ, Baumal CR, Hornegger J, Jayaraman V, Fujimoto JG, Duker JS, Waheed NK. Choroidal neovascularization analyzed on ultrahigh-speed swept-source optical coherence tomography angiography compared to spectral-domain optical coherence tomography angiography. Am J Ophthalmol. 2016;164:80–8.
5. Yoshida T, Ohno-Matsui K, Yasuzumi K, Kojima A, Shimada N, Futagami S, Tokoro T, Mochizuki M. Myopic choroidal neovascularization: a 10-year follow-up. Ophthalmology. 2003;110:1297–305.
6. Kojima A, Ohno-Matsui K, Teramukai S, Yoshida T, Ishihara Y, Kobayashi K, Shimada N, Yasuzumi K, Futagami S, Tokoro T, Mochizuki M. Factors associated with the development of chorioretinal atrophy around choroidal neovascularization in pathologic myopia. Graefes Arch Clin Exp Ophthalmol. 2004;242:114–9.
7. Boyer DS, Heier JS, Brown DM, Francom SF, Ianchulev T, Rubio RG. A phase IIIb study to evaluate the safety of ranibizumab in subjects with neovascular age-related macular degeneration. Ophthalmology. 2009;116:1731–9.
8. Bressler NM, Boyer DS, Williams DF, Butler S, Francom SF, Brown B, Di Nucci F, Cramm T, Tuomi LL, Ianchulev T, Rubio RG. Cerebrovascular accidents in patients treated for choroidal neovascularization with ranibizumab in randomized controlled trials. Retina. 2012;32:1821–8.
9. Rosenfeld PJ, Brown DM, Heier JS, Boyer DS, Kaiser PK, Chung CY, Kim RY. Ranibizumab for neovascular age-related macular degeneration. N Engl J Med. 2006;355:1419–31.
10. Verteporfin in Photodynamic Therapy Study Group. Photodynamic therapy of subfoveal choroidal neovascularization in pathologic myopia with verteporfin. 1-year results of a randomized clinical trial–VIP report no. 1. Ophthalmology. 2001;108:841–52.
11. Sarao V, Veritti D, Macor S, Lanzetta P. Intravitreal bevacizumab for choroidal neovascularization due to pathologic myopia: long-term outcomes. Graefes Arch Clin Exp Ophthalmol. 2016;254:445–54.
12. Ruiz-Moreno JM, Arias L, Montero JA, Carneiro A, Silva R. Intravitreal anti-VEGF therapy for choroidal neovascularisation secondary to pathological myopia: 4-year outcome. Br J Ophthalmol. 2013;97:1447–50.
13. Ruiz-Moreno JM, Montero JA, Araiz J, Arias L, Garcia-Layana A, Carneiro A, Figueroa MS, Silva R. Intravitreal anti-vascular endothelial growth factor therapy for choroidal neovascularization secondary to pathologic myopia: six years outcome. Retina. 2015;35:2450–6.
14. Yang HS, Kim JG, Kim JT, Joe SG. Prognostic factors of eyes with naïve subfoveal myopic choroidal neovascularization after intravitreal bevacizumab. Am J Ophthalmol. 2013;156(6):1201–10.
15. Ahn SJ, Park KH, Woo SJ. Subfoveal choroidal thickness changes following anti-vascular endothelial growth factor therapy in myopic choroidal neovascularization. Invest Ophthalmol Vis Sci. 2015;56:5794–800.
16. Shimada N, Ohno-Matsui K, Hayashi K, Yoshida T, Tokoro T, Mochizuki M. Macular detachment after successful intravitreal bevacizumab for myopic choroidal neovascularization. Jpn J Ophthalmol. 2011;55:378–82.
17. Vance SK, Khan S, Klancnik JM, Freund KB. Characteristic spectral-domain optical coherence tomography findings of multifocal choroiditis. Retina. 2011;31:717–23.
18. Kim YM, Yoon JU, Koh HJ. The analysis of lacquer crack in the assessment of myopic choroidal neovascularization. Eye (Lond). 2011;25:937–46.
19. Wakabayashi T, Ikuno Y, Oshima Y, Hamasaki T, Nishida K. Aqueous concentrations of vascular endothelial growth factor in eyes with high myopia with and without choroidal neovascularization. J Ophthalmol. 2013;2013:257381.

20. Wolf S, Balciuniene VJ, Laganovska G, Menchini U, Ohno-Matsui K, Sharma T, Wong TY, Silva R, Pilz S, Gekkieva M, RADIANCE Study Group. RADIANCE: a randomized controlled study of ranibizumab in patients with choroidal neovascularization secondary to pathologic myopia. Ophthalmology. 2014;121(3):682–92.

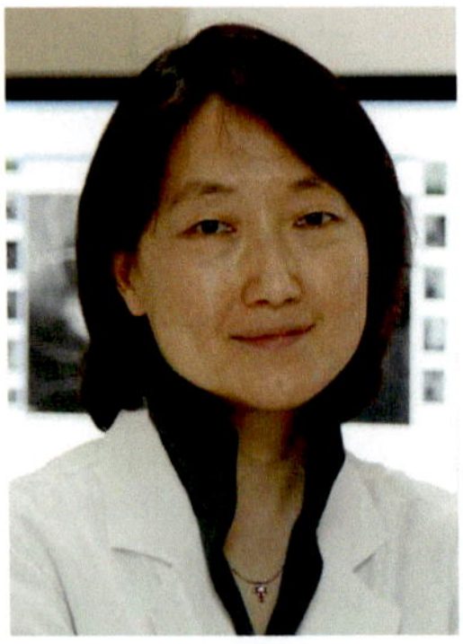

Seung-Young Yu, MD, PhD, is a current professor at the Department of Ophthalmology, Kyung Hee University Hospital. She has an in-depth understanding of the latest systems in retinal imaging, particularly in AMD and diabetic retinopathy, including OCT technologies and fundus autofluorescence systems.

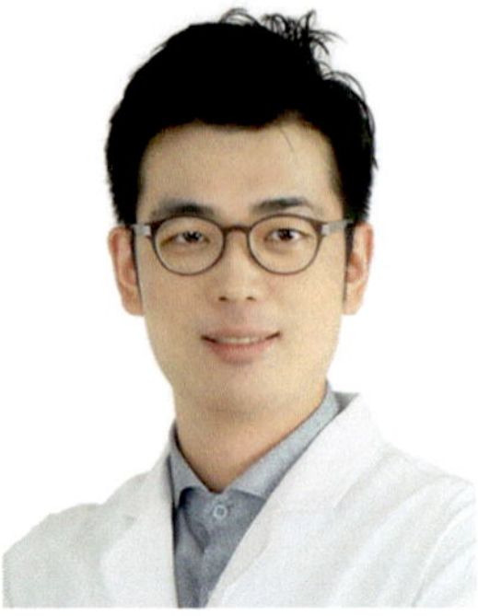

Kiyoung Kim, MD, PhD, is a current clinical associate professor at the Department of Ophthalmology, Kyung Hee University Hospital. His current research interests include updated retinal imaging in retinal vascular diseases and AMD. His recent published articles have focused on OCTA imaging in diabetic retinopathy.

Pachychoroid-Related Choroidal Neovascularization

10

Apoorva Ayachit and Jay Chhablani

10.1 Introduction

The word pachychoroid is derived from the Greek word παχύ (pachy—thick). The pachychoroid spectrum refers to a group of conditions that are characterized by a thickened choroid. The first disease described in this spectrum was pachychoroid pigment epitheliopathy (PPE) (Warrow and colleagues). PPE was described as a condition causing RPE changes similar to central serous chorioretinopathy (CSC) but without the attendant subretinal fluid. Subsequently CSC, neovasculopathy, and polypoidal choroidal vasculopathy characterized by the commonality of a thickened choroid were considered a part of the pachychoroid spectrum. Recently, Cheung et al. included focal choroidal excavation and peripapillary pachychoroid syndrome in the expanded spectrum of pachychoroid.

10.2 Pathophysiology of Pachychoroid

Increased choroidal thickness is considered a marker of pachychoroid. The thickening could be either diffuse or correspond spatially to pathological changes, focally. The choroidal thickness is normally thickest subfoveally, followed by temporal fovea and the nasal fovea. In peripapillary pachychoroid, however, the nasal choroid is thicker than the subfoveal and temporal choroid.

Choroidal thickness can be influenced by age, axial length, refractive error, blood pressure, and diurnal variation. It varies across ethnicities and the imaging platforms used. A wide range of values have hence been reported in normal subjects and there is no set threshold for thickness defining pachychoroid. Eyes with CSC and PNV have been noted to have choroidal thickness of 345–505 μm [1, 2] and 223–590 μm [3, 4], respectively. In these studies, the contralateral normal eyes also had increased choroidal thickness [2]. In view of the wide range of choroidal thickness, researchers often use the cutoff of 300 μm for subfoveal choroidal thickness for defining pachychoroid.

The key feature of pachychoroid, however, is not only the quantitative measurement of thickness. Focal/diffuse choriocapillaris effacement/attenuation is considered characteristic of pachychoroid. The attenuation is accompanied by dilatation of the outer choroid, i.e., the Haller's layer. The thinning of choriocapillaris may cause the outer choroid to occupy the full extent of the choroid [5]. Considering the various factors affecting choroidal thickness, pachychoroid phenotype may be identified in eyes even with normal or thinner choroid [5]. The increase in the volume of

A. Ayachit
Department of Vitreo-retina,
M M Joshi Eye Institute, Hubballi, Karnataka, India

J. Chhablani (✉)
Department of Ophthalmology, University of Pittsburgh Medical Center, Pittsburgh, PA, USA

J. Chhablani (ed.), *Choroidal Neovascularization*, https://doi.org/10.1007/978-981-15-2213-0_10

the outer choroid is also offset by a reduction of the choriocapillaris and inner choroid volume causing a given eye to have less than usual choroid thickness in pachychoroid phenotype [6]. Morphology of the choroid is thus more valuable than quantitative measurements alone. Whether the dilation of the Haller vessels (pachyvessels) occurs first or is secondary to the inner choroidal attenuation is still unknown. It has been hypothesized that the inner choroidal circulation suffers ischemic and inflammatory insults due to loss of volume and may result in hypoxic venous dilatation seen as pachyvessels.

Understanding of pachychoroid has spawned great interest in its clinical implications. Choroidal pathology causes RPE/Bruch's membrane irregularities, elevation, and thinning. The effacement and effective loss of the choriocapillaris due to expansion of Haller vessel volume induces damage to the RPE/Bruch's membrane complex. If the RPE can overcome the chronic fluid overload it is known as uncomplicated pachychoroid.

If the RPE however fails to overcome the choroidal congestion, features of pachychoroid pigment epitheliopathy (PPE) like RPE changes and outer retinal thinning occur, that signifies progressive dysfunction of RPE. With continuing RPE damage, breakdown of the RPE barrier and the accompanying choriocapillaris loss may lead to the development of sub-RPE and subretinal fluid, i.e., CSC. New vessels may develop in response to the ischemia causing pachychoroid neovasculopathy (PNV). Eyes with PPE lesions have been noted to have a higher risk of developing PNV [7, 8].

Finally, the ends of the neovessels develop aneurysms and convert to polypoidal choroidal vasculopathy (PCV). Thus, in eyes with PCV precursor lesions like PPE, CSC and even PNV may be present. Angiogenic factors that are overexpressed in these eyes due to loss of choriocapillaris may cause the development of PNV and subsequent PCV. Chronic inflammation involving choriocapillaris may also produce angiogenesis [9].

Terao et al. analyzed and compared the cytokine profiles in the aqueous humor of eyes with PNV, nAMD, and controls. Responses to intravitreal injection of aflibercept were also analyzed in the PNV and nAMD groups. In the PNV group, VEGF-A was significantly lower than in the nAMD group ($p = 0.03$) but was similar to that in the control group ($p = 0.86$). The nAMD group showed positive correlations between interleukin (IL-6 and IL-8 ($p < 0.001$), IL-6 and monocyte chemoattractant protein (MCP)-1 ($p = 0.002$) and IL-8 and MCP-1 ($p = 0.002$). There was a proportionate decrease in VEGF and PIGF after 1 month of aflibercept injection in dry maculae compared to wet maculae in the nAMD group. In PNV eyes however, there were no differences in the VEGF-A/PIGF levels between dry and wet maculae suggesting that other cytokines may be driving the neovascular activity in PNV [10].

Major AMD susceptibility genes ARMS2 and CFH4–7 has led to the understanding that AMD is a genetically homogenous disease. However, the differences in the phenotype of nAMD between Asians and Caucasians have led to speculation about the possible differences in genotype. Considering that PCV/polypoidal variant of nAMD is commoner in Asians, and soft drusen are less prevalent in Asians, susceptibilities for PCV and in turn AMD maybe differently driven [11]. Miyake et al. studied genetic susceptibilities in Japanese patients diagnosed with pachychoroid neovasculopathy and neovascular AMD. Pachychoroid neovasculopathy was observed in 39 individuals (19.5%). Their genetic susceptibility to AMD genes was significantly lower than that of neovascular AMD; ARMS2 ($p = 0.029$), CFH ($p = 0.013$), and genetic risk score calculated from 11 AMD susceptibility genes ($p = 0.0038$). These results showed that patients with pachychoroid neovasculopathy were genetically less susceptible to AMD [12].

Lehmann and associates have hypothesized that pachychoroid characteristics may have an autosomal dominant mode of inheritance [13].

10.2.1 Clinical Features

Patients with PNV are younger than those with CNVM due to wet AMD. Miyake and colleagues in their study of 200 patients with CNVM showed that patients with PNV were significantly younger than those with wet AMD (68.7 years vs. 75.6 years) [12]. Patients with PNV may present for the first time with symptoms of decreased vision, metamorphopsia, and/or central scotoma. However, more often history of CSC, i.e., repeated episodes of central scotomas, may be elicited. Patients on routine follow-up for chronic CSC may also have rebound fluid due to a subclinical neovascular membrane. Rarely, photopsias have been described in patients with extramacular PNV [14]. The hitherto described entity "CSC-associated CNVM" is increasingly being recognized as in fact PNV because of the shared features of choroidal hyperpermeability and congestion. Further, CSC-associated CNVM maybe declared an incorrect label because the exact mechanism of how CSC by itself causes CNVM has not been proven.

Acute onset vision loss may be noted if there is a hemorrhage or new-onset fluid in a patient without history of CSC who has now developed PNV. A quiescent PNV may also be detected incidentally in the fellow eyes of patients with established PNV/PCV. Quiescent PNVs are detected incidentally on OCT angiography or by FFA/ICGA.

10.2.2 Clinical Examination

Eyes with PNV exhibit features of pachychoroid such as reduced tessellation of fundus giving an orange appearance. RPE abnormalities are commonly seen. In patients with chronic CSC, descending tracts of hyperpigmentation may be seen. PNV usually presents as a small greenish membrane with subretinal hemorrhage and subretinal fluid.

10.2.3 Autofluorescence

The descending tracts of CSC may be more apparent. Tracts are generally hyperautofluorescent with or without hypoautofluorescent borders denoting chronicity (Fig. 10.1).

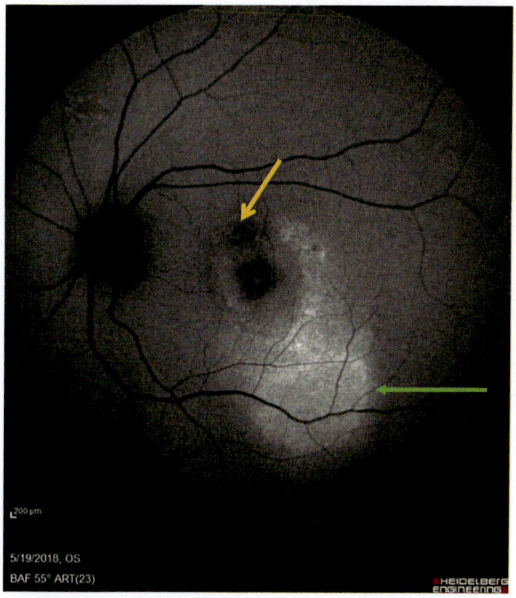

Fig. 10.1 AF image of a case of PNV showing hyperAF descending tracts owing to chronic CSC (green arrow). PNV was seen at the area showing hypoAF superior to the fovea (yellow arrow)

10.2.4 OCT

10.2.4.1 Cross-sectional OCT

As mentioned earlier, increased choroidal thickness with inner choroidal attenuation is the hallmark of pachychoroid on OCT. Querques et al. in their study on quiescent PNV found subfoveal choroidal thickness was 399 ± 72 microns in their series [15]. PNVs may also correspond spatially to areas of focal pachychoroid. Extramacular PNV may be due to extramacular foci of pachychoroid. Dansingani et al. in their study evaluating enface features of pachychoroid disorders found choroidal thickness of >300 microns subfoveally. In the eyes with normal subfoveal thickness, there was an extrafoveal focus of maximal choroidal thickness exceeding 300 µm [16]. In these cases, choroidal thickness mapping revealed that the extrafoveal focus of maximal choroidal thickness exceeded the choroidal thickness subfoveally by at least 50 µm. The importance of noting the area of maximal choroidal thickness was to correlate the disease foci with the distribution of the thickened choroidal vessels [16] (Fig. 10.2).

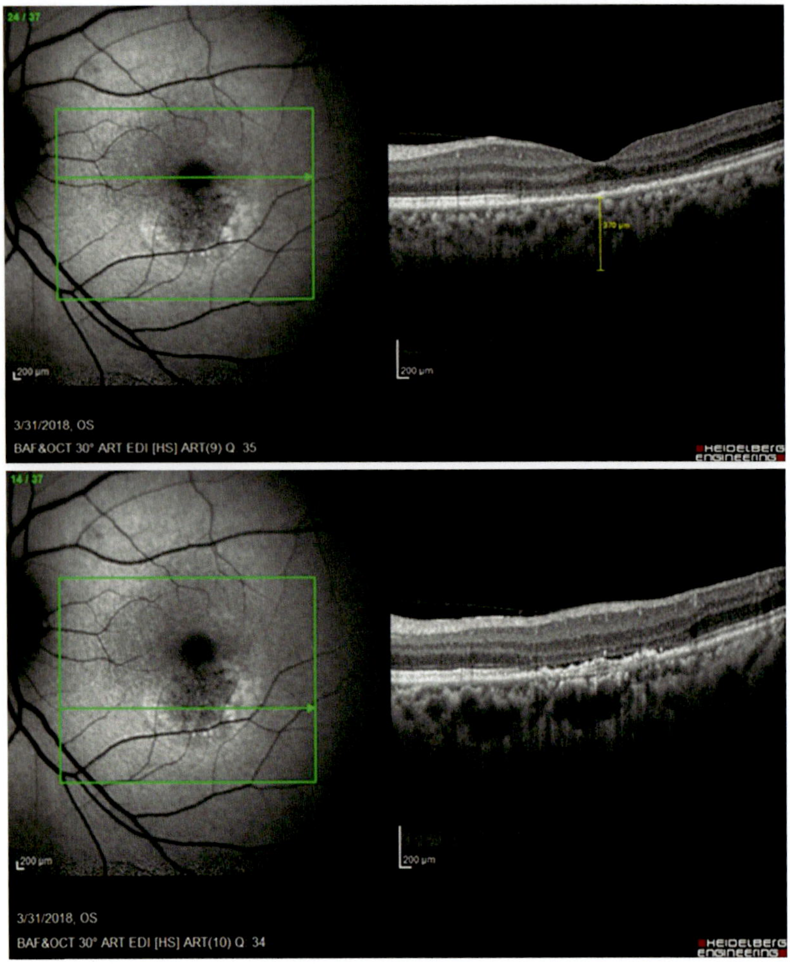

Fig. 10.2 AF + OCT image of a case of extrafoveal PNV. At the fovea (top), although the choroidal thickness is increased; the extrafoveal inferior focus with the flat irregular PED (DLS) has pachyvessels with effacement of choriocapillaris (bottom)

OCT may reveal areas of PPE, which is considered a forme-fruste of CSC. Pachydrusen may be apparent. PNV, being a type 1 CNVM, is usually noted as a flat irregular PED. This is referred to as a double layer sign (DLS) wherein there is a membrane insinuated between RPE and Bruch's membrane [17]. There may also be fluid accumulation between RPE and Bruch's membrane resulting from leakage from the network of abnormal vessels. Sheth et al. comprehensively evaluated EDI OCT images of patients with pachychoroid variant to discern various tomographic features of DLS to better characterize the pachychoroid disease spectrum. Of the 102 eyes of 79 patients analyzed, they found that none of the PPE eyes had DLS. Fifteen eyes with PNV had DLS (93.75%). In total, 32 of the 35 PCV eyes (91.43%) showed the presence of DLS, whereas DLS was seen in only 11 of the 35 eyes of CSC (31.43%). DLS was significantly associated with PCV and PNV as compared to CSC. Further in eyes with PNV and PCV, the DLS had a characteristic moderate hyperreflectivity in contrast to CSC eyes which had a hyporeflective DLS ($P < 0.001$). DLS height and width were significantly more in the PCV and PNV groups as compared with the CSC group. They concluded that the changes in the dimensions of DLS from one stage of pachychoroid spectrum (i.e., CSC) to the terminal stages (i.e., PNV and finally PCV) represents a progressive worsening of RPE–Bruch's membrane complex impairment. The DLS site also corresponded to the midphase choroidal hyperfluorescence, dilated choroidal veins, and abnormal network of vessels on ICGA [18] (Fig. 10.3).

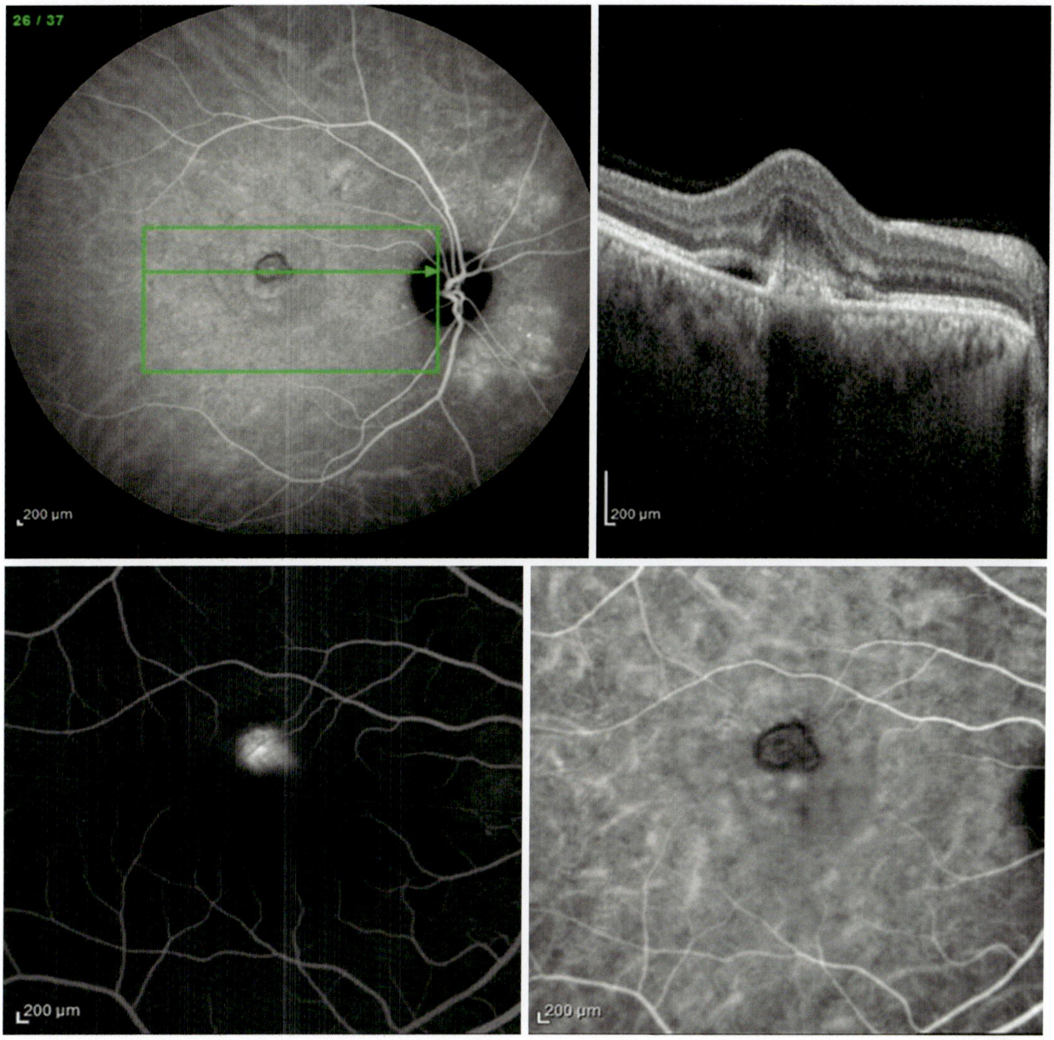

Fig. 10.3 ICGA + OCT (top)—hyperreflective DLS corresponding to a network seen on ICGA. The OCT also shows intraretinal edema with subretinal fluid. Simultaneous FFA and ICGA shows late leakage and an abnormal network, respectively

SRF in PNV maybe clear. However, if associated with CSC, the SRF may be associated with fibrin and a vacuole sign indicating the active leakage point of the CSC (Fig. 10.4). In this situation it is indeed difficult to attribute the fluid to either CSC or PNV alone. IRF and spongy edema are also frequently seen in the setting of PNV. Subretinal hemorrhage is seen as hyperreflectivity with back-shadowing. Subretinal hyperreflective material (SHRM) may be indicative of a PNV. Rarely intraretinal hyperreflective material may be present. In all, the presence of a hyperreflective DLS with SRF, SHRM is indicative of an active PNV (Fig. 10.4).

Frequently in patients on follow-up with chronic CSC with dry macula, there may be a hyperreflective DLS with no exudation (SRF/IRF). These are termed quiescent CNVs and do not meet the criteria for treatment. These may require frequent follow-up and an OCTA may be warranted (refer to the section on OCTA).

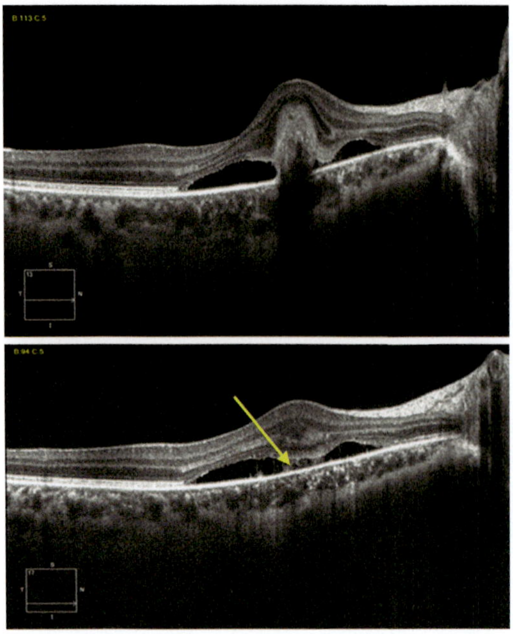

Fig. 10.4 Case of CSC with PNV showing subretinal membrane with subretinal hyperreflective material (top). In lower sections, line scans showing SRF with fibrin (yellow arrow) (bottom)

10.2.4.2 OCT Angiography

Freund et al. studied the enface features of eyes with pachychoroid. In 66 eyes of 33 patients including uncomplicated pachychoroid, PPE, CSC, PNV, and PCV, there was focal choriocapillaris atrophy with deep choroidal vessels occupying the entire choroidal thickness. Enface SS-OCT in all eyes demonstrated dilated outer choroidal vessels in the temporal quadrants, extending into the macular area. The dilation seen on the enface correlated spatially with the areas of maximal choroidal thickness. These were referred to as "pachyvessels." Diffuse pachyvessels were seen in only 5 eyes, whereas 28 eyes had focally distributed pachyvessels. The appearance of the choroidal vessels on the enface represented their inward displacement as a consequence of choriocapillaris thinning [16].

Freund et al. further stated that these dilated deep choroidal vessels retain their caliber as they traverse the macula. Unlike normal choroidal vessels, pachyvessels do not taper, and terminate at their posterior extent, and appear to terminate abruptly. This same property is appreciated on ICGA as well. The property of inward displacement of pachyvessels can be further confirmed by the corresponding cross-sectional OCT in which the choroidal vessels occupy the entire choroidal thickness.

The PNV network can be identified noninvasively using OCTA. PNV networks have been found to be corresponding to the hyperreflective DLS on OCT. Dansingiani et al. reported that in eyes with pachychoroid features, a hyperreflective DLS on OCT has more diagnostic value than dye-based angiography. Given the difficulty in detecting latent type 1 neovascularization in pachychoroid eyes using conventional retinal imaging and the fact that untreated PNVs can lead to hemorrhage, exudation, atrophy, and fibrosis; OCTA can be valuable in detecting a subclinical/ quiescent PNV. The frequency with which quiescent neovascularization evolves to clinical significance is unknown, but its presence may indicate a closer follow-up of the patient [19]. In conclusion, OCT angiography detection rate for type 1 neovascularization under a hyperreflective DLS or a flat irregular PED (FIPED) was found to be 95% compared to the dye angiography detection rate of 29% [19] (Fig. 10.5).

Querques et al. studied six eyes with quiescent PNV on OCTA. The diagnosis of treatment-naïve "quiescent" CNV was defined as a flat irregular PED (FIPED) with moderate reflectivity with no intraretinal or subretinal fluid on OCT, late-phase ill-defined hyperfluorescent lesion, leakage on fluorescein angiography, and hyperfluorescent network in the early and mid-phases of ICGA along with the presence of pachychoroid characteristics. The most frequently observed features on OCTA were irregular shape and well-defined margin. In addition, 100% of the vascular networks were seen on OCTA [15] (Fig. 10.6).

Querques et al. have noted in a study that quiescent CNVs enlarge over time with no consequent activity seen on OCT [20]. It remains to be seen if the same is true of PNV networks. It is easy to monitor PNV networks on OCTA noninvasively, including monitoring the area of CNV over time. In quiescent CNV secondary to AMD, Querques and group suggested that the absence

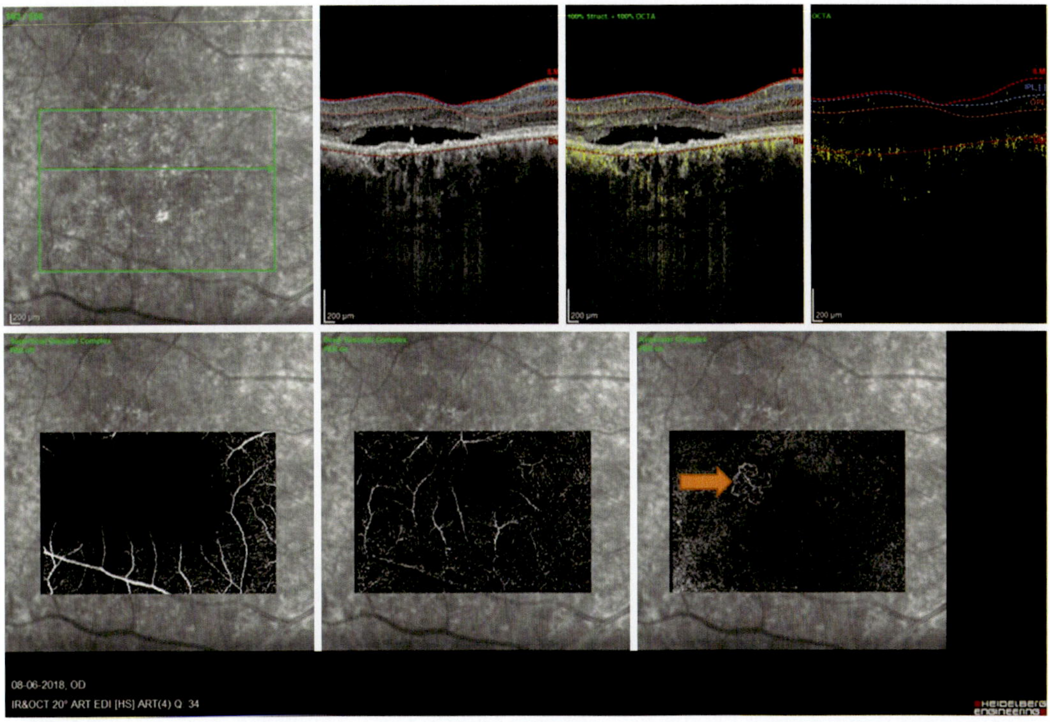

Fig. 10.5 OCTA in a case of PNV showing a well-defined network in the slab corresponding to the DLS (orange arrow)

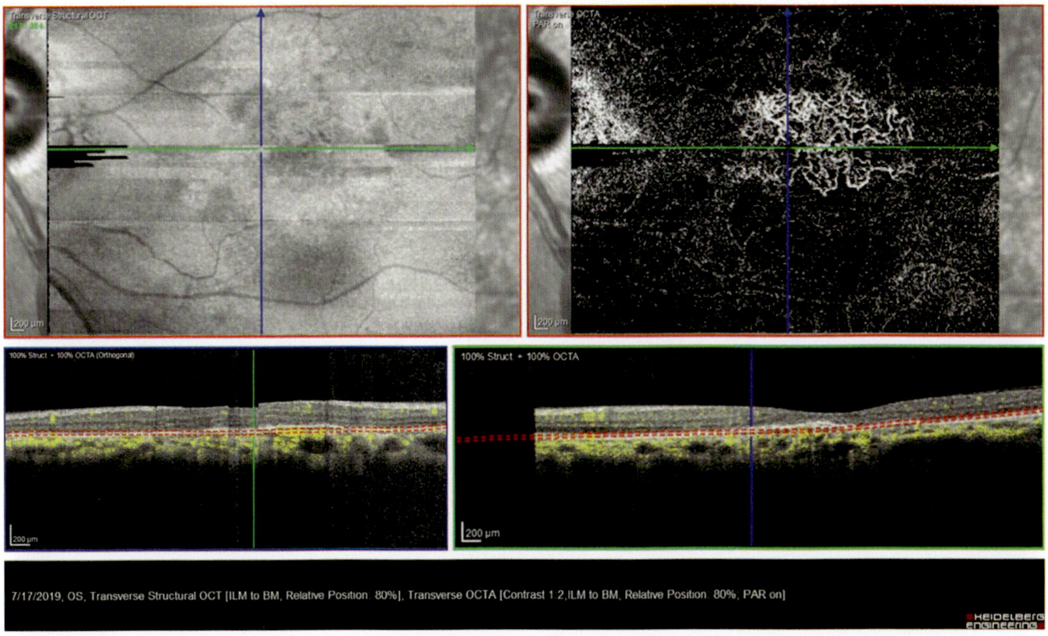

Fig. 10.6 A large quiescent CNV corresponding to the DLS in a case of PNV. There is no associated fluid

of a detectable core vessel may represent a protective factor against increased activity from quiescent CNV [21]. Thus, as an extrapolation, the higher prevalence of a detectable core vessel in quiescent pachychoroid neovasculopathy may be associated with a higher tendency to activation in pachychoroid neovasculopathy than AMD.

New fluid in a case of chronic CSC can be either a recurrence of CSC or due to the development of a PNV network. In cases of refractory CSCs not responding to conventional treatments, a subclinical PNV found on OCTA may be the cause of recurrent fluid. Identification of vascular networks assumes paramount importance in such cases.

10.2.4.3 FFA

Differentiating chronic CSC from AMD can be challenging as the two conditions may have very similar features on conventional angiography, characterized by RPE atrophy and diffuse leakage owing to diffuse retinal pigment epitheliopathy. Importantly, the areas of type 1 neovascularization are correlated spatially to areas displaying pachychoroid features. This OCT correlation is possible during simultaneous FFA + OCT [5]. Early stippled fluorescence with late leakage is the feature of PNV, being a sub-RPE membrane (Fig. 10.7). It may sometimes be difficult to differentiate between the diffuse stippling of hyperfluorescence of chronic CSC from

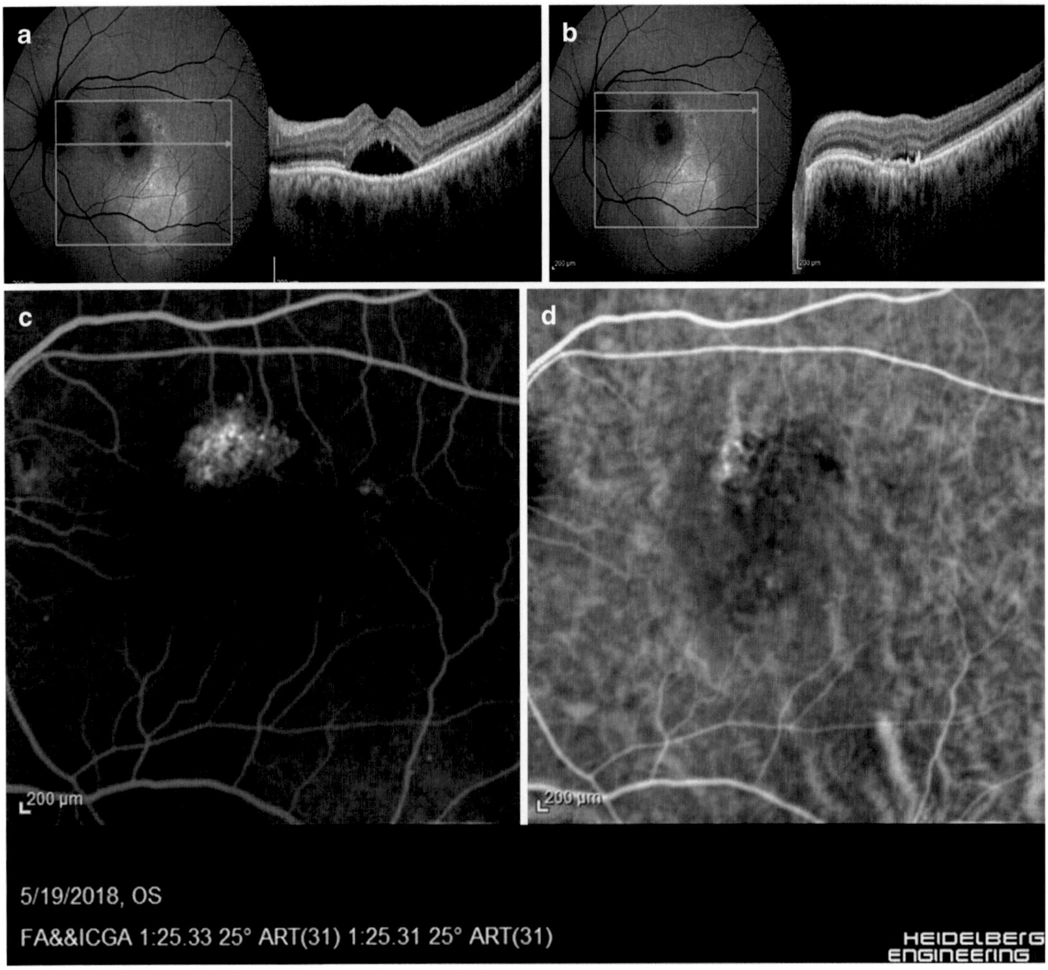

Fig. 10.7 The same eye as Fig. 10.1. (**a**) AF + OCT showing SRF at macula. (**b**) DLS corresponding to hypoAF. (**c**) late leakage on FFA and abnormal vascular network on ICGA (**d**)

the stippling of a PNV. The PNV would demonstrate late leakage in addition to the background of mottled hyperfluorescence due to diffuse retinal pigment epitheliopathy of chronic CSC. In CSC co-existing with PNV, there may be dot-block leaks/smokestack leaks suggesting acute on chronic CSC.

10.2.4.4 ICGA

Flash-based ICGA shows an early hypofluorescence followed by a late hot spot/plaque. With the advent of scanning laser ophthalmoscopy (SLO) imaging, networks of PNV are more obvious. A clear well-defined abnormal vascular network is apparent in the late phases of the angiogram. In addition, large caliber choroidal vessels are seen traversing the fundus. These do not taper toward the macula. Areas of choroidal hyperpermeability classical of pachychoroid are also seen on ICGA. These findings may be present in the apparently normal fellow eye as well (Fig. 10.8). Areas of hyperpermeability are characteristically seen in areas where there is intact choriocapillaris. This is also a feature seen on simultaneous ICGA + OCT [5]. This holds importance when planning photodynamic therapy for PNV/chronic CSC associated with PNV. Furthermore, unlike quiescent CNV in AMD characterized by late hyperfluorescence, in PNV eyes only the early-mid phases of ICGA show the quiescent neovascular network as these have late washout. This makes diagnosis challenging. Therefore, it is emphasized that OCTA is a better tool for diagnosing quiescent networks.

10.2.5 Treatment

10.2.5.1 Anti-VEGF therapy

Jung et al., in a retrospective study, compared the efficacy of intravitreal injection of ranibizumab and aflibercept for patients with PNV. Eyes were initially treated with 3 monthly loading injections of ranibizumab or aflibercept. They found that at 3 months, the rate of complete fluid absorption was higher in the aflibercept-treated group than in the ranibizumab-treated group ($p = 0.018$). The mean reduction of subfoveal choroidal thickness was also greater in the aflibercept group than in the ranibizumab group ($p = 0.013$). However, there was no difference in visual acuity or central macular thickness. Also, complete fluid absorption was noted after switching from ranibizumab to aflibercept in 13 of 15 eyes (86.7%). Adjunctive photodynamic therapy was required in six eyes. They concluded that anti-VEGF treatments helped improve visual acuity at 12 months. Aflibercept was better than ranibizumab in causing fluid resorption and reducing choroidal thickness at 3 months [22].

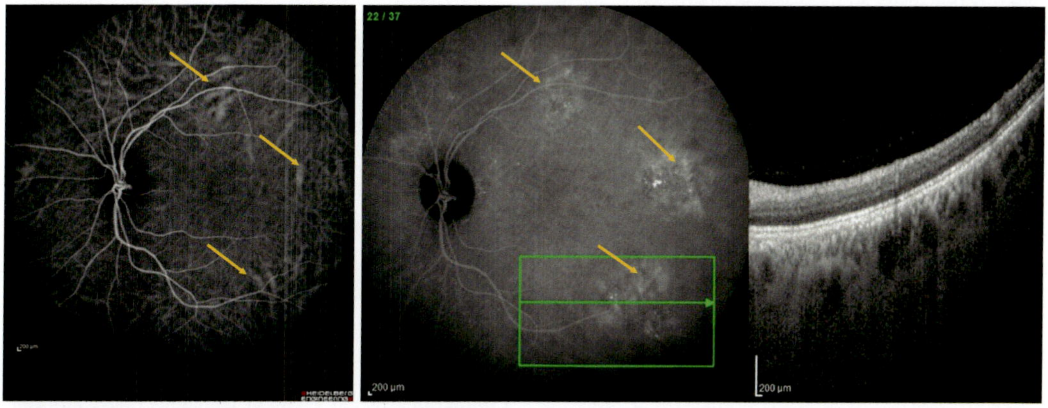

Fig. 10.8 Other eye of the patient depicted in Fig. 10.3. Early frames of ICGA show large caliber vessels in the midperiphery (yellow arrows) corresponding to areas of choroidal hyperpermeability in late phases. OCT line scans through these areas show enlarged choroidal vessels

Hata et al. reported lower intraocular VEGF levels in pachychoroid neovasculopathy than in nAMD [23]. Despite this, the authors noted favorable response to anti-VEGF therapy in eyes with PNV Almost 90% of patients responded with initial anti-VEGF therapy and only 11.1% needed adjunctive PDT therapy [24]. To minimize the deteriorating effects of repeated PDT, applying PDT as a deferred or rescue option has been suggested in PCV [24]. They suggested PNV may also need PDT only as a rescue option like PCV [25].

Azuma et al. investigated the effect of anti-VEGF therapy on choroidal structure of PNV and other types of neovascular age-related macular degeneration (non-PNV). Twenty-one eyes with PNV and 34 eyes with non-PNV who underwent anti-VEGF treatment were reviewed. CNV area at baseline was measured with FFA. The luminal and stromal areas in the choroid were measured at baseline and 1 month. The association between dry macula or visual acuity at 1 month and baseline values or changes in the luminal or stromal area at 1 month, baseline CNV area, were analyzed in patients with or without PNV. In non-PNV, change of luminal area ($p = 0.0001$), baseline CNV area ($p = 0.033$), and aflibercept versus ranibizumab ($p = 0.0048$) were shown to be predictors for dry macula [26].

A retrospective study of 46 eyes with PNV treated with intravitreal anti-VEGF therapy demonstrated improvement in visual acuity after a mean follow-up of 38.3 months [27]. In the MINERVA study, eyes with PNV treated with ranibizumab experienced a higher letter gain compared to the sham group at 2 months [28]. It has also been observed that PNV eyes have a longer retreatment-free interval compared to AMD eyes following loading doses. As mentioned earlier, this is due to lower dependence on VEGF levels in PNV eyes [12].

10.3 Conclusion

PNV is a distinct entity that is to be differentiated from other causes of CNVM. SD-OCT (EDI), SS-OCT, FFA, ICGA, and OCTA findings of PNV are distinct and help in the distinction from AMD-related and other secondary CNVMs. PNV is characterized by CNVM in younger patients along with features of thick choroid and choriocapillaris attenuation on imaging. Quiescent PNV is to be monitored closely for the development of activity. There is a lower dependence of PNV on VEGF levels, thus requiring a smaller number of injections and having longer retreatment-free intervals. PDT is a viable option as a rescue treatment for PNV unresponsive to anti-VEGF therapy.

Key Points

- PNV is commoner in Asian populations than Caucasians. Patients tend to be younger than AMD age group and have a distinct genetic susceptibility.
- PNV has lower dependence on VEGF levels compared to nAMD.
- Clinically, pigmentary alterations, reduced tessellation of the fundus, and features of CNVM like fluid and hemorrhage may be seen.
- EDI-OCT shows increased choroidal thickness (predominantly Haller layer expansion) with concomitant choriocapillaris attenuation. PNV corresponds spatially to the thickened choroid and has a double layer sign.
- FFA shows stippled fluorescence and may show diffuse changes of chronic CSC. AF may also show descending tracts.
- ICGA shows pachyvessels, areas of choroidal permeability along with hot spot/plaque of the PNV. PNV shows late washout phenomenon in contrast to nAMD.
- OCTA is a noninvasive modality that can detect active and quiescent PNV with high sensitivity and specificity.
- PNV has shown favorable response to anti-VEGF treatments and has a longer treatment-free interval. PDT may be used as a rescue option in cases refractory to anti-VEGF therapy.

Conflict of Interest None of the authors have any conflict of interest.

References

1. Imamura Y, Fujiwara T, Margolis R, Spaide RF. Enhanced depth imaging optical coherence tomography of the choroid in central serous chorioretinopathy. Retina. 2009;29:1469–73.
2. Fujiwara T, Imamura Y, Margolis R, Slakter JS, Spaide RF. Enhanced depth imaging optical coherence tomography of the choroid in highly myopic eyes. Am J Ophthalmol. 2009;148:445–50.
3. Koizumi H, Yamagishi T, Yamazaki T, Kinoshita S. Relationship between clinical characteristics of polypoidal choroidal vasculopathy and choroidal vascular hyperpermeability. Am J Ophthalmol. 2013;155:305–13. e301
4. Gupta P, Ting DSW, Thakku SG, et al. Detailed characterization of choroidal morphologic and vascular features in age-related macular degeneration and polypoidal choroidal vasculopathy. Retina. 2017;37:2269–80.
5. Dansingani KK, Balaratnasingam C, Naysan J, Freund KB. Enface imaging of pachychoroid spectrum disorders with swept source optical coherence tomography. Retina. 2016;36:499–516.
6. Balaratnasingam C, Lee WK, Koizumi H, Dansingani K, Inoue M, Freund KB. Polypoidal choroidal vasculopathy: a distinct disease or manifestation of many? Retina. 2016;36:1–8.
7. Roisman L, Zhang Q, Wang RK, et al. Optical coherence tomography angiography of asymptomatic neovascularization in intermediate age-related macular degeneration. Ophthalmology. 2016;123: 1309–19.
8. Yanagi Y, Mohla A, Lee WK, et al. Prevalence and risk factors for nonexudative neovascularization in fellow eyes of patients with unilateral age-related macular degeneration and polypoidal choroidal vasculopathy. Invest Ophthalmol Vis Sci. 2017;58:3488–95.
9. Peiretti E, Ferrara DC, Caminiti G, Mura M, Hughes J. Choroidal neovascularization in caucasian patients with longstanding central serous chorioretinopathy. Retina. 2015;35:1360–7.
10. Terao N, Koizumi H, Kojima K, Yamagishi T, Yamamoto Y, Yoshii K, et al. Distinct aqueous humour cytokine profiles of patients with pachychoroid neovasculopathy and neovascular age-related macular degeneration. Sci Rep. 2018;8(1):1–10.
11. Coscas G, et al. Comparison of exudative age-related macular degeneration subtypes in Japanese and French Patients: multicenter diagnosis with multimodal imaging. Am J Ophthalmol. 2014;158:309–318e2.
12. Miyake M, Ooto S, Yamashiro K, Takahashi A, Yoshikawa M, Akagi-Kurashige Y, et al. Pachychoroid neovasculopathy and age-related macular degeneration. Sci Rep. 2015;5:1–11.
13. Lehmann M, Bousquet E, Beydoun T, Behar-Cohen F. PACHYCHOROID: an inherited condition? Retina. 2015;35:10–6.
14. Kiss S, Rusu I, Seidman C, Orlin A, D'amico D, Gupta M. Pachychoroid neovasculopathy in extramacular choroidal neovascularization. Clin Ophthalmol. 2016;10:1275–82.
15. Carnevali A, Capuano V, Sacconi R, Querques L, Marchese A, Rabiolo A, et al. OCT angiography of treatment-Naïve quiescent Choroidal neovascularization in Pachychoroid Neovasculopathy. Ophthalmology Retina. 2017;1(4):328–32.
16. Dansingani K, Balaratnasingam C, Naysan J, Freund K. En face imaging of pachychoroid spectrum disorders with swept-source optical coherence tomography. Retina. 2016;36(3):499–516.
17. Sato T, Kishi S, Watanabe G, et al. Tomographic features of branching vascular networks in polypoidal choroidal vasculopathy. Retina. 2007;27:589–94.
18. Sheth J, Anantharaman G, Chandra S, Sivaprasad S. "Double-layer sign" on spectral domain optical coherence tomography in pachychoroid spectrum disease. Indian J Ophthalmol. 2018;66(12):1796.
19. Dansingani K, Balaratnasingam C, Klufas M, Sarraf D, Freund K. Optical coherence tomography angiography of shallow irregular pigment epithelial detachments in pachychoroid spectrum disease. Am J Ophthalmol. 2015;160(6):1243–1254.e2.
20. Querques G, Srour M, Massamba N, et al. Functional characterization and multimodal imaging of treatment-naïve "quiescent" choroidal neovascularization. Invest Ophthalmol Vis Sci. 2013;54:6886e6892.
21. Carnevali A, Cicinelli MV, Capuano V, et al. Optical coherence tomography angiography: a useful tool for diagnosis of treatment-naïve quiescent choroidal neovascularization. Am J Ophthalmol. 2016;169:189e198.
22. Jung B, Kim J, Lee J, Baek J, Lee K, Lee W. Intravitreal aflibercept and ranibizumab for pachychoroid neovasculopathy. Sci Rep. 2019;9:1–7.
23. Hata M, et al. Intraocular vascular endothelial growth factor levels in pachychoroid neovasculopathy and neovascular age-related macular degeneration. Invest Ophthalmol Vis Sci. 2017;58:292–8.
24. Lee JH, Lee WK. One-year results of adjunctive photodynamic therapy for type 1 neovascularization associated with thickened choroid. Retina. 2016;36:889–95.
25. Gomi F, et al. Initial versus delayed photodynamic therapy in combination with ranibizumab for treatment of polypoidal choroidal vasculopathy: the fujisan study. Retina. 2015;35:1569–76.
26. Azuma K, Tan X, Asano S, Shimizu K, Ogawa A, Inoue T, et al. The association of choroidal structure and its response to anti-VEGF treatment with the short-time outcome in pachychoroid neovasculopathy. PLoS One. 2019;14(2):e0212055.

27. Chhablani J, Kozak I, Pichi F, et al. Outcomes of treatment of choroidal neovascularization associated with central serous chorioretinopathy with intravitreal antiangiogenic agents. Retina. 2015;35:2489–97.

28. Lai TYY, Staurenghi G, Lanzetta P, et al. Efficacy and safety of ranibizumab for the treatment of choroidal neovascularization due to uncommon cause: twelve-month results of the MINERVA study. Retina. 2017 Jul 12;38(8):1464–77.

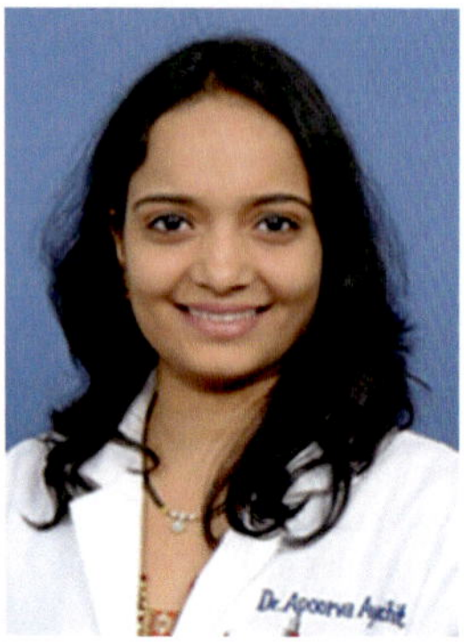

Dr. Apoorva Ayachit
Qualifications

1. MS Ophthalmology (Delhi University—2015)
2. Fellow of International Council of Ophthalmology (FICO), ICO—London 2016
3. Diplomate of National Board—2016
4. Fellowship in Vitreoretinal Surgery (FVRS—RGUHS affiliated)—M M Joshi Eye Institute, Hubballi
5. FAICO—vitreoretina 2018—Awarded at AIOC Coimbatore

Current post Consultant, Department of Vitreoretina, M M Joshi Eye Institute

She has multiple publications, book chapters to her credit. Special interest in macular imaging.

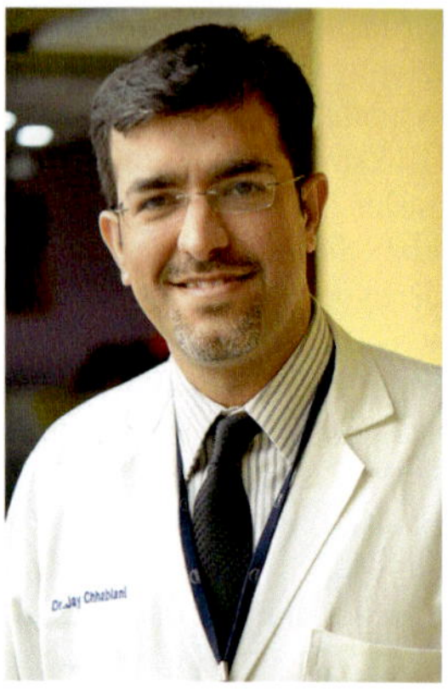

Dr. Jay Chhablani is a Vitreo-Retina Specialist at the University of Pittsburgh Eye Center. He completed a clinical vitreo-retina fellowship at Sankara Nethralaya, Chennai, India, and was an International Council of Ophthalmology (ICO) fellow at Jules Gonin Eye Hospital, Switzerland, in 2009. He was a Clinical Instructor at the Jacobs Retina Center at Shiley Eye Center, University of California, San Diego, USA (2010–2012) before joining the faculty at L V Prasad Eye Institute, Hyderabad, India (2012–2019). His areas of interest are macular disorders and recent imaging techniques. He has published more than 300 articles in peer-reviewed journals with a focus on the field of the choroid. He is the editor of the books *Choroidal Disorders* and *Central Serous Chorioretinopathy*, and he is on the review boards of all the high-impact ophthalmology journals. He is also on the editorial board of several specialty journals, including the *American Journal of Ophthalmology*. He is a member of the American Academy of Ophthalmology's Global ONE network committee. He has won several national and international awards and delivered the inaugural Ian Constable lecture at the Asia-Pacific Vitreo-Retina Society in 2016. He received the Inaugural Namperumalsamy Young Researcher Award in 2018, presented by the Vitreo-Retina Society of India.

11 Inflammatory Choroidal Neovascularization

Alvaro Olate-Perez, Carolina Bernal-Morales,
Aina Moll-Udina, Alfredo Adan,
and Javier Zarranz-Ventura

11.1 Introduction

Inflammatory choroidal neovascularization (CNV) membranes are generated in the choriocapillaris in the context of local inflammation and frequently sprout to the retina through defects in the retinal pigment epithelium (RPE)–Bruch's membrane complex, that are commonly seen in infectious and noninfectious uveitis [1]. After age-related macular degeneration (AMD) and myopia, uveitis syndromes appear as the third leading cause for CNVs and are frequently present in specific clinical conditions such as punctate inner choroidopathy (PIC), multifocal choroiditis (MFC), multiple evanescent white dot syndromes (MEWDS), serpiginous choroiditis (SC), presumed ocular histoplasmosis (POHS), toxoplasma retinochoroiditis, and Vogt–Koyanagi–Harada's disease (VKH) [2]. The exact pathophysiology of inflammatory CNVs is yet to be elucidated, and there are mainly two mechanisms that may concur, an inflammatory mediated angiogenic stimulus and the abovementioned frequent disruption in the RPE–Bruch's membrane complex seen in these clinical conditions, among other complex processes [1, 2].

The diagnostic tools and treatment options for inflammatory CNV have experienced significant advances in the last decade. As in other fields, the development of new noninvasive imaging techniques such as optical coherence tomography angiography (OCTA) beyond the structural optical coherence tomography (OCT) scans has complemented the classic fluorescein angiography (FA) and autofluorescence examination techniques and has provided new insights to diagnose and monitor CNV progression. Currently, the first-line therapy for inflammatory CNVs is intravitreal anti-VEGF drugs, although beneficial outcomes have also been reported for other treatment options such as corticosteroids and immunosuppressive agents [3].

11.2 Epidemiology

Inflammatory CNVs represent a severe complication which may cause irreversible central visual loss. Uveitis syndromes are more frequent in young people, often in active working-age, and

A. Olate-Perez · C. Bernal-Morales
Institut Clínic de Oftalmología, Hospital Clínic, Barcelona, Spain

A. Moll-Udina · A. Adan · J. Zarranz-Ventura (✉)
Institut Clínic de Oftalmología, Hospital Clínic, Barcelona, Spain

Institut de Investigacions Biomediques August Pi i Sunyer (IDIBAPS), Barcelona, Spain

J. Chhablani (ed.), *Choroidal Neovascularization*, https://doi.org/10.1007/978-981-15-2213-0_11

Table 11.1 Prevalence and incidence of main infectious and noninfectious uveitis

Infectious uveitis		Noninfectious uveitis		
	Prevalence		Prevalence	Incidence
POHS	Frequent	Vogt–Koyanagi–Harada	0.3% [7]; 9–15% cases [2]	6.4% [7]
Toxoplasmosis	0.3–19% [2]	Multifocal choroiditis	4.6% [7]; 33–50% cases [2]	3.6% [7]
West Nile virus chorioretinitis	Few cases reported	Punctate inner choroidopathy	11.8% [7] 76–100% cases [2]	13.2% [7]
Intraocular Tuberculosis	Uncommon	Serpiginous choroiditis	4.7% [7] 10–25% cases [2]	2.7% [7]

for this reason early detection and timely treatment of CNV is essential to reduce the risk of permanent irreversible visual loss which could be invalidating for their daily activities [3, 4].

With regards to the etiology, two groups of inflammatory CNV are described, those secondary to noninfectious or infectious uveitis. The main causes of infectious uveitis-associated CNVs are toxoplasma and presumed ocular histoplasmosis syndrome (POHS). Toxoplasma is a relatively common type of uveitis and the only protozoan affecting the eye which has been associated with inflammatory CNV. POHS is produced by histoplasma capsulatum, a species of dimorphic fungi, which occurs mainly in central and eastern United States CNV [4]. The prevalence of these two features varies according to geographical area. According to previously published data, toxoplasmosis presents higher rates in South Asia and POHS in North America [2]. Other infectious uveitis types are rarely associated with CNV development and only single case reports and small case series have been reported. This is the case of inflammatory CNV secondary to Tuberculosis, Toxocara, West Nile virus, Congenital Rubella Retinopathy, Candida albicans, Cryptococcus neoformans, and Aspergillus fumigatus [5]. Interestingly, some cases have also been reported secondary to endophthalmitis [2].

The prevalence and incidence of inflammatory CNV secondary to noninfectious uveitis is higher, according to more robust epidemiological data. The main conditions associated to inflammatory CNVs are PIC, MFC, MEWDS, SC, and VKH disease. Baxter et al. reported in a multicenter study of 15,137 noninfectious uveitis eyes that 2% of posterior uveitis or panuveitis cases had a history of CNV (active or past) at the moment of diagnosis, being rarely found in anterior and intermediate uveitis patients. Moreover, in this same series posterior uveitis presented a higher prevalence of CNV (2.7%) compared to panuveitis (0.8%) [6]. Another study reported a cumulative incidence of inflammatory CNV in noninfectious uveitis of 2.7% at 2 years, presenting the majority of the cases within the first 6 months after diagnosis [7]. In this series, no significant difference was found in terms of incidence between panuveitis and posterior uveitis, but VKH and PIC were associated with increased risk of developing CNV than other noninfectious uveitis syndromes [7]. Prevalence and incidence of CNV at presentation are summarized in Table 11.1. Finally, the main risk factors for the development of inflammatory CNV in uveitis syndromes include active inflammation status, concomitant retinal neovascularization, and previous CNV diagnosis in the fellow eye [3, 4].

11.3 Diagnosis

11.3.1 Signs and Symptoms

Symptoms may be different in each specific case and may ultimately depend on the location of the inflammatory CNV complex. According to this, subfoveal CNVs are usually more symptomatic, causing visual loss, metamorphopsia or central scotoma, and extrafoveal CNV are less symptomatic or even asymptomatic, and may often be detected incidentally by direct examination or ancillary tests such as OCT or OCTA in routine clinical exams.

On clinical examination concomitant signs of posterior uveitis or panuveitis are often seen, and

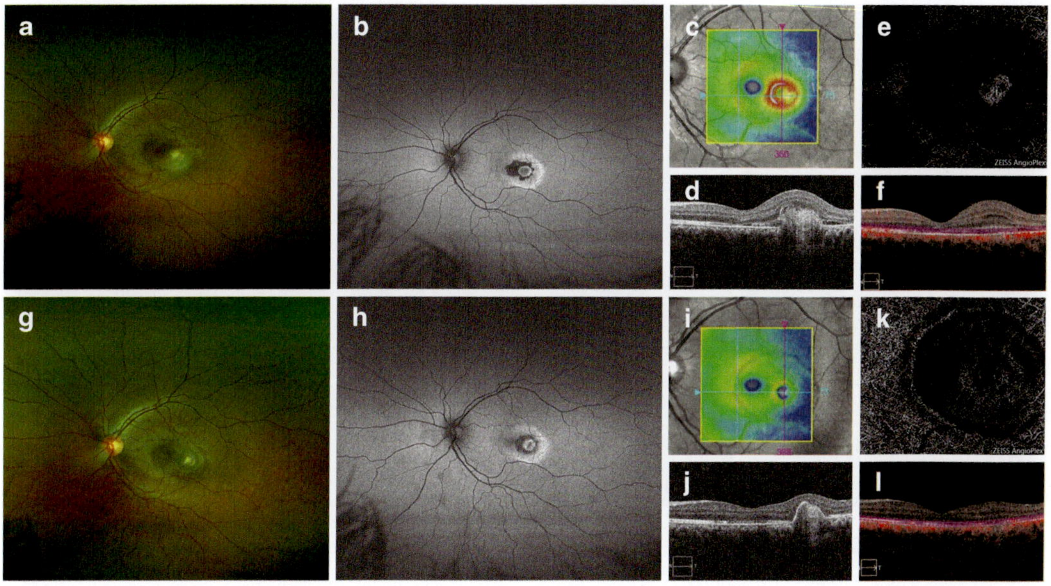

Fig. 11.1 A 29-year-old male with LE choroidal neovascularization adjacent to an old toxoplasma macular scar. Fundus picture (**a**) shows a juxtafoveal inferotemporal subretinal hemorrhage, represented by a hypofluorescent area in the fundus autofluorescence (FAF) image (**b**) surrounded by a hyperfluorescent halo. A focal area of retinal thickening is seen in the thickness map of the structural OCT scan (**c**), corresponding to a dense hyperreflective material lesion with associated subretinal fluid detected in the cross-sectional image of the b-scan (**d**). OCTA (**e**, **f**) shows a choroidal neovascularization of glomerular pattern in the avascular plexus. One month after the second injection of Aflibercept (Eylea®) the macular hemorrhage disappeared (**g**), FAF showed a mild decrease of the hypoautofluorescent halo (**h**), structural OCT revealed complete resolution of subretinal fluid and a residual solid pigment epithelium detachment lesion compatible with the old scar (**i**, **j**), and OCTA (**k**, **l**) showed complete regression of the glomerular-shape CNV in the avascular plexus

more rarely intermediate uveitis. In funduscopy, findings suggestive of CNV include green-gray subretinal discoloration areas, intra- and subretinal fluid, hemorrhages, and scars.

The main clinical characteristics are described below disclosed by etiologies [1–3]:

- **Presumed ocular histoplasmosis syndrome (POHS):** Three classic findings are described, which include peripapillary atrophy, focal oval-shaped chorioretinal lesions (histo spots), and no vitreous inflammation. CNVs appear usually in the peripapillary or subfoveal regions, frequently in the edges of preexisting chorioretinal scars.
- **Ocular toxoplasmosis:** It commonly appears as an oval whitish focal retinochoroiditis area adjacent to atrophic scar lesions, with dense overlying vitritis. CNV is located at the edge of old lesions and may be associated to hemorrhages and intra- or subretinal fluid (Fig. 11.1).
- **Multifocal choroiditis (MC):** Multiple yellow-white punched-out lesions are located peripapillary and in the mid-periphery with minimal vitritis. CNV is usually associated with active inflammatory retinal lesions, which may be located in the foveal or extrafoveal macular regions.
- **Punctate inner choroidopathy (PIC):** Multiple, small, round, yellow-white lesions are seen in the posterior pole with no signs of vitreous inflammation. CNV frequently is associated with the inflammatory lesions located in the subfoveal region (Fig. 11.2).
- **Serpiginous choroiditis (SC):** Gray-white lesions with a geographical distribution affecting the posterior pole. CNV lesions may appear in the edges of chorioretinal atrophy plaques distributed in the peripapillary, subfoveal, and/or extrafoveal regions (Fig. 11.3).
- **Vogt–Koyanagi–Harada (VKH) disease:** Multiple exudative retinal detachments are

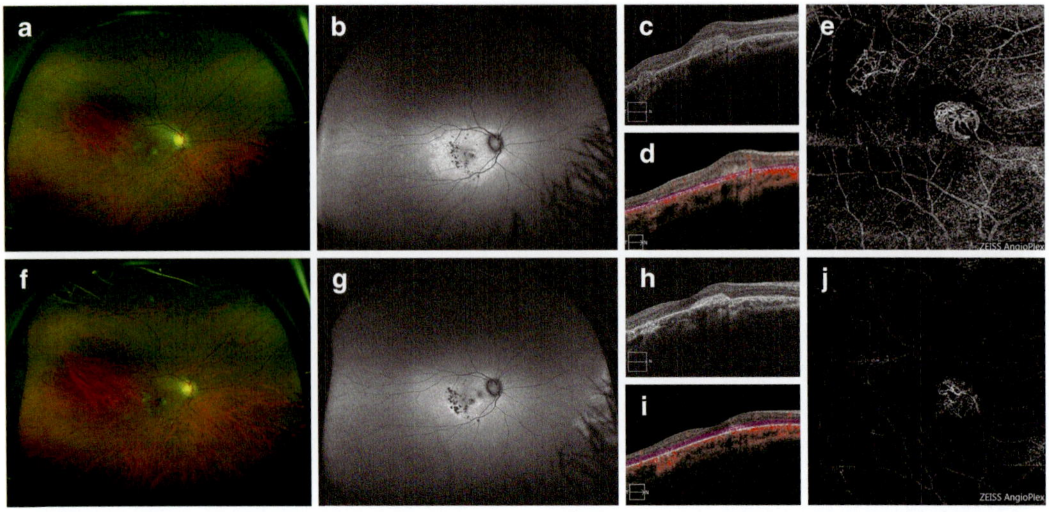

Fig. 11.2 A 34-year-old female diagnosed with punctate inner choroidopathy and previous history of CNV treated with two intravitreal injections of anti-VEFG 2 years ago. She presented with a new relapse of her disease with new white dots in the posterior pole adjacent to old atrophic scars (**a**). Fundus autofluorescence (**b**) showed a hyperautofluorescent diffuse pattern in the posterior pole with hyperautofluorescent lesions corresponding to the white dots in mid periphery seen in funduscopy. Structural OCT (**c**) showed two subretinal hyperreflective material lesions with poorly defined edges in two different areas, corresponding to two independent active CNVs. OCTA confirmed both CNV lesions (superotemporal and inferonasal to fovea) in the avascular plexus level (**d**, **e**). Five months after an intravitreal implant of dexamethasone (Ozurdex®) (**f**), autofluorescence showed hypoautofluorescence of the posterior pole and isolated lesions (**g**), and regression of the CNV lesions with well-defined edges in the structural OCT (**h**) and OCTA (**i**, **j**) images. Of note, OCTA images showed a reduction in the lesion size and vessel density of both neovascular complexes compared to baseline images

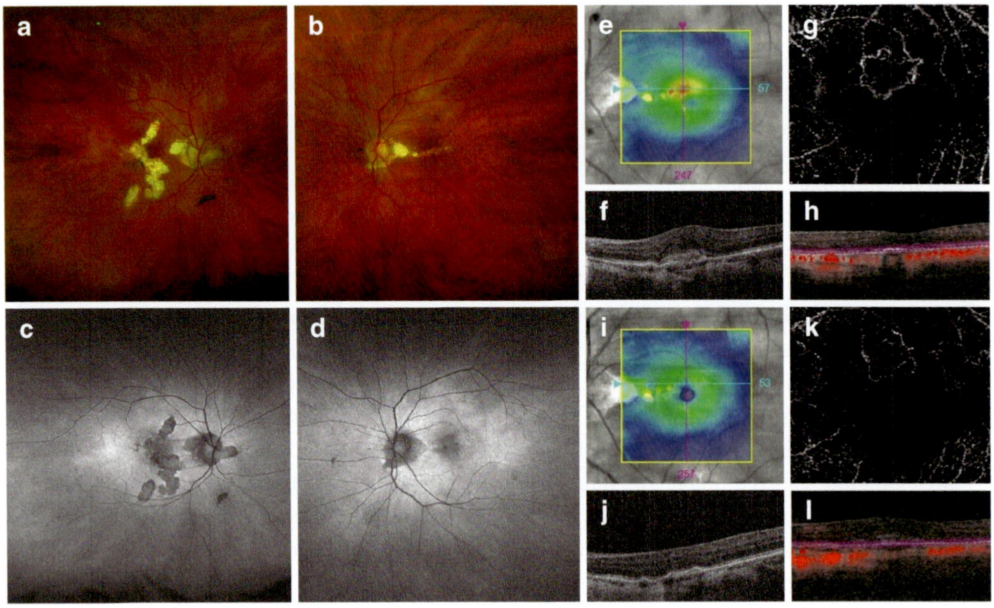

Fig. 11.3 A 76-year-old female with serpiginous choroiditis associated to tuberculosis. Fundus retinographies (**a**, **b**) showed chorioretinal atrophy lesions in both eyes. Fundus autofluorescence showed hypoautofluorescent lesion corresponding to the atrophy areas (**c**, **d**). In the LE, a lacy wheel-shaped CNV was seen in both the structural OCT (**e**, **f**) and OCTA (**g**, **h**). Three months after a single aflibercept (Eylea®) injection a reduction in the lesion thickness and size is seen in the structural OCT (**i**, **j**) and regression of the CNV is observed in the OCTA (**k**, **l**)

seen, often associated with granulomatous anterior uveitis. CNV is usually extrafoveal and associated with hemorrhages and exudation.

11.3.2 Fluorescein Angiography

Fluorescein angiography (FA) has classically been the principal technique employed for CNV diagnosis. Inflammatory CNV lesions typically show early hyperfluorescence and late leakage, as other types of CNV. In selected cases, it is often difficult to differentiate between CNV and uveitic lesions and additional tests are required. Active chorioretinal lesions commonly show an early hypofluorescent pattern with late leakage, whereas inactive lesions show early hypofluorescence without leakage [8].

11.3.3 Fundus Autofluorescence

Fundus autofluorescence (FAF) may also be helpful in differentiating active CNV from inflammatory lesions. Active inflammatory lesions often show a hyperautofluorescent pattern, whereas inflammatory CNVs frequently appear with a more patchy hypoautofluorescent signal, especially if these are adjacent to chorioretinal atrophy patches [2]. In these situations, FAF may also be useful to differentiate areas of intact RPE from subretinal hemorrhages (hyper- and hypoautofluorescent, respectively).

11.3.4 Indocyanine green angiography

Indocyanine green (ICG) angiography is frequently used to evaluate the status of the choroid, due to the higher molecular weight and greater binding ability to proteins than fluorescein. For these reasons, it is an exceptional tool to identify CNV but also to evaluate other choroidal findings as granulomas, choriocapillaris hypoperfusion, and choroiditis, being really helpful in the differential diagnosis of such conditions in case of diagnostic dilemmas [9].

11.3.5 Optical Coherence Tomography

Optical coherence tomography (OCT) is essential for the diagnosis and management of inflammatory CNV lesions due to its noninvasive nature and high reproducibility in sequential follow-up scans [10]. Inflammatory CNVs frequently appear in OCT as hyperreflective lesions in the subretinal space, between the neurosensory retina and the RPE following a type 2 CNV pattern [11]. In some occasions, multiple hyperreflective projections extending from the CNV may appear ("pitchfork sign"). This sign has been suggested as a distinctive characteristic of inflammatory CNV by some authors [12]. OCT activity signs for inflammatory CNV include subretinal and/or intraretinal fluid, as well as increased retinal thickness or blurry margins of the lesion edges. These parameters can also be helpful in the follow-up of these lesions [10].

11.3.6 Optical Coherence Tomography Angiography

Optical coherence tomography angiography (OCTA) is an evolution of structural OCT that allows the reconstruction of the retinal vascular plexuses by sequential image captures and image processing algorithms, based on the detection of blood movement without the need of dye injection [13]. Thanks to this ability to identify perfused and non-perfused structures, inflammatory CNV can be diagnosed and differentiated from inflammatory lesions as these do not present vascular flow [14]. This is especially important and helpful to inform treatment decisions in such circumstances, in other to decide whether intravitreal corticosteroids or anti-VEGF drugs should be administered in each individual case. Moreover, in comparison with other multimodal image techniques, OCTA is able to detect structural and functional changes [15].

Recent publications have highlighted the role of OCTA in the diagnosis and follow-up of CNV secondary to PIC [16], multifocal choroiditis [17], and serpiginous choroiditis [18], among other inflammatory causes. Zahid et al. published the first case of CNV diagnosed by OCTA in a multifocal choroiditis patient, demonstrating that OCTA may be useful also during the follow-up of these lesions revealing decreases in flux and size after treatment [19]. Nevertheless, the most frequent OCTA finding related with inflammatory CNV is hypoperfusion of the choriocapillaris adjacent to the neovascular membrane (perilesional hypointense halo), which diminishes with anti-VEGF treatment. However, OCTA has some significant limitations. For example, the edges of an active CNV are often not well defined in OCTA images, which may well be a consequence of real changes in the CNV vascular structure or an artifact produced by the hyperreflective material that often surrounds the neovascular lesion, a frequent finding in mature CNVs. These features may be a significant limitation to obtain helpful information about CNV activity with OCTA. Finally, manual segmentation of OCTA images is very often required to avoid artifact and segmentation errors, especially in cases with abnormal retinal anatomy as in inflammatory CNVs associated to posterior uveitis syndromes [15].

11.4 Comparing AMD-Associated CNV and Inflammatory CNV

Most knowledge of inflammatory CNV is extrapolated from AMD studies. According to the OCT-based classification, AMD-associated CNV can be classified as type 1 (subretinal pigment epithelium), type 2 (subretinal), or type 3 (retinal angiomatous proliferation). Inflammatory CNV presents a higher percentage of type 2 membranes [2]. In both type 2 AMD-associated and inflammatory CNVs the alteration occurs at the RPE level, leading to abnormal new vessels growth from the choriocapillaris toward the subretinal space. However, RPE defects are usually focal in inflammatory CNV and diffuse in AMD-associated CNV [20]. In the pathogenesis of AMD, several factors contribute to CNV development such as inflammation, complement cascade activation, macrophage dysregulation, and abnormal growth factors levels [20]. These factors and a healthier RPE related to the younger age of uveitis patients could explain why AMD-associated CNVs normally require repeated and prolonged treatments with anti-VEGF therapies, whereas inflammatory CNV typically requires a lower number of injections and shorter duration treatments, as described in several different case series.

11.5 Management

11.5.1 Anti-VEGF

It is known that a pro-inflammatory environment in the retina (as occurs in uveitis) could generate the release of VEGF, a mediator of angiogenesis [1, 21]. Despite this, clinical studies show controversial results. Paroli et al. reported higher VEGF levels in the aqueous humor of VKH patients compared to healthy controls [22]; however, this could not be confirmed by Banerjee et al. in CNV secondary to PIC [23].

Several recent case series have reported successful outcomes with anti-VEGF therapy in inflammatory CNV lesions secondary to infectious and noninfectious uveitis. In the first group, Schadlu et al. demonstrated visual improvement or stabilization in 85% of eyes treated with intravitreal bevacizumab in cases with POHS [24]. Korol et al. demonstrated clinical improvement in CNV secondary to toxoplasmosis with intravitreal aflibercept [25]. Other cases successfully treated with anti-VEGF include ocular tuberculosis and toxocariasis [26]. With regards to noninfectious CNV, cases successfully treated with intravitreal anti-VEGF in multifocal choroiditis [27–33], PIC [26, 31, 34, 35], serpiginous choroiditis [18, 33, 36, 37], and VKH [26, 28, 31] have been published. Table 11.2 summarizes the main studies of inflammatory CNV treated with anti-angiogenic therapy.

11.5.2 Corticosteroids

Systemic and local corticosteroids have been widely used in the treatment of CNV secondary to uveitis due to its anti-inflammatory effects.

Table 11.2 Summary of studies showing antiangiogenic therapy in inflammatory CNV. *MC* Multifocal choroiditis, *PIC* Punctate inner choroidopathy, *SC* Serpiginous choroiditis, *VKH* Vogt–Koyanagi–Harada syndrome, *Toxo* Ocular toxoplasmosis, *POHS* Presumed ocular histoplasmosis syndrome, *SO* Sympathetic ophthalmia, *Sarco* Ocular sarcoidosis, *VA Stab* Number of patients with visual acuity stabilization at the end of follow-up, *Mean IVT* Mean intravitreal therapy injections in the study

Study (year)	Etiology							Follow-up	VA Stab	Mean IVT	Bevacizumab	Ranibizumab	Aflibercept	Study Type
	MC	PIC	SC	VKH	Toxo	POHS	Others							
Adan et al. (2007); Spain [27]	X	X	X			X	Birdshot	7.1 m	8/9	1	X			Retrospective
Schadlu et al. (2008); USA [24]						X		22.43 w	24/28	1.8	X			Retrospective
Tran et al. (2008); France [28]	X		X	X			SO	7.5 m	10/10	2.5	X			Retrospective
Fine et al. (2009); USA [29]	X							6 m	5/6	2.3	X	X		Retrospective
Doctor et al. (2009); USA [30]	X			X			Birdshot, SO	15.3 m	4/6	2.7	X			Retrospective
Lott et al. (2009); USA [26]	X	X	X	X	X	X	Toxocara, Sarco	7 m	15/21	2	X			Retrospective
Kramer et al. (2010); Israel [31]	X	X			X	X		12 m	10/10	2	X			Retrospective
Menezo et al. (2011); Spain [34]		X						12.5 m	9/10	1.9		X		Retrospective
Cornish et al. (2011); UK [35]		X						14.9 m	8/9	2.9	X	X		Retrospective
Julian et al. (2011); France [32]	X						Ampiginous	15 m	12/15	4.25	X			Retrospective
Rouvas et al. (2011); Greece [33]	X	X	X		X			17.6 m	16/16	2.3		X		Retrospective
Ianetti et al. (2013); Italy [36]		X	X	X	X		Birdshot	19.25 m	7/8	3.75	X			Prospective
Mansour et al. (2012); Lebanon [37]	X	X	X	X	X	X		36 m	67/81	3	X			Retrospective
Parodi et al. (2014); Italy [18]			X					12 m	4/7	1	X			Prospective
Korol et al. (2017); Ukraine [25]					X			12 m	15/15	1.7			X	Prospective
Roy et al. (2017); India [46]			X	X	X			17.93	24/30	2.76	X	X		Retrospective

There is evidence to suggest that inflammatory cytokines produced in uveitis could promote the development of CNV [38]. Flaxel et al. described in a series of subfoveal CNV secondary to MFC and PIC vision stabilization in 83% of patients that were treated with 1 mg/kg/day of oral corticosteroid for 3–5 days followed by a tapering dose period [39]. Martidis et al. compared the effect of oral prednisone versus a single sub-Tenon triamcinolone acetonide injection for subfoveal CNV secondary to POHS. Oral prednisone group resulted in a greater initial VA improvement at 2 weeks that remain stable at 3 months, but no differences were observed in the final VA between both treatment options [40]. In another study of CNV secondary to POHS, Rechtman et al. reported VA improvement in 30% and stabilization in 50% of eyes treated with intravitreal triamcinolone alone [41].

11.5.3 Laser Photocoagulation

Laser photocoagulation causes the destruction of the CNV, and for this reason it is not utilized for subfoveal CNV due to the development of permanent scotomas. The macular photocoagulation study (MPS) showed post laser therapy benefits for juxtafoveal and extrafoveal CNV in POHS, with reduced relative risk of visual acuity loss of six lines at 5 years [1, 2]. However, since the advent of anti-VEGF therapies, laser photocoagulation treatment has been relegated even in these cases and it is no longer used for CNV.

11.5.4 Photodynamic Therapy

Photodynamic therapy (PDT) with verteporfin causes vascular damage and occlusion after laser photoactivation. PDT has been used as monotherapy or in combination with other treatments (anti-VEGF, corticosteroids, and immunosuppression) in inflammatory CNV associated to MC, PIC, SC, VKH syndrome, toxoplasmic retinochoroiditis, and POHS. Stabilization of lesions was common in most of the studies [3].

11.5.5 Immunosuppressive Treatment

Immunosuppressive agents have been introduced as an alternative treatment for noninfectious CNV, mainly for patients where corticosteroid treatment is contraindicated.

Systemic immunosuppressive therapies can be effective in the resolution of inflammatory CNV as demonstrated by Dees et al. in a series of CNV in posterior uveitis cases treated with cyclosporin [42]. Immunosuppressive therapies may be also used in combination with other treatments. Hogan et al. showed that a combination treatment with oral mycophenolate and photodynamic therapy achieved good disease control in patients with inflammatory CNV associated to posterior uveitis for a relatively long follow-up period [43]. Combination therapies with systemic methotrexate and anti-VEGF drugs have also been reported with positive outcomes in inflammatory CNV [44]. The use of intravitreal methotrexate has also been reported in inflammatory CNV related to multifocal choroiditis [45].

Key Points

- Choroidal neovascularization (CNV) is a severe complication of uveitis.
- CNV may be present at diagnosis or appear with the evolution of the disease, so home-monitoring with Amsler grid charts, high awareness, and close follow-up are required despite the stability of the associated uveitis syndrome.
- OCT and OCTA appear as the most employed retinal imaging techniques for the diagnosis and follow-up of CNV lesions.
- Anti-VEGF therapy is the first-line treatment for both infectious and noninfectious CNV membranes.

References

1. Dhingra N, Kelly S, Majid MA, Bailey CB, Dick AD. Inflammatory choroidal neovascular membrane in posterior uveitis-pathogenesis and treatment. Indian J Ophthalmol. 2010;58(1): 3–10.

2. Agarwal A, Invernizzi A, Singh RB, Foulsham W, Aggarwal K, Handa S, Agrawal R, Pavesio C, Gupta V. An update on inflammatory choroidal neovascularization: epidemiology, multimodal imaging, and management. J Ophthalmic Inflamm Infect. 2018;8(1):13.
3. Miller DG, Singerman LJ. Vision loss in younger patients: a review of choroidal neovascularization. Optom Vis Sci. 2006;83(5):316–25.
4. Walia HS, Shah GK, Blinder KJ. Treatment of CNV secondary to presumed ocular histoplasmosis with intravitreal aflibercept 2.0 mg injection. Can J Ophtalmol. 2016;51(2):91–6.
5. Neri P, Lettieri M, Fortuna C, et al. Inflammatory choroidal neovascularization. Middle East Afr J Ophthalmol. 2009;16:245–51.
6. Symons RCA, Shah SM, Do DV, Hanout M, Sepah YJ, Nguyen QD. Neovascularization. In: Zierhut M, editor. Intraocular inflammation. 1st ed. Berlin: Springer; 2016. p. 471–83.
7. Baxter SL, Pistilli M, Pujari SS, Liesegang TL, Suhler EB, Thorne JE, Foster CS, Jabs DA, Levy-Clarke GA, Nussenblatt RB, Rosenbaum JT, Kempen JH. Risk of choroidal neovascularization among the uveitides. Am J Ophthalmol. 2013;156(3):468–77.e2.
8. Kotsolis AI, Killian FA, Ladas ID, Yannuzzi LA. Fluorescein angiography and optical coherence tomography concordance for choroidal neovascularisation in multifocal choroidtis. Br J Ophthalmol. 2010;94(11):1506–8.
9. Atmaca LS, Batioğlu F, Atmaca P. Evaluation of choroidal neovascularization in age-related macular degeneration with fluorescein and indocyanine green videoangiography. Ophthalmologica. 1996;210(3):148–51.
10. Drexler W, Fujimoto JG. State-of-the-art retinal optical coherence tomography. Prog Retin Eye Res. 2008;27(1):45–88.
11. Wu K, Zhang X, Su Y, Ji Y, Zuo C, Li M, Wen F. Clinical Characteristics of Inflammatory Choroidal Neovascularization in a Chinese Population. Ocul Immunol Inflamm. 2016;24(3):261–7.
12. Hoang QV, Cunningham ET Jr, Sorenson JA, Freund KB. The "pitchfork sign" a distinctive optical coherence tomography finding in inflammatory choroidal neovascularization. Retina. 2013;33(5):1049–55.
13. Yu S, Lu J, Cao D, Liu R, Liu B, Li T, Luo Y, Lu L. The role of optical coherence tomography angiography in fundus vascular abnormalities. BMC Ophthalmol. 2016;16:107.
14. Cheng L, Chen X, Weng S, Mao L, Gong Y, Yu S, Xu X. Spectral-domain optical coherence tomography angiography findings in multifocal choroiditis with active lesions. Am J Ophthalmol. 2016;169:145–61.
15. Adan A, Llorens V, Mesquida M, Carreño E. OCTA en neovascularizaci6n coroidea inflamatoria. In: Adan A, Zarranz-Ventura J, editors. Angiografía por Tomografía de Coherencia Óptica (OCTA). Mesa Redonda 93 Congreso Sociedad Española de Oftalmología. 1st ed. Madrid: Sociedad Española de Oftalmología; 2017. p. 133–40.
16. Levison AL, Baynes KM, Lowder CY, Kaiser PK, Srivastava SK. Choroidal neovascularization on optical coherence tomography angiography in punctate inner choroidopathy and multifocal choroiditis. Br J Ophthalmol. 2017;101(5):616–22.
17. Amer R, Priel E, Kramer M. Spectral-domain optical coherence tomographic features of choroidal neovascular membranes in multifocal choroiditis and punctate inner choroidopathy. Graefes Arch Clin Exp Ophthalmol. 2015;253(6):949–57.
18. Parodi MB, Iacono P, La Spina C, Knutsson KA, Mansour A, Arevalo JF, Bandello F. Intravitreal bevacizumab for choroidal neovascularisation in serpiginous choroiditis. Br J Ophthalmol. 2014;98(4):519–22.
19. Zahid S, Chen KC, Jung JJ, Balaratnasingam C, Ghadiali Q, Sorenson J, Rofagha S, Freund KB, Yannuzzi LA. Optical coherence tomography angiography of chorioretinal lesions due to idiopathic multifocal choroiditis. Retina. 2017;37(8):1451–63.
20. D'Ambrosio E, Tortorella P, Iannetti L. Management of uveitis-related choroidal neovascularization: from the pathogenesis to the therapy. J Ophthalmol. 2014;2014:450428.
21. Xiong M, Elson G, Legarda D, Leibovich SJ. Production of vascular endothelial growth factor by murine macrophages: regulation by hypoxia, lactate, and the inducible nitric oxide synthase pathway. Am J Pathol. 1998;153(2):587–98.
22. Paroli MP, Teodori C, D'Alessandro M, Mariani P, Iannucci G, Paroli M. Increased vascular endothelial growth factor levels in aqueous humor and serum of patients with quiescent uveitis. Eur J Ophthalmol. 2007;17(6):938–42.
23. Banerjee S, Savant V, Scott RA, Curnow SJ, Wallace GR, Murray PI. Multiplex bead analysis of vitreous humor of patients with vitreoretinal disorders. Invest Ophthalmol Vis Sci. 2007 May;48(5):2203–7.
24. Schadlu R, Blinder KJ, Shah GK, Holekamp NM, Thomas MA, Grand MG, Engelbrecht NE, Apte RS, Joseph DP, Prasad AG, Smith BT, Sheybani A. Intravitreal bevacizumab for choroidal neovascularization in ocular histoplasmosis. Am J Ophthalmol. 2008;145(5):875–8.
25. Korol AR, Zborovska O, Kustryn T, Dorokhova O, Pasyechnikova N. Intravitreal aflibercept for choroidal neovascularization associated with chorioretinitis: a pilot study. Clin Ophthalmol. 2017;11: 1315–20.
26. Lott MN, Schiffman JC, Davis JL. Bevacizumab in inflammatory eye disease. Am J Ophthalmol. 2009;148(5):711–7.e2.
27. Adan A, Mateo C, Navarro R, Bitrian E, Casaroli-Marano RP. Intravitreal bevacizumab (avastin) injection as primary treatment of inflammatory choroidal neovascularization. Retina. 2007;27(9):1180–6.
28. Tran TH, Fardeau C, Terrada C, Ducos De Lahitte G, Bodaghi B, Lehoang P. Intravitreal bevacizumab for refractory choroidal neovascularization (CNV) secondary to uveitis. Graefes Arch Clin Exp Ophthalmol. 2008 Dec;246(12):1685–92.

29. Fine HF, Zhitomirsky I, Freund KB, Barile GR, Shirkey BL, Samson CM, Yannuzzi LA. Bevacizumab (avastin) and ranibizumab (lucentis) for choroidal neovascularization in multifocal choroiditis. Retina. 2009 Jan;29(1):8–12.
30. Doctor PP, Bhat P, Sayed R, Foster CS. Intravitreal bevacizumab for uveitic choroidal neovascularization. Ocul Immunol Inflamm. 2009 Mar–Apr;17(2):118–26.
31. Kramer M, Axer-Siegel R, Jaouni T, Reich E, Hemo I, Priel E, Averbukh E, Ehrlich R, Chowers I, Weinberger D, Amer R. Bevacizumab for choroidal neovascularization related to inflammatory diseases. Retina. 2010 Jun;30(6):938–44.
32. Julián K, Terrada C, Fardeau C, Cassoux N, Français C, LeHoang P, Bodaghi B. Intravitreal bevacizumab as first local treatment for uveitis-related choroidal neovascularization: long-term results. Acta Ophthalmol. 2011;89(2):179–84.
33. Rouvas A, Petrou P, Douvali M, Ntouraki A, Vergados I, Georgalas I, Markomichelakis N. Intravitreal ranibizumab for the treatment of inflammatory choroidal neovascularization. Retina. 2011;31(5):871–9.
34. Menezo V, Cuthbertson F, Downes SM. Positive response to intravitreal ranibizumab in the treatment of choroidal neovascularization secondary to punctate inner choroidopathy. Retina. 2010;30(9):1400–4.
35. Cornish KS, Williams GJ, Gavin MP, Imrie FR. Visual and optical coherence tomography outcomes of intravitreal bevacizumab and ranibizumab in inflammatory choroidal neovascularization secondary to punctate inner choroidopathy. Eur J Ophthalmol. 2011;21(4):440–5.
36. Iannetti L, Paroli MP, Fabiani C, Nardella C, Campanella M, Pivetti-Pezzi P. Effects of intravitreal bevacizumab on inflammatory choroidal neovascular membrane. Eur J Ophthalmol. 2013;23(1):114–8.
37. Mansour AM, Arevalo JF, Fardeau C, Hrisomalos EN, Chan WM, Lai TY, Ziemssen F, Ness T, Sibai AM, Mackensen F, Wolf A, Hrisomalos N, Heiligenhaus A, Spital G, Jo Y, Gomi F, Ikuno Y, Akesbi J, LeHoang P, Adan A, Mahendradas P, Khairallah M, Guthoff R, Ghandour B, Küçükerdönmez C, Kurup SK. Three-year visual and anatomic results of administrating intravitreal bevacizumab in inflammatory ocular neovascularization. Can J Ophthalmol. 2012;47(3):269–74.
38. Reddy VM, Zamora RL, Kaplan HJ. Distribution of growth factors in subfoveal neovascular membranes in age-related macular degeneration and presumed ocular histoplasmosis syndrome. Am J Ophthalmol. 1995;120(3):291–301.
39. Flaxel CJ, Owens SL, Mulholland B, Schwartz SD, Gregor ZJ. The use of corticosteroids for choroidal neovascularisation in young patients. Eye (Lond). 1998;12(Pt 2):266–72.
40. Martidis A, Miller DG, Ciulla TA, Danis RP, Moorthy RS. Corticosteroids as an antiangiogenic agent for histoplasmosis-related subfoveal choroidal neovascularization. J Ocul Pharmacol Ther. 1999;15(5):425–8.
41. Rechtman E, Allen VD, Danis RP, Pratt LM, Harris A, Speicher MA. Intravitreal triamcinolone for choroidal neovascularization in ocular histoplasmosis syndrome. Am J Ophthalmol. 2003;136(4):739–41.
42. Dees C, Arnold JJ, Forrester JV, Dick AD. Immunosuppressive treatment of choroidal neovascularization associated with endogenous posterior uveitis. Arch Ophthalmol. 1998;116(11):1456–61.
43. Hogan A, Behan U, Kilmartin DJ. Outcomes after combination photodynamic therapy and immunosuppression for inflammatory subfoveal choroidal neovascularisation. Br J Ophthalmol. 2005;89(9):1109–11.
44. Kolomeyer AM, Roy MS, Chu DS. The use of intravitreal ranibizumab for choroidal neovascularization associated with Vogt-Koyanagi-Harada syndrome. Case Rep Med. 2011;2011:747648.
45. Mateo-Montoya A, Baglivo E, de Smet MD. Intravitreal methotrexate for the treatment of choroidal neovascularization in multifocal choroiditis. Eye (Lond). 2013;27(2):277–8.
46. Roy R, Saurabh K, Bansal A, Kumar A, Majumdar AK, Paul SS. Inflammatory choroidal neovascularization in Indian eyes: Etiology, clinical features, and outcomes to anti-vascular endothelial growth factor. Indian J Ophthalmol. 2017;65(4):295–300.

Dystrophy-Related Choroidal Neovascularization

12

Pierluigi Iacono, Stefano Da Pozzo,
Alessandro Papayannis, Francesco Romano,
Alessandro Arrigo, and Maurizio Battaglia Parodi

12.1 Introduction

Choroidal neovascularization (CNV) can complicate the clinical course of chorioretinal dystrophies. In the forms with primary involvement of the macular area, the occurrence of the CNV adds a high and significant risk of rapid deterioration of the function of central vision and overall the age of onset is very early compared to the more common form associated with age-related macular degeneration (AMD) [1, 2]. To date, there is no precise data on the prevalence of CNV in retinal dystrophies and most of our knowledge related to this topic derives from case series or single case reports. As observed in the more frequent forms of CNV associated with age-related macular degeneration or pathological myopia, the advent of anti-VEGF drug therapy has provided a more reassuring perspective on the evolution of the disease and the efficacy of the therapy. Below we will examine the most recent studies on CNV associated with retinal dystrophies and the available treatment options.

12.2 Retinitis Pigmentosa

Retinitis Pigmentosa (RP) is an inherited retinal dystrophy caused by the loss of photoreceptors and characterized by retinal pigment deposits visible on fundus examination. The prevalence of RP is approximately 1/5000 worldwide, so that RP is the most common inherited disease of the retina. The most common form of RP is a rod-cone dystrophy and it is initially characterized by night blindness, followed by the progressive loss in the peripheral visual field in daylight, and eventually leading to blindness after several decades. The course of the disease may be frequently complicated by cataract formation in young age and cystoid macular edema. The exact prevalence of CNV in RP is unknown. Two interesting and recent studies explored in retrospective analysis the morphological alterations of the macular area by mean of optical coherence tomography in a large sample of patients affected

P. Iacono (✉)
IRCCS-Fondazione Bietti, Rome, Italy

TS-RETINA, Trieste, Italy

S. Da Pozzo
TS-RETINA, Trieste, Italy

A. Papayannis
Azienda Sanitaria Universitaria Giuliano Isontina, S.O.C. di Oculistica di Monfalcone e Gorizia, Monfalcone, Italy

F. Romano
Eye Clinic, Department of Biomedical and Clinical Science, Luigi Sacco Hospital, University of Milan, Milan, Italy

A. Arrigo
Department of Ophthalmology of San Raffaele Scientific Institute, University Vita-Salute, Milan, Italy

M. B. Parodi
TS-RETINA, Trieste, Italy

Department of Ophthalmology of San Raffaele Scientific Institute, University Vita-Salute, Milan, Italy

J. Chhablani (ed.), *Choroidal Neovascularization*, https://doi.org/10.1007/978-981-15-2213-0_12

by RP at different stages of evolution [3, 4]. Triolo et al. identified three cases of CNV in a group of 176 eyes with a calculated prevalence of 1.7%; no evidence of CNV was demonstrated in the cohort of 183 eyes examined by Braima et al.

The low prevalence of this uncommon complication is clearly reflected in the scarce literature available with reference to this topic. To date and according to our research, only a few case reports have been published which, however, offer some interesting considerations.

Ivakiri et al. report data on the natural history in two patients with CNV associated with RP and followed for a period of 14 and 15 years, respectively [5]. The lesions were juxtafoveal and subfoveal and received no type of treatment. In the first case, the visual acuity was 0.3 at the first visit and was reduced to 0.04 at 14 years of follow-ups. In the second case, visual acuity passed from 0.03 at the first visit to hand motion at 15 years of follow-ups. As expected, the visual function declined progressively.

Marano et al. describes a single case with CNV subfoveal, followed for 15 months and receiving a partial laser treatment of the CNV. The patient showed a stabilization of visual acuity that was equal to 0.1 with some phases of CNV reactivation and bleeding in the follow-up period [1].

Cheng et al. reported the results of PDT with verteporfin in two patients [6]. In the first case, a 63-year-old female, with extrafoveal predominantly, classic CNV, subretinal hemorrhage and visual acuity 6/15 received a single session of PDT. Her visual acuity improved to 6/9 at 3-months examination with slow resolution of the subretinal hemorrhage and after 2 years of follow-up showed no recurrence. A second case, a 72-year-old male, presented a subfoveal predominantly classic CNV and a baseline visual acuity of 6/120. The patient received a single session of PDT with a subsequent improvement of visual acuity, a progressive resolution of the CNV, and no recurrence.

The last treatment option considered for CNV related to RP is anti-VEGF. The first experience on the use of bevacizumab was reported by Malik et al. A 40-year-old male with subfoveal classic CNV and a serious visual acuity decline, counting finger at 2 m, received an initial single intravitreal bevacizumab 1.25 mg injection [7]. One month later, the CNV regressed with a complete resolution of the serous detachment, a meaningful decrease in central retinal thickness, passing from 415 to 290 μm, and no leakage on fluorescein angiography. Although a single injection achieved a complete stabilization of the neovascular lesion with no recurrence in the following 12 months of follow-up, no benefit on visual acuity could be recorded.

Bevacizumab was also employed as a first-line treatment for juxtafoveal CNV associated with RP by Battaglia Parodi et al. [8]. A 66-year-old woman with baseline visual acuity of 20/200 in the left eye, classic juxtafoveal CNV evidenced on fluorescein angiography, neurosensory detachment overlying the hyperreflective lesion corresponding to the CNV as demonstrated on OCT examination, received intravitreal injections of bevacizumab (1.25 mg) during a monthly monitoring planned of follow-up. At 1 month of examination, the visual acuity improved to 20/100 and a complete resolution of neurosensory detachment was demonstrated on OCT. During the 1-year follow-up, the patient experienced reactivation of the CNV with recurrent neurosensory detachment and visual acuity deterioration and received four additional injections. The patient was monitored for visual field and electroretinogram responses which turned out to be stable during the follow-up. Finally, at 12 months of examination, visual acuity was stable at 20/100 and no sign of CNV activity was demonstrated, especially with no subfoveal extension. Compared with the case presented by Malik, Battaglia Parodi et al. demonstrated the importance to customize the monitoring of the neovascular lesion as it is possible to observe a frequent reactivation of the CNV. Another important observation provided by Battaglia Parodi et al. concerns the safety of the treatment. In particular, the neuroprotective effect of VEGF on retinal ganglion cells and the role for endogenous VEGF in the maintenance and function of Muller cells and photoreceptors is well known; these findings should be particularly taken into consideration in RP, characterized by progressive anatomical damage involving the same cell populations. In this single case, the visual field and the electrooculogram responses did not get worse during the 1-year follow-up; this suggests that a limited anti-VEGF therapy may not lead to further damage.

A similar conclusion was achieved in a report presented by Miyata et al. A 56-year-old woman received an anti-VEGF treatment in a pro-re-nata regimen for multiple recurrences of CNV activity over a 2-year follow-up. Despite a tailored monitoring, the patient experienced a visual acuity deterioration to a value of 20/100 starting from the baseline value of 20/50. Subsequently the case was treated in a fixed bimonthly regimen that continued for 6 years with 34 anti-VEGF injections administered in the whole period. During the follow-up a slight decline in the central visual field was registered without a difference between the treated and untreated eye, with a mean deviation reduction of 0.32 and 0.68 dB/year, in the treated and untreated eye. At the final visit the CNV did not show activity and the visual acuity was stable at a solid 20/100.

Finally, an additional interesting case report was described by Sayadi et al. [9]. In this case OCT angiography was applied to describe a type 3 neovascularization, formerly defined retinal angiomatous proliferation, in a patient with RP and cystoid macular edema and receiving 8 intravitreal ranibizumab injections over a 1-year follow-up. Unfortunately, the authors did not report the effects of anti-VEGF therapy for the type 3 neovascularization, the change in the visual acutiy, the comparison of the OCT angiography image with conventional fluorescein, or indocyanine green angiography. In particular, no description was provided with regard to the evaluation of type 3 neovascularization in association with cystoid macular edema and which methodology was applied during the anti-VEGF therapy monitoring to differentiate the retinal fluid originating from the neovascularization and the fluid collection secondary to the cystoid macular edema.

12.3 Best Vitelliform Macular Dystrophy

CNV is a possible complication of Best vitelliform macular dystrophy (BVMD). CNV may show exudative manifestations, with subretinal fluid and subretinal hemorrhages, leading to a visual acuity worsening [10]. Typically exudative CNV develops in the initial stages of the disease, before the vitelliruptive evolution. On the other hand, CNV without exudation is detectable in almost 90% of eyes affected by BVMD in the more advanced stages of the disease [11]. Focal choroidal excavation can be associated with the CNV growth, probably due to the mechanical contraction secondary to the CNV [12].

Identification of the CNV can be achieved by means of conventional techniques including fluorescein and indocyanine green angiography but also using optical coherence tomography [13]. Optical coherence tomography angiography can effectively visualize CNV associated with BVMD, depicting the whole neovascular extension (Figs. 12.1, 12.2, 12.3, and 12.4) [11].

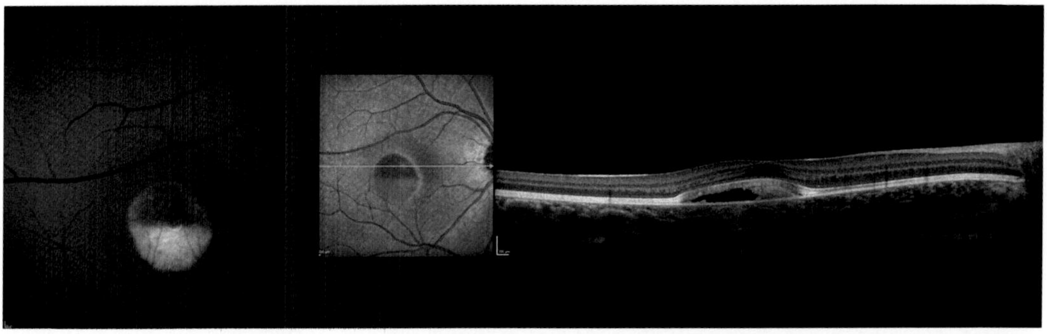

Fig. 12.1 Choroidal neovascularization in Best vitelliform macular dystrophy. Nine-year-old male in Best pseudohypopyon stage on blue-light fundus autofluorescence and on optical coherence tomography

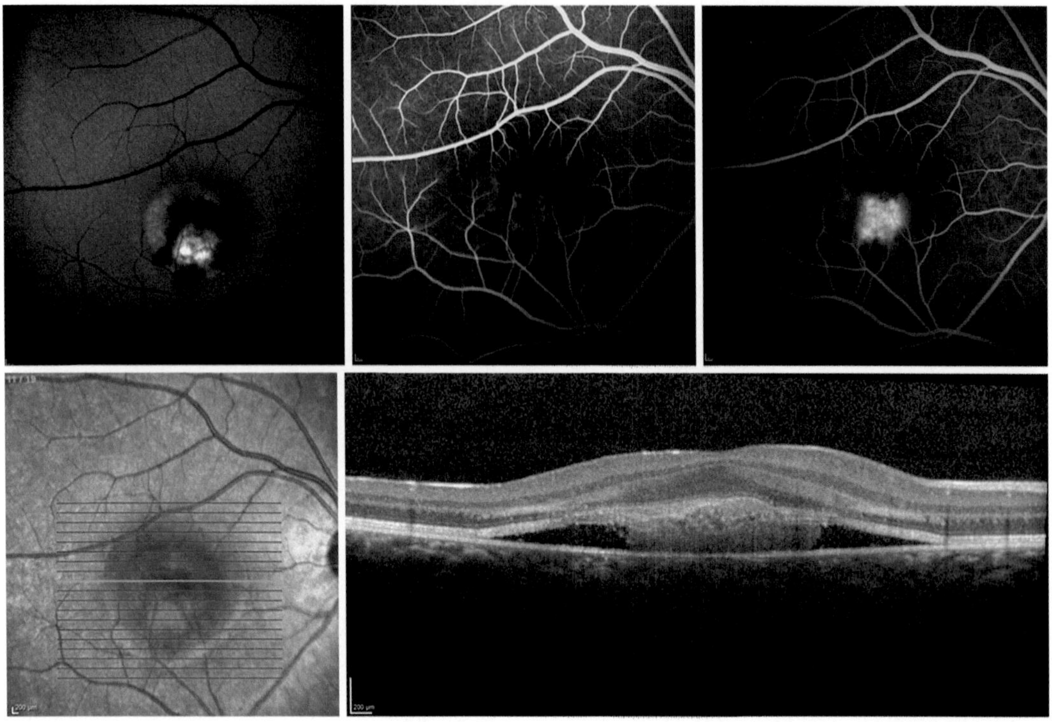

Fig. 12.2 Choroidal neovascularization in Best vitelliform macular dystrophy. Same case as Fig. 12.1, 1 year later, when choroidal neovascularization developed. Blue-light fundus autofluorescence revealed a blocked fluorescence due to subretinal hemorrhage. OCT disclosed a wide subretinal detachment. Fluorescein angiography clearly showed a type II choroidal neovascularization in the early phase, with dye leakage in more advanced phases

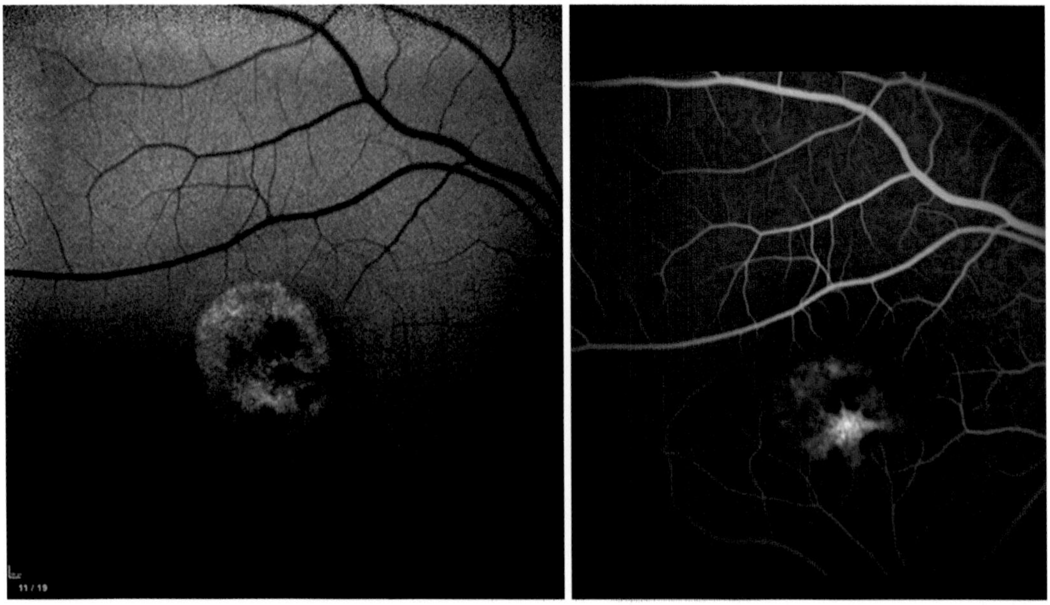

Fig. 12.3 Choroidal neovascularization in Best vitelliform macular dystrophy. Same case as Fig. 12.1, same patient 6 months after a single ranibizumab injection. Blue-light fundus autofluorescence shows an irregular hyperreflective signal. OCT scan reveals the subretinal fluid resolution, whereas fluorescein angiography discloses no dye leakage from the scar

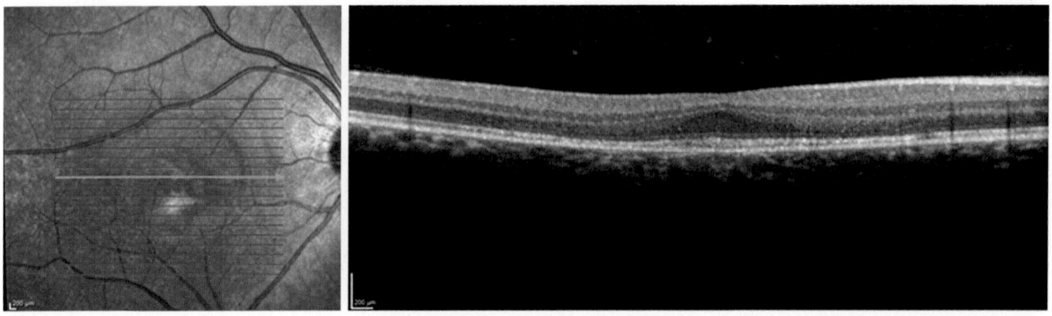

Fig. 12.3 (continued)

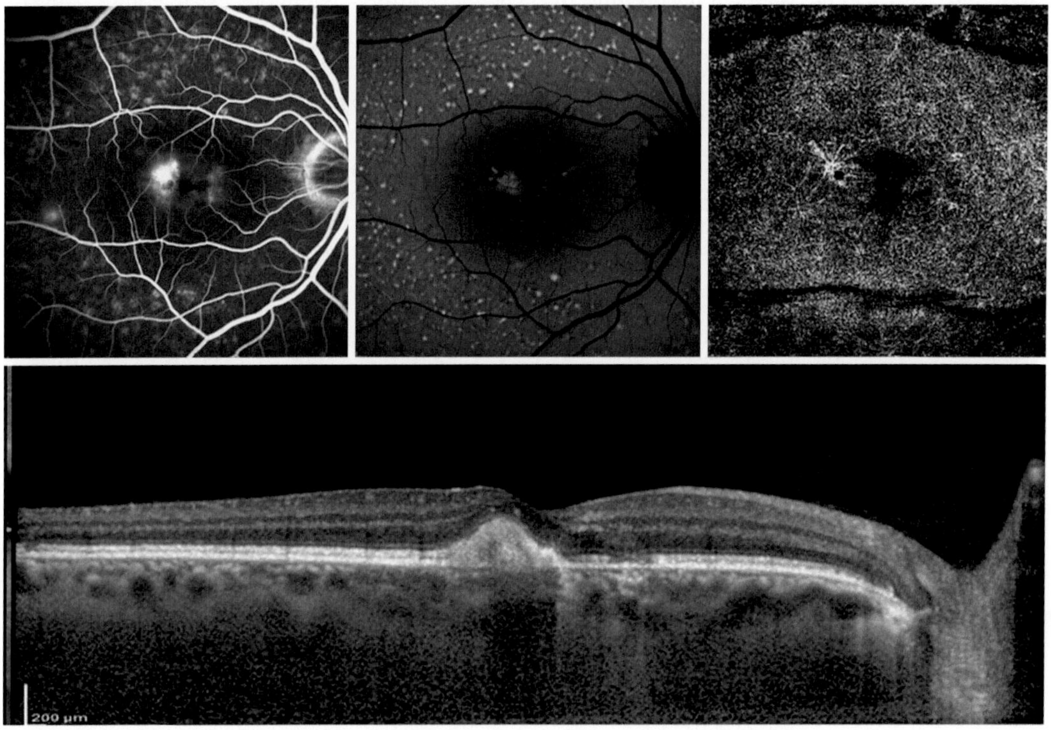

Fig. 12.4 Choroidal neovascularization in Stargardt disease/fundus flavimaculatus. Fluorescein angiography clearly shows leakage from choroidal neovascularization on a background of "silent" choroid and multiple hyperfluorescent pisciform flecks. Blue-light fundus autofluorescence reveals the characteristic hyperautofluorescence in areas of lipofuscin accumulation at the posterior pole. Optical coherence tomography angiography well identifies the neovascular network. B-scan OCT demonstrates the CNV with small amount of intraretinal fluid

Compared with fluorescein angiography, OCT-A allows a better characterization of the CNV, clearly delineating the CNV network in at least four patterns, namely, dense net, loose net, unidentifiable, and in a pattern more recently defined as "ring-shape." Additional advantages of OCT-A are represented by a better visualization of the CNV and a more precise quantification of the CNV area also in the presence of vitelliform deposits able to mask the CNV borders; OCT-A depicts more clearly the vasculature across the different retinal layers. However, OCT-A presents some limitations, the main being the inability to detect the leakage and as a consequence it fails to provide suitable information on the activity of the CNV [14, 15].

The management of CNV secondary to BVMD is still unclear. Overall, treatment, especially with intravitreal anti-VEGF, is associated with better functional outcomes with respect to observation alone [10]. At present, possible treatment options include photodynamic therapy and intravitreal anti-VEGF. Photodynamic therapy is effective in stopping the neovascular growth, but it may bring about atrophic changes and subretinal fibrosis causing functional damage over the follow-up. Anti-VEGF approach is currently the most used treatment, requiring a number of intravitreal injections from 1 to 2, and leading to the stabilization of the CNV activity [16].

12.4 Stargardt Disease/Fundus Flavimaculatus

Since its first report in medical literature, the clinical spectrum of Stargardt disease (SD) has enriched increasingly. Usually, in early stages, patients sustain a progressive visual loss, presenting in childhood or early adulthood with normal fundus appearance [17]. Later in life, the disease progresses toward macular atrophy and the appearance of yellowish retinal flecks. The final result is a visual acuity deterioration up to 20/200 or worse. SD transmission is autosomal recessive and it is due to mutations in ABCA4 gene (OMIM 601691), which encodes an adenosine triphosphate-binding cassette transporter [18, 19]. In the absence of normal ABCA4 function, photoreceptor metabolism is compromised and A2E, a component of lipofuscin, accumulates in photoreceptors and the retinal pigment epithelium (RPE), causing injury to both.

Laboratory and hystopathologic findings described the essence of SD to be a diffuse lipofuscin deposits at the RPE level. On fluorescein angiography, choroidal details are frequently masked by these deposits, a sign also known as "dark" choroid.

In more recent years, optical coherence tomography (OCT) provided meaningful information regarding the location and progression of the pathologic lesions involving the photoreceptors, the retinal pigment epithelium (RPE) and the retinal–choroidal vascularization [20, 21]. In particular, it has been demonstrated that the loss of the inner and outer segments of the photoreceptors precedes the degenerative damage involving the RPE [22]. The presence of hyperreflective foci (HF) is an additional morphological element to be taken into account in the evolutionary processes of Stargardt's disease. In detail, the HF turns out to be more frequent in the pathological edge compared with the healthy edge of the atrophy. In addition, HF number in the outer retina of the pathological edge significantly decreases during the different stages of evolution with an enlargement of the area as the HF number progressively reduces [23]. OCT-A has further contributed to the understanding of degenerative mechanisms affecting retinal and choroidal vascular laminae. Guduru et al. have shown that alterations in the RPE appear to be significantly larger than the choriocapillaris layer vessel loss, which suggests that RPE damage might precede that of choriocapillaris [24]. Battaglia Parodi et al. demonstrated a progressive vascular impairment with an early involvement of the superficial and the deep retinal plexuses. In eyes with advanced atrophic changes a greater reduction in choriocapillaris density was demonstrated in comparison with eyes without atrophy. Mastropasqua et al. convey to similar conclusions. Eyes with advanced Stargardt's disease showed a meaningful reduction of the vascular density of the superficial capillary plexus, deep capillary plexus, and choriocapillaris related to a progressive reduction of the macular thickness [25]. The morphological characterization of the retinal alterations in the Stargardt's disease needs further study. However, numerous potential biomarkers have been made available as sensitive anatomic outcome measures for defining the more appropriate endpoints for clinical trials.

Another clinical entity, defined as fundus flavimaculatus (FFM) is an SD-like phenotype, first described by Franceschetti and François. It is characterized by late-onset of symptoms with slow deterioration, but still presenting a progressive central atrophy and late loss of visual acuity

[26]. SD and FFM are terms frequently used interchangeably in the literature, but probably it is more proper to consider them as different phenotypes of a single, heterogeneous disease.

Degenerative changes involving the RPE may extend to the Bruch's membrane, paving the way to subsequent choroidal neovascularization (CNV). On average, CNV is an infrequent complication in late stages of retinal dystrophies, In the available literature there are only a few case series and case reports about CNV associated with SD/FFM.

CNV is a rare complication in SD/FFM (up to 2% according to Armstrong et al. [27]), but associated with a rapid progression and poor prognosis (Fig. 12.4) [27–29]. More recently even retinal angiomatous proliferation or type 3 CNV was described in a case of FF [30].

Natural history in terms of final visual acuity has been described [27, 31] and resulted to be unfavorable. Data about treatment options are strictly dependent on the time period of the reports. Laser photocoagulation was proposed but is now abandoned.

Photodynamic therapy (PDT) with verteporfin was then proposed and administered [32–36]. Only case series with a maximum of three eyes or single case reports are available. On average a stabilization in visual acuity was achieved with one or more PDT sessions. However, the rarity of SD/FFM and CNV association did not allow to plan a controlled study. Encouraging results can be obtained also administering intravitreal injection with anti-VEGF drugs. As well as with PDT only small case series or single case reports were reported, both with ranibizumab [30, 37–40] and bevacizumab [41]. Battaglia Parodi et al. reported that the frequency of injections did not differ significantly from corresponding values described for CNV in age-related macular degeneration (7 per year). Anti-VEGF usually can halt CNV activity but visual acuity does not improve [40]. In the same paper, the authors pointed out some potential drawbacks of anti-VEGF treatment. Enlargement of the atrophic changes and development of outer retinal tubulation may indicate that anti-VEGF treatment may aggravate the growth of atrophy in SD/FFM. Lipofuscin-filled RPE cells may be more vulnerable to further degenerative processes secondary to the effects of anti-VEGF molecules. on RPE and choriocapillaris. Also the high retreatment rate may imply that ranibizumab may control the CNV activity only in part. OCT detection of subretinal hyperreflective material associated with hyperreflective dots may be interpreted as the indirect manifestation of an inflammatory reaction related to these biochemical alterations [41, 42].

In conclusion, even if CNV complicating SD/FF is quite rare, available protocols of treatment provide suboptimal results in terms of visual acuity preservation.

12.5 Pattern Dystrophy

The definition of pattern dystrophy (PD) of the retinal pigment epithelium (RPE) includes a heterogeneous group of inherited retinal diseases with a natural history that is not entirely known. These disorders are characterized by abnormal pigment distribution in the RPE due to the accumulation of lipofuscin [15, 43, 44].

Overall, five main PD subforms can be identified on the basis of the RPE alterations [15, 43, 45]:

- Adult-Onset Foveomacular Vitelliform Dystrophy (AOFVD)
- Butterfly-shaped pigment dystrophy
- Reticular dystrophy (RD)
- Multifocal PD simulating fundus flavimaculatus
- Fundus pulverulentus

Mutations in the peripherin/RDS gene and a high phenotypic variability have been observed between individuals. Although the natural history of PD is not clearly known the prognosis is generally favorable. The visual function is generally preserved for a long time and the patients usually have their visual acuity maintained until the sixth decade. The onset of atrophy or CNV may complicate the clinical course, leading to a progressive visual acuity deterioration. Nevertheless, some cases with subfoveal CNV may show a relatively stable visual function in the short-term follow-up, with a visual loss in the long run [43, 46, 47].

Variable therapeutic options have been proposed for the management of subfoveal CNV related to PD including laser photocoagulation, photodynamic therapy with verteporfin (vPDT), and anti-VEGF therapy. vPDT has been used in the treatment of subfoveal CNV secondary to PD in some studies obtaining a temporary short-term functional stabilization, followed subsequently by a progressive long-term visual acuity deterioration [48, 49]. More specifically, Battaglia Parodi et al. demonstrated a visual acuity decline of 3 lines in 70% of treated cases at the 3-year examination. Laser photocoagulation may bring about a functional deterioration, due to the following scar enlargement, as described in a single case of extrafoveal CNV secondary to fundus pulverulentus treated with conventional laser photocoagulation [50].

A larger number of studies are available with regard to anti-VEGF therapy for CNV associated with different PD subtypes. In spite of the limitations related to the administration of different drugs, study design, and treatment protocols, the clinical reports describe overall positive anatomical and functional effects, with resolution of the CNV activity, visual acuity stabilization or improvement in 87–92% of cases, over a 12–24-month follow-up [51–56]. Owing to the rarity of CNV complicating PD, the studies share similar and obvious limitations including the small number of patients, short follow-up, uneven genetic characterization, and absence of a control group. Nevertheless, the anti-VEGF approach represents the most promising treatment for the management of CNV secondary to PD.

12.6 Bietti Crystalline Corneoretinal Dystrophy

Bietti crystalline dystrophy (BCD) is a rare autosomal recessive chorioretinal degeneration first described by Bietti in 1939 and characterized by the presence of yellow-white crystals deposits in the retina and in about one-third of cases also into the cornea [57]. Progressive atrophy and degeneration of the retinal pigment epithelium and choroid are observed as BCD evolves; symptoms are similar to those of RP with reduced visual acuity, hemeralopia, visual field loss, and impaired color vision. It is caused by mutations in the CYP4V2 gene, which encodes for a protein whose structure suggests that it may play an active role in fatty acid metabolism [58]. CNV may occur during the first stages of course disease and in young age [59–63]. Two hypotheses are currently formulated to explain the pathogenetic mechanisms leading to the CNV formation. One theory proposes that the CNV might be caused by the chronic irritation of Bruch's membrane by the crystals deposits [64, 65]. The second theory suggests a main role of the drusen-like deposits characterizing the BCD [59]. Le Tien and Nachiappan described two young patients, 29- and 33-years old, receiving intravitreal ranibizumab [60, 63]. In both cases ranibizumab stabilized the CNV after a course of 3 monthly intravitreal injections with a visual acuity improvement from 20/50 to 20/32 in a case and a visual acuity stabilization at 6/9 in the second case.

12.7 Miscellaneous

CNV may be an uncommon complication in very rare retinal disorders including choroideremia, gyrate atrophy, cone dystrophy, enhanced S-cone syndrome, congenital retinoschisis, and only a handful of case reports are presented in the current literature [66–76]. Although the occurrence of CNV can be considered infrequent, clinicians should always bear in mind this possible complication that generally appears at a younger age and in subjects with a more unfavorable functional prognosis. Intravitreal anti-VEGF therapy seems to be a valid treatment option; however, there are no guidelines for therapeutic drug monitoring related to a specific retinal disorder and each subject should receive a tailored approach.

References

1. Marano F, Deutman AF, Leys A, Aandekerk AL. Hereditary retinal dystrophies and choroidal neovascularization. Graefes Arch Clin Exp Ophthalmol. 2000;238:760–4.
2. Battaglia Parodi M, Iacono P, Bandello F. Antivascular endothelial growth factor in hereditary dystrophies. Dev Ophthalmol. 2010;46:107–10.
3. Triolo G, Pierro L, Parodi MB, De Benedetto U, Gagliardi M, Manitto MP, Bandello F. Spectral domain optical coherence tomography findings in patients with retinitis pigmentosa. Ophthalmic Res. 2013;50:160–4.
4. Braimah IZ, Dumpala S, Chhablani J. Outer retinal tubulation in retinal dystrophies. Retina. 2017;37:578–84.
5. Iwakiri R, Okinami S, Hirata A. [Two cases of retinitis pigmentosa associated with choroidal neovascularization]. Nippon Ganka Gakkai Zasshi. 2007;111:606–611.
6. Cheng JY, Adrian KH. Photodynamic therapy for choroidal neovascularization in stargardt disease and retinitis pigmentosa. Retin Cases Brief Rep. 2009;3:388–90.
7. Malik A, Sood S, Narang S. Successful treatment of choroidal neovascular membrane in retinitis pigmentosa with intravitreal bevacizumab. Int Ophthalmol. 2010;30:425–8.
8. Battaglia Parodi M, De Benedetto U, Knutsson KA, Scotti F, Librando A, Bandello F, Iacono P. Juxtafoveal choroidal neovascularization associated with retinitis pigmentosa treated with intravitreal bevacizumab. J Ocul Pharmacol Ther. 2012;28:202–4.
9. Sayadi J, Miere A, Souied EH, Cohen SY. Type 3 neovascularization associated with retinitis pigmentosa. Case Rep Ophthalmol. 2017;8:245–9.
10. Khan KN, Mahroo OA, Islam F, et al. Functional and anatomical outcomes of choroidal neovascularization complicating BEST1-related retinopathy. Retina. 2017;37:1360–70.
11. Battaglia Parodi M, Romano F, Cicinelli MV, et al. Retinal vascular impairment in best vitelliform macular dystrophy assessed by means of optical coherence tomography angiography. Am J Ophthalmol. 2018;187:61–70.
12. Battaglia Parodi M, Casalino G, Iacono P, et al. The expanding clinical spectrum of choroidal excavation in macular dystrophies. Retina. 2018;38:2030–4.
13. Battaglia Parodi M, Iacono P, Romano F, Bandello F. Spectral domain optical coherence tomography features in different stages of best vitelliform macular dystrophy. Retina. 2018;38:1041–6.
14. Guduru A, Gupta A, Tyagi M, Jalali S, Chhablani J. Optical coherence tomography angiography characterisation of best disease and associated choroidal neovascularisation. Br J Ophthalmol. 2018;102(4):444–7.
15. Shahzad R, Siddiqui MA. Choroidal neovascularization secondary to best vitelliform macular dystrophy detected by optical coherence tomography angiography. J AAPOS. 2017;21(1):68–70.
16. Padhi TR, Anderson BJ, Abbey AM, et al. Choroidal neovascular membrane in paediatric patients: clinical characteristics and outcomes. BJO. 2018;102:1232–7.
17. Battaglia Parodi M. Eredodistrofie Corioretiniche. Rome: Verduci Editore; 2002. p. 21–60.
18. Allikmets R, Singh N, Sun H, et al. A photoreceptor cell specific ATP-binding transporter gene (ABCR) is mutated in recessive Stargardt macular dystrophy. Nat Genet. 1997;15:236–46.
19. Koenekoop RK. The gene for Stargardt disease, ABCA4, is a major retinal gene: a mini review. Ophthalmic Genet. 2003;24:75–80.
20. Jampol LM, Shankle R, Tornambe P, et al. Diagnostic and therapeutic challenges. Retina. 2006;26:1072–6.
21. Margolis R, Mukkamala SK, Jampol LM, et al. The expanded spectrum of focal choroidal excavation. Arch Ophthalmol. 2011;129:1320Y5.
22. Alabduljalil T, Patel RC, Alqahtani AA, Gao SS, Gale MJ, Zhang M, Jia Y, Huang D, Chiang PW, Chen R, Wang J, Weleber RG, Pennesi ME, Yang P. Correlation of outer retinal degeneration and choriocapillaris loss in Stargardt disease using en face optical coherence tomography and optical coherence tomography angiography. Am J Ophthalmol. 2019;202:79–90.
23. Guduru A, Lupidi M, Gupta A, Jalali S, Chhablani J. Comparative analysis of autofluorescence and OCT angiography in Stargardt disease. Br J Ophthalmol. 2018;102(9):1204–7.
24. Battaglia Parodi M, Sacconi R, Romano F, Bandello F. Hyperreflective foci in Stargardt disease: 1-year follow-up. Graefes Arch Clin Exp Ophthalmol. 2019;257(1):41–8.
25. Mastropasqua R, Toto L, Borrelli E, Di Antonio L, Mattei PA, Senatore A, Di Nicola M, Mariotti C. Optical coherence tomography angiography findings in Stargardt disease. PLoS One. 2017;12(2):e0170343.
26. Franceschetti A, François J. Fundus flavimaculatus. Arch Ophthalmol. 1965;25:505–30.
27. Armstrong J, Meyer D, Xu S, Elfervig J. Long-term follow-up of Stargardt's disease and fundus flavimaculatus. Ophthalmology. 1998;105:448–58.
28. Klein R, Lewis RA, Meyers SM, Myers FL. Subretinal neovascularization associated with fundus flavimaculatus. Arch Ophthalmol. 1978;96:2054–7.
29. Pawlak D, Souied E, Mimoun G, et al. Fundus flavimaculatus and choroidal neovascularisation. J Fr Ophtalmol. 2006;29:188–94.
30. Quijano C, Querques C, Massamba N, Soubrane G, Souied EH. Type 3 choroidal neovascularization associated with fundus flavimaculatus. Ophthalmic Res. 2009;42:152–4.
31. Rotenstreich Y, Fishman GA, Anderson RJ. Visual acuity loss and clinical observations in a large series

of patients with Stargardt disease. Ophthalmology. 2003;110:1151–8.
32. Valmaggia C, Niederberger H, Helbig H. Photodynamic therapy for choroidal neovascularisation in fundus flavimaculatus. Retina. 2002;22:111–3.
33. Souied EH, Pawlak D, Algan M, Sayag D, Coscas G, Soubrane G. Photodynamic therapy for choroidal neovascularization on late-onset fundus flavimaculatus. Am J Ophthalmol. 2005;140:312–4.
34. Japiassù RM, Ferreira Moura Brasil O, Soares Maia H, Soares Maia A, Moura Brasil O. Photodynamic therapy for bilateral and simultaneous choroidal neovascularization in Stargardt disease. Retin Cases Brief Rep. 2008;2:9–11.
35. Kim HH, Carvounis PE, Albini TA, Eric R, Holz ER, Mieler WF. Photodynamic therapy for bilateral subfoveal choroidal neovascularization complicating Stargardt macular dystrophy. Retin Cases Brief Rep. 2008;2:6–8.
36. Cheng JY, Koh HCA. Photodynamic therapy for choroidal neovascularization in Stargardt disease and retinitis pigmentosa. Retin Cases Brief Rep. 2009;3:388–90.
37. Querques G, Bocco MC, Soubrane G, Souied EH. Intravitreal ranibizumab (Lucentis) fr choroidal neovascularization associated with Stargardt's disease. Graefes Arch Clin Exp Ophthalmol. 2008;246:319–21.
38. Tejerina A, García-Pous M, Palacios Pozos E, Desco Esteban MC, Mataix Boronat J. Ranibizumab for choroidal neovascularization in fundus flavimaculatus. Retin Cases Brief Rep. 2008;2:250–2.
39. Koh V, Naing T, Chee C. Fundus flavimaculatus and choroidal neovascularization in a young patient with normal electroretinography: case report. Can J Ophthalmol. 2012;47:e3–5.
40. Battaglia Parodi M, Munk MR, Iacono P, Bandello F. Ranibizumab for subfoveal choroidal neovascularisation associated with Stargardt disease. Br J Ophthalmol. 2015;99:1268–70.
41. Roy R, Kumar A, Ghosh S, Lobo A, Agarwal P. All that glitters are not flecks: inflammatory choroidal neovascularization in fundus flavimaculatus. Ocul Immunol Inflamm. 2015;23(2):188–90.
42. Radu RA, Hu J, Yuan Q, et al. Complement system dysregulation and inflammation in the retinal pigment epithelium of a mouse model for Stargardt macular degeneration. J Biol Chem. 2011;286:18593–601.
43. Gass JDM. Stereoscopic atlas of macular diseases: diagnosis and treatment. 4th ed. St. Louis: CV Mosby; 1997. p. 314–25.
44. Francis PJ, Schultz DW, Gregory AM, et al. Genetic and phenotypic heterogeneity in pattern dystrophy. Br J Ophthalmol. 2005;89:1115–9.
45. Marmor MF, Byers B. Pattern dystrophy of the retinal pigment epithelium. Am J Ophthalmol. 1976;13:112–6.
46. Taillanter-Francoz N, Remy C, Bonnet M, Baserer T. Choroidal neovessels associated with reticular dystrophy of the pigment epithelium: case report (in French). Bull Soc Ophtalmol Fr. 1981;81:539–41.
47. Marano F, Deutman AF, Pinckers AJ, et al. Reticular dystrophy of the retinal pigment epithelium and choroidal neovascularization: a fluorescein and ICGV study. Acta Ophthalmol Scand. 1997;75:22–7.
48. Parodi MB, Da Pozzo S, Ravalico G. Photodynamic therapy for choroidal neovascularization associated with pattern dystrophy. Retina. 2003;23:171–6.
49. Parodi MB, Liberali T, Pedio M, et al. Photodynamic therapy of subfoveal choroidal neovascularization secondary to reticular pattern dystrophy: three-year results of an uncontrolled, prospective case series. Am J Ophthalmol. 2006;141:1152–4.
50. Parodi MB. Choroidal neovascularization in fundus pulverulentus. Acta Ophthalmol Scand. 2002;80:559–60.
51. Parodi MB, Iacono P, Cascavilla M, Zucchiatti I, Kontadakis DS, Bandello F. Intravitreal bevacizumab for subfoveal choroidal neovascularization associated with pattern dystrophy. Invest Ophthalmol Vis Sci. 2010;51:4358–61.
52. Schutt F, Davies S, Kopitz J, et al. Photodamage to human RPE cells by A2-E, a retinoid component of lipofuscin. Invest Ophthalmol Vis Sci. 2000;41:2303–8.
53. Mimoun G, Caillaux V, Querques G, et al. Ranibizumab for choroidal neovascularization associated with adult-onset foveomacular vitelliform dystrophy: one-year results. Retina. 2013;33:513–21.
54. Empeslidis T, Vardarinos A, Deane J, Banerjee S. Intravitreal ranibizumab in the treatment of butterfly-shaped pattern dystrophy associated with choroidal neovascularization: a case report. Case Rep Ophthalmol. 2012;3:77–82.
55. Vaclavik V, Tran HV, Gaillard MC, et al. Pattern dystrophy with high intrafamilial variability associated with Y141C mutation in the peripherin/RDS gene and successful treatment of subfoveal CNV related to multifocal pattern type with anti-VEGF (ranibizumab) intravitreal injections. Retina. 2012;32:1942–9.
56. Montero JA, Ruiz-Moreno JM, De La Vega C. Intravitreal bevacizumab for adult-onset vitelliform dystrophy: a case report. Eur J Ophthalmol. 2007;17:983–6.
57. Bietti G. Ueber familiaercs vorkommen von 'retinitis punctata albescens' (verbunden mit 'dystrophia marginalis cristallinea corneae'), glitzern des glaskoerpers und anderen degenerativen augenveraenderungen. Klin Monatsbl Augenheilkd. 1939;99: 737–57.
58. Li A, Jiao X, Munier FL, Schorderet DF, Yao W, Iwata F, Hayakawa M, Kanai A, Shy Chen M, Alan Lewis R, Heckenlively J, Weleber RG, Traboulsi EI, Zhang Q, Xiao X, Kaiser-Kupfer M, Sergeev YV, Hejtmancik JF. Bietti crystalline corneoretinal dystrophy is caused

by mutations in the novel gene CYP4V2. Am J Hum Genet. 2004;74(5):817–26.
59. Li Q, Li Y, Zhang X, Xu Z, Zhu X, Ma K, She H, Peng X. Utilization of fundus autofluorescence, spectral domain optical coherence tomography, and enhanced depth imaging in the characterization of Bietti crystalline dystrophy in different stages. Retina. 2015;35:2074–84.
60. Le Tien V, Atmani K, Querques G, Massamba N, Souied EH. Ranibizumab for subfoveal choroidal neovascularization in Bietti crystalline retinopathy. Eye (Lond). 2010;24:1728–9.
61. Gupta B, Parvizi S, Mohamed MD. Bietti crystalline dystrophy and choroidal neovascularisation. Int Ophthalmol. 2011;31:59–61.
62. Atmaca LS, Muftuoglu O, Atmaca-Sonmez P. Peripapillary choroidal neovascularization in Bietti crystalline retinopathy. Eye (Lond). 2007;21:839–42.
63. Nachiappan K, Krishnan T, Madhavan J. Ranibizumab for choroidal neovascular membrane in a rare case of Bietti's crystalline dystrophy: a case report. Indian J Ophthalmol. 2012;60:207–9.
64. Yin X, Yang L, Chen N, Cui H, Zhao L, Feng L, Li A, Zhang H, Ma Z, Li G. Identification of CYP4V2 mutation in 36 Chinese families with Bietti crystalline corneoretinal dystrophy. Exp Eye Res. 2016;146:154–62.
65. Mamatha G, Umashankar V, Kasinathan N, Krishnan T, Sathyabaarathi R, Karthiyayini T, Amali J, Rao C, Madhavan J. Molecular screening of the CYP4V2 gene in Bietti crystalline dystrophy that is associated with choroidal neovascularization. Mol Vis. 2011;17:1970–7.
66. Inanc M, Tekin K, Teke MY. Bilateral choroidal neovascularization associated with gyrate atrophy managed with intravitreal bevacizumab. Int Ophthalmol. 2018;38:1351–5.
67. Gulkilik G, Erdur SK, Eliacik M, Odabasi M, Ozsutcu M, Demirci G, Kocabora MS. A case of cone dystrophy associated with choroidal neovascularization. Retin Cases Brief Rep. 2018;12:111–4.
68. Chatziralli I, Theodossiadis G, Emfietzoglou I, Theodossiadis P. Intravitreal ranibizumab for choroidal neovascularization secondary to gyrate atrophy in a young patient: a multimodal imaging analysis. Eur J Ophthalmol. 2015;25:e119–22.
69. Marano F, Deutman AF, Pinckers AJ, Aandekerk AL. Gyrate atrophy and choroidal neovascularization. Arch Ophthalmol. 1996;114:1295.
70. Campos-Pavón J, Torres-Peña JL. Choroidal neovascularization secondary to choroideremia. Arch Soc Esp Oftalmol. 2015;90:289–91.
71. Palejwala NV, Lauer AK, Weleber RG. Choroideremia associated with choroidal neovascularization treated with intravitreal bevacizumab. Clin Ophthalmol. 2014;8:1675–9.
72. Endo K, Yuzawa M, Ohba N. Choroideremia associated with subretinal neovascular membrane. Acta Ophthalmol Scand. 2000;78:483–6.
73. Robinson D, Tiedeman J. Choroideremia associated with a subretinal neovascular membrane. Case Rep Retina. 1987;7:70–4.
74. Bertoli F, Pignatto S, Rizzetto F, Lanzetta P. A 5-year-old case of choroidal neovascularization in enhanced S-cone syndrome treated with ranibizumab. Case Rep Ophthalmol. 2018;9:510–5.
75. Broadhead GK, Grigg JR, McCluskey P, Korsakova M, Chang AA. Bevacizumab for choroidal neovascularisation in enhanced S-cone syndrome. Doc Ophthalmol. 2016;133:139–43.
76. Ranchod TM, Faia LJ, Drenser KA. Peripapillary choroidal neovascularization in congenital retinoschisis. Retin Cases Brief Rep. 2011;5:336–8.

Choroidal Neovascularization Associated with Angioid Streaks

13

Christof Hänsli and Sandrine A. Zweifel

13.1 Angioid Streaks and Associated Diseases

13.1.1 Introduction

Angioid streaks (AS) are a clinical finding with linear or branching patterns in the posterior pole. They were first described in 1889 [1], named "angioid" in 1892 [2] according to their vessel-like appearance, and found to be a pathology of Bruch's membrane (BM) in 1917 [3, 4].

Angioid streaks are a frequent finding in pseudoxanthoma elasticum (PXE), with an incidence of 59–87% of patients. After 20 years of disease, almost all patients with PXE have AS [3]. They also occur in 8–15% of patients with Paget's disease, and can occur in Ehlers–Danlos syndrome, Marfan syndrome, sickle cell hemoglobinopathies, and hypercalcemia. They have also been described in an enlarging list of other diseases including chronic congenital hyperphosphatemia and Sturge–Weber syndrome. A systemic association can be identified in at least 50% of patients, of which PXE is the most frequent, but AS are also observed as an isolated ocular finding (idiopathic) [3].

C. Hänsli · S. A. Zweifel (✉)
University Hospital Zurich, Zurich, Switzerland

University of Zurich, Zurich, Switzerland
e-mail: christof.haensli@usz.ch;
sandrine.zweifel@usz.ch

Secondary choroidal neovascularization (CNV) occurs in up to 65% of patients with AS [5]. Prognosis of untreated secondary CNV due to AS is poor. Development of a disciform scar, typically at the posterior pole, leads to a relevant vision loss with a best corrected visual acuity (BCVA) of 20/200 or less at the fourth to fifth decade of life [6].

13.1.2 Pseudoxanthoma Elasticum: Incidence, Genetics, and Histopathology

Pseudoxanthoma elasticum is an autosomal recessive disorder, with a prevalence of 1:25,000 to 1:100,000 [7]. It is caused by a mutation of the ABCC6 gene, a part of the subclass C of the ATP-binding cassette transporter (ABC). The gene ABCC6 is highly expressed in kidney and liver, with lower expression rates in skin, retina, and vessel walls, which are the clinically affected tissues in PXE [7, 8].

Histologic findings of the skin in PXE classically include elastin abnormalities in the mid-epidermis with swelling, granular degeneration, and fragmentation. The first detectable sign is calcification of elastin fibers in electron microscopy [8]. Similar alterations are found in the BM of the eye. Calcification and thickening make BM brittle, leading to breaks in BM, clinically appearing as AS [8]. Later, ingrowth of fibrovascular

J. Chhablani (ed.), *Choroidal Neovascularization*, https://doi.org/10.1007/978-981-15-2213-0_13

tissue from the choriocapillaris may occur, leading to CNV and development of a disciform scar with subretinal fibrosis and atrophy, especially when CNV remains untreated [7, 8]. In small and medium-sized vasculature of the body, calcification of elastic fibers seems to resemble normal atherosclerosis [8].

Signaling cascades leading to these changes are complex, and not yet fully understood. The substrate of ABCC6 and its role in the pathogenesis of PXE are largely unknown [9]. The pathologic mechanism is possibly not due to a single gene, but modulated by many genetic modifiers [9]. Main important pathways seem to involve transforming growth factor beta (TGF-β), bone morphogenetic proteins (BMPs), and inorganic phosphates (PPi). All are known factors in the homeostasis of extracellular matrix, its mineralization, and vascular calcification [9].

First clinical signs of PXE are asymptomatic small yellow papules on the skin, beginning at the neck and shoulder in the adolescence [7]. Cardiovascular involvement of the disease can lead to early-onset atherosclerosis, coronary or valvular heart disease, and restrictive cardiomyopathy, with unknown prevalence but possibly resulting in death [7]. The systemic manifestations with possibly life-threatening vascular complications and the vision-threatening ocular complications make the knowledge of the disease important. Early recognition enables an appropriate screening for systemic or ocular complications and thus treatment in early stages leads to better treatment outcomes.

13.1.3 Paget's Disease

Juvenile Paget's disease is a rare recessively inherited disorder, associated with accelerated bone turnover, long bone deformity, growth impairment, and fractures in early life. It is associated with progressive retinopathy characterized by the development of AS. Retinal abnormalities increase with age. The underlying mutation leads to a loss of function of osteoprotegerin. This glycoprotein has an important function in regulating bone turnover and may inhibit calcification of elastic fibers. Thus, its deficiency may lead to BM calcification and BM cracks, apparent as AS [10]. Secondary CNV is a possible complication causing visual loss in young patients [10].

13.1.4 Hemoglobinopathies

Elastic tissue disorders, similar to PXE, with ocular involvement are a frequent finding in hemoglobinopathies. Angioid streaks have been reported in 1–22% of patients with sickle cell disease, depending on patients' age, in 20% with β-thalassemia, and in 10% with sickle thalassemia [11]. The changes seem to be acquired as a consequence of the underlying disease, with a generally milder clinical course and later onset, compared to PXE [11].

13.1.5 Other Causes

Other mechanisms have been proposed in the formation of AS or provoking secondary CNV in preexisting AS. For example, acceleration/deceleration trauma may cause hyperextension of the eyeball in its equator line, leading to ruptures of BM and/or the secondary formation of CNV in preexisting AS [12].

13.2 Clinical Features

13.2.1 Incidence and Visual Loss

Angioid streaks, independent of underlying disease, usually occur bilaterally and are equally distributed in men and women [5]. They affect younger patients of average 43–57 years [5, 13]. Secondary CNV occurs in 67.5% of patients with AS, and is bilaterally in 31.2% of patients with AS. Prior to the anti-VEGF era, a decreased BCVA less than 20/200 was shown in 40.4% of eyes with AS. In younger patients with AS without CNV, BCVA can be normal [14]. Most (86%) of the CNV lesions are macular or both macular and extramacular, only 14% of lesions were extramacular [5].

In PXE, 94% of patients have associated AS, with macular involvement in more than half of the eyes (Fig. 13.1). Sixty percent of patients have bilateral BCVA > 20/50 on presentation. Visual loss increases with age. Best corrected visual acuity <20/50 in at least one eye occurs in 20% of younger patients, but increases to 75% of patients older than 52 years. Visual impairment with bilateral BCVA <20/50 occurs in 17% of patients with PXE.

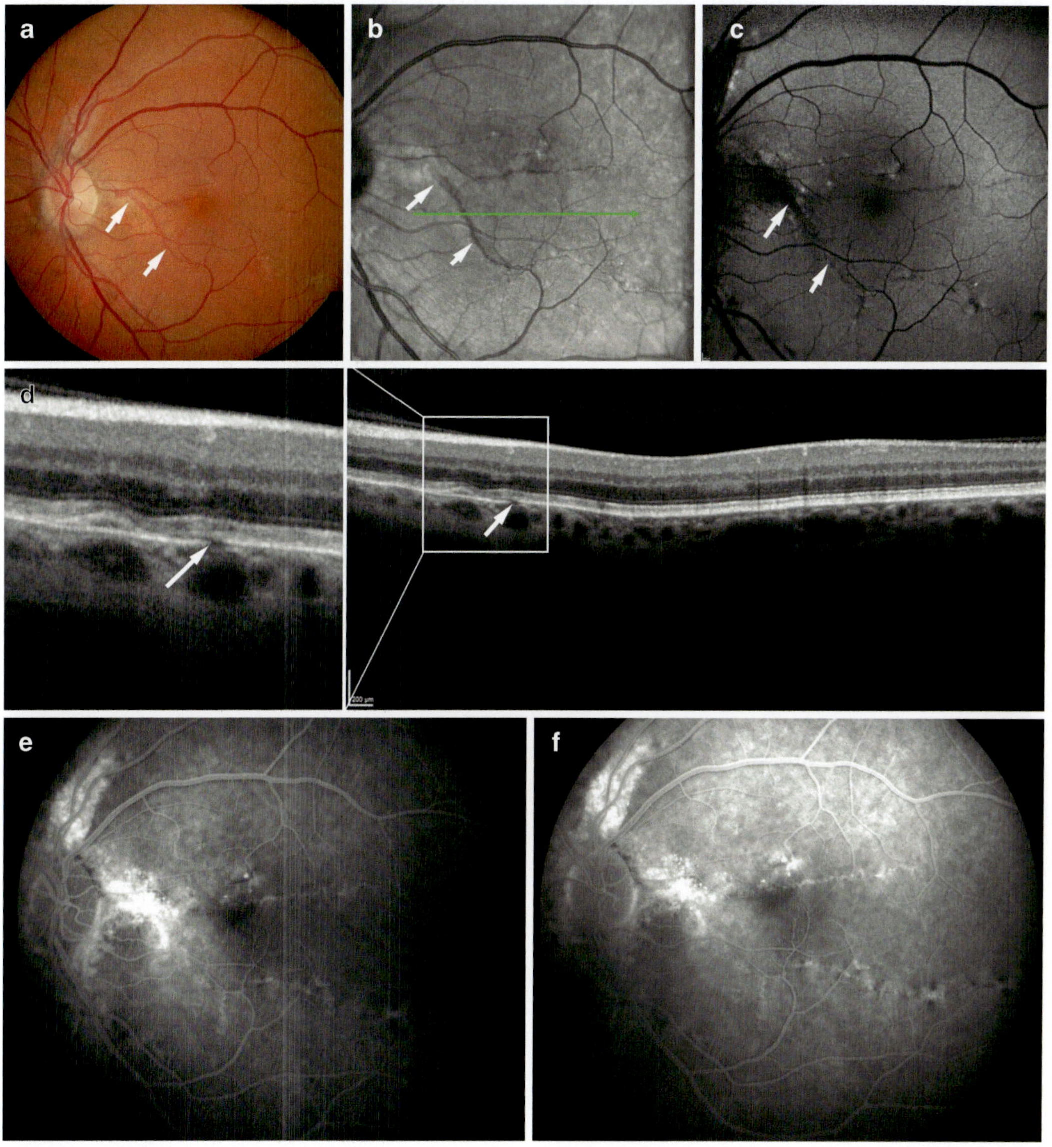

Fig. 13.1 Multimodal imaging findings of angioid streaks (AS). Multimodal imaging of the left eye of a 50-year-old patient with histologically proven pseudoxanthoma elasticum with AS without secondary choroidal neovascularization. BCVA was 20/30 in the left eye. Angioid streaks emanating from the optic disc in the posterior pole appear reddish-brown in fundus photography (**a**, white arrows), hyporeflective on confocal scanning laser ophthalmoscopy (cSLO) (**b**) with indication of corresponding OCT scan (green line) and hypoautofluorescent (**c**). The corresponding OCT image with its enlarged section (**d**) demonstrates Bruch's membrane break (white arrow). Fluorescein angiography shows window defect with hyperfluorescence in the arteriovenous phase (**e**) and late staining (**f**)

13.2.2 Ocular Imaging Findings

Diagnosis and treatment monitoring of complications associated with AS is based on multimodal imaging including color fundus photography, near-infrared imaging (NIR), fundus autofluorescence (FAF), fluorescein-angiography (FA), indocyanine green angiography (ICG), optical coherence tomography (OCT), and OCT angiography (OCTA).

13.2.2.1 Angioid Streaks

Angioid streaks appear as linear crack-like lines in the posterior pole, emanating radially from the optic disc with a diminishing width toward the periphery [15]. The color of AS is brown in 50%, but can also appear gray or reddish-brown (Fig. 13.1a) [5].

Angioid streaks are best visualized using NIR or confocal scanning laser ophthalmoscopy (cSLO) imaging (Fig. 13.1b) [16]. They appear as dark hyporeflective linear bands in the posterior pole with sharp borders. The lesions correspond to BM breaks in OCT (Fig. 13.1d).

Fundus autofluorescence can reveal larger areas of retinal pigment epithelium (RPE) damage than visible on clinical examination or color fundus photography [17, 18]. Angioid streaks appear as hypoautofluorescent lines, even though not as distinct as in NIR imaging (Fig. 13.1c) [16]. A hyperautofluorescent margin of the streak can occur, called the parastreak phenomenon. It is thought to result from RPE cell proliferation and secondary lipofuscin accumulation. This parastreak phenomenon is more often observed in patients without CNV. The mechanism for this distribution remains unknown [17].

Spectral domain (SD-) OCT offers the possibility to show retinal architecture in a near-histological resolution. Angioid streaks are visualized as breaks in BM (Fig. 13.1d). The overlying RPE can remain intact, be altered, focally detached, or completely absent [16]. Additional OCT findings are BM undulations (Fig. 13.1d) and large dehiscences of BM [19]. Over time, BM undulations can progress to BM breaks, especially at vortexes and margins of BM undulations [19]. Eyes with CNV due to AS show a higher prevalence of BM undulations, suggesting a continuous disease progress from BM undulations to BM breaks and later secondary CNV [19, 20]. Subretinal hyperreflective material above and beneath RPE/BM complex can indicate CNV. This sign of CNV often occurs at locations of larger BM breaks, suggesting the development of CNV at locations of BM breaks [19].

Smaller defects in BM may be difficult to detect in OCT B-scans or appear obscured by complications such as hemorrhages. In these cases, en-face reconstruction of BM layer from OCT may visualize breaks in BM which are not visible in other imaging modalities [21].

Angioid streaks appear as hyperfluorescent window defects in early frames with sharp borders and without leakage in later frames in FA (Figs. 13.1e and f) and ICG [15]. Typically they seem to appear more prominent in ICG, even though few cases are better highlighted by other modalities [15].

Optical coherence tomography angiography (OCTA) offers the possibility to visualize choriocapillaris vessels underlying RPE in a very high resolution, not achievable with other modalities. In OCTA, AS without CNV typically shows underlying choriocapillaris rarefication, corresponding to the dark areas in NIR imaging and RPE/BM hyporeflectivity in SD-OCT [22]. These findings are irrelevant of the underlying disease (PXE, sickle cell disease, or idiopathic). A minor part of AS, with a bright and adjacent dark appearance in NIR imaging and subretinal hyperreflective material in OCT, shows irregular choriocapillaris vascular network, for which fibrovascular tissue remodeling is hypothesized [22].

Changes in the choriocapillaris vascular network can be analyzed using flow voids in OCTA. Choriocapillaris changes can be detected in AS, even in the absence of RPE atrophy. Besides remarkable structural differences in the appearance of the choriocapillaris layer, higher proportions of larger flow voids (areas greater than 10,000 or 40,000 μm^2 with lack of flow signal) can be measured, compared to normal eyes [23].

13.2.2.2 Peau d'Orange and Reticular Pseudodrusen

Peau d' orange is usually the first ocular sign, preceding AS for 1–8 years [7]. It is a non-confluent yellowish granular finding located predominantly in the temporal macula, resembling the skin of an orange: in French "peau d'orange" [24] (Fig. 13.3a). It is best visualized as small dark flecks in NIR imaging, appearing as isoreflective non-confluent spots in NIR imaging in an area of hyperreflectivity (Fig. 13.3b) [25], with corresponding round hypocyanescent spots in ICG [15]. Areas of peau d'orange show hyperreflectivity of the outer band of the RPE/BM complex in SD-OCT (Fig. 13.3f) [14, 16, 26].

Posteriorly adjacent to peau d'orange, a yellow confluent area can be seen, with a reduced visualization of underlying choroidal vessels [26]. Angioid streaks are located within this area and stretching to its borders. It is thought to be the representation of calcium deposits in the BM layer [16, 26]. Cracks of BM may propagate within this hypercalcified and thus brittle layer, just as in a shell of an egg. Hence, the French term "coquille d'œuf" has been proposed for this phenomenon [26]. This area can be highlighted by separating color channels of a fundus photograph and multiplying red and green channel with an image processing software.

Reticular pseudodrusen (subretinal drusenoid deposits) [27] may look similar to peau d'orange in fundoscopy and color fundus photography. They are located more posteriorly than peau d'orange and appear as hyporeflective non-confluent spots in NIR [25]. Optical coherence tomography shows multiple small subretinal hyperreflective accumulations leading to undulations of the outer retinal layers, appearing in 50% of PXE patients with AS [25, 28].

13.2.2.3 Crystalline Bodies and Comet Lesions

Crystalline bodies are small chorioretinal atrophies, appearing as nodular crystalline or white bodies, and can be associated with a white tail of RPE atrophy extending posteriorly, resembling a comet [29]. FA reveals early transmission and late staining hyperfluorescence [14]. Crystalline bodies show round irregularly shaped hyperreflective borders with a hyporeflective space within interrupted retinal layers in SD-OCT [14, 30]. Underlying RPE is altered or atrophic, creating a hypertransmission artifact in SD-OCT [14].

13.2.2.4 Optic Disc Drusen

Optic disc drusen can be diagnosed in 8–25% of patients with PXE; they are often only visualized using FAF [7].

13.2.2.5 Pattern Dystrophy-Like Changes

Multiple irregular hyperautofluorescent lines and spots can cause various presentations of pattern dystrophy-like appearance, visible in FAF [16, 28, 31, 32]. These changes seem to occur more often in patients with CNV in at least one eye, and may thus be a risk factor for the development of CNV [17]. Fundus pulverulentus is a rare subform of pattern dystrophy. In patients with PXE who show fundus pulverulentus, subretinal fibrosis is more often present than without fundus pulverulentus (34.6 vs. 4.2%, respectively). This subretinal fibrosis often leads to vision loss due to macular atrophy and/or CNV [33].

13.2.2.6 Atrophy

In atrophic areas, underlying choroidal vessels are visible in color fundus photography, but AS under atrophic areas are less visible. Atrophy as a sign of additional RPE damage appears hypoautofluorescent in FAF. In eyes with AS, atrophy can appear as RPE rips, sharply demarcated multilobular RPE atrophy, or poorly defined RPE atrophy [17, 18]. Most eyes with AS and atrophy show small dot-like hyperautofluorescent patterns in the perilesional area (Fig. 13.5b). Atrophy shows the loss of the ellipsoid and RPE bands with choroidal hypertransmission and hyperreflective spots within the outer retinal layers in SD-OCT [34, 35]. Angioid streaks appear as breaks in BM in SD-OCT, which also shows underlying choroidal thinning [34].

Atrophy of the RPE is detectable in 32% of patients with PXE [34]. In 7% it occurs without concomitant CNV, most commonly between 60 and 70 years of age. Being relatively rare below

40 years, the incidence of atrophy increases with age to virtually all patients over 70 years. In most of the patients with AS and RPE atrophy, secondary CNV is adjacent or within the atrophic area.

Before the development of atrophy, eyes typically show pattern dystrophy-like changes, reticular pseudodrusen, and reduced subfoveal choroidal thickness [34]. Typically, separate atrophic areas develop individually and later coalesce, sparing the fovea until advanced stages [34]. The progression rate of RPE atrophy and its size increasingly vary with age. In eyes with PXE and pattern dystrophy, progression is faster [34]. Visual deterioration depends on the precise location [36].

Quantitative analysis of FAF is reduced in patients with PXE, compared to normal eyes, especially in the nasal macula, with a more pronounced effect in advanced disease [31].

13.2.2.7 Choroidal Neovascularization Secondary to Angioid Streaks

Choroidal neovascularizations in the era of SD-OCT can be graded as type 1–3 neovascularizations (NV) based on their anatomic location, first described in age-related macular degeneration (AMD). Type 1 NV was defined as the growth of new vessels below the RPE, type 2 NV as the growth of vessels in the subretinal space, and type 3 NV within the retina. Polypoidal choroidal vasculopathy (PCV) is considered as a specific subform of type 1 NV in AMD [37].

Choroidal neovascularization in AS can be of types 1 or 2, or PCV [38]. In classic CNV (type 2 NV), FA typically shows early well-defined hyperfluorescence with dye leakage in later frames (Figs. 13.2a–e). Occult CNV (type 1 NV) may be hidden in FA but can be detected with early hypercyanescence and late leakage using ICG [15]. OCT can show intra- and subretinal fluid as a sign of CNV activity and/or subretinal hyperreflective material (Figs. 13.2e, 13.3, and 13.4).

Polypoidal choroidal vasculopathy may appear as a primary lesion [38] or may develop during the follow-up in association with other types of neovascularizations [39]. Over time type 1 CNV can develop into type 2 CNV [38]. The clinical course of eyes with AS and secondary CNV shows progressive visual loss, compared to eyes without CNV. Vision loss is more pronounced in patients with type 2 NV, and even more with fibrotic scars secondary to previous CNV [38].

Eyes with type 2 CNV also have more secondary complications compared to type 1 CNV, such as subretinal hemorrhage (75 vs. 25%, respectively) or cystoid retinal fluid (78 vs. 13%, respectively) [38]. But severe visual loss due to hemorrhage may also occur in type 1 CNV [40]. Thus, it may be a continuous disease progress of CNV developing under AS before crossing the RPE, which increases morbidity.

Subretinal detachment or subretinal fluid may be signs of CNV activity. However, subretinal fluid can occur in patients without evidence of CNV in FA [28, 41]. In these cases, subretinal fluid is not responsive to treatment with anti-VEGF. Additionally, subretinal fluid can appear at remote locations without connection to active CNV, which also may not be responding to anti-VEGF treatment or cause visual deterioration [28, 41].

Hyperreflective foci are discrete, dot-shaped, hyperreflective lesions solely identifiable on SD-OCT imaging (Fig. 13.4) [42]. Hyperreflective foci are more present in patients with active CNV. They may be an early sign before the recurrence of CNV activity under anti-VEGF treatment in a pro re nata (PRN) regimen. Hyperreflective foci thus may possibly be used as a marker for monitoring CNV activity [42].

Subretinal detachments are less frequent in CNV due to AS than in CNV due to AMD (17 vs. 59%) [20]. Intraretinal or subretinal fluid thus is not a necessary finding in secondary CNV [43]. Outer retinal tubulations are tubular structures, visible in SD-OCT, and first described in AMD [44]. The incidence of outer retinal tubulations is higher in secondary CNV due to AS (71%), compared to CNV due to AMD (34%) [20]. Most (74%) of them appear at the border of a CNV lesion. Submacular choroidal thickness and volume remain normal in patients with AS without CNV. But they are increased in patients with

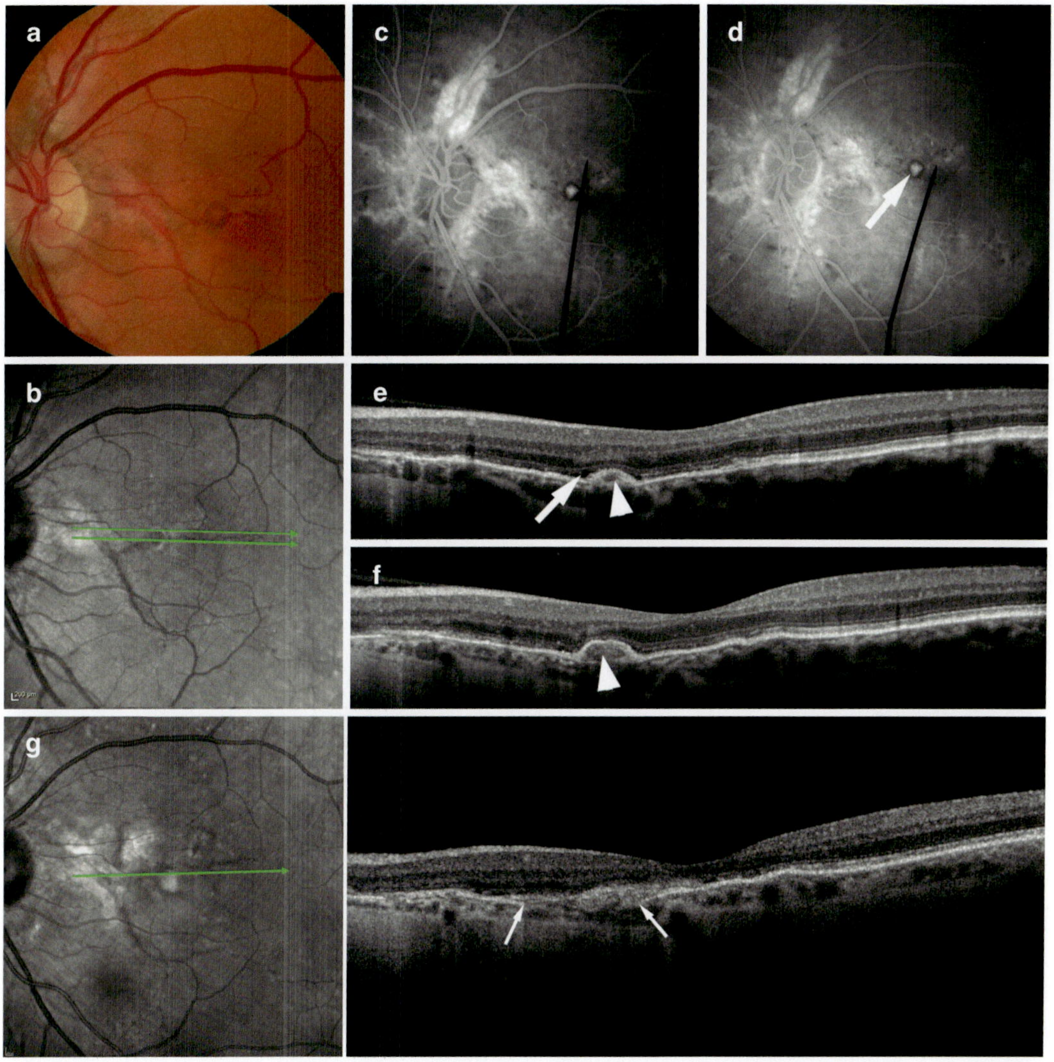

Fig. 13.2 Choroidal neovascularization associated with angioid streaks. Fundus photography (**a**), near-infrared imaging (**b**), middle (**c**) and late (**d**) frames of fluorescein angiography (FA) of the same patient as shown in Fig. 13.1 three years later after initial presentation, now demonstrating a secondary choroidal neovascularization (CNV). BCVA was 20/20, but the patient was symptomatic and reported metamorphopsia. Note the fibrovascular pigment epithelial detachment on OCT (**e**, **f** arrowheads) associated with subretinal fluid (**e**, white arrow) corresponding with the hyperfluorescent lesion on FA. Ten years later under close monitoring and continuous anti-VEGF therapy vision remained 20/20. In the OCT (**g**) larger dehiscences in the Bruch's membrane (between white arrows), advanced CNV with fibrotic tissue, but no subretinal fluid could be detected

secondary CNV due to AS, independently of previous treatment or treatment modality [45].

Optical Coherence Tomography Angiography

Optical coherence tomography angiography offers the possibility to visualize retinal vessels including CNV membranes at very high resolution, and without the need for dye injection. Due to its noninvasive properties and relatively small recording time, OCTA can be used more frequently compared to FA. This provides the basis for a potential use in regular follow-up and treatment monitoring CNV.

Optical coherence tomography angiography is able to detect the majority of, but not all, CNV

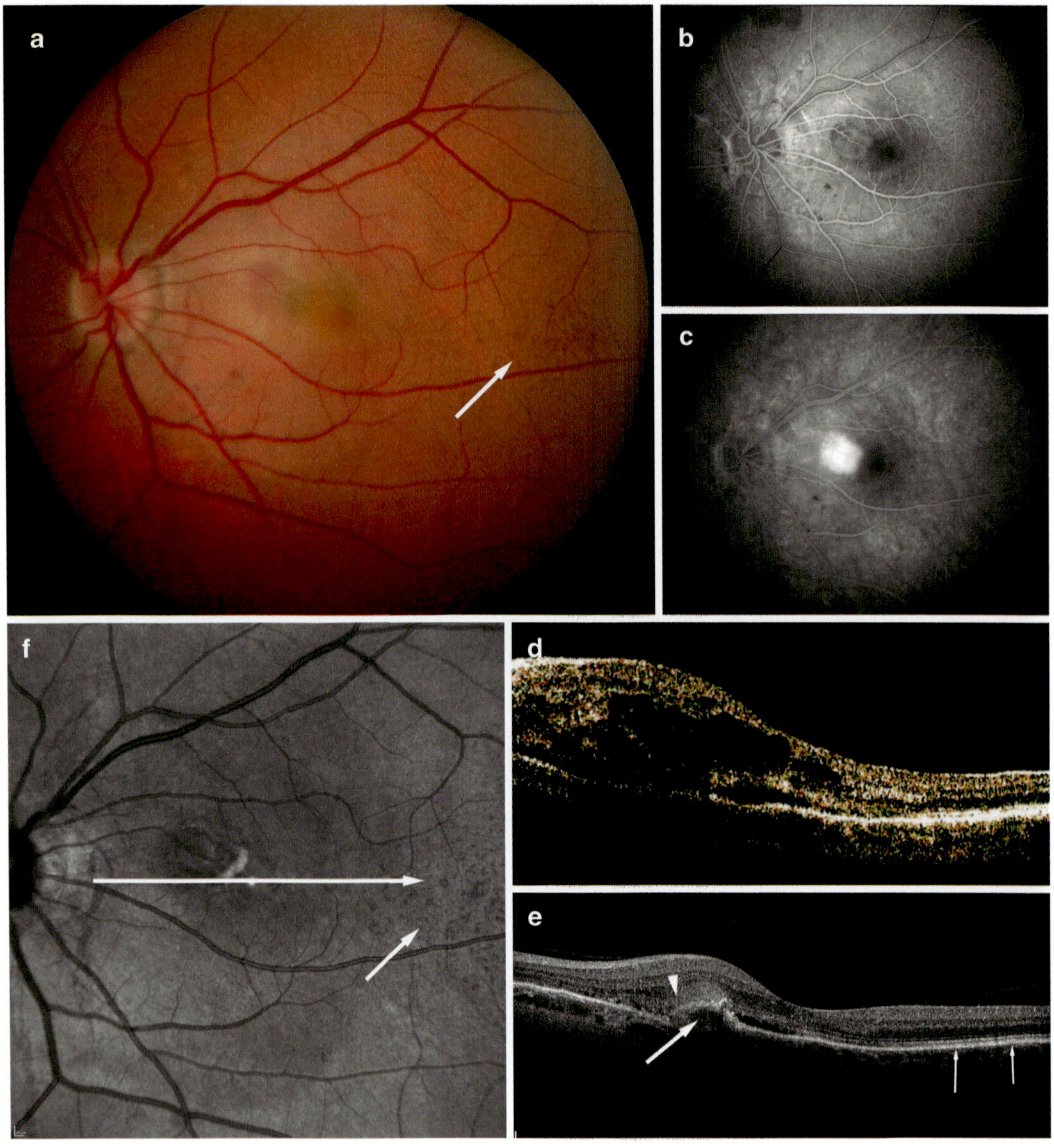

Fig. 13.3 Peau d'orange, angioid streaks, and CNV in a patient with pseudoxanthoma elasticum. Left eye of a 52-year-old female with secondary choroidal neovascularization (CNV) due to angioid streaks (AS) with pseudoxanthoma elasticum (PXE). BCVA at baseline was 20/200, she has been noticing a central scotoma since a few days. Fundus photography (**a**) showing macular hemorrhage associated with a neovascular membrane, AS and peau d'orange (white arrow), fluorescein angiography showing (**b**) early well-defined hyperfluorescence and (**c**) late leakage, and OCT (**d**, time domain at the baseline visit) showing macular thickening with intra- and subretinal fluid. Spectral-domain (SD)-OCT imaging 1 year later under treatment with four anti-VEGF injections with bevacizumab: note the fibrovascular pigment epithelial detachment (**e**, white arrow), subretinal fluid and subretinal hyperreflective material (**e**, white arrowhead). Hyperreflectivity of the outer retinal pigment epithelium/ Bruch's membrane complex appears in SD-OCT in the areas of peau d'orange (**e**, small arrows). Near-infrared image (**f**) indicating the location of B-scan and showing peau d'orange (white arrow)

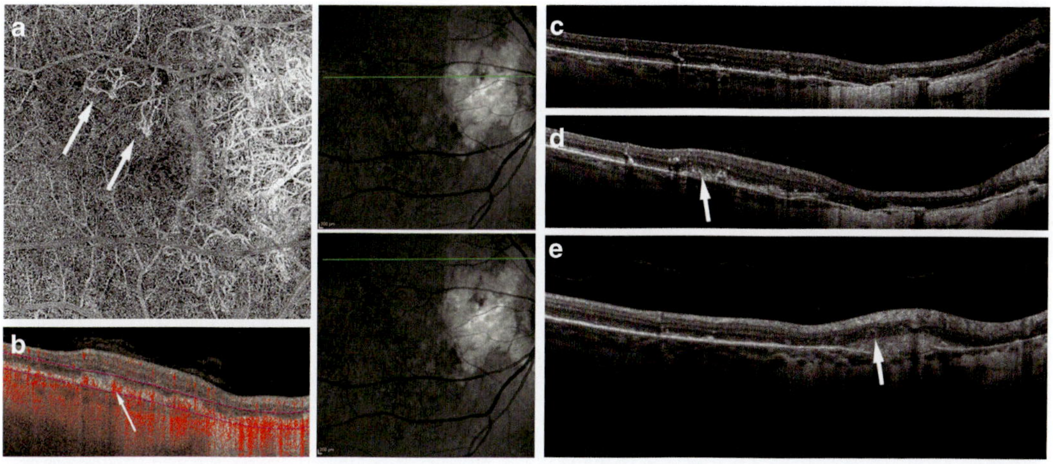

Fig. 13.4 OCT angiography of secondary CNV due to idiopathic angioid streaks. Right eye of a 58-year-old female patient with secondary choroidal neovascularization (CNV) due to idiopathic angioid streaks (AS). Recurrency occurred 6 months after anti-VEGF therapy was paused with the development of CNV in the macular area. At this time point the patient had still good visual acuity (20/20, 91 ETDRS letters) but noticed metamorphopsia. In the en face OCTA slab of the outer retina and choriocapillaris (**a**) there was evidence of a neovascular network (white arrows), corresponding to flow on the B-Scan (**b**, white arrow). In the structural OCT subretinal hyperreflective material (SHRM), suggestive for active CNV could be observed (**d**, white arrow). Note that 2 months prior SHRM was not present (**c**). Outer retinal tubulation overlying a mature neovascular complex can be observed suprapapillary (**e**, white arrow)

proven by FA or ICG (Figs. 13.4, 13.5) [43]. On the other hand, OCTA may be able to detect and monitor the growth of CNV without signs of leakage in FLA or fluid in OCT [40].

In patients after initiation of anti-VEGF treatment, the CNV membrane may appear as a "tangled vascular network" also named "pruned vascular tree" with a loose lace appearance with filamentous vessels and few large branches or vascular trunks. Alternatively, CNV can appear "interlacing" with a densely ramified vascular hyperintensity with a convoluted or cobweb shape, multiple and tortuous thin vessels, and sometimes a perilesional halo. A mixed form is also described [22, 43]. The majority of CNV show foveal or juxtafoveal involvement in OCTA [22, 43].

The interlacing or mixed network is more often associated with CNV activity, and with previous treatment in the last 6 months and activity signs in multimodal imaging using SD-OCT and FA. The interlacing pattern could therefore itself be a possible sign of activity [43]. In the tangled appearing CNV, no activity was described [22].

Of note, the mentioned classification is based on qualitative criteria and its reproducibility and applicability in a clinical setting and treatment decisions remain to be proven.

13.3 Treatment and Monitoring Regimen

Treatment initiation is mainly based on FA and ICG, but OCTA can add additional guidance in treatment initiation and control, as mentioned above. It may also be a suitable tool to exclude active CNV in the case of possibly misleading findings in other imaging modalities, such as subretinal fluid. Due to the lack of larger studies, in

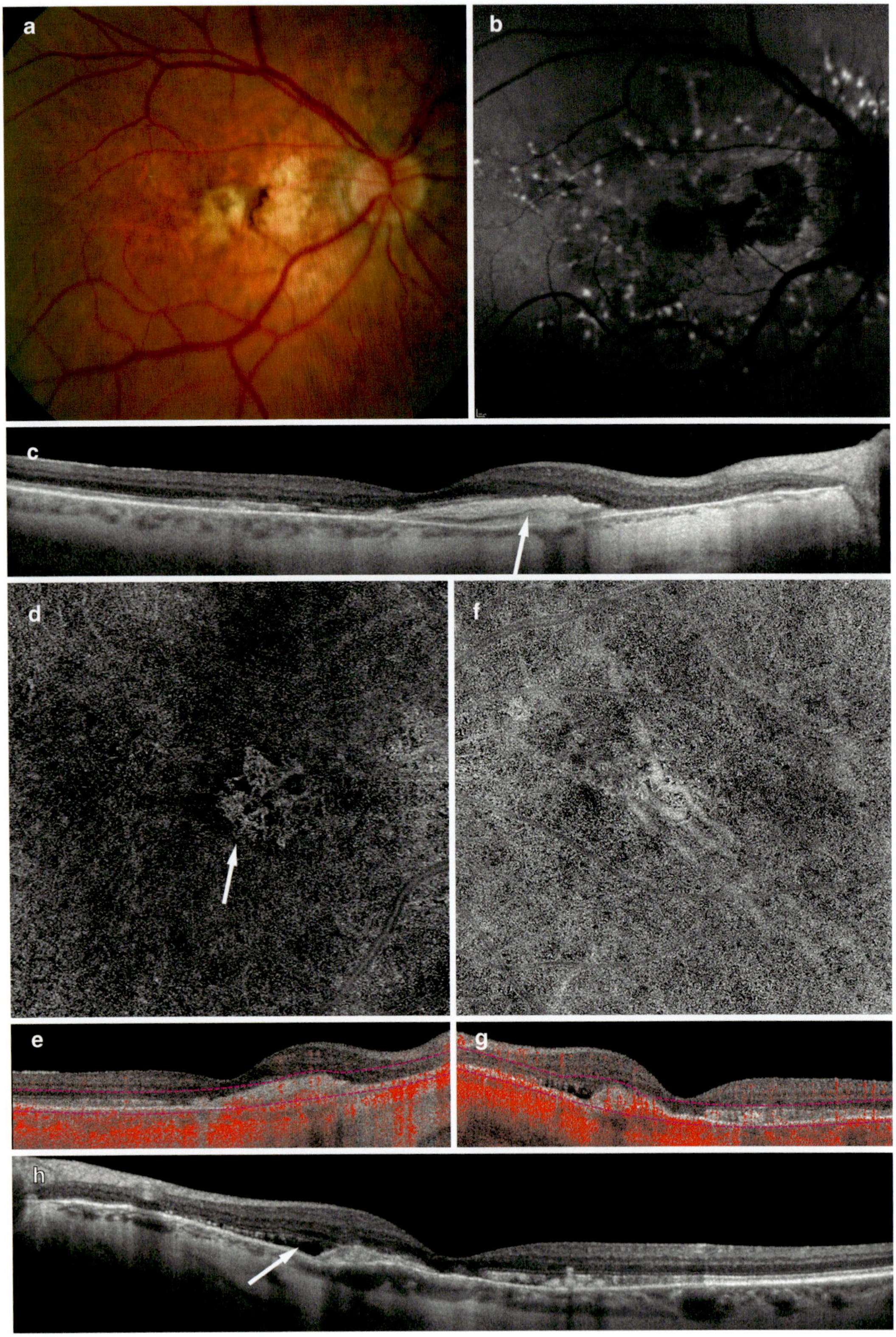
a
b
c
d
f
e
g
h

Fig. 13.5 Long-term follow-up of CNV associated with angioid streaks. Same patient as shown in Fig. 13.3, 10 years later undergoing anti-VEGF therapy in both eyes with an average of six injections per year due to persistent activity. Six weeks after the last injection in the right eye, BCVA was 20/32. Fundus photography (**a**) and fundus autofluorescence (**b**) of the right eye show extrafoveal atrophy and pigment clumping and hyperautofluorescent spots surrounding the atrophy and fibrovascular lesion (**b**). The OCT of the right eye (**c**) shows an advanced (mature) CNV without intra- or subretinal fluid, en face OCTA slab of the outer retina and choriocapillaris (**d**), B-scan with flow overlay in red (**e**), confirms the neovascular network (white arrow). The OCT of the left eye (**h**) 6 weeks after the last injection, shows subretinal hyperreflective material and adjacent subretinal fluid (white arrow), but no definite sign of a neovascular network in the en face OCTA slab of the outer retina and choriocapillaris (**f**), (**g**) B-scan with flow overlay (**g**), BCVA was 20/50. In the right eye, treatment was continued in an extended interval, in the left eye, findings remained stable without treatment

borderline cases, an individual treatment decision will be based on multimodal imaging interpreted by experienced ophthalmologists.

13.3.1 Ranibizumab

13.3.1.1 MINERVA Trial

The efficacy of intravitreal ranibizumab in the treatment of secondary CNV due to AS has been shown in a phase 3 randomized controlled trial. A significant and clinically relevant treatment effect after 2 months using a pro re nata (PRN) regimen, compared to sham in CNV because of an uncommon cause could be shown [46]. In the subgroup of secondary CNV due to AS, after 2 months a BCVA gain (in early treatment of diabetic retinopathy study letters) of +11.0 letters in the ranibizumab arm versus –3.5 letters in the sham arm was found. After 2 months, all patients received open-label ranibizumab according to PRN.

In the overall study population, after 12 months with ranibizumab according to PRN, the change of BCVA was +11.0 letters compared to baseline, with a mean of 5.8 injections. Gain of 15 ETDRS letters occurred in 48.7%, and loss of more than 15 ETDRS in 2.7%. Central subfield thickness as a marker of disease activity decreased by −77.0 μm after month 2, compared to +9.8 μm in the sham group. After 12 months the effect remained stable in the original treatment group with −102.7 μm [46]. Thus, ranibizumab is the only medication with level 1 evidence for treatment of secondary CNV due to AS, yet. Functional and anatomic effects with a PRN regimen are similar to reported monthly treatment for 1 year [47, 48].

A cost-effectiveness analysis of the study population in the MINERVA trial proved PRN intravitreal ranibizumab to be a highly cost-effective intervention in patients with secondary CNV due to other causes than AMD and myopia [49] with costs of 1363£ per quality-adjusted life year in a 2018 United Kingdom setting.

13.3.1.2 Long-Term Treatment Outcomes

Long-term treatment outcomes exist with level 2 evidence from previous non-randomized real-life trials.

The PIXEL study was a retro- and prospective non-randomized trial to evaluate the long-term efficacy of ranibizumab in a real-life setting with a follow-up time of up to 4 years in 29% of patients (mean 39.2 months, SD ±27.3) [50]. In 98 eyes of 72 patients, mean BCVA remained stable from baseline to 4 years of follow-up [50]. The proportion of patients with BCVA stabilization within 15 ETDRS letters from baseline was 77.3% after 2 years and 52% after 4 years. Best corrected visual acuity loss of more than 15 ETDRS letters occurred in 11.4% after 2 years, and 26.3% after 4 years. The proportions of eyes with CNV dropped from 68.4% at baseline to 32.1% after four years, and the proportion of CNV leakage from 39.8% to 14.3%, respectively [50]. The mean annual number of injections was 4.1 in the first and 2.7 in the second year [50]. Other levels 2 and 3 studies and case reports show similar long-term outcomes for up to 6 years [51–53].

13.3.2 Bevacizumab

A series of retrospective or non-randomized smaller studies or case series using bevacizumab showed similar results. Best corrected visual acuity stabilization within 2 ETDRS lines or BCVA increase compared to baseline, were shown in 65.2–100% of eyes with a follow-up time of 12–100 months [20, 54–58]. Signs of disease activity or recurrence were frequent even after treatment. Eyes with early disease showed significantly better visual gain than with advanced disease [56]. An initial gain of mean BCVA could not always be maintained over 24 or 36 months, but mean BCVA remained stable compared to the initial baseline [59]. In younger patients, CNV seems to behave more aggressively [60].

A retrospective analysis of 52 eyes of 39 patients treated with both ranibizumab and bevacizumab showed an overall deterioration in mean BCVA of an average of 6.8 ETDRS letters with a mean follow-up of 33.8 months (SD 19.6) [61]. Within this group, the patients with subfoveal CNV had higher BCVA loss, compared to non-subfoveal, with a loss of 11 versus 3 ETDRS letters per year [61]. Summing up, there is a level 2 evidence for bevacizumab in CNV due to AS.

13.3.3 Aflibercept

Intravitreal injections with aflibercept using a PRN regimen has been reported as an effective therapy in treatment-naïve CNV due to AS in case reports [42, 62]. In a case report treat and extend (T&E) regimen using aflibercept has been reported as being effective after 1 year with a total of six injections [63].

Whether a PRN regimen is superior to T&E remains an object of clinical reasoning based on the understanding of the disease. Most studies, among the MINERVA trial, used PRN [64].

Aflibercept has shown functional and anatomic improvement in treating refractory visual loss and CNV activity after previous bevacizumab and ranibizumab treatment in CNV due to AS in case reports, possibly offering the potential as a second-line treatment option. To date, this evidence remains level 3 [65, 66].

13.3.4 Historic Treatment Regimens

13.3.4.1 Laser Photocoagulation and Transpupillary Thermotherapy

Thermal photocoagulation was aimed to coagulate CNV to stop vessel hyperpermeability and disease progression. It was historically the first treatment for AMD-related CNV [6]. Results of various reports in secondary CNV due to AS overall were not convincing, at best leading to stabilization or slowing down of visual loss in most cases [6]. Frequent retreatments were necessary with a delay of the natural history of the disease being the best achievable outcome. Additionally, laser photocoagulation leads to an immediate drop in retinal function at the treated area. Thus, it is frequently resulting in vision loss and central scotoma, due to the central localization of CNV.

Transpupillary thermotherapy was tried intending to obliterate CNV vessels, without a positive or lasting effect [6].

13.3.4.2 Surgical Treatments

Subretinal CNV extraction and macular translocation surgery have been reported to treat CNV secondary to AS [6]. Short-term stabilization of visual acuity was achieved, but recurrences and complications were frequent.

13.3.4.3 Photodynamic Therapy

Photodynamic therapy (PDT) with verteporfin is more selectively destroying CNV with less collateral tissue damage and proved favorable over the natural history of the disease in AMD-related CNV [6]. Most conducted studies showed slowing down of disease progression and visual deterioration. The effect was independent of standard 3-monthly or more frequent treatment protocols. A meta-analysis from 2013 showed an overall visual loss after PDT, compared to baseline [6]. Lesion size also increased under PDT treatment in all studies which reported this outcome parameter. The same meta-analysis showed the benefit of anti-VEGF agents compared to PDT prior to the randomized controlled trial [6]. Combination therapy of PDT and anti-VEGF did not show a benefit over anti-VEGF alone.

13.4 Summary

Angioid streaks are a rare ophthalmologic finding. They are frequently associated with systemic disease. Pseudoxanthoma elasticum is the most frequent association and, besides ocular morbidity, carries a cardiovascular risk. Secondary CNV occur in a large proportion of patients with AS. Untreated, they have an unfavorable course with progredient vision loss in young patients. Thus, regular examinations of patients with AS is recommended, yearly or biyearly under 40 years of age, and twice a year thereafter [13].

The current mainstay of treatment of secondary CNV due to AS are intravitreal anti-VEGF agents using a PRN regimen with level 1 evidence for ranibizumab, level 2 evidence for bevacizumab, and level 3 evidence for aflibercept [6, 46]. Treatment outcome is better at early stages of disease. Together with the progressive natural course of the disease this prompts for regular screening and early treatment of affected patients with AS and secondary CNV, respectively. Using Anti-VEGF, an early BCVA gain of mean 2 ETDRS lines after 2 months has been reported, remaining stable for 12 months with a mean of 5.8 injections [46]. Stabilization within 15 ETDRS letters was retrospectively shown in 77.3% after 2 years and 52% after 4 years [50].

Multimodal imaging is necessary for diagnosis, treatment decision, and monitoring. AS are best visualized with NIR. FAF additionally shows atrophy and pattern dystrophy-like changes, which can be precursors of vision loss and CNV. Active CNVs demonstrate leakage in angiography and are often associated with hyperreflective foci, subretinal hyperreflective material, and intra- or subretinal fluid in OCT. Optical coherence tomography angiography offers additional guidance in therapy, specifically in detecting the growth of otherwise inactive CNV. It may also be of help in cases of isolated subretinal fluid without concomitant CNV, and thus refractory to treatment (Figs. 13.4, 13.5).

13.5 Key Learning Points

- Angioid streaks have a complex pathogenesis, can be related to many clinical conditions, of which PXE is the most frequent, but are also observed as an isolated ocular finding (idiopathic).
- Deformation and ruptures of BM are associated with angioid streaks as shown by histology and OCT.
- The development of CNV is suggested to occur at locations of BM breaks. Secondary CNV can lead to severe visual loss in relatively young patients.
- Type 1 and 2 CNV seem to be a continuous disease progress emanating at locations of BM breaks.
- In active CNV treatment is recommended using intravitreal anti-VEGF agents in a pro re nata regimen. A treat and extend regimen might be a good alternative; however, there is only limited evidence supporting this.
- OCT angiography can provide additional information in less active CNV or subretinal fluid without CNV. Classification of CNV activity using OCTA has been based on qualitative criteria; however, its reproducibility remains to be proven.
- Multimodal imaging is important in the diagnosis and treatment of CNV associated with AS.

References

1. Doyne R. Choroidal and retinal changes. The results of blows on the eyes. Trans Ophthalmol Soc UK. 1889;9:128.
2. Knapp H. On formation of dark angiod streaks as an unusual metamorphosis of retinal hemorrhage. Arch Ophthalmol (Chicago, Ill: 1960). 1892;21:289.
3. Chatziralli I, Saitakis G, Dimitriou E, Chatzirallis A, Stoungioti S, Theodossiadis G, et al. ANGIOID streaks: a comprehensive review from pathophysi-

ology to treatment. Retina (Philadelphia, PA). 2019;39(1):1–11.
4. Kumudhan D, Wallace EJ, Roxburgh ST. Angioid streaks in identical twins. Br J Ophthalmol. 2004;88(6):837–8.
5. Abujamra S, Negretto AD, Saraceno JJ, Oliveira TL, Gomes AM. Angioid streaks: fundoscopic analysis of 317 cases. Arq Bras Oftalmol. 2008;71(6):819–21.
6. Gliem M, Finger RP, Fimmers R, Brinkmann CK, Holz FG, Charbel IP. Treatment of choroidal neovascularization due to angioid streaks: a comprehensive review. Retina (Philadelphia, PA). 2013;33(7):1300–14.
7. Finger RP, Charbel Issa P, Ladewig MS, Gotting C, Szliska C, Scholl HP, et al. Pseudoxanthoma elasticum: genetics, clinical manifestations and therapeutic approaches. Surv Ophthalmol. 2009;54(2):272–85.
8. Hu X, Plomp AS, van Soest S, Wijnholds J, de Jong PT, Bergen AA. Pseudoxanthoma elasticum: a clinical, histopathological, and molecular update. Surv Ophthalmol. 2003;48(4):424–38.
9. Van Gils M, Nollet L, Verly E, Deianova N, Vanakker OM. Cellular signaling in pseudoxanthoma elasticum: an update. Cell Signal. 2019;55:119–29.
10. Kerr NM, Cassinelli HR, DiMeglio LA, Tau C, Tuysuz B, Cundy T, et al. Ocular manifestations of juvenile Paget disease. Arch Ophthalmol (Chicago, Ill: 1960). 2010;128(6):698–703.
11. Aessopos A, Farmakis D, Loukopoulos D. Elastic tissue abnormalities resembling pseudoxanthoma elasticum in beta thalassemia and the sickling syndromes. Blood. 2002;99(1):30–5.
12. Fajardo Sanchez J, Chau Ramos CE, Mazagatos Used PJ, Aparicio Hernandez-Lastras MJ. The effect of the acceleration/deceleration trauma in angioid streaks: a pathogenic hypothesis. Archivos de la Sociedad Espanola de Oftalmologia. 2016;91(9):446–9.
13. Orssaud C, Roche O, Dufier JL, Germain DP. Visual impairment in pseudoxanthoma elasticum: a survey of 40 patients. Ophthalmic Genet. 2015;36(4):327–32.
14. Ari Yaylali S, Akcakaya AA, Erbil HH, Salar S, Karakurt Y. Optical coherence tomography findings in pseudoxanthoma elasticum. Eur J Ophthalmol. 2010;20(2):397–401.
15. Arvas S, Akar S, Yolar M, Yetik H, Kizilkaya M, Ozkan S. Optical coherence tomography (OCT) and angiography in patients with angioid streaks. Eur J Ophthalmol. 2002;12(6):473–81.
16. Charbel Issa P, Finger RP, Holz FG, Scholl HP. Multimodal imaging including spectral domain OCT and confocal near infrared reflectance for characterization of outer retinal pathology in pseudoxanthoma elasticum. Invest Ophthalmol Vis Sci. 2009;50(12):5913–8.
17. Finger RP, Charbel Issa P, Ladewig M, Gotting C, Holz FG, Scholl HP. Fundus autofluorescence in pseudoxanthoma elasticum. Retina (Philadelphia, PA). 2009;29(10):1496–505.
18. Sawa M, Ober MD, Freund KB, Spaide RF. Fundus autofluorescence in patients with pseudoxanthoma elasticum. Ophthalmology. 2006;113(5):814–20.e2.
19. Marchese A, Parravano M, Rabiolo A, Carnevali A, Corbelli E, Cicinelli MV, et al. Optical coherence tomography analysis of evolution of Bruch's membrane features in angioid streaks. Eye. 2017;31(11):1600–5.
20. Ellabban AA, Hangai M, Yamashiro K, Nakagawa S, Tsujikawa A, Yoshimura N. Tomographic fundus features in pseudoxanthoma elasticum: comparison with neovascular age-related macular degeneration in Japanese patients. Eye (Lond). 2012;26(8):1086–94.
21. Hanhart J, Greifner H, Rozenman Y. Locating and characterizing angioid streaks with en face optical coherence tomography. Retin Cases Brief Rep. 2017;11(3):203–6.
22. Corbelli E, Carnevali A, Marchese A, Cicinelli MV, Querques L, Sacconi R, et al. Optical coherence tomography angiography features of angioid streaks. Retina (Philadelphia, PA). 2018;38(11):2128–36.
23. Spaide RF. Choriocapillaris signal voids in maternally inherited diabetes and deafness and in pseudoxanthoma elasticum. Retina (Philadelphia, PA). 2017;37(11):2008–14.
24. Smith JL, Gass JD, Justice J Jr. Fluorescein fundus photography of angioid streaks. Br J Ophthalmol. 1964;48:517–21.
25. Gliem M, Hendig D, Finger RP, Holz FG, Charbel IP. Reticular pseudodrusen associated with a diseased bruch membrane in pseudoxanthoma elasticum. JAMA Ophthalmology. 2015;133(5):581–8.
26. Spaide RF. Peau d'orange and angioid streaks: manifestations of Bruch membrane pathology. Retina (Philadelphia, PA). 2015;35(3):392–7.
27. Zweifel SA, Spaide RF, Curcio CA, Malek G, Imamura Y. Reticular pseudodrusen are subretinal drusenoid deposits. Ophthalmology. 2010;117(2):303–12.e1.
28. Zweifel SA, Imamura Y, Freund KB, Spaide RF. Multimodal fundus imaging of pseudoxanthoma elasticum. Retina (Philadelphia, PA). 2011;31(3):482–91.
29. Gass JD. "Comet" lesion: an ocular sign of pseudoxanthoma elasticum. Retina (Philadelphia, PA). 2003;23(5):729–30.
30. Barteselli G, Viola F. Comet lesions in pseudoxanthoma elasticum: a spectral domain optical coherence tomography analysis. Retina (Philadelphia, PA). 2015;35(5):1051–3.
31. Gliem M, Muller PL, Birtel J, McGuinness MB, Finger RP, Herrmann P, et al. Quantitative fundus autofluorescence in pseudoxanthoma elasticum. Invest Ophthalmol Vis Sci. 2017;58(14):6159–65.
32. Agarwal A, Patel P, Adkins T, Gass JD. Spectrum of pattern dystrophy in pseudoxanthoma elasticum. Arch Ophthalmol (Chicago, Ill: 1960). 2005;123(7):923–8.
33. Ebran JM, Martin L, Leftheriotis, Navasiolava N, Ferre M, Milea D, et al. Subretinal fibrosis is associated with fundus pulverulentus in pseudoxanthoma

elasticum. Graefes Arch Clin Exp Ophthalmol. 2018;256(4):699–707.
34. Gliem M, Muller PL, Birtel J, Hendig D, Holz FG, Charbel IP. Frequency, phenotypic characteristics and progression of atrophy associated with a diseased Bruch's membrane in pseudoxanthoma elasticum. Invest Ophthalmol Vis Sci. 2016;57(7):3323–30.
35. Sadda SR, Guymer R, Holz FG, Schmitz-Valckenberg S, Curcio CA, Bird AC, et al. Consensus definition for atrophy associated with age-related macular degeneration on OCT: classification of atrophy report 3. Ophthalmology. 2018;125(4):537–48.
36. Schoenberger SD, Agarwal A. Geographic chorioretinal atrophy in pseudoxanthoma elasticum. Am J Ophthalmol. 2013;156(4):715–23.
37. Freund KB, Zweifel SA, Engelbert M. Do we need a new classification for choroidal neovascularization in age-related macular degeneration? Retina (Philadelphia, PA). 2010;30(9):1333–49.
38. Nakagawa S, Yamashiro K, Tsujikawa A, Otani A, Tamura H, Ooto S, et al. The time course changes of choroidal neovascularization in angioid streaks. Retina (Philadelphia, PA). 2013;33(4):825–33.
39. Baillif-Gostoli S, Quaranta-El Maftouhi M, Mauget-Faysse M. Polypoidal choroidal vasculopathy in a patient with angioid streaks secondary to pseudoxanthoma elasticum. Graefes Arch Clin Exp Ophthalmol. 2010;248(12):1845–8.
40. Andreanos KD, Rotsos T, Koutsandrea C, Kymionis GD, Georgalas I, Ladas ID. Detection of nonexudative choroidal neovascularization secondary to angioid streaks using optical coherence tomography angiography. Eur J Ophthalmol. 2017;27(5):e140–e3.
41. Hansen MS, Klefter ON, Larsen M. Retinal degeneration and persistent serous detachment in the absence of active choroidal neovascularization in pseudoxanthoma elasticum. Acta Ophthalmol. 2014;92(2):e156–7.
42. Parodi MB, Arrigo A, Romano F, Aragona E, Marchese A, Cicinelli MV, et al. Hyperreflective foci number correlates with choroidal neovascularization activity in angioid streaks. Invest Ophthalmol Vis Sci. 2018;59(8):3314–9.
43. Chapron T, Mimoun G, Miere A, Srour M, El Ameen A, Semoun O, et al. Optical coherence tomography angiography features of choroidal neovascularization secondary to angioid streaks. Eye. 2018;33:385–91.
44. Zweifel SA, Engelbert M, Laud K, Margolis R, Spaide RF, Freund KB. Outer retinal tubulation: a novel optical coherence tomography finding. Arch Ophthalmol (Chicago, Ill: 1960). 2009;127(12):1596–602.
45. Ellabban AA, Tsujikawa A, Matsumoto A, Ogino K, Hangai M, Ooto S, et al. Macular choroidal thickness and volume in eyes with angioid streaks measured by swept source optical coherence tomography. Am J Ophthalmol. 2012;153(6):1133–43.e1.
46. Lai TYY, Staurenghi G, Lanzetta P, Holz FG, Melissa Liew SH, Desset-Brethes S, et al. Efficacy and safety of ranibizumab for the treatment of choroidal neovascularization due to uncommon cause: twelve-month results of the MINERVA study. Retina (Philadelphia, PA). 2018;38(8):1464–77.
47. Finger RP, Charbel Issa P, Hendig D, Scholl HP, Holz FG. Monthly ranibizumab for choroidal neovascularizations secondary to angioid streaks in pseudoxanthoma elasticum: a one-year prospective study. Am J Ophthalmol. 2011;152(4):695–703.
48. Heier JS, Brown D, Ciulla T, Abraham P, Bankert JM, Chong S, et al. Ranibizumab for choroidal neovascularization secondary to causes other than age-related macular degeneration: a phase I clinical trial. Ophthalmology. 2011;118(1):111–8.
49. McCarthy G, Fenu E, Bennett N, Almond C. Intravitreal Ranibizumab for the treatment of visual impairment due to choroidal neovascularization associated with rare diseases: cost-effectiveness in the UK. Adv Ther. 2019;36(3):632–44.
50. Mimoun G, Ebran JM, Grenet T, Donati A, Cohen SY, Ponthieux A. Ranibizumab for choroidal neovascularization secondary to pseudoxanthoma elasticum: 4-year results from the PIXEL study in France. Graefes Arch Clin Exp Ophthalmol. 2017;255(8):1651–60.
51. Tilleul J, Mimoun G, Querques G, Puche N, Zerbib J, Lalloum F, et al. Intravitreal ranibizumab for choroidal neovascularization in angioid streaks: four-year follow-up. Retina (Philadelphia, PA). 2016;36(3):483–91.
52. Zebardast N, Adelman RA. Intravitreal ranibizumab for treatment of choroidal neovascularization secondary to angioid streaks in pseudoxanthoma elasticum: five-year follow-up. Semin Ophthalmol. 2012;27(3-4):61–4.
53. Savastano MC, Minnella AM, Zinzanella G, Falsini B, Caporossi A. Successful long-term management of choroidal neovascularization secondary to angioid streaks in a patient with pseudoxanthoma elasticum: a case report. J Med Case Rep. 2014;8:458.
54. Lekha T, Prasad HN, Sarwate RN, Patel M, Karthikeyan S. Intravitreal bevacizumab for choroidal neovascularization associated with Angioid streaks: long-term results. Middle East Afr J Ophthalmol. 2017;24(3):136–42.
55. El Matri L, Kort F, Bouraoui R, Karim B, Chebil A, Chaker N. Intravitreal bevacizumab for the treatment of choroidal neovascularization secondary to angioid streaks: one year of follow-up. Acta Ophthalmol. 2011;89(7):641–6.
56. Finger RP, Charbel Issa P, Schmitz-Valckenberg S, Holz FG, Scholl HN. Long-term effectiveness of intravitreal bevacizumab for choroidal neovascularization secondary to angioid streaks in pseudoxanthoma elasticum. Retina (Philadelphia, PA). 2011;31(7):1268–78.
57. Mimoun G, Tilleul J, Leys A, Coscas G, Soubrane G, Souied EH. Intravitreal ranibizumab for choroidal neovascularization in angioid streaks. Am J Ophthalmol. 2010;150(5):692–700.e1.
58. Sawa M, Gomi F, Tsujikawa M, Sakaguchi H, Tano Y. Long-term results of intravitreal bevacizumab injec-

tion for choroidal neovascularization secondary to angioid streaks. Am J Ophthalmol. 2009;148(4):584–90.e2.
59. Iacono P, Battaglia Parodi M, La Spina C, Bandello F. Intravitreal bevacizumab for nonsubfoveal choroidal neovascularization associated with angioid streaks: 3-year follow-up study. Am J Ophthalmol. 2016;165:174–8.
60. Alagoz C, Alagoz N, Ozkaya A, Celik U, Turan MF, Yazici AT, et al. Intravitreal bevacizumab in the treatment of choroidal neovascular membrane due to angioid streaks. Retina (Philadelphia, PA). 2015;35(10):2001–10.
61. Giacomelli G, Finocchio L, Biagini I, Sodi A, Murro V, Introini U, et al. Long-term follow-up of choroidal neovascularization due to angioid streaks with pro re nata intravitreal anti-VEGF treatment. Ophthalmologica. 2017;238(1-2):44–51.
62. Vaz-Pereira S, Collaco L, De Salvo G, van Zeller P. Intravitreal aflibercept for choroidal neovascularisation in angioid streaks. Eye (Lond). 2015;29(9):1236–8.
63. Diago T. Treat and extend regimen with aflibercept for choroidal neovascularization in angioid streaks. Eye (Lond). 2016;30(4):637–9.
64. Vaz-Pereira S, Collaco L, De Salvo G, van Zeller P. Intravitreal aflibercept for choroidal neovascularisation in angioid streaks. Eye (Lond). 2016;30(4):639.
65. Tetikoglu M, Sagdik HM, Aktas S, Ozcura F. Intravitreal aflibercept for refractory choroidal neovascularization secondary to angioid streaks. Eye (Lond). 2016;30(6):894–5.
66. Esen E, Sizmaz S, Demircan N. Intravitreal aflibercept for management of subfoveal choroidal neovascularization secondary to angioid streaks. Indian J Ophthalmol. 2015;63(7):616–8.

Idiopathic Choroidal Neovascularization

14

Faisal A. Almarek and Sulaiman M. Alsulaiman

14.1 Introduction

Choroidal neovascularization (CNV) per se is a description of a pathological entity rather than a diagnostic term, when it is attributed to an ocular or systemic cause such as age-related macular degeneration (AMD), degenerative myopia, inflammatory/infectious causes, pseudoxanthoma elasticum, etc., a diagnosis is reached. More than 30 ocular conditions have been associated with choroidal neovascularization [1].

Formerly named hemorrhagic macular choroidopathy, idiopathic focal subretinal neovascularization, or focal macular choroidopathy, idiopathic CNV is considered a diagnosis of exclusion in which no primary ocular or systemic disease is identified. It has been described to occur in healthy patients under the age of 50 years [2–4]. The majority of the ophthalmic research on choroidal neovascularization is focused on age-related macular degeneration, which is considered the most common cause of CNV. In comparison, studies on idiopathic CNV are scarce. This could be attributed to the relatively limited number of patients with this condition [5]. Because it affects younger patients in their working age, a significant impact on visual function over a longer life span may ensue.

14.2 Pathogenesis

The pathogenesis of CNV is speculated to be a nonspecific healing mechanism to a specific stimulus that is the underlying ocular or systemic disease. It is characterized by new vessel formation that passes through stages of activity and involution [6]. Gass has classified the neovascular formation based on biomicroscopic and histopathologic findings from surgical specimens to type 1 lesion, that is under the retinal pigment epithelium (RPE), which is usually found in AMD, or type 2 lesion located under the retina, that is usually associated with presumed ocular histoplasmosis (POHS) [7]. Histopathological studies were conducted on surgically excised subfoveal idiopathic CNV and were compared to other specimens in patients with CNV secondary to AMD and POHS. The microscopic examination identified the presence of RPE cells, vascular endothelial cells, photoreceptors, macrophages, myofibroblasts, glial cells, and erythrocytes. The histopathological findings in idiopathic CNV were similar to those of AMD and POHS with the exception of basal laminar linear deposits found in membranes from patients with AMD [8].

F. A. Almarek
College of medicine, Imam Mohammad bin Saud Islamic University, Riyadh, Saudi Arabia

S. M. Alsulaiman (✉)
Vitreoretinal Division, King Khaled Eye Specialist Hospital, Riyadh, Saudi Arabia
e-mail: ssulaiman@kkesh.med.sa

J. Chhablani (ed.), *Choroidal Neovascularization*, https://doi.org/10.1007/978-981-15-2213-0_14

Although histopathological studies did not show a significant difference among CNV samples from different etiologies, Ho et al. [2] proposed that subfoveal idiopathic CNV could be focal in nature and these membranes are enveloped with a bilayer of RPE similar to those seen in POHS type 2 CNV membranes that result in smaller lesions and greater preservation of the photoreceptors, and hence a more favorable outcome compared to CNV secondary to AMD.

Idiopathic CNV has the tendency toward affecting the posterior pole rather than the peripheral retina. The cause of this remains speculative. Bottoni and associates [4] proposed that the nature of the choroidal vasculature in the macular area plays a role. As a watershed area of end arterial supply (branches of short posterior arteries) to this area has a temporally diminished blood supply which secondarily affects the Bruch's membrane, RPE and causes neovascularization. Although no abnormality in the lobular choroidal filling of the macular area was established in their study.

Lee and colleagues [9] further studied the topographical relation between choroidal watershed zones (CWZs) and idiopathic CNV. Based on indocyanine green angiography (ICGA) findings of previous studies by Hayashi and de Laey [10], CWZs were classified into four categories: I, nasal filling; II-A, temporal filling; II-B, temporal filling with delayed fluorescence in the foveal area; III, upper or lower temporal quadrant filling; and IV, scattered dye filling. They found that CWZs involving the fovea were seen in more patients with idiopathic CNV than in the control group, suggesting that CWZs were related to idiopathic CNV topographically, and CWZ classification was a predictor of the functional outcomes. This indicates that choroidal perfusion could play a role in the development of CNV in young to middle-age patients.

Subfoveal choroidal thickness (SCT) in patients with unilateral idiopathic CNV was compared to the fellow normal eyes and was found to be significantly thicker. Furthermore, treatment with intravitreal anti-vascular endothelial growth factor (VEGF) led to a decrease in the SCT, and reactivation of idiopathic CNV was associated with increased SCT. Thicker subfoveal choroid may be related to choroidal hyperpermeability, which is associated with the development of idiopathic CNV, and SCT changes may reflect disease activity [11].

Although no systemic diseases are usually identified in idiopathic CNV, one study by Sasahara and colleagues [12] looked into the circulating hematopoietic stem cells (HSCs) in patients with idiopathic CNV, which was compared to a control group with no CNV or systemic disease. HSCs play a role in normal and pathological postnatal angiogenesis. These cells are derived from bone marrow and can differentiate into various cells, which are thought to play an important role in tissue injury repair. In their study, HSCs were collected from peripheral blood, followed by an evaluation of the functional activity of these cells between the groups. They found that some of the functional activities were reduced in patients with idiopathic CNV especially in patients with progressing lesions. Based on these findings, they concluded that the functional activity of circulating HSCs may be a novel biomarker for idiopathic CNV.

Choroidal inflammation is a known cause of CNV. Many uveitic entities such as Vogt–Koyanagi–Harada disease, serpiginous choroiditis, white dot syndromes, and others could be complicated by choroidal neovascular membrane formation. In idiopathic CNV, no apparent signs of inflammation are detectable by clinical examination but some investigators proposed that subclinical inflammation might play a role, whether it is localized to the choroid [13] or systemic. Yang et al. [14] reported in their study of serum inflammatory markers in patients with idiopathic CNV that serum VEGF was significantly higher in patients with idiopathic CNV compared to healthy subjects. This might lead to an increased VEGF in the macula through circulation given the nature of rich blood supply by the fenestrated choriocapillaris. This finding was consistent with studies on patients with CNV secondary to AMD [15, 16]. On the other hand, local (intraocular) inflammatory markers are believed to be contributing to the pathogenesis of CNV in AMD [17–

20]. In eyes with idiopathic CNV, multiple studies looked at the inflammatory markers of samples obtained from the aqueous humor. Yin et al. [21] studied the level of multiple inflammatory markers in patients with idiopathic CNV including 27 cytokines. Compared to a control group, there was a significantly higher level of IL-2, IL-10, IL-15, IL-17, basic FGF, and GM-CSF. After adjusting for the axial length between the groups, IL-17 was the only significantly higher cytokine in the idiopathic CNV group. IL-17 is an inflammatory cytokine that plays a role in multiple autoimmune and inflammatory diseases. It is also known to promote the angiogenesis effect of VEGF.

14.3 Clinical Features, Multimodal Imaging, and Differential Diagnosis

As mentioned earlier, idiopathic CNV usually affects the posterior pole. The proposed theory could be related to the nature of the choroidal circulation in the macular area [4, 10]. Fundus examination often reveals a grayish membrane in the macula with or without sub-macular hemorrhage. It is usually unilateral but bilateral cases have been reported (Fig. 14.1) [3, 22, 23].

Fluorescein angiography (FA) and ICGA are commonly used for diagnosing CNV of various etiologies. FA usually shows an early phase

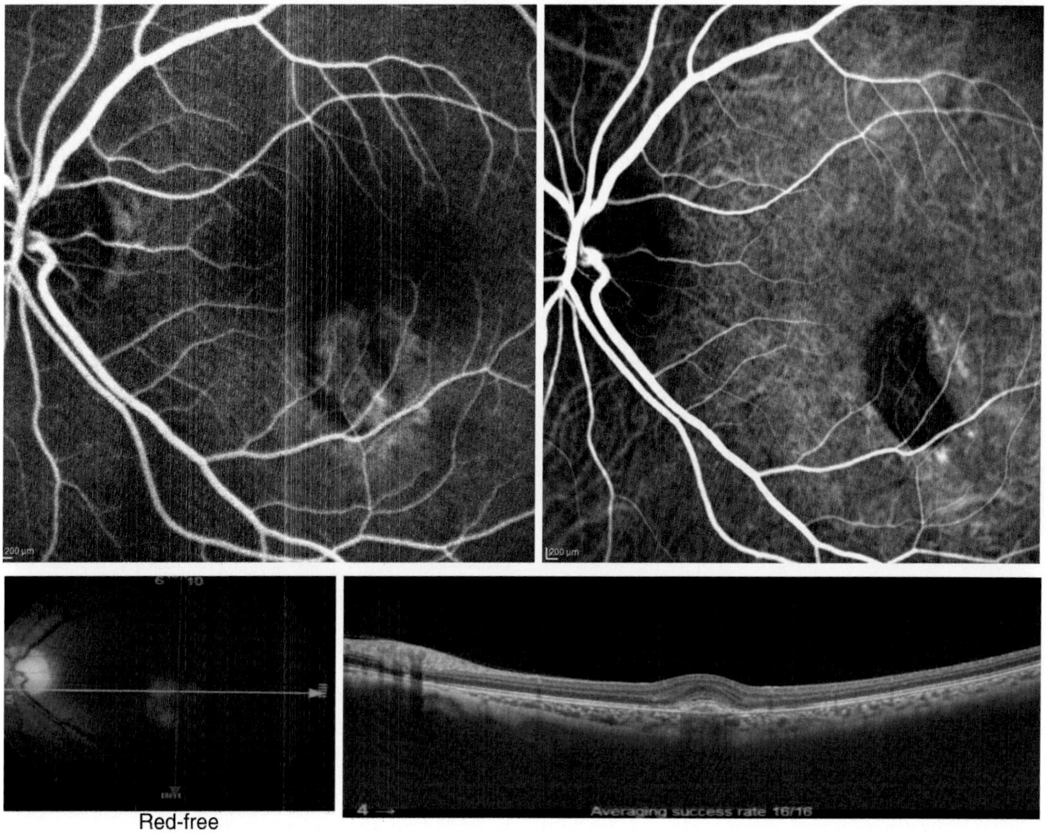

Fig. 14.1 A 36-year old female presented with diminution of vision since 2 months in her left eye. Clinical examination revealed the presence of choroidal neovascular membrane (CNV) with subretinal heamorrhage and subretinal fluid. Late venous phase of the fluorescein angiogram (top left) and early phase of the indocyanine green angiogram(top right) showed a well defined classic CNV. Optical coherence tomography (middle) passing through the lesion showed a type 2 CNV with subretinal fluid. The optical coherence tomography angiography shows the presence of neovascular network in the outer retina and choriocapillaris segments (bottom). A diagnosis of idiopathic CNV was made based on exclusion and the patient received three monthly anti-VEGF injections following which her vision improved significantly. Courtesy Dr. Vishal Gowindhari, LV Prasad Eye Institute, Bhubhaneswar, India

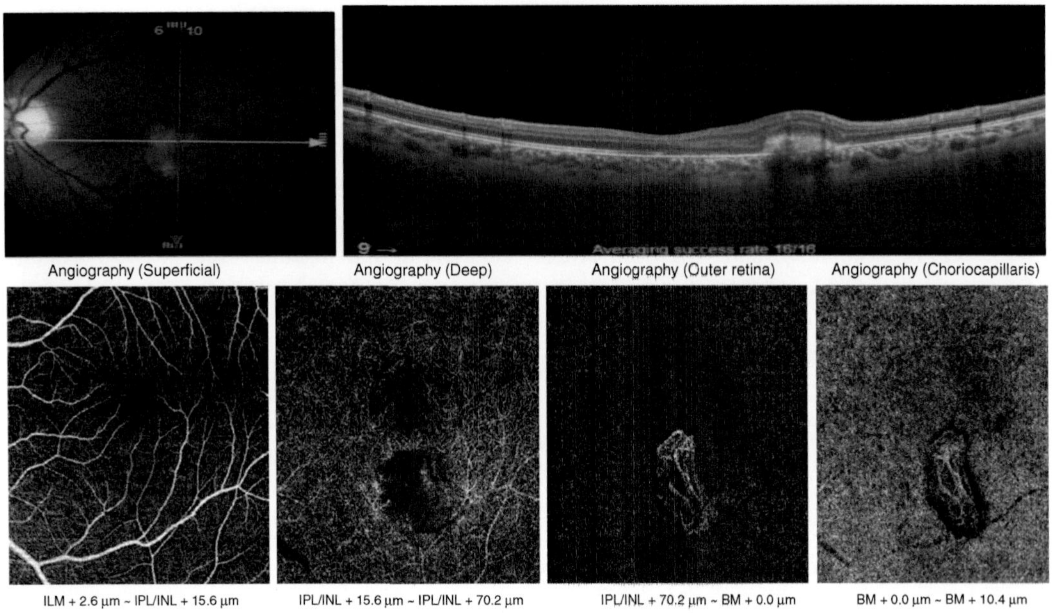

Fig. 14.1 (continued)

hyperfluorescence that increases with time and progresses to leakage in the late phase. Given that idiopathic CNV is usually a type 2 CNV and is expected to behave as a classic CNV on FA. ICGA is used if the diagnosis is not certain after FA and optical coherence tomography (OCT). It is of higher value in cases of occult CNV, polypoidal choroidal vasculopathy, retinal angiomatous proliferation, or in cases associated with RPE detachment. Kumar et al. [24] reported ICGA findings of seven eyes with type 2 idiopathic CNV. ICGA showed a patch of diffuse hyperfluorescence in three of seven eyes, a network of abnormal vessels in four of seven eyes, and all eyes showed a hypofluorescent halo around the CNV. The ring of hypofluorescence was also observed in all of the 12 eyes with idiopathic CNV reported by Toju et al. [25].

OCT is now the gold standard in diagnosing and monitoring treatment response in CNV. Subretinal hyper-reflectivity is usually observed that might be associated with other findings such as subretinal or intraretinal hyporeflective signal corresponding to intraretinal or subretinal fluid.

Optical coherence tomography angiography (OCTA) is a noninvasive dye-less imaging modality. The use of OCTA in clinical settings has been increasing in the last few years. Few studies evaluated OCTA in idiopathic CNV [24, 26–28]. An irregular close-knit formation of intertwined and convoluted vessels was observed at the level of the outer retina that is normally supposed to be avascular so any flow at that layer could be interpreted as a neovascularization. Factors that might affect the quality of the OCTA images such as pigment epithelial detachment, high refractive error, posterior staphyloma, or poor fixation are usually not encountered in patients with idiopathic CNV, which makes it a useful tool in evaluating these lesions [24].

Chen et al. [27] studied the OCTA features of 17 eyes with idiopathic CNV and monitored the response after treatment with anti-VEGF. They found that the most common morphological structure in idiopathic CNV was "tree-in-bud" morphology that differs from AMD-related CNV, in which a large central trunk of "sea fan" vessels is commonly seen. The authors speculated that the difference in the morphological structures might play a role in the prognosis and response to treatment. Interestingly, these membranes were monitored at day 1 post treatment with intravitreal anti-VEGF (ranibizumab) with OCT and OCTA images. Selected areas of flow in the CNV were significantly smaller on OCTA but no change in fluid with B-scan OCT images was observed. Based on this finding, OCTA could be a more sensitive tool in predicting outcome instead of relying on OCT and visual acuity solely.

Near-infrared autofluorescence (IR-AF) has been investigated as an imaging tool in CNV. Keilhauer et al. [29] proposed that images of IR-AF are derived from the melanin in RPE and choroid. IR-AF features in 12 eyes with idiopathic CNV were studied by Toju and colleagues [25]. In six of the studied eyes, a well-defined ring of hyperautofluorescence surrounding the hypoautofluorescent CNV lesion at baseline was noted before treatment with bevacizumab. After treatment, all eyes showed a ring of hyperautofluorescence that became more prominent as the lesions regressed which was confirmed by the absence of leakage on FA. Three of the treated eyes showed signs of recurrence of CNV activity that were observed by leakage on FA and accumulation of subretinal fluid on OCT. The hyperautofluorescent ring became partially obscured and became clearly visible after retreatment. The hyperautofluorescent ring corresponded with a hypofluorescent halo or dark rim on ICGA during the regression of the lesions. It has been proposed that this well-defined hyperautofluorescent ring represents the melanin in the proliferating RPE cells at the outer margin of the CNV lesion as the lesions involute which also appear as a hypofluorescent rim on ICGA.

Certain entities with subtle or atypical clinical findings or prior to the appearance of the full clinical picture may be mistakenly labeled as idiopathic CNV. Some eyes enrolled in the macular photocoagulation study for the idiopathic CNV arm [30, 31] manifested the clinical picture of senile macular degeneration with more than minimal drusen or atrophic histoplasmosis scar during the first year of follow-up. Other conditions that may be complicated by CNV and could be overlooked in clinical examination include punctate inner choroidopathy, central serous chorioretinopathy, multifocal choroiditis, subtle angioid streaks, and buried optic nerve head drusens. Laser-induced CNV has been reported with the use of handheld laser pointers and cosmetic laser devices [32, 33]. The history of exposure to handheld laser devices in young children is usually difficult to elicit and the diagnosis may be significantly delayed [34].

14.4 Natural History and Prognosis

Data on the natural history of CNV is derived from the era prior to anti-VEGF for lesions that are mainly located sub-foveally in which laser photocoagulations was not applied based on the criteria of the macular photocoagulation study [30]. Eyes with idiopathic CNV that were assigned to observation had three times the risk of severe vision loss compared to the treated eyes after one year of follow-up. Lesions that spared the center of foveal avascular zone had progressed during the one-year follow-up to involve the center in 33% of untreated eyes. Ho et al. [2] retrospectively studied the natural history of 19 patients with unilateral idiopathic CNV located in the center of the foveal avascular zone, with a follow-up period ranging from 5 to 230 months. They found that patients with idiopathic CNV had a significantly better long-term visual prognosis compared to patients with POHS or AMD with subfoveal CNV. Up to 90% of patients with idiopathic subfoveal CNV had improved or maintained vision in the follow-up period. This was not the same for patients with POHS or AMD subfoveal CNV, where vision was maintained or improved in 29 and 15%, respectively. The size of CNV was the only parameter associated with the final visual acuity, lesions less than or equal to 1 disc diameter in size were associated with better final visual acuity of 20/60 or better. It is speculated that favorable prognosis of idiopathic CNV compared to AMD might be related to the age of the affected patients; younger patients have a more active RPE that is more successful in enveloping the CNV and promoting auto-involution of the lesion. Another reason could be related to the nature of the subretinal neovascular membrane which is focal in nature in idiopathic CNV rather than the diffuse form, which is seen with AMD, thus affecting a smaller area and allowing preservation of the photoreceptors.

In another study, Lindblom et al. [3] concluded that idiopathic CNV carries a more favorable prognosis compared to AMD and treatment recommendations, at that time, with laser photocoagulation (prior to the availability of anti-VEGF) should be reconsidered given the possible complications of laser treatment including inadvertent foveal burn, RPE tear, or creeping laser scars.

Although the natural history of idiopathic CNV is more favorable compared to AMD and POHS, individual variations still exist and cases with irreversible visual loss have been observed [2].

14.5 Treatment

14.5.1 Laser Photocoagulation

Laser photocoagulation to macular CNV is considered a historical treatment after the introduction of less destructive treatment modalities such as photodynamic therapy and anti-VEGF therapy. Macular photocoagulation study (MPS) was a multicenter randomized clinical trial that evaluated the effect of argon laser [30] and krypton laser [31] photocoagulation in the treatment of CNV associated with AMD, POHS, or idiopathic CNV versus observation in preventing or delaying severe vision loss defined by the study as six or more lines decrease in visual acuity. Lesions eligible for treatment based on study criteria included lesions located 200–2500 μm from the center of the foveal avascular zone for argon laser trial; lesions within 1–199 μm for the krypton laser trial were treated with laser photocoagulation. After 1 year, up to three times of untreated eyes compared to treated eyes had lost six or more lines of visual acuity. Further randomization of patients with idiopathic CNV was halted based on the recommendation of the data reviewing committee, as it was unlikely that a sufficient number of subjects would be recruited during the expected study lifetime. However, accumulated data showed a pattern of treatment benefit in idiopathic CNV similar to that seen in AMD and POHS. Treatment complications reported by MPS study included hemorrhage, perforation of Bruch's membrane, retinal hole, too extensive treatment, extension of laser scar (runoff) to the center of foveal avascular zone, and wrinkling of the internal limiting membrane.

14.5.2 Photodynamic Therapy

Photodynamic therapy (PDT) has the ability to selectively occlude the abnormal CNV with minimal effect on the overlying retina. A diode laser with low energy is used to activate the verteporfin dye and initiate a photochemical reaction that leads to occlusion of the abnormal CNV. PDT for CNV has been proven effective in patients with AMD, pathological myopia, and POHS [35–37]. Its efficacy in preventing moderate to severe vision loss in predominantly classic CNV secondary to AMD has been established [35]. Idiopathic CNV usually is a classic CNV angiographically and PDT may be effective in occluding CNV as in predominantly classic CNV seen in AMD. Chan and associates [23] prospectively studied 17 eyes with idiopathic CNV. Eyes were treated with PDT for subfoveal and juxtafoveal lesions. There was a mean of 2.3 lines improvement in best-corrected visual acuity (BCVA) at the end of 12 months follow-up with most gain noticed in the first 3 months. At 12-month visit, 41% had a BCVA of 20/40 or better, and 82% had a BCVA of 20/100 or better. These results were better compared to the natural history in the observational study reported by Ho et al. [2]. The need for retreatment was assessed every 3 months, 47% of eyes needed retreatment with a mean number of 1.8 treatments per eye in 1 year, which is less than 3.4 treatments for AMD and pathological myopia, and 2.9 treatments for POHS. Factors associated with better final visual outcome were: active lesions on presentation, smaller lesion size, and lesions that underwent only one PDT treatment. Reported complications included blurry of vision in one case and submacular hemorrhage in three cases. No serious systemic complications were encountered.

Kang and colleagues [22] retrospectively studied the long-term effect of PDT on 30 eyes with idiopathic CNV. At 5-year follow-up period, 46.7% gained vision, whereas 20% lost vision when compared to baseline. Comparing this to the natural history reported by Ho et al. [2] where only 5% of eyes showed significant vision loss, long-term effect of PDT for idiopathic CNV appears to be limited. Eyes with juxtafoveal lesions lost more gain compared to subfoveal ones despite better visual acuity at baseline. The author proposed that the harmful effect of PDT on foveal center and RPE cells could explain the limited long-term outcome especially in juxtafoveal CNV lesions.

Inflammation of the choroid has been proposed as an underlying cause of idiopathic CNV [13]. Steroids are frequently used to control non-infectious uveitis and choroidal inflammation. Combining PDT with systemic steroids in the treatment of idiopathic CNV was studied by Giovannini and associates [38]. Two groups of 10 eyes each with idiopathic CNV were assigned to either PDT alone or PDT after a course of systemic steroids. Steroid regimen was given as 1-gram methylprednisolone intravenously for 3 days followed by oral prednisolone of 1 mg/kg per day and tapered according to individual basis. The group with combination therapy had a better reduction of CNV size, better final BCVA, and less number of PDT treatments. Hyperplastic fibrotic scars were observed in the PDT only treatment group. This suggests that steroids have a suppressing effect on fibroblast activity.

14.5.3 Anti-vascular Endothelial Growth Factors

With the introduction of anti-VEGF for the treatment of CNV, clinical practice has changed dramatically. It is considered the mainstay treatment of CNV with a proven benefit observed in many studies, the majority of these looked into AMD-related CNV. Idiopathic CNV has been studied to a lesser extent. The main outcome of treatment at the time of laser photocoagulation was to prevent or delay severe visual loss as defined by the MPS [30] while with anti-VEGF, a significant improvement in visual acuity is observed compared to previous treatment modalities (Fig. 14.2).

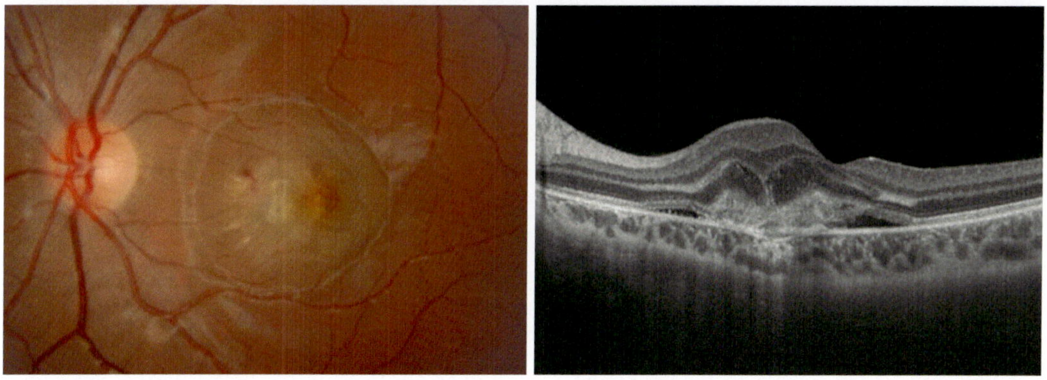

Fig. 14.2 Fundus photograph showing a choroidal neovascular membrane (CNV) involving the fovea. Optical Coherence Tomography (OCT) through the lesion revealed a type 2 CNV with subretinal and intraretinal fluid. Optical Coherence Tomography Angiography (OCTA) confirmed the presence of a vascular network. Following treatment (lower images), resolution of intraretinal and subretinal fluid was observed with restoration of the foveal contour, although a pigment epithelial detachment persisted. OCTA showed a less prominent vascular network. Courtesy Dr. Sumit Randhir Singh, LV Prasad Eye Institute, Visakhapatnam, India

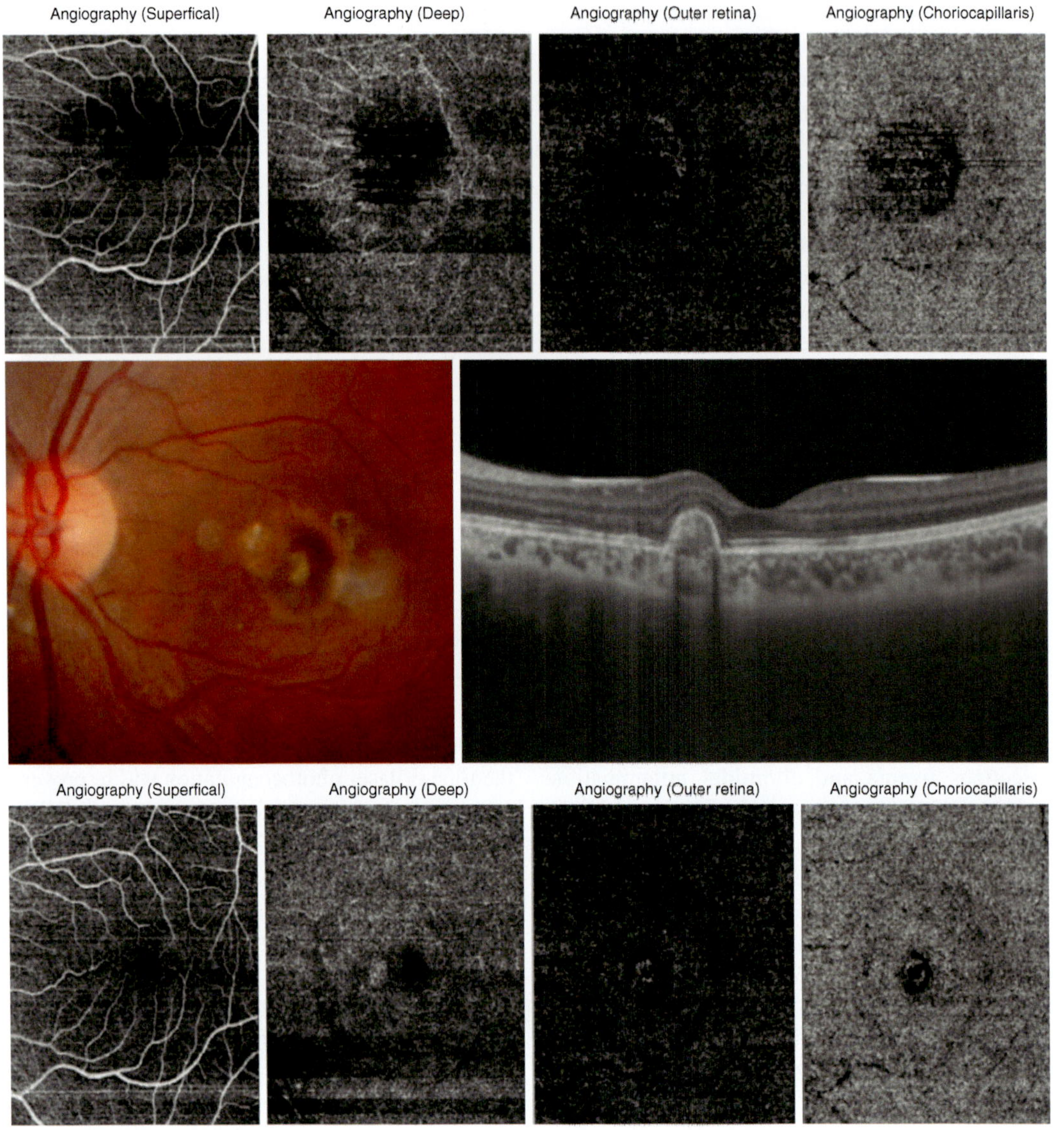

Fig. 14.2 (continued)

14.5.4 Bevacizumab

A number of studies investigated the efficacy of different anti-VEGF agents in the treatment of idiopathic CNV. Mandal and colleagues [39] reported their findings in treating 32 eyes with idiopathic CNV using bevacizumab 1.25 mg/0.05 ml. The need for reinjection was assessed monthly based on the reduction of subretinal fluid, central macular thickness (CMT), or resolution of pigment epithelial detachment (PED) on OCT images. Maximum reduction of CMT and maximum improvement of visual acuity was observed in the first 4 weeks. Subretinal fluid resolved faster than intraretinal fluid whereas PED resolved last. At the end of 12 weeks follow-up, 59% eyes had improved BCVA, 34% remained stable, and 6% had dropped BCVA. The mean number of injections was 1.7 per eye with 12 patients requiring 2 injections, 4 patients requiring 3 injections, and 1 patient requiring 4 injections over a mean follow-up period of 4.2 months.

Zhang et al. [40] prospectively evaluated 40 eyes with subfoveal idiopathic CNV treated using intravitreal bevacizumab 1.25 mg/0.05 ml once then as needed (PRN) regimen. At 1-year follow-up, 70% showed improvement in vision while 30% remained stable and none lost vision. Of note, 60% of eyes needed reinjection with a mean of two injections per eye, all were performed within 3 months of the initial treatment with no recurrence on follow-up. At 12-month follow-up, all lesions were cicatrized. Although there is no consensus on the frequency or the number of injections in idiopathic CNV, the authors proposed that given the nature of idiopathic CNV being smaller in size and affecting younger patients with healthier RPE a single injection followed by PRN approach may be more effective in comparison to monthly injection. Inou et al. [41] reported similar findings for seven eyes with subfoveal and juxtafoveal idiopathic CNV. All eyes either improved or remained stable at 1-year follow-up. The mean number of bevacizumab injections was 2.7 per eye.

A larger retrospective study by Qi H-J et al. [42] in 77 Chinese patients with idiopathic CNV (subfoveal and juxtafoveal) who were treated with bevacizumab found that 79% gained vision, 20% remained stable, and 1% lost > 2 lines of vision. Reinjection was needed in 81% of eyes with a mean of 2.47 injections per eye over a mean follow-up period of 14.3 months.

14.5.5 Ranibizumab

Unlike bevacizumab that is used as off-label for the treatment of CNV, ranibizumab is approved by the United States Food and Drug Administration for the treatment of wet AMD. The evidence on the safety of one medication over the other remains contradictory.

In a prospective study by Yin and associates [21], 39 eyes with idiopathic CNV received intravitreal ranibizumab 0.5 mg/0.05 ml. Aqueous humor samples were obtained and inflammatory cytokines were assessed prior and after treatment. Twenty-four eyes (61.5%) required retreatment during the 1-year follow-up period with a mean of 2.1 injections per eye. All eyes gained vision at the end of follow-up. Although the aqueous level of VEGF was not higher compared to the control group prior to treatment, its level was significantly decreased compared to pretreatment. Subgroup analysis of inflammatory cytokines comparing the single injection group with the multiple injections group showed a significantly higher level of IL-10 and macrophage inflammatory protein 1b (MIP-1b) in the multiple injection group. The authors suggested that other molecules besides VEGF may play a crucial role in idiopathic CNV formation.

14.5.6 Comparative Studies

Multiple studies compared between bevacizumab and ranibizumab for the treatment of wet AMD [43–46]. Both medications were equally effective; however, there are concerns that bevacizumab may have a worse side effect profile due to its greater systemic bioavailability.

In a retrospective study by Zhou et al. [47], 60 eyes with idiopathic CNV were treated with either ranibizumab or bevacizumab with 30 eyes in each group. At 2-year follow-up, both drugs were effective in the treatment of CNV with no significant difference in the clinical outcome between the groups. Most patients required three or more injections in both groups (90% of bevacizumab group and 97% in the ranibizumab group) with a mean number of 3.20 and 3.13 injections in bevacizumab and ranibizumab, respectively. Central retinal thickness was significantly less in the ranibizumab group but no difference in the final visual acuity compared to the bevacizumab group was observed. Both medications were equally safe with no reported systemic or ocular complications.

Similar findings in a retrospective comparative study of 47 eyes with idiopathic CNV by Sudhalkar et al. [48] were reported. Both medications were equally effective in improving visual acuity with no difference in final central macular thickness between the treated groups. The mean number of injections was 2.4 injections over a 1-year period. No ocular or systemic complications were observed.

From the previous studies, it is noted that the mean number of injections is significantly lower compared to that reported for the treatment of wet AMD [44]. There is no consensus on the best treatment regimen for idiopathic CNV. Several studies with relatively small numbers reported using monthly injections while others used treatment as needed. Further prospective controlled studies on idiopathic CNV to assess the best regimen are needed.

14.5.7 Surgical Treatment

Submacular surgery and macular translocation are possible options for the treatment of subfoveal idiopathic CNV. Few studies looked into surgical options in idiopathic CNV as well as other non-AMD related CNV such as POHS, pathological myopia, or uveitis. [49, 50] As part of the submacular surgery trials (SST), surgical removal versus observation of subfoveal CNV associated with ocular histoplasmosis or idiopathic form trial found no benefit or a smaller benefit to surgery than the trial was designed to detect. The risk of retinal detachment was 5% and the risk of recurrence of CNV was ≥50% [50].

Surgical treatment for CNV in the era of anti-VEGF is limited. The disadvantages of surgery include being invasive and requiring more complex surgical skills. Complications such as retinal detachment, cataract progression, and high incidence of recurrence have been reported. The benefit over risk is difficult to be established especially in idiopathic CNV which usually has a favorable prognosis and good response to less invasive treatment options such as anti-VEGF therapy.

14.6 Key Learning Points

1. Idiopathic CNV usually affects the posterior pole in patients younger than 50 years of age.
2. It is usually unilateral but could be bilateral.
3. It is a diagnosis of exclusion. Findings related to other etiologies may appear over time.
4. It carries a better prognosis when compared to age-related macular degeneration.
5. It requires significantly less number of intravitreal anti-VEGF injections to achieve quiescence when compared to wet AMD.

References

1. Green WR, Wilson DJ. Choroidal neovascularization. Ophthalmology. 1986;93:1169–76.
2. Ho AC, Yannuzzi LA, Pisicano K, Derosa J. The natural history of idiopathic subfoveal choroidal neovascularization. Ophthalmology. 1995;102:782–9.
3. Lindblom B, Andersson T. The prognosis of idiopathic choroidal neovascularization in persons younger than 50 years of age. Ophthalmology. 1998;105:1816–20.
4. Bottoni FG, Deutman AF. Idiopathic sub-retinal neovascular membranes in the macula (hemorrhagic macular choroidopathy of young adults). Doc Ophthalmol. 1987;64:311–43.
5. Cohen SY, Laroche A, Leguen Y, Soubrane G, Coscas GJ. Etiology of choroidal neovascularization in young patients. Ophthalmology. 1996;103:1241–4.
6. Grossniklaus HE, Green W. Choroidal neovascularization. Am J Ophthalmol. 2004;137:496–503.
7. Gass JDM. Biomicroscopic and histopathologic considerations regarding the feasibility of surgical excision of subfoveal Neovascular membranes. Am J Ophthalmol. 1994;118:285–98.
8. Thomas JW, Grossniklaus HE, Lambert HM, Aaberg TM, L'hernault N. Ultrastructural features of surgically excised idiopathic subfoveal neovascular membranes. Retina. 1993;13:93–8.
9. Lee JE, Shin MK, Chung IY, Lee JE, Kim HW, Lee SJ, Park SW, Byon IS. Topographical relationship between the choroidal watershed zone and submacular idiopathic choroidal neovascularisation. Br J Ophthalmol. 2015;100:652–9.
10. Hayashi K, Laey JD. Indocyanine green angiography of submacular choroidal vessels in the human eye. Ophthalmologica. 1985;190:20–9.
11. Ahn SJ, Kim TW, Ahn J, Woo SJ, Park KH, Lee BR. Subfoveal choroidal thickness in idiopathic choroidal neovascularization. Ophthalmology. 2014;121(7):1486–7.
12. Sasahara M, Otani A, Yodoi Y, Yoshimura N. Circulating hematopoietic stem cells in patients

with idiopathic choroidal neovascularization. Invest Ophthalmol Vis Sci. 2009;50:1575.
13. Giovannini A, Scassellati-Sforzolini B, Mariotti C, D'Altobrando E. Indocyanine green angiographic findings in idiopathic choroidal neovascularization. Int Ophthalmol. 1996;20(4):171–9.
14. Yang F, Dou H-L, Ma Z, Li Y-L, Lu X-R, Wang X, He P-P. Serum inflammatory factors in patients with idiopathic choroidal neovascularization. Ocul Immunol Inflamm. 2010;18:390–4.
15. Tsai D-C, Charng M-J, Lee F-L, Hsu W-M, Chen S-J. Different plasma levels of vascular endothelial growth factor and nitric oxide between patients with choroidal and retinal neovascularization. Ophthalmologica. 2006;220:246–51.
16. Lip P-L, Blann AD, Hope-Ross M, Gibson JM, Lip GY. Age-related macular degeneration is associated with increased vascular endothelial growth factor, hemorheology and endothelial dysfunction. Ophthalmology. 2001;108:705–10.
17. Stefansson E, Geirsdottir A, Sigurdsson H. Metabolic physiology in age related macular degeneration. Prog Retinal Eye Res. 2011;30(1):72–80.
18. Wankun X, Wenzhen Y, Min Z, Weiyan Z, Huan C, Wei D, et al. Protective effect of paeoniflorin against oxidative stress in human retinal pigment epithelium in vitro. Mol Vis. 2011;17:3512–22.
19. Zhao M, Bai Y, Xie W, Shi X, Li F, Yang F, et al. Interleukin-1beta level is increased in vitreous of patients with neo- vascular age-related macular degeneration (nAMD) and polypoidal choroidal vasculopathy (PCV). PLoS One. 2015;10(5):e0125150.
20. Miao H, Tao Y, Li XX. Inflammatory cytokines in aqueous humor of patients with choroidal neovascularization. Mol Vis. 2012;18:574–80.
21. Yin H, Fang X, Ma J, et al. Idiopathic choroidal neovascularization: intraocular inflammatory cytokines and the effect of intravitreal Ranibizumab treatment. Scientific Reports. 2016;25(6):31880.
22. Kang HM, Koh HJ. Five-year visual outcome and visual prognostic factors after photodynamic therapy with verteporfin for idiopathic choroidal neovascularization. ARC J Ophthalmol. 2016;1:12–8.
23. Chan W-M, Lam DS, Wong T-H, Lai TY, Kwok AK, Tam BS, Li KK. Photodynamic therapy with verteporfin for subfoveal idiopathic choroidal neovascularization. Ophthalmology. 2003;110:2395–402.
24. Kumar A, Vohra R, Agrawal S, Chawla R, Azad SV, Venkatesh P, Sharma A. Characterization of idiopathic choroidal neovascularization using fluorescein angiography, indocyanine green angiography, and optical coherence tomography angiography. Ophthal Surg Lasers Imaging Retina. 2018;49:516–22.
25. Toju R, Iida T, Sekiryu T, Saito M, Maruko I, Kano M. Near-infrared autofluorescence in patients with idiopathic submacular choroidal neovascularization. Am J Ophthalmol. 2012;153:314–9.
26. Wang Q, Chan SY, Jonas JB, Wei WB. Optical coherence tomography angiography in idiopathic choroidal neovascularization. Acta Ophthalmol. 2015;94:415–7.
27. Chen Q, Yu X, Sun Z, Dai H. The application of OCTA in assessment of anti-VEGF therapy for idiopathic choroidal neovascularization. J Ophthalmol. 2016;2016:1–8.
28. Liu B, Bao L, Zhang J. Optical coherence tomography angiography of pathological myopia sourced and idiopathic choroidal neovascularization with follow-up. Medicine. 2016;95(14):e3264.
29. Keilhauer CN, Delori FC. Near-infrared autofluorescence imaging of the fundus: visualization of ocular melanin. Invest Ophthalmol Vis Sci. 2006;47:3556.
30. Macular Photocoagulation Study Group. Argon laser photocoagulation for idiopathic neovascularization. Arch Ophthalmol. 1983;101:1358.
31. Krypton laser photocoagulation for idiopathic neovascular lesions. Arch Ophthalmol. 1990;108:832.
32. Veronese C, Maiolo C, Huang D, Jia Y, Armstrong GW, Morara M, Ciardella AP. Optical coherence tomography angiography in pediatric choroidal neovascularization. Am J Ophthalmol Case Rep. 2016;2:37–40.
33. Wang R, Wykoff CC, Christie L, Croft DE, Major JC, Fish RH, Brown DM. Choroidal neovascularization secondary to alexandrite laser exposure. Retinal Cases Brief Rep. 2016;10:244–8.
34. Raoof N, Bradley P, Theodorou M, Moore AT, Michaelides M. The new pretender: a large UK case series of retinal injuries in children secondary to handheld lasers. Am J Ophthalmol. 2016;171:88–94.
35. Group1A VI. Photodynamic therapy of subfoveal choroidal neovascularization in age-related macular degeneration with verteporfin. Arch Ophthalmol. 1999;117:1329.
36. Bressler NM. Photodynamic therapy of subfoveal choroidal neovascularization in pathologic myopia with verteporfin. Ophthalmology. 2001;108:841–52.
37. Saperstein DA, Rosenfeld PJ, Bressler NM, Rosa RH, Sickenberg M, Sternberg P, Aaberg TM, Aaberg TM, Reaves TA. Photodynamic therapy of subfoveal choroidal neovascularization with verteporfin in the ocular histoplasmosis syndrome. Ophthalmology. 2002;109:1499–505.
38. Giovannini A, Neri P, Mercanti L, Brue C. Photodynamic treatment versus photodynamic treatment associated with systemic steroids for idiopathic choroidal neovascularisation. Br J Ophthalmol. 2007;91:620–3.
39. Mandal S. Intravitreal bevacizumab for subfoveal idiopathic choroidal neovascularization. Arch Ophthalmol. 2007;125:1487.
40. Zhang H, Liu Z-L, Sun P, Gu F. Intravitreal bevacizumab for treatment of subfoveal idiopathic choroidal neovascularization: results of a 1-year prospective trial. Am J Ophthalmol. 2012;153(2):300–6.

41. Inoue M, Kadonosono K, Watanabe Y, Sato S, Kobayashi S, Yamane S, Ito R, Arakawa A. Results of 1-year follow-up examinations after intravitreal bevacizumab administration for idiopathic choroidal neovascularization. Retina. 2010;30:733–8.
42. Qi H-J, Li X-X, Tao Y. Outcome of intravitreal bevacizumab for idiopathic choroidal neovascularization in a Chinese population. Can J Ophthalmol. 2010;45:381–5.
43. CATT Research Group. Ranibizumab and bevacizumab for neovascular age-related macular degeneration. N Engl J Med. 2011;364:1897–908.
44. Chakravarthy U, Harding SP, Rogers CA, Downes SM, Lotery AJ, Wordsworth S, Reeves BC. Ranibizumab versus bevacizumab to treat neovascular age-related macular degeneration. Ophthalmology. 2012;119:1399–411.
45. Krebs I, Schmetterer L, Boltz A, Told R, Vécsei-Marlovits V, Egger S, Schönherr U, Haas A, Ansari-Shahrezaei S, Binder S. A randomised double-masked trial comparing the visual outcome after treatment with ranibizumab or bevacizumab in patients with neovascular age-related macular degeneration. Br J Ophthalmol. 2013;97:266–71.
46. Kodjikian L, Souied EH, Mimoun G, Mauget-Faÿsse M, Behar-Cohen F, Decullier E, Huot L, Aulagner G. Ranibizumab versus bevacizumab for neovascular age-related macular degeneration: results from the GEFAL noninferiority randomized trial. Ophthalmology. 2013;120:2300–9.
47. Zhou P, Yang L, Jin X. Ranibizumab versus bevacizumab for the treatment of idiopathic choroidal neovascularization: 2-year results. Eur J Ophthalmol. 2015;26:262–7.
48. Sudhalkar A, Yogi R, Chhablani J. Anti-vascular endothelial growth factor therapy for naive idiopathic choroidal neovascularization. Retina. 2015;35:1368–74.
49. Essex RW, Tufail A, Bunce C, Aylward GW. Two-year results of surgical removal of choroidal neovascular membranes related to non-age-related macular degeneration. Br J Ophthalmol. 2007;91:649–54.
50. Submacular Surgery Trials Research Group. Surgical removal vs observation for subfoveal choroidal neovascularization, either associated with the ocular histoplasmosis syndrome or idiopathic: I. ophthalmic findings from a randomized clinical trial: submacular surgery trials (SST) group H trial: SST report no. 9—correction. Arch Ophthalmol. 2005;123:28.

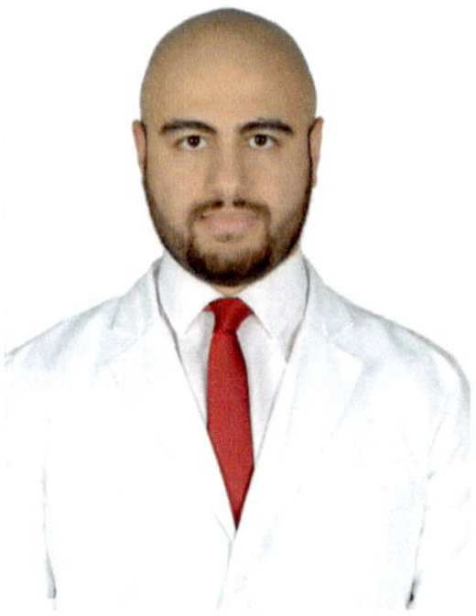

Faisal A. Almarek, MD received his medical degree in 2010. Completed residency training in ophthalmology at King Khaled Eye Specialist Hospital and King Saud University, Riyadh, Saudi Arabia. He then joined the vitreoretinal surgery fellowship at King Khaled Eye Specialist Hospital. Dr. Almarek is currently an assistant professor at the department of ophthalmology, Imam Mohammed Bin Saud Islamic University, Riyadh, Saudi Arabia.

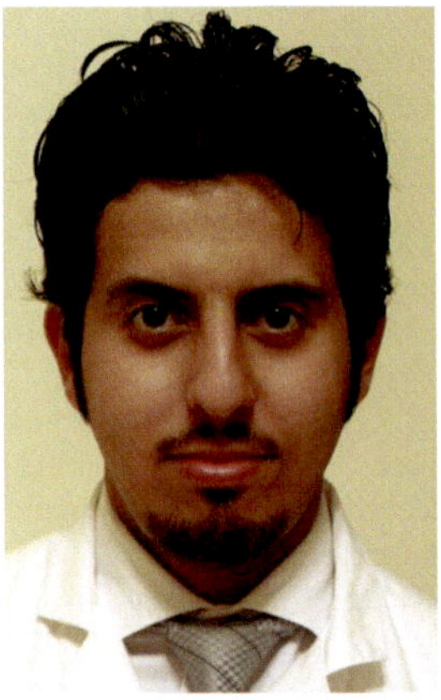

Sulaiman M. Alsulaiman, MD received his medical degree in 2006 and completed residency in ophthalmology at King Khaled Eye Specialist Hospital and King Saud University, Riyadh, Saudi Arabia. He then completed vitreoretinal surgery and uveitis fellowships at King Khaled Eye Specialist Hospital followed by pediatric retina fellowship at the Eye and Ear infirmary, University of Illinois, Chicago. Dr Alsulaiman is currently an attending vitreoretinal surgeon at the King Khaled Eye Specialist Hospital.

15 Subretinal Neovascularization Associated with Idiopathic Juxtafoveal Telangiectasia

Matthew R. Starr and Sophie J. Bakri

15.1 Introduction

Macular telangiectasia (MacTel) or idiopathic juxtafoveal telangiectasia includes several phenotypic subtypes of retinal vascular disease that primarily affect the posterior pole. Gass published an extensive classification system on the various subtypes of macular telangiectasia in 1993 [1], but despite the complex classification systems, there are in essence two forms. One has a congenital abnormality that is typically unilateral and may be a part of the Coats disease spectrum, referred to as MacTel type 1, and an acquired form that is typically bilateral found in middle-aged adults that is referred to as MacTel type 2. The classification system was further refined by Yanuzzi in 2006 using multimodal imaging analyses [2]. Yanuzzi and colleagues classified the original MacTel type 1 as an aneurysmal macular telangiectasia, while MacTel type 2 was labeled as an idiopathic macular telangiectasia. This chapter will focus on the subretinal neovascularization associated with idiopathic juxtafoveal telangiectasia or MacTel type 2.

The vascular changes in MacTel are thought to affect the capillaries of the temporal fovea first, hence the term juxtavofeal telangiectasia [3, 4]. These abnormalities were initially thought to be vasculature in origin, but as newer imaging modalities and postmortem studies have become available, it is now believed that MacTel is possibly a neurodegenerative disorder affecting the perifoveal Müller cells and photoreceptors. The atrophy of these cells, in turn, leads to the vascular abnormalities and retinal changes seen in MacTel type 2 [3, 5–8].

There are two population-based studies examining the incidence and prevalence of MacTel type 2 in primarily Caucasian populations [9, 10]. The Beaver Dam Eye Study, found a prevalence of MacTel type 2 of 0.1% [10], while the Melbourne Collaborative Cohort study found a prevalence of 0.0045–0.022% [9]. The prevalence of MacTel in a primarily African population of nearly 8600 patients was found to be 0.06%, similar to the other two studies [11]. Although no specific gene has been identified, it is widely accepted that the condition is autosomal dominant with an incomplete penetrance [12, 13].

15.2 Clinical Exam and History

Patients with MacTel tend to present with mild visual complaints or even a central scotoma in their fifth or sixth decades of life [3]. The characteristic fundus findings include the loss of retinal transparency, and the presence of capillary dilatation and telangiectasias, right-angle vessels, and

M. R. Starr · S. J. Bakri (✉)
Department of Ophthalmology, Mayo Clinic, Rochester, MN, USA
e-mail: bakri.sophie@mayo.edu

J. Chhablani (ed.), *Choroidal Neovascularization*, https://doi.org/10.1007/978-981-15-2213-0_15

retinal pigment epithelial (RPE) hyperplasia. The earliest manifestation of MacTel type 2 tends to be loss of the retinal transparency (Fig. 15.1a), which begins temporal to the fovea, but eventually extends to involve the entire perifoveal area [10]. Involvement of both the inner and the outer capillary plexuses has been described [2]. The hard exudates seen on funduscopic examination

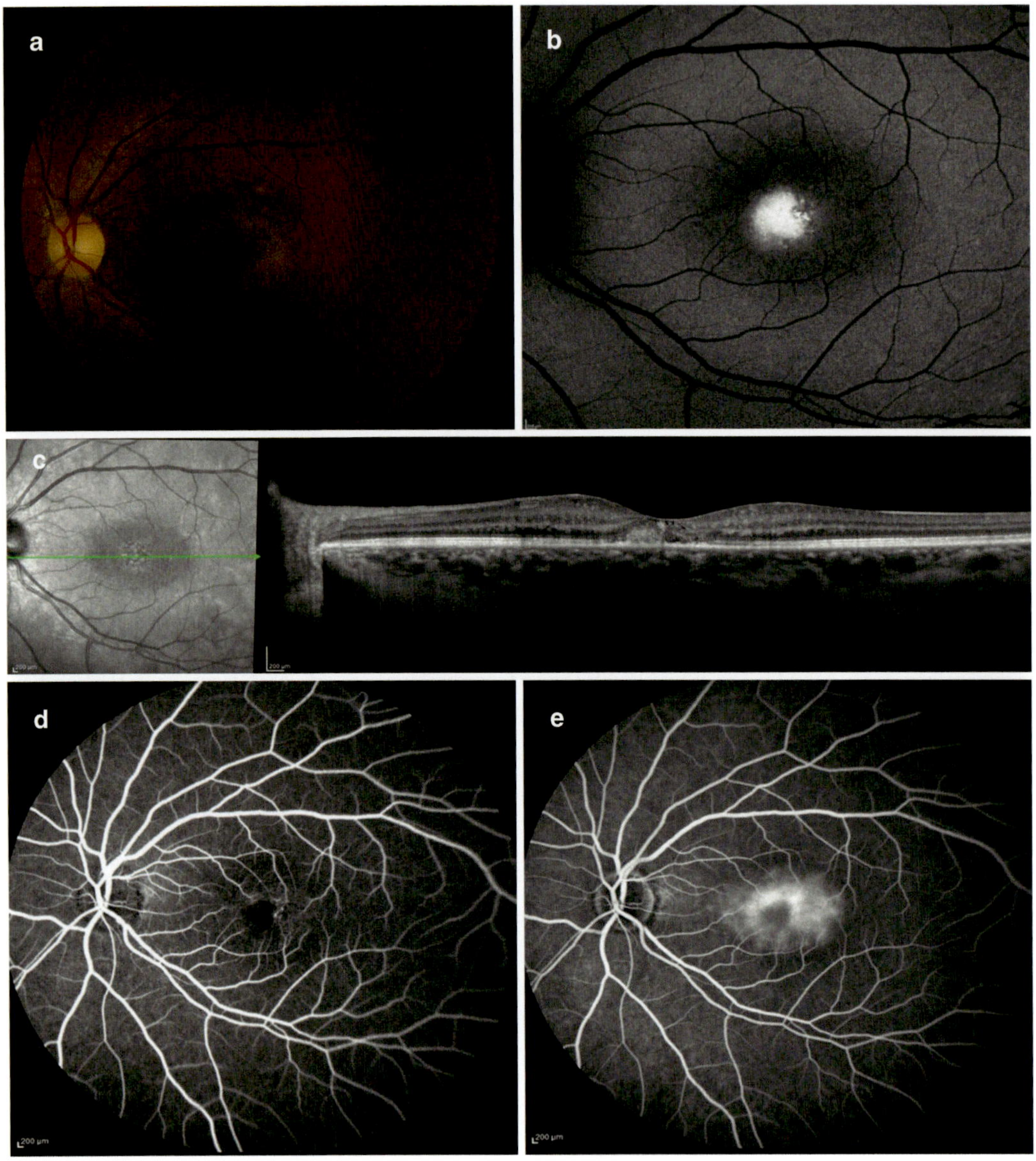

Fig. 15.1 Left eye imaging of a 41 year-old female with macular telangiectasia type 2 with associated vitelliform-like lesion in the left eye. On fundus photography (**a**) there is evidence of decreased retinal transparency with blunted retinal vessels and yellow foveal depositis. Fundus autofluoresence revealed loss of the central hypo-autofluorescent fovea with a hyper-autofluorescent lesion at the fovea and a stippled hyperautofluorescent area temporal to fovea (**b**). Optical coherence tomography revealed a flat-top atrophic cyst, bullseye pattern ellipsoid zone layer loss, and scattered intraretinal cysts (**c**). On early phase fluorescein angiography at 34 s there is evidence of telangiectatic vasculature just temporal to the fovea (**d**) with diffuse late leakage of these vessels on late phase fluorescein angiography at 9 minutes (**e**)

of those patients with MacTel type 1 are typically not seen in patients with MacTel type 2, however, crystalline deposits can be seen in the vitreoretinal interface in those patients with MacTel type 2 [14]. As venules course toward the fovea in patients with MacTel type 2, they dilate and make right-angle turns into the deeper retinal layers. RPE hyperplasia is also noted along the courses of these right-angle venules and lastly, atrophic retinal changes occur [2]. This atrophy can potentially lead to the formation of full-thickness macular holes [15–17].

Subretinal neovascularization may occur in patients with MacTel, and is typically preceded by the right-angle venules with subsequent RPE hyperplasia [1]. These patients will typically manifest with acute vision changes, loss of vision, metamorphopsia, or with a central scotoma. The neovascularization is retinal in origin as evidenced by the feeder vessels from the retinal arteries draining into the venules [18]. Lastly, a disciform scar can manifest as the advanced stage of the neovascularization process, leading to a significant decline in visual acuity.

15.3 Diagnostic Imaging

On fundus autofluorescence, there is a loss of the foveal hypoautofluorescent center, thought to be due to the depletion of the retinal pigment at the fovea (Fig. 15.1b) [19]. On optical coherence tomography (OCT), patients may frequently present with temporal enlargement of the foveal pit, hyporeflective cavities of the inner and outer retina, normal retinal thickness despite angiographic evidence of leakage, disruption of the inner and outer photoreceptor segments, increased reflectivity of the inner retinal layers, hyperreflective intraretinal lesions, and outer retinal atrophy late in the disease. Infrequently, patients may present with lamellar or full-thickness macular holes, foveal detachments, or subfoveal debris (Fig. 15.1c) [2, 3, 20]. Fluorescein angiography (FA) reveals early telangiectatic capillaries in the temporal fovea in the early phase of the FA (Fig. 15.1d). During the early stages of the disease, there may be a mild hyperfluorescence in the absence of abnormal capillaries thought to be staining of the outer retina [1], but this might actually be a window defect due to loss of the macular pigment in the perifoveal region [21]. Over the course of the disease, the telangiectatic vessels will eventually involve the entire parafoveal region. During the later stages of the FA, there is diffuse hyperfluorescence presumed due to the abnormal vasculature in the absence of choroidal neovascularization (CNV, Fig. 15.1e). OCT angiography (OCTA) reveals the abnormally dilated vessels tend to be drawn to a temporal focal point in the fovea and can highlight the point where venules dive down to the deeper vasculature [22]. Newer studies have identified retinal–choroidal anastomoses that develop before subretinal neovascularization and in concordance with the development of right-angle venules. Spaide et al. postulated that the abnormal vessels moved posterior toward the choroid, rather than into the vitreous, due to the metabolic derangements these patients have; one of which is potentially high cholesterol [22].

15.4 Associated Systemic Medical Conditions

Recent studies have found that patients with MacTel type 2 have a higher prevalence of systemic vascular comorbidities such as diabetes mellitus, hyperlipidemia, hypertension, obesity, and cancer [3, 23, 24]. Additionally, it appears that patients with MacTel may be more likely to have a history of smoking [3]. It is very possible that diabetes and hypertension lead to increased susceptibility of the macular vasculature to develop the abnormalities seen in MacTel patients. Due to the associations with these diseases, it is plausible other vascular diseases could be associated with MacTel, but no other systemic medical risk factors have been identified. Recently, there was no association found between MacTel and obstructive sleep apnea [25], while there remain no definitive ocular associations that have been found with macular telangiectasia.

15.5 Subretinal Neovascularization Associated with Idiopathic Macular Telangiectasia

Subretinal neovascular complexes are a late manifestation of MacTel type 2 and are thought to be distinct from the CNV lesions seen in patients with age-related macular degeneration (AMD) and neovascularization elsewhere of diabetes [23]. These lesions may present at any time during the natural course of the disease [1], but are typically preceded by the right-angle venules and RPE hyperplasia [22]. Gass classified the neovascularization seen these patients as type 2 subretinal neovascularization that developed from the proliferation and remodeling of the outer capillary plexus and extended underneath the retina and RPE but above Bruch's membrane [1]. Yanuzzi in 2006 proposed that the subretinal neovascularization originated from the deep retinal circulation and in his study observed retinal to retinal and retinal to subretinal anastomoses [2]. Yanuzzi and colleagues felt the subretinal neovascularization in MacTel was similar to that of retinal angiomatous proliferation lesions with proliferation of the deep capillary circulation served by these abnormal anastomoses [2]. Gass also noted that certain end-stage eyes were noted to have anastomoses between these subretinal neovascular complexes and the choroid [1]. These choroidal anastomoses were also found in a separate study by Engelbrecht and colleagues [18]. These anastomoses and neovascular complexes were difficult to image, though, due to the leaky nature of both the neovascular complexes and abnormally dilated venules that typically were overlying them. OCTA imaging, however, nicely is able to delineate these subretinal neovascular complexes [26]. These findings were further explained by Spaide et al. who noted the presence of retinal choroidal anastomoses in 65% of eyes with MacTel type 2 and that these anastomoses occur before and independent to the development of the subretinal neovascular complexes associated with late-stage MacTel type 2 [22]. This led the group to conclude that MacTel type 2 may not be a pure neurodegenerative process with secondary retinal and vascular changes, as the choroid appears to be involved as well (Fig. 15.2).

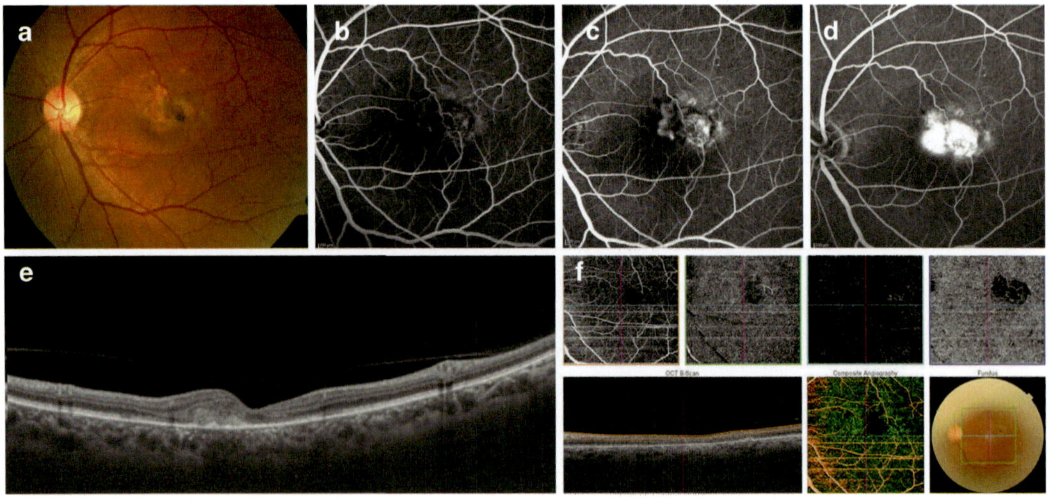

Fig. 15.2 A 68-year-old male with subretinal neovascularization presumed due to idiopathic macular telangiectasia type 2. Color fungus photograph (**a**) of the left eye with loss of retinal transparency, retinal pigment epithelial changes, and blunted retinal vasculature. Fluorescein angiography of the left eye (B-D) with the early phase (**b**) at 28 s revealing a retinal neovascular network temporal to the fovea. This lesion progressive leaked through the course of the angiography, evidenced at both 51 s (**c**) and on the late phase angiogram at 7 min (**d**). Optical coherence tomography (**e**) of the left eye of the same patient with subretinal hyper-reflective material consistent with a potential neovascular network. Optical coherence tomography angiography (**f**) of the left eye reveals a fine network or retinal neovascularization temporal to the fovea. Photographs courtesy of Dr. Avantika Dogra, LV Prasad Eye Institute, Hyderabad, India

15.6 Treatment of Subretinal Neovascularization in Macular Telangiectasia Type 2

As previously mentioned, the subretinal neovascular complexes in eyes with macular telangiectasia type 2 are very different from the CNV lesions seen in patients with AMD. Park and colleagues in 1996 described the natural history of these fibrovascular lesions in 11 eyes. The cohort had an average follow up of 44 months and only 2 eyes lost 2 or more lines of vision after the detection of the subretinal neovascularization [27]. Additionally, Park et al. studied the effects of grid laser photocoagulation in patients with macular edema and subretinal neovascularization and found no benefits in improving or stabilizing long-term visual acuity in a cohort of 10 eyes compared to a control population [28]. Park concluded that perhaps focal laser photocoagulation may not be beneficial as the vision does not tend to worsen over time. Given that the average follow-up in both studies was around 5 years, they may not adequately represent the eyes that will deteriorate much later in the course of the disease. Regardless, both studies reflect how different these fibrovascular complexes are compared to typical CNV lesions.

Other studies have examined the use of photodynamic therapy (PDT) in MacTel patients with macular edema, but without subretinal neovascularization lesions which found mixed results [29, 30]. All are small case reports or case series which make it difficult to glean the clinical utility of these studies for nonproliferative MacTel. MacTel associated with subretinal neovascularization complexes, though, seems to respond well to PDT. Several small case series have shown improvement or stability in visual acuity over time in eyes with subretinal neovascularization treated with PDT [31–35]. The first report of visual improvement was a case report by Potter and colleagues in 2002 that noted visual improvement that was stable 7 months after treatment. Interestingly, the fluorescein leakage from the telangiectatic vessels persisted, but the leakage from the subretinal neovascularization stopped [33]. There were two series of 6 patients each, both with follow up less than 2 years, that found the majority of eyes maintained visual acuity through the course of their respective studies [32, 34]. Snyers et al. reported that one eye in their series of 5 had vision loss persist after PDT with persistent fluorescein leakage without enlargement of the neovascular lesion [35]. Hershberger and colleagues also noted that in their series of eyes, there was rapid refilling of the neovascular lesions thought to be due to the choroidal–retinal anastomoses that develop during the natural course of the disease [31]. These anastomoses perhaps can lead to treatment failure if eyes are followed long enough. In the series by Hussain, all 6 eyes had evidence of associated retinal pigment epithelial damage [32] and in another report, there was atrophy of the RPE following PDT [36]. There is reasonable concern that the verteporfin may leak from the telangiectatic vessels and cause direct toxic damage to the surrounding neurosensory retina and RPE [3]. Given the small reported numbers with minimal follow-up, potentially toxic side effects, and in the setting of newer antiangiogenic medications, PDT may play a limited role in the management of subretinal neovascularization associated with MacTel type 2, but perhaps can be reserved for certain, refractory neovascular lesions.

With the success intravitreal anti-VEGF injections have had on visual recovery and stabilization with other causes of CNV [37, 38], several studies evaluated the visual and anatomical outcomes in MacTel patients with subretinal neovascularization (Table 15.1) [39–47]. Jorge and colleagues were the first to show an improvement in visual acuity in a patient with subretinal neovascularization in 2006 [41]. This led to larger case series and retrospective studies that all showed an improvement in visual acuity and a decrease in retinal thickness over the treatment course. In the series of 9 eyes by Roller and colleagues, eyes needed an average of 4.9 injections over a mean period of approximately 1.5 years [46]. In a similar study by Narayanan et al. who evaluated 16 eyes over a 1 year time period, eyes only required on average 1.9 injections. These reports conclude that these subretinal neovascu-

Table 15.1 Summary of studies examining the use of intravitreal anti-vascular endothelial growth factor injections for the treatment of idiopathic macular telangiectasia type 2

Study	Number of eyes	Intravitreal agent	Mean number of intravitreal injections	Baseline visual acuity (Snellen acuity)	Final visual acuity (Snellen acuity)	Mean follow-up (years)
Charbel et al. [39]	6	Bevacizumab	2	20/80	20/50	1.5
Do et al. [40]	10	Ranibizumab	6	20/64	20/50	0.5
Jorge et al. [41]	1	Bevacizumab	1	20/40	20/20	2
Kovach and Rosenfeld [43]	5	Bevacizumab	2.8	20/86	20/48	1.3
Mandal et al. [44]	6	Bevacizumab	1	20/200	20/100	0.5
Narayanan et al. [45]	16	Bevacizumab and Ranibizumab	1.9	20/120	20/70	1
Roller et al. [46]	9	Bevacizumab	4.9	20/80	20/63	1.5
Toygar et al. [47]	25	Bevacizumab	8.4	20/91	20/62	3.3

lar complexes appear to respond well to intravitreal anti-VEGF therapy with fewer injections than their AMD counterparts. The study with the longest follow-up period was reported by Toygar and colleagues on 25 eyes with an average follow-up of 3.5 years [47]. These eyes required a mean of 8.4 injections over that time frame with an improvement in visual acuity and reduction in retinal thickness that was maintained over the study period. Conversely, intravitreal anti-VEGF for the management of macular edema without subretinal neovascularization in MacTel patients has been largely unsuccessful with no functional or visual benefit [48]. Thus, the preferred treatment for patients with MacTel who experience a sudden decline in visual acuity due to subretinal neovascularization is with intravitreal anti-VEGF therapy. Compared to other diseases causing CNV, patients with MacTel may require fewer injections in order to maintain visual acuity gains and retinal thickness reduction.

Other modalities that have been tried for these subretinal neovascular complexes include transpupillary thermotherapy (TTT), combination PDT with both triamcinolone and anti-VEGF agents, and even surgical removal of the lesions. The report on TTT followed 13 eyes over a mean period of 8.6 months with 11 eyes that had stable visual acuity, 1 eye with improved vision, and 1 eye with a decrease in visual acuity [49]. Both combination PDT with triamcinolone and PDT with anti-VEGF have been reported successfully [29, 50, 51], but the same concerns with PDT in these eyes persists and thus the data is limited regarding combination PDT therapy. Lastly, surgical removal of the subretinal neovascular membranes has been tried in two separate reports, both of which report difficulty removing the subretinal complexes without damaging or removing the adjacent neurosensory retina making surgery obsolete in the management of subretinal neovascularization associated with macular telangiectasia [52, 53].

Key Learning Points

1. Patients with macular telangiectasia type 2 may develop subretinal neovascular complexes that originate from the retinal vasculature.
2. These complexes almost always form after the development of right-angle venules and RPE hyperplasia.
3. The neovascularization may develop independently from the formation of retinal–choroidal

anastomoses seen in patients with macular telangiectasia.
4. Nonproliferative macular telangiectasia does not respond to anti-VEGF therapy.
5. The subretinal neovascular complexes in macular telangiectasia do not respond to well to focal laser or photodynamic therapy.
6. Anti-VEGF for the management of neovascular complexes in macular telangiectasia patients maintains visual acuity gains and reductions in retinal thickness.
7. Patients with macular telangiectasia may require fewer anti-VEGF injections than other patients with typical choroidal neovascular lesions.

References

1. Gass JD, Blodi BA. Idiopathic juxtafoveolar retinal telangiectasis. Update of classification and follow-up study. Ophthalmology. 1993;100(10):1536–46.
2. Yannuzzi LA, Bardal AM, Freund KB, Chen KJ, Eandi CM, Blodi B. Idiopathic macular telangiectasia. Arch Ophthalmol. 2006;124(4):450–60.
3. Charbel Issa P, Gillies MC, Chew EY, et al. Macular telangiectasia type 2. Prog Retin Eye Res. 2013;34:49–77.
4. Tikellis G, Gillies MC, Guymer RH, McAllister IL, Shaw JE, Wong TY. Retinal vascular caliber and macular telangiectasia type 2. Ophthalmology. 2009;116(2):319–23.
5. Eliassi-Rad B, Green WR. Histopathologic study of presumed parafoveal telangiectasis. Retina. 1999;19(4):332–5.
6. Gass JD. Histopathologic study of presumed parafoveal telangiectasis. Retina. 2000;20(2):226–7.
7. Powner MB, Gillies MC, Zhu M, Vevis K, Hunyor AP, Fruttiger M. Loss of Muller's cells and photoreceptors in macular telangiectasia type 2. Ophthalmology. 2013;120(11):2344–52.
8. Wubben TJ, Zacks DN, Besirli CG. Retinal neuroprotection: current strategies and future directions. Curr Opin Ophthalmol. 2019;30(3):199–205.
9. Aung KZ, Wickremasinghe SS, Makeyeva G, Robman L, Guymer RH. The prevalence estimates of macular telangiectasia type 2: the Melbourne collaborative cohort study. Retina. 2010;30(3):473–8.
10. Klein R, Blodi BA, Meuer SM, Myers CE, Chew EY, Klein BE. The prevalence of macular telangiectasia type 2 in the Beaver Dam eye study. Am J Ophthalmol. 2010;150(1):55–62. e52
11. Sallo FB, Leung I, Mathenge W, et al. The prevalence of type 2 idiopathic macular telangiectasia in two African populations. Ophthalmic Epidemiol. 2012;19(4):185–9.
12. Parmalee NL, Schubert C, Figueroa M, et al. Identification of a potential susceptibility locus for macular telangiectasia type 2. PLoS One. 2012;7(8):e24268.
13. Ronquillo CC, Wegner K, Calvo CM, Bernstein PS. Genetic penetrance of macular telangiectasia type 2. JAMA Ophthalmol. 2018;136(10):1158–63.
14. Moisseiev J, Lewis H, Bartov E, Fine SL, Murphy RP. Superficial retinal refractile deposits in juxtafoveal telangiectasis. Am J Ophthalmol. 1990;109(5):604–5.
15. Charbel Issa P, Scholl HP, Gaudric A, et al. Macular full-thickness and lamellar holes in association with type 2 idiopathic macular telangiectasia. Eye (Lond). 2009;23(2):435–41.
16. Patel B, Duvall J, Tullo AB. Lamellar macular hole associated with idiopathic juxtafoveolar telangiectasia. Br J Ophthalmol. 1988;72(7):550–1.
17. Karth PA, Raja SC, Brown DM, Kim JE. Outcomes of macular hole surgeries for macular telangiectasia type 2. Retina. 2014;34(5):907–15.
18. Engelbrecht NE, Aaberg TM Jr, Sung J, Lewis ML. Neovascular membranes associated with idiopathic juxtafoveolar telangiectasis. Arch Ophthalmol. 2002;120(3):320–4.
19. Solberg Y, Dysli C, Wolf S, Zinkernagel MS. Fluorescence lifetime patterns in macular telangiectasia type 2. Retina. 2020; https://doi.org/10.1097/IAE.0000000000002411.
20. Sallo FB, Leung I, Clemons TE, Peto T, Bird AC, Pauleikhoff D. Multimodal imaging in type 2 idiopathic macular telangiectasia. Retina. 2015;35(4):742–9.
21. Gillies MC, Zhu M, Chew E, et al. Familial asymptomatic macular telangiectasia type 2. Ophthalmology. 2009;116(12):2422–9.
22. Spaide RF, Yannuzzi LA, Maloca PM. Retinal-choroidal anastomosis in macular telangiectasia type 2. Retina. 2018;38(10):1920–9.
23. Chew EY, Murphy RP, Newsome DA, Fine SL. Parafoveal telangiectasis and diabetic retinopathy. Arch Ophthalmol. 1986;104(1):71–5.
24. Clemons TE, Gillies MC, Chew EY, et al. Medical characteristics of patients with macular telangiectasia type 2 (MacTel Type 2) MacTel project report no. 3. Ophthalmic Epidemiol. 2013;20(2):109–13.
25. Lee MG, Marshall NS, Clemons TE, et al. No association between sleep apnoea and macular telangiectasia type 2 and its markers of severity and progression: a case-control study and retrospective cohort study. Clin Exp Ophthalmol. 2019; https://doi.org/10.1111/ceo.13363.
26. Balaratnasingam C, Yannuzzi LA, Spaide RF. Possible choroidal neovascularization in macular telangiectasia type 2. Retina. 2015;35(11):2317–22.
27. Park D, Schatz H, McDonald HR, Johnson RN. Fibrovascular tissue in bilateral juxtafoveal telangiectasis. Arch Ophthalmol. 1996;114(9):1092–6.

28. Park DW, Schatz H, McDonald HR, Johnson RN. Grid laser photocoagulation for macular edema in bilateral juxtafoveal telangiectasis. Ophthalmology. 1997;104(11):1838–46.
29. De Lahitte GD, Cohen SY, Gaudric A. Lack of apparent short-term benefit of photodynamic therapy in bilateral, acquired, parafoveal telangiectasis without subretinal neovascularization. Am J Ophthalmol. 2004;138(5):892–4.
30. Kotoula MG, Chatzoulis DZ, Karabatsas CH, Tsiloulis A, Tsironi EE. Resolution of macular edema in idiopathic juxtafoveal telangiectasis using PDT. Ophthalmic Surg Lasers Imaging. 2009;40(1):65–7.
31. Hershberger VS, Hutchins RK, Laber PW. Photodynamic therapy with verteporfin for subretinal neovascularization secondary to bilateral idiopathic acquired juxtafoveolar telangiectasis. Ophthalmic Surg Lasers Imaging. 2003;34(4):318–20.
32. Hussain N, Das T, Sumasri K, Ram LS. Bilateral sequential photodynamic therapy for sub-retinal neovascularization with type 2A parafoveal telangiectasis. Am J Ophthalmol. 2005;140(2):333–5.
33. Potter MJ, Szabo SM, Chan EY, Morris AH. Photodynamic therapy of a subretinal neovascular membrane in type 2A idiopathic juxtafoveolar retinal telangiectasis. Am J Ophthalmol. 2002;133(1):149–51.
34. Potter MJ, Szabo SM, Sarraf D, Michels R, Schmidt-Erfurth U. Photodynamic therapy for subretinal neovascularization in type 2A idiopathic juxtafoveolar telangiectasis. Can J Ophthalmol. 2006;41(1): 34–7.
35. Snyers B, Verougstraete C, Postelmans L, Leys A, Hykin P. Photodynamic therapy of subfoveal neovascular membrane in type 2A idiopathic juxtafoveolar retinal telangiectasis. Am J Ophthalmol. 2004;137(5):812–9.
36. Shanmugam MP, Agarwal M. RPE atrophy following photodynamic therapy in type 2A idiopathic parafoveal telangiectasis. Indian J Ophthalmol. 2005;53(1):61–3.
37. Brown DM, Michels M, Kaiser PK, et al. Ranibizumab versus verteporfin photodynamic therapy for neovascular age-related macular degeneration: two-year results of the ANCHOR study. Ophthalmology. 2009;116(1):57–65. e55
38. Rosenfeld PJ, Brown DM, Heier JS, et al. Ranibizumab for neovascular age-related macular degeneration. N Engl J Med. 2006;355(14):1419–31.
39. Charbel Issa P, Finger RP, Holz FG, Scholl HP. Eighteen-month follow-up of intravitreal bevacizumab in type 2 idiopathic macular telangiectasia. Br J Ophthalmol. 2008;92(7):941–5.
40. Do DV, Bressler SB, Cassard SD, et al. Ranibizumab for macular telangiectasia type 2 in the absence of subretinal neovascularization. Retina. 2014;34(10):2063–71.
41. Jorge R, Costa RA, Calucci D, Scott IU. Intravitreal bevacizumab (Avastin) associated with the regression of subretinal neovascularization in idiopathic juxtafoveolar retinal telangiectasis. Graefes Arch Clin Exp Ophthalmol. 2007;245(7):1045–8.
42. Karagiannis D, Georgalas I, Ladas I, Eustratios P, Mitropoulos P. A case of subretinal neovascularization treated with intravitreal ranibizumab in a patient with idiopathic juxtafoveal retinal telangiectasis. Clin Interv Aging. 2009;4:63–5.
43. Kovach JL, Rosenfeld PJ. Bevacizumab (avastin) therapy for idiopathic macular telangiectasia type II. Retina. 2009;29(1):27–32.
44. Mandal S, Venkatesh P, Abbas Z, Vohra R, Garg S. Intravitreal bevacizumab (Avastin) for subretinal neovascularization secondary to type 2A idiopathic juxtafoveal telangiectasia. Graefes Arch Clin Exp Ophthalmol. 2007;245(12):1825–9.
45. Narayanan R, Chhablani J, Sinha M, et al. Efficacy of anti-vascular endothelial growth factor therapy in subretinal neovascularization secondary to macular telangiectasia type 2. Retina. 2012;32(10):2001–5.
46. Roller AB, Folk JC, Patel NM, et al. Intravitreal bevacizumab for treatment of proliferative and non-proliferative type 2 idiopathic macular telangiectasia. Retina. 2011;31(9):1848–55.
47. Toygar O, Guess MG, Youssef DS, Miller DM. Long-term outcomes of intravitreal bevacizumab therapy for subretinal neovascularization secondary to idiopathic macular telangiectasia type 2. Retina. 2016;36(11):2150–7.
48. Charbel Issa P, Finger RP, Kruse K, Baumuller S, Scholl HP, Holz FG. Monthly ranibizumab for nonproliferative macular telangiectasia type 2: a 12-month prospective study. Am J Ophthalmol. 2011;151(5):876–86. e871
49. Shukla D, Singh J, Kolluru CM, Kim R, Namperumalsamy P. Transpupillary thermotherapy for subfoveal neovascularization secondary to group 2A idiopathic juxtafoveolar telangiectasis. Am J Ophthalmol. 2004;138(1):147–9.
50. Rishi P, Shroff D, Rishi E. Combined photodynamic therapy and intravitreal ranibizumab as primary treatment for subretinal neovascular membrane (SRNVM) associated with type 2 idiopathic macular telangiectasia. Graefes Arch Clin Exp Ophthalmol. 2008;246(4):619–21.
51. Smithen LM, Spaide RF. Photodynamic therapy and intravitreal triamcinolone for a subretinal neovascularization in bilateral idiopathic juxtafoveal telangiectasis. Am J Ophthalmol. 2004;138(5):884–5.
52. Berger AS, McCuen BW 2nd, Brown GC, Brownlow RL Jr. Surgical removal of subfoveal neovascularization in idiopathic juxtafoveolar retinal telangiectasis. Retina. 1997;17(2):94–8.
53. Davidorf FH, Pressman MD, Chambers RB. Juxtafoveal telangiectasis-a name change? Retina. 2004;24(3):474–8.

Peripapillary Choroidal Neovascularization

16

Sumit Randhir Singh and Jay Chhablani

16.1 Introduction

Peripapillary choroidal neovascular membrane (CNVM) is a distinct terminology used to describe CVNM that is located near the optic nerve head. Broadly speaking, any CNVM a portion of which is located within one disc diameter is considered as peripapillary CVNM [1]. Approximately 10% of all CNVM are peripapillary in a location with a female predilection [1–3].

Description of peripapillary CNVM includes the number of clock hours, quadrants, size of CNVM complex, and distance from fovea. Ruben et al. devised a grading system to classify the CNVM in different zones. Each zone centered around the disc covers 60 degrees. Zone 1 extends 30 degrees above and below a straight line connecting optic disc and fovea [2]. Although no consensus exists, few authors have defined large peripapillary CNVM as lesions with size more than 3.5 disc areas or involving >50% of disc circumference [4]. These large lesions may show unpredictable growth and may harbor a predominantly occult component [4]. Fellow eye involvement is common in up to 20–62% of cases in patients more than 70 years of age [5, 6]. This event can happen either concomitantly or after a gap of several years [5].

Most common location of CMVM is nasal to the optic disc in up to 40% of the cases [7], however, these patients may be asymptomatic whereas the most common location in symptomatic patients is temporal due to involvement of papillomacular bundle [8]. Histopathological studies show the presence of these CNVM lesions in apparently normal eyes suggestive of a higher prevalence of peripapillary CNVM as previously thought [8, 9].

Peripapillary CNVM has certain differences with respect to subfoveal CNVM. There is a variation in terms of etiology, location of the lesions. A majority (up to 2/3rd) of peripapillary CNVM may be asymptomatic for long duration [7], and therefore treatment may not be warranted in contrast to subfoveal CNVM, which invariably needs treatment. The site of CNVM formation in PCNVM is through the breaks in Bruch's membrane (57%) or through the end of Bruch's membrane at the edge of the optic disc (43%) more commonly on nasal side [8].

16.2 Etiologies

A myriad of ocular diseases can lead to the formation of peripapillary CNVM, the most common being neovascular age-related macular degeneration (AMD), inflammatory chorioretinal disorders,

S. R. Singh
Smt. Kanuri Santhamma Centre for Vitreo-Retinal Diseases, L V Prasad Eye Institute, Hyderabad, India

J. Chhablani (✉)
Department of Ophthalmology, University of Pittsburgh Medical Center, Pittsburgh, PA, USA

J. Chhablani (ed.), *Choroidal Neovascularization*, https://doi.org/10.1007/978-981-15-2213-0_16

angioid streaks, and optic disc anomalies [10]. No identifiable cause can be ascertained in a significant proportion (up to 40%) of these eyes, hence termed idiopathic [6]. While AMD and idiopathic causes predominate in elderly, inflammatory, optic disc anomalies, and angioid streaks are more commonly seen in younger age groups [11].

16.3 Chorioretinal Degenerations

Neovascular AMD AMD is characterized by drusen of size more than 63 μ, retinal pigment epithelial (RPE) atrophy, fibrovascular pigment epithelial detachments (FVPED), and/or disciform scars in the macular area with reports suggesting an association of peripapillary CNVM with advanced stages of AMD [7, 12]. However, these macular changes in the form of RPE atrophy and drusen (including subretinal drusenoid deposits, SDD) can be present in the peripapillary area also which may be a harbinger of peripapillary CNVM similar to macular CNVM. Overall, 45.2–84.6% of all cases of peripapillary CNVM are caused due to AMD [6, 13]. Wilde et al. reported the prevalence of peripapillary CNVM secondary to AMD as 3.9% (9 eyes among 231 neovascular AMD cases) [3]. Fellow eye involvement was seen in 19.8% and 54% patients with AMD-related peripapillary CNVM over 2 and 7 years, respectively [5, 6]. Bilaterality up to 62% was more common in patients with age more than 70 years [5].

Angioid Streaks CNVM is a rare complication in eyes with angioid streaks that are characterized by a break in brittle and calcified Bruch's membrane [14]. There can be systemic associations such as pseudoxanthoma elasticum, Ehlers–Danlos syndrome, Paget's disease of bone, sickle cell disease, or other hemoglobinopathies in half of the cases whereas in remaining cases, the cause is not identifiable [15]. The risk of CNVM formation increases with age and also appears related to the width, length, and location of angioid streaks, especially in close proximity to disc [16, 17]. The reported incidence of CNVM in these eyes has been as high as 72–86% [18, 19]. CNVM in these eyes, however, are small and have a higher probability of being asymptomatic.

Pathological Myopia It is defined as degenerative changes in eyes with high myopia (≥6 D, diopters) [20]. Often termed as myopic maculopathy or myopic macular degeneration, a consensus definition according to META analysis for Pathologic Myopia (META-PM) study includes the presence of diffuse/patchy chorioretinal atrophy or macular atrophy or presence of staphyloma [21]. There is sparse literature on peripapillary CNVM in myopic eyes with one case series reporting the incidence as 4.2% (11 of 260 myopic CNVM) [22]. This is despite a high overall incidence (5–11%) of myopic CNVM in eyes with pathological myopia [23]. These CNVM are known to develop at the edge of conus around the optic disc and more commonly seen with large conus [22]. Their source of origin is possible through a defect in Bruch's membrane at the site of lacquer cracks near the myopic conus. Moreover, they tend to regress even without treatment [22].

Post Laser Photocoagulation Though laser photocoagulation has been used to treat CNVM in multiple clinical scenarios, the risk of recurrence and CNVM formation at the edge of the lesion is well documented. Govindhari et al. have shown exacerbation of CNVM after 3 months of laser in a case of angioid streak [24].

16.4 Inflammatory

A host of inflammatory chorioretinal disorders can lead to CNVM formation. Common causes include infectious (toxoplasma retinochoroiditis, presumed ocular tuberculosis) and inflammatory pathologies (sarcoidosis, serpiginous-like choroiditis (SLC), Punctate inner choroidopathy (PIC), multifocal choroiditis and panuveitis (MCP), presumed ocular histoplasmosis syndrome (POHS), Vogt–Koyanagi–Harada (VKH) syndrome and other inflammatory chorioretinopathies) [10, 25–28]. The background inflammatory pathology may or may not be active once clinical manifestations of CNVM ensue. Animal models suggest that neovascularization can occur even in the absence of disease activity [29].

The etiologies vary widely according to geographic location. For instance, POHS is commonly reported from Ohio and Mississippi river valleys and is very rare outside this endemic zone [30]. POHS is the most common cause of inflammatory CNVM in children in Western literature [31]. Ocular tuberculosis is more commonly seen in the Indian subcontinent [25, 27].

Perentes et al. have reported a prevalence of 1.9% (12/648 patients) of subretinal membranes [10]. In contrast to other causes, the primary treatment for ocular inflammation in the form of local or systemic steroid or immunomodulatory therapy needs to be continued as they may complement and help reduce inflammation.

16.5 Idiopathic

This category where no underlying choroidal or retinal pathology can be established is a diagnosis of exclusion and includes 5–40% of patients with peripapillary CNVM [6, 32]. Idiopathic CNVM similar to AMD-related CNVM are predominantly occult in majority of eyes (64.1%) [6]. Although the recurrence rates appear comparable between idiopathic and AMD CNVM, the visual outcomes in idiopathic cases are relatively better [6].

16.6 Optic Disc Anomalies

Optic nerve head drusen (ONHD) are an incidental finding in majority of the patients with an estimated prevalence of 3.4–24 individuals per 1000 population [33]. These originate due to disturbed axonal metabolism in association with a small scleral canal [33, 34]. Duncan et al. have reported a 25% (24 of 98 eyes) incidence rate of CNVM in pediatric population with ONHD. The majority (21 out of 24) were located nasal to disc while the remaining 3 were located temporally [34].

Idiopathic intracranial hypertension (IIH) has also been rarely associated with CNVM (0.53%) [35–38]. The proposed mechanism is a combination of hypoxia due to axonal swelling combined with pressure deformity of Bruch's membrane at the edge of optic nerve head leading to localized discontinuity. These events lead to the process of angiogenesis and formation of CNVM [36, 39].

Morning glory syndrome is a congenital condition associated with retinal dysplasia, and excavation of optic disc filled with glial tissue and pigment ring. Few case reports have shown an association of CNVM with morning glory syndrome and tilted disc syndrome in peripapillary location [40–43]. CNVM have also been reported in eyes with retinochoroidal coloboma in peripapillary location, optic nerve coloboma, congenital optic disc pit, or optic neuritis [44–48].

16.7 Dystrophies

Pozzoni et al. reported a case in a 12-year male with peripapillary CNVM in a case of Best disease. Vitelliform lesion was present at macula with subretinal heme and CNVM adjacent to optic disc margin [49]. Browning et al. reported 3 eyes of peripapillary CNVM due to pattern dystrophy among which 2 and 1 were occult and classic CNVM, respectively [6].

16.8 Congenital/Benign/Malignant Lesions of Retina and Choroid

Very rarely, choroidal neoplastic lesions can be associated with CNVM. Less than 1% of giant choroidal nevi (≥10 mm basal dimension) develop CNVM over a mean period of 61 months [50]. Peripapillary CNVM associated with choroidal nevi was seen in a total of 4 eyes (17%) among 24 eyes with choroidal nevi associated CNVM [51]. Tuncer et al. reported a case of peripapillary CNVM in a 16-year female with choroidal nevus [52]. Optic disc melanocytoma and choroidal osteoma also are associated with CNVM [6, 53–56]. Kase et al. reported a case of retinoblastoma with peripapillary CNVM in a 1-year old who underwent enucleation [57].

Congenital, benign lesions like combined hamartoma of the retina and retinal pigment epithelium (CHRRPE) are also associated with CNVM in 6% of eyes which characteristically exude and leak less compared to CNVM due to other causes [58–60]. The descriptions in previous reports, however, had no mention of exact location of CNVM lesions. They are usually present at the junction of abnormal hamartomatous and normal retina. OCT angiography, therefore, plays an important role in identifying CNVM in these eyes [60].

16.9 Multimodal Imaging

Optical Coherence Tomography Optical Coherence Tomography (OCT) plays an important role in establishing the diagnosis and determining the disease activity during the follow-up. AMD-related and idiopathic CNVM are usually located below RPE (type 1) whereas inflammatory CNVM are above RPE level (type 2). Subretinal hyper-reflectivity in the form of hemorrhage, exudation or neovascular membrane, or sub-RPE hyper-reflectivity such as FVPED can be identified using structural OCT b scans.

Fundus Fluorescein Angiography Fundus Fluorescein Angiography (FFA) is an invasive modality and is able to determine the location of CNVM either at subretinal (classic) or sub RPE (occult) level. FFA in classic CNVM shows well-defined margins of CNVM with hyperfluorescence in the early phase followed by a late leakage. Occult CNVM is characterized by irregular hyperfluorescence, ill-defined margins in early phase and late leakage. AMD-related and idiopathic variety CNVM are predominantly occult whereas inflammatory CNVM are commonly classic [61]. Choroidal nevi associated CNVM are predominantly classic (20 eyes, 83%) [51]. Kies and Bird reported a higher predominance of occult lesions (93%) in their cohort [62]. This is explained by higher incidence of AMD and idiopathic causes of peripapillary CNVM in their sample.

Indocyanine Angiography Indocyanine Angiography (ICGA) like FFA is an invasive diagnostic modality and is a gold standard test in the diagnosis of polypoidal choroidal vasculopathy (PCV). PCV is characterized by the presence of branching vascular networks with terminal, aneurysmal polypoidal dilatations called polyps. ICGA may be particularly helpful in cases with occult or type 1 CNVM, and assess choroidal perfusion status in inflammatory choroidal disorders.

OCT Angiography OCT Angiography (OCTA) in recent years has evolved as an alternative to dye-based imaging techniques. Based on identification of motion contrast and sequential OCT b scans to estimate the decorrelation signals, OCTA can identify blood flow in the retinal and choroidal vessels up to choriocapillaris [63]. This can be especially useful in identifying CNVM in conditions such as choroidal osteoma, CHRRPE, inflammatory CNVM where FFA may not identify CNVM due to diffuse RPE or choroidal changes [55, 60].

16.10 Natural History

Visual prognosis and natural history are influenced by underlying etiology, proximity to papillomacular bundle, and involvement of a number of clock hours of the optic disc. Reports show contrasting results with few showing that visual prognosis is poor if left untreated [5, 11]. In contrast, Lin et al. have shown that in eyes with peripapillary CNVM post AMD, observation with prompt treatment using anti-VEGF agents is a good strategy. Up to 42% of patients with fovea sparing SRF or exudation were observed for periods ranging from months to years (median 16 months) [13]. Spontaneous regression of peripapillary CNVM due to pathological myopia was seen in five eyes with a reduction in visual acuity in only one eye due to chorioretinal atrophy around the regressed CNVM [22].

Though previous authors have suggested a conservative approach in cases with extrafoveal lesions, these studies were done prior to the widespread availability of anti-VEGF agents [5]. Silvestri et al. reported the natural history of peripapillary CNVM in a cohort of 20 eyes. Causes of vision loss were extension of membrane at subfoveal level, exudation, subretinal fluid, and hemorrhage involving the fovea [5]. They also proposed that younger patients (<40 years) of age had unilateral disease and showed better visual prognosis compared to older patients.

As a general rule, inflammatory CNVM tend to fare better compared to CNVM related to AMD. The possible reasons could be small sized, classic nature of CNVM in otherwise young, healthy individuals with overall good health of RPE–Bruch's complex [27, 64, 65].

16.11 Treatment

Multiple treatment options have been described in the literature including close observation, laser photocoagulation, photodynamic therapy (PDT), anti-vascular endothelial growth factors (VEGF), and rarely, surgical extraction.

Observation Condition such as IIH where the papilledema is controlled adequately using medical or surgical techniques, spontaneous regression of CNVM has been reported. This approach of close follow-up is especially useful in cases with localization of CNVM to peripapillary area alone with no subfoveal extension [35]. Peripapillary CNVM extending more than 750 μ from fovea, not involving 1.5 clock hours of temporal peripapillary region may be carefully observed [66]. However, one should bear in mind that these CNVM are known to show unpredictable growth patterns [62].

Laser Photocoagulation This was the first modality used in clinical practice. A pre-anti-VEGF era report suggests no significant difference of visual acuity with respect to position or size of CNVM complex [2]. On the other hand, Cialdini et al. reported maintained or improved visual acuity in 20 eyes (80%) post laser photocoagulation [67]. According to macular photocoagulation study (MPS) guidelines, temporal 1.5 clock hours of temporal retina need to be spared to avoid iatrogenic damage to papillomacular bundle. A total of 14% of patients treated with laser photocoagulation lost 6 or more lines of visual acuity compared to 26% of untreated eyes, the difference was however not significant ($p = 0.29$) [68]. In view of the high recurrence rates with laser and possibility of missing the extent of CNVM, especially in occult lesions, Kies and Bird proposed to treat a wide margin of normal-looking retina around CNVM [62].

Laser photocoagulation using argon laser in angioid streaks has been associated with either persistence or recurrence [19]. Shah et al. showed efficacy of laser in a case of Inflammatory CNVM in sarcoidosis [69]. Smaller CNVM located outside the vascular arcades if treated promptly carry a good prognosis. There is no significant utility in treating eyes with large lesion or associated large subretinal hemorrhage. Laser is a treatment of choice in pregnancy when PDT and anti-VEGF agents are not considered safe [70]. However, this is associated with multiple adverse effects and carries a risk of permanent scotoma, increase risk of scar expansion, damage to papillomacular bundle, vitreous hemorrhage, and branch retinal artery occlusion [11, 71]. There is also a high risk of recurrence (19–50%) in literature [6, 62, 67, 72]. In view of no significant reduction of recurrence, side effect profile, and availability of better alternatives, laser photocoagulation is no longer the main treatment modality.

Photodynamic Therapy Various reports have shown the utility of PDT with verteporfin (Visudyne; Novartis Pharmaceuticals Corporation, New Jersey) in eyes with peripapillary CNVM secondary to AMD, POHS, and idiopathic CNVM [73, 74]. PDT appears to cause a lesser tissue damage compared to laser [75]. Some authors suggest avoiding PDT in cases with CNVM in close proximity to the optic disc (within 200 μ) whereas others have refuted this proposition and reported no obvious damage to optic nerve even after including the optic nerve within the field of PDT application [73, 74, 76]. Pozzoni et al. successfully treated a case of peripapillary CNVM with best disease with repeated sessions of reduced fluence PDT [49].

Rosenblatt et al. reported at least 2 line visual acuity gain in 6 out of 7 eyes with CNVM due to AMD, POHS, and a follow-up ranging from 6 to 13.5 months [74]. Long-term visual acuity, however, is not known and it is likely that short-term gain may not be maintained over long term. Moreover, there is an additional need for multiple sessions of PDT along with a risk of iatrogenic damage to the optic disc. It is therefore advisable to use PDT in cases nonresponsive to anti-VEGF agents.

Submacular Surgery and Macular Translocation Introduced in 1991 by Thomas and Kaplan, submacular surgery was attempted initially in cases with foveal CNVM [77]. Submacular surgery in peripapillary CNVM remained an option in large CNVM with extensive exudation where PDT and laser were relatively contraindicated.

Atebara et al. reported successful visual outcomes in peripapillary CNVM secondary to POHS confined to extrafoveal location (3 eyes, 20/20) and 14 eyes with extension involving subfoveal location as well. A total of 7 eyes reached 20/40 visual acuity. Recurrence was noted in 4/17 eyes at 32 months [78]. Other authors have also reported visual and anatomical outcomes with CNVM related to histoplasmosis, AMD, and idiopathic nature [79, 80]. Bains et al. in their study of 17 eyes with age > 55 years showed that only one-third patients had improvement or stabilization of visual acuity [80]. Tran et al. reported a successful excision of CNVM in case of melanocytoma with visual acuity of 20/25 at 14 months [54].

However, with a host of complications, variable outcomes (35% to 88% patients maintain or gain visual acuity) and easy availability of anti-VEGF agents, these surgical techniques have fallen out of favor [76, 80–84].

Anti-VEGF Agents Multiple anti-VEGF agents including intravitreal bevacizumab, ranibizumab, aflibercept, and ziv-aflibercept have been used to treat CNVM with successful outcomes [69, 85, 86]. Representative cases are shown as (Figs. 16.1 and 16.2). One major drawback, however, is the need for multiple injections due to short-term action of these agents. Though various landmark studies showed the importance of anti-VEGF agents in subfoveal CNVM, Nguyen et al. reported the anatomical resolution and outcomes of intravenous bevaziumab in patients with peripapillary CNVM due to AMD and myopia [87]. Pederson et al. showed anatomical resolution with maintained visual acuity in one eye with peripapillary CNVM [88]. Lin et al. treated eyes with AMD related peripapillary CNVM with a median of 3 anti-VEGF injections to obtain complete resolution of SRF [13]. This is comparable to previous reports of 3.96 injections in macular CNVM due to AMD [89].

Mansour et al. reported results of bevacizumab in eyes with inflammatory CNVM through 3 months. Though this study had only 8 eyes with peripapillary CNVM, the visual outcomes were encouraging in the short term [26]. Figueroa et al. studied 6 eyes of peripapillary CNVM treated with bevacizumab. Five eyes showed complete anatomical resolution with a mean improvement of 4 lines [90]. Hoeh et al. reported that among 4 eyes treated with intravitreal bevacizumab (mean ± SD:3.5 ± 3.1) through 34 weeks, two lost visual acuity while one maintained vision [91].

Anti VEGF agents can help in resolution of CNVM with no damage to papillomacular bundle. However, need for frequent injections, absence of level I evidence in eyes with peripapillary CNVM can pose questions in using anti-VEGF agents as first-line agents.

Very few reports exist in literature, which questions the efficacy of anti-VEGF agents and prove better outcomes with laser photocoagulation [69]. Munie et al. reported the successful outcomes of bevacizumab in eyes with CNVM due to choroidal nevi. Though their cohort had 4 eyes with peripapillary CNVM, these eyes were not analyzed separately [51]. Other authors have reported similar successful outcomes in eyes with CNVM due to melanocytoma with bevacizumab [53]. Mansour et al. reported successful outcomes using bevacizumab (2 eyes) and ranibizumab (one eye) in cases with peripapillary CNVM due to choroidal osteoma. Two patients had an improvement in vision while one maintained visual acuity [56].

Combination Therapy Studies have also shown a beneficial effect of combination treatment comprising laser photocoagulation and anti-VEGF agents [92]. Adrean et al. have reported significant visual and anatomical

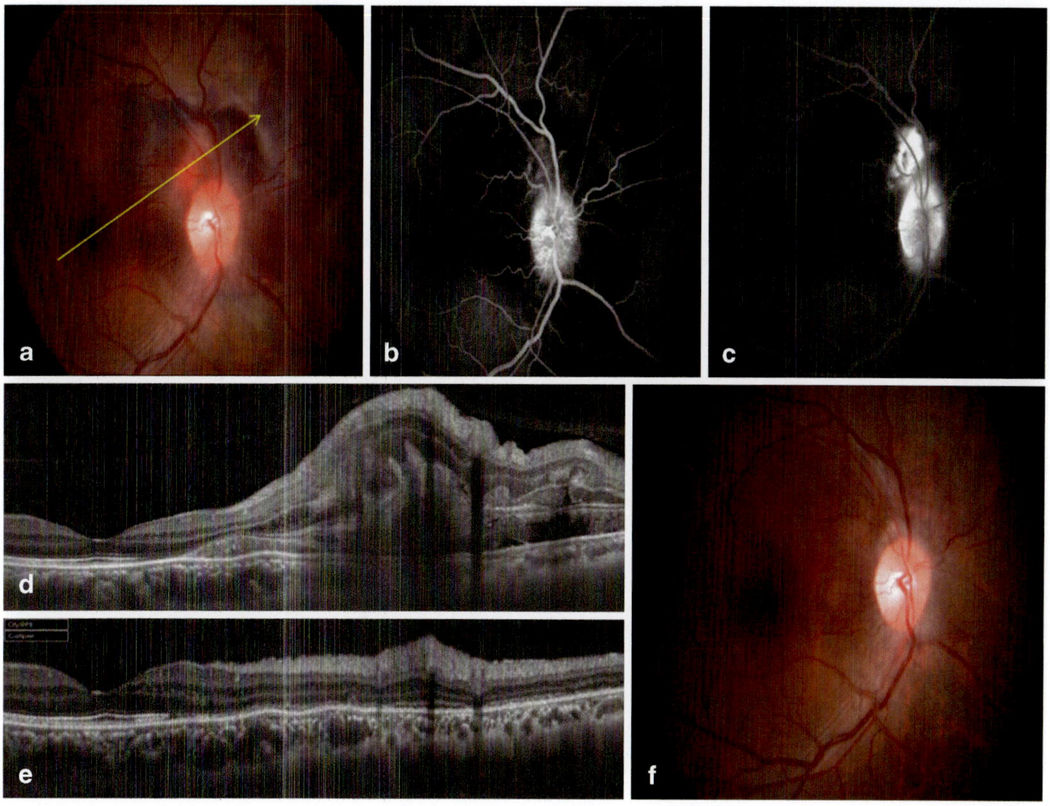

Fig. 16.1 Multimodal imaging of a 58-year-old male with acute onset diminution of vision and a best-corrected visual acuity (BCVA) of 20/25. Fundus examination revealed peripapillary subretinal heme and subretinal yellowish lesion superior to disc (**a**). Fundus fluorescein angiography early and late phase showed early hyperfluorescence and late leak suggestive of classic CNVM (**b**, **c**). Optical coherence tomography (OCT, line scan) through the lesion and fovea revealed the presence of intraretinal and subretinal fluid and subretinal hyperreflectivity suggestive of type 2 CNVM (**d**). A diagnosis of idiopathic CNVM was made and patient was treated with intravitreal bevacizumab (IVB). Post 2 IVB injections, BCVA improved to 20/20. OCT showed resolution of SRF/IRF with fundus photography showing resolution of subretinal heme (**e**, **f**)

improvement in 5 eyes with peripapillary CNVM treated with combination treatment of intravitreal bevacizumab and laser therapy [92].

Inflammatory CNVM deserve special mention because underlying inflammation may remain active in up to 40% of individuals at the time of CNVM diagnosis. Therefore, a combination of steroids (either oral or periocular) may be helpful to counteract the inflammation along with anti-VEGF agents [25]. Tables 16.1 and 16.2 list the etiologies leading to peripapillary CNVM formation and a brief review of literature respectively.

16.12 Conclusions

Anti-VEGF agents form the first line of therapy for the treatment of peripapillary CNVM. Laser photocoagulation and PDT can be used in isolation or as a combination therapy in select conditions only. Recurrences are common, depend on the underlying pathology and may need prolonged treatment leading to an overall fair visual prognosis. Young age and inflammatory CNVM fare better compared to CNVM in elderly secondary to AMD.

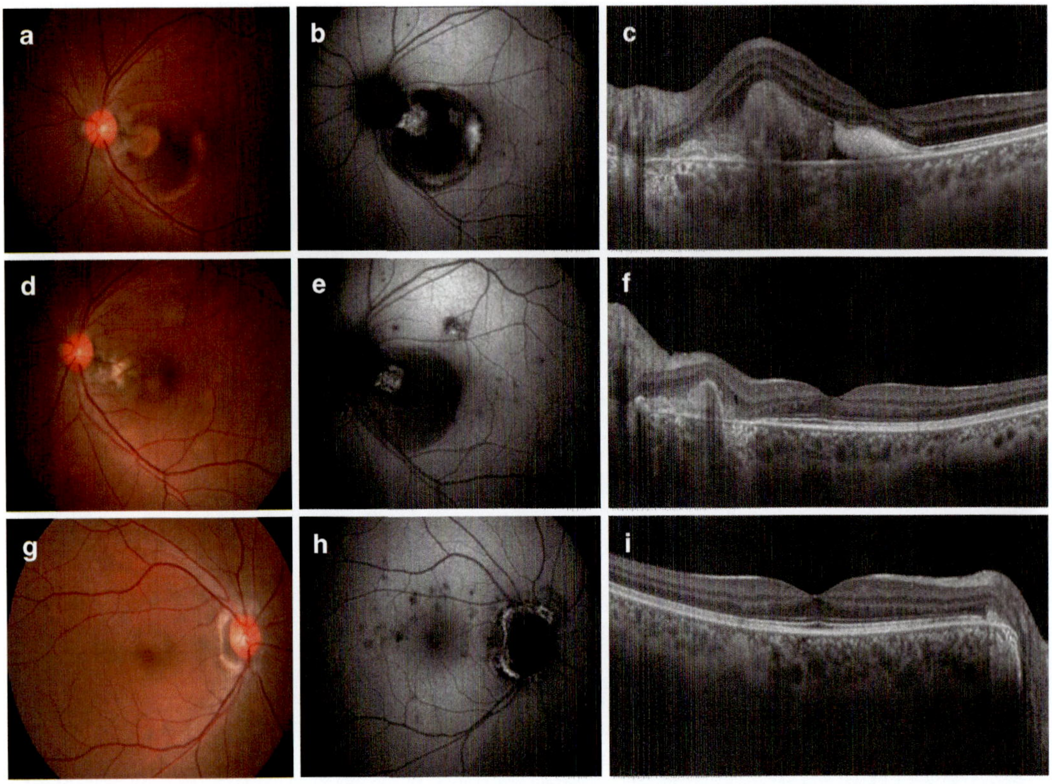

Fig. 16.2 Multimodal imaging of 39-year male with diminution of vision in left eye (20/50) and fundus showing subretinal heme and lesion temporal to optic disc (**a**). Autofluorescence (AF) showed blocked fluorescence due to heme, hyperautofluorescence corresponding to lesion and multiple small, dot-like hypoAF suggestive of focal RPE loss (**b**). OCT confirmed the presence of type 2 CNVM (**c**). A presumptive diagnosis of punctate inner choroidopathy (PIC) with secondary CNVM in left eye was made. Post five intravitreal bevacizumab injections over 24 months, visual acuity improved to 20/20. Fundus photograph and AF showed peripapillary atrophy, multiple hypoAF lesion over posterior pole which was better delineated on AF (**d**, **e**) along with subretinal scar temporal to disc which was confirmed on OCT (**f**). Right eye showed peripapillary scarring and multiple small, hypoAF lesions (**g**, **h**) with OCT showing a normal foveal contour (**i**)

Table 16.1 List of conditions leading to formation of peripapillary choroidal neovascular membrane (CNVM)

Degenerative
Age-related macular degeneration (AMD)
Pathological myopia
Angioid streaks
Post-laser photocoagulation
Idiopathic
Inflammatory
Presumed ocular histoplasmosis syndrome (POHS)
Presumed ocular tuberculosis (POTB)
Vogt–Koyanagi–Harada syndrome (VKH)
Sarcoidosis
Multifocal Choroiditis with Panuveitis (MFC)
Punctate inner choroidopathy (PIC)
Eales/Vasculitis
Serpiginous choroiditis/Serpiginous-like choroiditis
Birdshot retinochoroidopathy
Pars planitis
Optic disc anomalies
Optic disc drusen
Idiopathic intracranial hypertension (IIH)
Optic nerve coloboma

Table 16.1 (continued)

Morning glory syndrome
Optic disc pit
Optic neuritis
Tilted disc syndrome
Traumatic choroidal ruptures
Dystrophies
Best disease
Pattern dystrophy

Table 16.1 (continued)

Congenital/benign/malignant lesions of retina and choroid
Choroidal nevus
Choroidal osteoma
Malignant melanoma Retinoblastoma
Combined Hamartoma of the Retina and Retina Pigment Epithelium (CHRRPE)

Table 16.2 Compilation of previous studies on peripapillary choroidal neovascular membrane (CNVM) treated using various modalities

Author (year)	Number of eyes	Pathology	Change in BCVA (logMAR/ Snellen)	Follow-up (mean, months)	Treatment (mean ± SD)	Outcomes
Kies and Bird (1988) [62]	55	AMD and Idiopathic		23 ± 6	Laser	Recurrence seen in 10 eyes (76.9%) post laser and in some eyes outside the treatment area.
Cialdini et al. (1989) [67]	27	AMD (17) and Idiopathic (10)	Maintained/ improved (80%)	37.7	Laser	Out of 25 treated eyes, anatomical resolution in 23 eyes (92%) and recurrence in 7 eyes (28%).
Ruben et al. (1994) [2]	20	Idiopathic	NA	20	Laser (2 sessions)	Final BCVA not dependent on size/ location of CNV or treatment status (lasered or not)
Blinder et al. (2005) [83]	11	AMD	Maintained/ improved (64%)	23	Surgical removal of CNVM	Surgical removal may be helpful in cases ineligible for PDT and laser treatment.
Rosenblatt et al. (2005) [74]	7	AMD and Inflammatory (POHS)	20/200–20/150 to 20/20–20/80	6–13.5	PDT	At least 2 line BCVA gain was noted in 6 eyes while one eye maintained 20/20 vision.
Wendel et al. (2005) [35]	6	IIH	NA	11[a]	Obs (3), laser (2), PDT(1)	Prevalence was 6 (out of 1140; 0.53%), no recurrence was seen after resolution of papilledema.
Aisenbrey et al. (2007) [76]	8	AMD	20/63–20/40	26	Surgical removal of CNVM	Surgical extraction in eyes with extensive CNVM can be helpful to prevent subfoveal extension.
Bernstein et al. (2008) [73]	7	AMD	0.63 ± 0.31–0.41 ± 0.43	3–33	PDT	Inclusion of optic nerve in treatment zone of standard-dose verteporfin PDT may not lead to optic nerve damage.

(continued)

Table 16.2 (continued)

Author (year)	Number of eyes	Pathology	Change in BCVA (logMAR/ Snellen)	Follow-up (mean, months)	Treatment (mean ± SD)	Outcomes
Mansour et al. (2008) [26]	8[b]	Inflammatory	0.82 ± 0.36–0.47 ± 0.38[b]	3	IVB (1.1 ± 0.4)	IVB showed anatomical resolution of CNVM over short term (3 months) in varying etiology of inflammatory CNVM.
Almony et al. (2008) [84]	40	Inflammatory (POHS)	20/200–20/50 (median)	68	Surgical removal of CNVM	Surgical removal of CNVM may be an alternative in eyes with extensive CNVM when laser may be contraindicated.
Hoeh et al. (2008) [91]	4		0.65 ± 0.52 to 0.5 ± 0.44	8.5 ± 5	IVB (3.5 ± 3.1)	Two patients lost BCVA, while one each improved and maintained BCVA.
Hamoudi et al. (2011) [93]	12	AMD (3) and Idiopathic (9)	59–66 letters	15.9	IVR (6.2)	Seven eyes (58%) achieved complete inactivation of CNVM using IVR.
Nagaoka et al. (2011) [22]	11	Pathological myopia	0.47 ± 0.32–0.49 ± 0.45	28.3 ± 35.8	Obs (5), TA (1), PDT(1), IVB (4)	Incidence of 4.2% (11/260 eyes), 5 out of 11 regressed with no treatment without any future recurrence.
Davis et al. (2012) [32]	20	AMD (12), Inflammatory (6), Trauma (1), and Idiopathic (1)	20/40–20/30	13.5	IVB (5.6)	Anatomical resolution seen in 17 (85%) with a mean of 1 line gain of visual acuity.
Mansour et al. (2014) [56]	3	Choroidal osteoma	0.82 ± 0.42–0.53 ± 0.68	15.3	IVB, IVR (2.67)	Significant visual recovery using monotherapy of anti-VEGF agents.
Duncan et al. (2016) [34]	24	ONH drusen	20/15–20/25[c]	Cross-sectional	Not mentioned	Among 24 eyes, 21 eyes (87.5%) had nasal CNVM whereas remaining 3 eyes (12.5%) showed temporal CNVM.
Grewal et al. (2017) [94]	8	Coloboma		21.4 ± 12.1	IVB (2), laser (1)	CNVM was seen as a temporal grayish membrane at a temporal margin of coloboma.
Roy et al. (2017) [27]	4	Inflammatory	0.60 ± 0.49–0.40 ± 0.49[c]	17.93 ± 14.28	IVB, IVR (2.76)	Monotherapy of anti-VEGF agents appears to have an acceptable response in inflammatory CNVM.
Adrean et al. (2017) [92]	5	AMD (4)	20/50–20/30 (median)	31	IVB (3.8) + laser	Combination of IVB and laser led to no recurrence in 5 eyes through mean follow-up of 31 months.

Table 16.2 (continued)

Author (year)	Number of eyes	Pathology	Change in BCVA (logMAR/ Snellen)	Follow-up (mean, months)	Treatment (mean ± SD)	Outcomes
D'souza et al. (2018) [25]	8	Inflammatory	0.82 ± 0.96–0.51 ± 0.44	19 ± 15.6	IVB (5 eyes), IVR (3 eyes), 2.8 ± 1.3	Anti-VEGF need to be supplemented with immunosuppression in cases of active inflammation.
Lin et al. (2018) [13]	33	AMD	0.34 ± 0.32–0.60 ± 0.51	6–165	IVB/IVA (6, 3)[d]	Ten eyes (out of 24; 42%) had dry fovea throughout follow-up.
Ozgonul et al. (2019) [95]	13	IIH		8	IVB, IVR, IVA	Seven eyes were observed, and 6 eyes were given anti-VEGF agents. All patients received oral acetazolamide.

[a]Only for the three eyes treated with laser and PDT
[b]Analysis of 8 eyes of peripapillary CNVM among a cohort of 84 eyes with inflammatory CNVM
[c]BCVA of the entire cohort
[d]Median number of injection at year 1 and 2 respectively; 10 eyes (out of 23) were switched to IVA in view of nonresponse to IVB
BCVA best-corrected visual acuity; *logMAR* logarithm of minimum angle of resolution; *SD* standard deviation; *AMD* age-related macular degeneration; *NA* not available; *CF* counting fingers; *PDT* photodynamic therapy; *IVB* intravitreal bevacizumab; *POHS* presumed ocular histoplasmosis syndrome; *IVR* intravitreal ranibizumab; *IIH* idiopathic intracranial hypertension; *IVA* intravitreal aflibercept; *ONH* optic nerve head; *Obs* observation; *TA* triamcinolone acetonide

Key Learning Points

- Peripapillary CNVM are a rare cause of CNVM with an incidence of 10% and a female preponderance.
- Age-related macular degeneration (AMD), pathological myopia, inflammatory ocular pathologies, and angioid streaks are the most common pathologies leading to the formation of peripapillary CNVM.
- Etiology is not established in up to 40% of eyes, therefore labeled as idiopathic CNVM.
- Anti-VEGF agents are the first-line of drug in these cases. Laser photocoagulation and PDT can be used as an adjunct in select cases either as monotherapy or combination.
- Inflammatory CNVM and IIH need treatment of underlying disease with corticosteroids and/ or immunosuppressive agents or acetazolamide if disease active is still present.

References

1. Lopez PF, Green WR. Peripapillary subretinal neovascularization. A review. Retina. 1992;12:147–71.
2. Ruben S, Palmer H, Marsh RJ. The visual outcome of peripapillary choroidal neovascular membranes. Acta Ophthalmol (Copenh). 1994;72:118–21.
3. Wilde C, Patel M, Lakshmanan A, et al. The diagnostic accuracy of spectral-domain optical coherence tomography for neovascular age-related macular degeneration: a comparison with fundus fluorescein angiography. Eye (Lond). 2015;29:602–9. quiz 610
4. Flaxel CJ, Bird AC, Hamilton AM, et al. Partial laser ablation of massive peripapillary subretinal neovascularization. Ophthalmology. 1996;103:1250–9.
5. Silvestri G, Archer DB, Johnston PB. Peripapillary subretinal neovascular membranes: the natural history. Eye (Lond). 1993;7(Pt 3):398–402.
6. Browning DJ, Fraser CM. Ocular conditions associated with peripapillary subretinal neovascularization, their relative frequencies, and associated outcomes. Ophthalmology. 2005;112:1054–61.

7. Wilde C, Poostchi A, Mehta RL, et al. Prevalence of peripapillary choroidal neovascular membranes (PPCNV) in an elderly UK population-the Bridlington eye assessment project (BEAP): a cross-sectional study (2002-2006). Eye (Lond). 2019;33:451–8.
8. Sarks SH. New vessel formation beneath the retinal pigment epithelium in senile eyes. Br J Ophthalmol. 1973;57:951–65.
9. Curcio CA, Saunders PL, Younger PW, et al. Peripapillary chorioretinal atrophy: Bruch's membrane changes and photoreceptor loss. Ophthalmology. 2000;107:334–43.
10. Perentes Y, Van Tran T, Sickenberg M, et al. Subretinal neovascular membranes complicating uveitis: frequency, treatments, and visual outcome. Ocul Immunol Inflamm. 2005;13:219–24.
11. Jutley G, Jutley G, Tah V, et al. Treating peripapillary choroidal neovascular membranes: a review of the evidence. Eye (Lond). 2011;25:675–81.
12. Ambati J, Ambati BK, Yoo SH, et al. Age-related macular degeneration: etiology, pathogenesis, and therapeutic strategies. Surv Ophthalmol. 2003;48:257–93.
13. Lin T, Dans K, Meshi A, et al. Age-related macular degeneration-associated peripapillary choroidal neovascularization in the era of anti-vascular endothelial growth factor therapy. Retina. 2018; https://doi.org/10.1097/IAE.0000000000002272.
14. Shields JA, Federman JL, Tomer TL, et al. Angioid streaks. I. Ophthalmoscopic variations and diagnostic problems. Br J Ophthalmol. 1975;59:257–66.
15. Clarkson JG, Altman RD. Angioid streaks. Surv Ophthalmol. 1982;26:235–46.
16. Mansour AM, Ansari NH, Shields JA, et al. Evolution of angioid streaks. Ophthalmologica. 1993;207:57–61.
17. Shilling JS, Blach RK. Prognosis and therapy of angioid streaks. Trans Ophthalmol Soc U K. 1975;95:301–6.
18. Georgalas I, Papaconstantinou D, Koutsandrea C, et al. Angioid streaks, clinical course, complications, and current therapeutic management. Ther Clin Risk Manag. 2009;5:81–9.
19. Lim JI, Bressler NM, Marsh MJ, et al. Laser treatment of choroidal neovascularization in patients with angioid streaks. Am J Ophthalmol. 1993;116:414–23.
20. Cheung CMG, Arnold JJ, Holz FG, et al. Myopic choroidal neovascularization: review, guidance, and consensus statement on management. Ophthalmology. 2017;124:1690–711.
21. Ohno-Matsui K, Kawasaki R, Jonas JB, et al. International photographic classification and grading system for myopic maculopathy. Am J Ophthalmol. 2015;159:877–883.e877.
22. Nagaoka N, Shimada N, Hayashi W, et al. Characteristics of periconus choroidal neovascularization in pathologic myopia. Am J Ophthalmol. 2011;152:420–427.e421.
23. Wong TY, Ferreira A, Hughes R, et al. Epidemiology and disease burden of pathologic myopia and myopic choroidal neovascularization: an evidence-based systematic review. Am J Ophthalmol. 2014;157:9–25.e12.
24. Govindhari V, Chhablani J. To laser or not? Indian J Ophthalmol. 2018;66:463–6.
25. D'Souza P, Ranjan R, Babu U, et al. Inflammatory choroidal neovascular membrane: long-term visual and anatomical outcomes after intravitreal anti-vascular endothelial growth factor therapy. Retina. 2018;38:1307–15.
26. Mansour AM, Mackensen F, Arevalo JF, et al. Intravitreal bevacizumab in inflammatory ocular neovascularization. Am J Ophthalmol. 2008;146:410–6.
27. Roy R, Saurabh K, Bansal A, et al. Inflammatory choroidal neovascularization in Indian eyes: etiology, clinical features, and outcomes to anti-vascular endothelial growth factor. Indian J Ophthalmol. 2017;65:295–300.
28. Fine SL, Owens SL, Haller JA, et al. Choroidal neovascularization as a late complication of ocular toxoplasmosis. Am J Ophthalmol. 1981;91:318–22.
29. Forrester JV, Liversidge J, Dua HS, et al. Comparison of clinical and experimental uveitis. Curr Eye Res. 1990;9(Suppl):75–84.
30. Parnell JR, Jampol LM, Yannuzzi LA, et al. Differentiation between presumed ocular histoplasmosis syndrome and multifocal choroiditis with panuveitis based on morphology of photographed fundus lesions and fluorescein angiography. JAMA Ophthalmol. 2001;119:208–12.
31. Shakarchi FI. Ocular tuberculosis: current perspectives. Clin Ophthalmol. 2015;9:2223–7.
32. Davis AS, Folk JC, Russell SR, et al. Intravitreal bevacizumab for peripapillary choroidal neovascular membranes. Arch Ophthalmol. 2012;130:1073–5.
33. Auw-Haedrich C, Staubach F, Witschel H. Optic disk drusen. Surv Ophthalmol. 2002;47:515–32.
34. Duncan JE, Freedman SF, El-Dairi MA. The incidence of neovascular membranes and visual field defects from optic nerve head drusen in children. J AAPOS. 2016;20:44–8.
35. Wendel L, Lee AG, Boldt HC, et al. Subretinal neovascular membrane in idiopathic intracranial hypertension. Am J Ophthalmol. 2006;141:573–4.
36. Sathornsumetee B, Webb A, Hill DL, et al. Subretinal hemorrhage from a peripapillary choroidal neovascular membrane in papilledema caused by idiopathic intracranial hypertension. J Neuroophthalmol. 2006;26:197–9.
37. Belliveau MJ, Xing L, Almeida DR, et al. Peripapillary choroidal neovascular membrane in a teenage boy: presenting feature of idiopathic intracranial hypertension and resolution with intravitreal bevacizumab. J Neuroophthalmol. 2013;33:48–50.
38. Lee IJ, Maccheron LJ, Kwan AS. Intravitreal bevacizumab in the treatment of peripapillary choroidal neovascular membrane secondary to idiopathic intracranial hypertension. J Neuroophthalmol. 2013;33:155–7.
39. Morse PH, Leveille AS, Antel JP, et al. Bilateral juxtapapillary subretinal neovascularization associated with pseudotumor cerebri. Am J Ophthalmol. 1981;91:312–7.
40. Sobol WM, Bratton AR, Rivers MB, et al. Morning glory disk syndrome associated with subretinal neovascular membrane formation. Am J Ophthalmol. 1990;110:93–4.

41. Chuman H, Nao-i N, Sawada A. A case of morning glory syndrome associated with contractile movement of the optic disc and subretinal neovascularization. Nippon Ganka Gakkai Zasshi. 1996;100:705–9.
42. Cennamo G, Rossi C, Velotti N, et al. Ranibizumab in the treatment of choroidal neovascularization associated with morning glory syndrome. Acta Ophthalmol (Copenh). 2015;93:e516–7.
43. Özkaya A, Yilmaz I, Alkin Z, et al. Intravitreal ranibizumab in the treatment of choroidal neovascularization secondary to morning glory syndrome in a child. Saudi J Ophthalmol. 2016;30:140–3.
44. Dailey JR, Cantore WA, Gardner TW. Peripapillary choroidal neovascular membrane associated with an optic nerve coloboma. Arch Ophthalmol. 1993;111:441–2.
45. Guirgis MF, Lueder GT. Choroidal neovascular membrane associated with optic nerve coloboma in a patient with CHARGE association. Am J Ophthalmol. 2003;135:919–20.
46. Shaikh S, Trese M. Infantile choroidal neovascularization associated with choroidal coloboma. Retina. 2003;23:585–6.
47. Duchnowski E, Rodman JA. Juxtapapillary choroidal neovascular membrane following optic neuritis. Clin Exp Optom. 2010;93:91–4.
48. Borodic GE, Gragoudas ES, Edward WO, et al. Peripapillary subretinal neovascularization and serous macular detachment. Association with congenital optic nerve pits. Arch Ophthalmol. 1984;102: 229–31.
49. Pozzoni MC, Fine HF, Ferrara DC, et al. Peripapillary choroidal neovascularization in best disease. Retin Cases Brief Rep. 2012;6:176–8.
50. Li HK, Shields CL, Mashayekhi A, et al. Giant choroidal nevus clinical features and natural course in 322 cases. Ophthalmology. 2010;117:324–33.
51. Munie MT, Demirci H. Management of choroidal neovascular membranes associated with choroidal nevi. Ophthalmol Retina. 2018;2:53–8.
52. Tuncer S, Tugal-Tutkun I. Choroidal neovascularization secondary to choroidal nevus simulating an inflammatory lesion. Indian J Ophthalmol. 2013;61:305–6.
53. Al-Halafi AM. Successful treatment of melanocytoma associated choroidal neovascular membrane with intravitreal bevacizumab. Saudi J Ophthalmol. 2013;27:117–9.
54. Tran HV, Bovey EH, Uffer S, et al. Peripapillary choroidal neovascularization associated with melanocytoma of the optic disc: a clinicopathologic case report. Graefes Arch Clin Exp Ophthalmol. 2006;244:1367–9.
55. Szelog JT, Bonini Filho MA, Lally DR, et al. Optical coherence tomography angiography for detecting choroidal neovascularization secondary to choroidal osteoma. Ophthalmic Surg Lasers Imaging Retina. 2016;47:69–72.
56. Mansour AM, Arevalo JF, Al Kahtani E, et al. Role of intravitreal antivascular endothelial growth factor injections for choroidal neovascularization due to choroidal Osteoma. J Ophthalmol. 2014;2014: 210458.
57. Kase S, Parikh JG, Rao NA. Peripapillary subretinal neovascularization in retinoblastoma. Graefes Arch Clin Exp Ophthalmol. 2008;246:931–4.
58. Shields CL, Thangappan A, Hartzell K, et al. Combined hamartoma of the retina and retinal pigment epithelium in 77 consecutive patients visual outcome based on macular versus extramacular tumor location. Ophthalmology. 2008;115:2246–2252.e2243.
59. Echevarria L, Villena O, Nievas T, et al. Combined hamartoma of the retina and retinal pigment epithelium. Anti-VEGF treatment of the associated choroidal neovascular membranes. Arch Soc Esp Oftalmol. 2015;90:87–93.
60. Gupta R, Pappuru R, Dave V, et al. Choroidal neovascularization associated with combined hamartoma of retina and retinal pigment epithelium: multimodal imaging. Indian J Ophthalmol. 2018;66:1866–8.
61. Wolf S, Wald KJ, Remky A, et al. Evolving peripapillary choroidal neovascular membrane demonstrated by indocyanine green choroidal angiography. Retina. 1994;14:465–7.
62. Kies J, Bird A. Juxtapapillary choroidal neovascularization in older patients. Am J Ophthalmol. 1988;105:11–9.
63. de Carlo TE, Romano A, Waheed NK, et al. A review of optical coherence tomography angiography (OCTA). Int J Retina Vitreous. 2015;1:5.
64. Chan WM, Lai TY, Lau TT, et al. Combined photodynamic therapy and intravitreal triamcinolone for choroidal neovascularization secondary to punctate inner choroidopathy or of idiopathic origin: one-year results of a prospective series. Retina. 2008;28:71–80.
65. Cohen SY, Laroche A, Leguen Y, et al. Etiology of choroidal neovascularization in young patients. Ophthalmology. 1996;103:1241–4.
66. Reddy H, Loewenstein J, Lane A, et al. Peripapillary choroidal neovascularization. Invest Ophthalmol Vis Sci (Suppl). 2004;45:3077.
67. Cialdini AP, Jalkh AE, Trempe CL, et al. Argon green laser treatment of peripapillary choroidal neovascular membranes. Ophthalmic Surg. 1989;20:93–9.
68. Macular Photocoagulation Study Group. Laser photocoagulation for neovascular lesions nasal to the fovea. Results from clinical trials for lesions secondary to ocular histoplasmosis or idiopathic causes. Arch Ophthalmol. 1995;113:56–61.
69. Shah SP, Hubschman JP, Bourges JL, et al. Limited long-term efficacy of intravitreous anti-VEGF pharmacotherapy in sarcoidosis complicated by peripapillary choroidal neovascular membrane. Acta Ophthalmol. 2010;88:e243–4.
70. Schmidt-Erfurth U, Chong V, Loewenstein A, et al. Guidelines for the management of neovascular age-related macular degeneration by the European Society of Retina Specialists (EURETINA). Br J Ophthalmol. 2014;98:1144–67.
71. Lee J, Ferrucci S. Peripapillary subretinal neovascular membranes: a review. Optometry. 2011;82:681–8.
72. Annesley WH Jr, Shah HG, Mansour AM, et al. Krypton red laser photocoagulation of peripapillary subretinal neovascular membranes. Graefes Arch Clin Exp Ophthalmol. 1986;224:101–5.

73. Bernstein PS, Horn RS. Verteporfin photodynamic therapy involving the optic nerve for peripapillary choroidal neovascularization. Retina. 2008;28:81–4.
74. Rosenblatt BJ, Shah GK, Blinder K. Photodynamic therapy with verteporfin for peripapillary choroidal neovascularization. Retina. 2005;25:33–7.
75. Blumenkranz MS, Bressler NM, Bressler SB, et al. Verteporfin therapy for subfoveal choroidal neovascularization in age-related macular degeneration: three-year results of an open-label extension of 2 randomized clinical trials – TAP Report no. 5. Arch Ophthalmol. 2002;120:1307–14.
76. Aisenbrey S, Gelisken F, Szurman P, et al. Surgical treatment of peripapillary choroidal neovascularisation. Br J Ophthalmol. 2007;91:1027–30.
77. Thomas MA, Kaplan HJ. Surgical removal of subfoveal neovascularization in the presumed ocular histoplasmosis syndrome. Am J Ophthalmol. 1991;111:1–7.
78. Atebara NH, Thomas MA, Holekamp NM, et al. Surgical removal of extensive peripapillary choroidal neovascularization associated with presumed ocular histoplasmosis syndrome. Ophthalmology. 1998;105:1598–605.
79. Kertes PJ. massive peripapillary subretinal neovascularization: an indication for submacular surgery. Retina. 2004;24:219–25.
80. Bains HS, Patel MR, Singh H, et al. Surgical treatment of extensive peripapillary choroidal neovascularization in elderly patients. Retina. 2003;23:469–74.
81. Connor TB Jr, Wolf MD, Arrindell EL, et al. Surgical removal of an extrafoveal fibrotic choroidal neovascular membrane with foveal serous detachment in age-related macular degeneration. Retina. 1994;14:125–9.
82. Kokame GT, Yamaoka S. Subretinal surgery for peripapillary subretinal neovascular membranes. Retina. 2005;25:564–9.
83. Blinder KJ, Shah GK, Thomas MA, et al. Surgical removal of peripapillary choroidal neovascularization associated with age-related macular degeneration. Ophthalmic Surg Lasers Imaging. 2005;36: 358–64.
84. Almony A, Thomas MA, Atebara NH, et al. Long-term follow-up of surgical removal of extensive peripapillary choroidal neovascularization in presumed ocular histoplasmosis syndrome. Ophthalmology. 2008;115:540–545.e545.
85. Nochez Y, Le Lez ML, Pisella PJ. Intravitreal injections of ranibizumab in treatment of large peripapillary choroidal neovascularization. J Fr Ophtalmol. 2009;32:25–31.
86. Soliman W, Lund-Andersen H, Larsen M. Resolution of subretinal haemorrhage and fluid after intravitreal bevacizumab in aggressive peripapillary subretinal neovascularization. Acta Ophthalmol Scand. 2006;84:707–8.
87. Nguyen QD, Shah S, Tatlipinar S, et al. Bevacizumab suppresses choroidal neovascularisation caused by pathological myopia. Br J Ophthalmol. 2005;89:1368–70.
88. Pedersen R, Soliman W, Lund-Andersen H, et al. Treatment of choroidal neovascularization using intravitreal bevacizumab. Acta Ophthalmol Scand. 2007;85:526–33.
89. Carneiro AM, Mendonça LS, Falcão MS, et al. Comparative study of 1+PRN ranibizumab versus bevacizumab in the clinical setting. Clin Ophthalmol. 2012;6:1149–57.
90. Figueroa MS, Noval S, Contreras I. Treatment of peripapillary choroidal neovascular membranes with intravitreal bevacizumab. Br J Ophthalmol. 2008;92:1244–7.
91. Hoeh AE, Schaal KB, Ach T, et al. Treatment of peripapillary choroidal neovascularization with intravitreal bevacizumab. Eur J Ophthalmol. 2009;19:163–5.
92. Adrean SD, Grant S, Chaili S. Bevacizumab (avastin) and thermal laser combination therapy for peripapillary choroidal neovascular membranes. J Ophthalmol. 2017;2017:5.
93. Hamoudi H, Sørensen TL. Effect of intravitreal ranibizumab in the treatment of peripapillary choroidal neo vascularisation. J Ophthalmol. 2011;2011:602729.
94. Grewal DS, Tran-Viet D, Vajzovic L, et al. Association of Pediatric Choroidal Neovascular Membranes at the Temporal Edge of Optic Nerve and Retinochoroidal Coloboma. Am J Ophthalmol. 2017;174:104–12.
95. Ozgonul C, Moinuddin O, Munie M, et al. Management of Peripapillary Choroidal Neovascular Membrane in Patients With Idiopathic Intracranial Hypertension. J Neuroophthalmol. 2019;39:451–7.

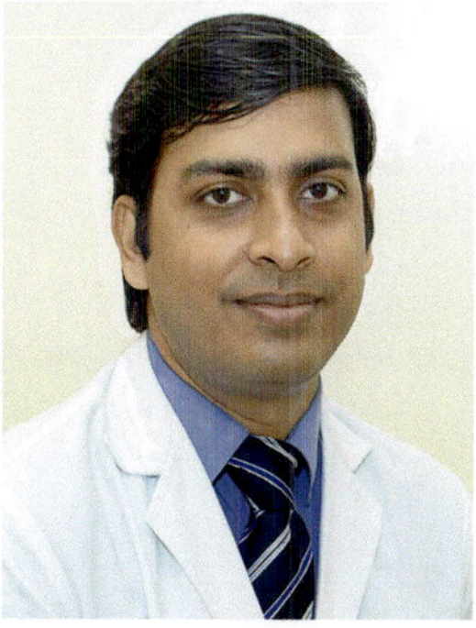

Sumit completed his basic medical degree and Master of Surgery (MS) in Ophthalmology from Jawaharlal Institute of Postgraduate Medical Education & Research (JIPMER), Puducherry and was awarded a gold medal as the best outgoing student in his postgraduation examination. He also won the best paper award in clinical sciences in JIPMER scientific society (JSS awards 2015-16). He subsequently completed a two-year fellowship in vitreoretina and uveitis at LVPEI, Hyderabad.

His main areas of clinical interest include diseases of the macula and newer imaging modalities such as OCT angiography, wide-field OCT, FFA, and imaging biomarkers for various retinal and choroidal diseases. He has to his credit more than 30 indexed publications in various national and international journals. He has co-authored 3 book chapters and 7 non-peer-reviewed publications with presentations at national and international meetings.

17 Choroidal Neovascularization in Pediatric Population

Şengül Özdek and Hatice Tuba Atalay

Choroidal neovascularization (CNV) is quite rare in children and adolescents. In this young population, CNV has been reported in association with infection, inflammation, optic disc anomalies, retinal dystrophies, disruption of Bruch's membrane, choroidal tumors, and trauma. Often, no cause is found and the CNV is said to be idiopathic (Table 17.1) [1–3].

17.1 Etiology

17.1.1 Inflammatory/Infectious

Inflammatory CNV is the most common type of CNV among children and adolescents. The most common cause of CNV secondary to inflammation is presumed ocular histoplasmosis syndrome (POHS) [4]. The clinical syndrome is most common in the United States, which is endemic for *Histoplasma capsulatum*. The classical triad of POHS is atrophic chorioretinal spots, peripapillary atrophy, and CNV. The CNV may manifest at multiple sites, mostly at peripapillary and subfoveal locations. The pathogenesis of CNV in POHS is thought to be nonspecific. Focal infection or inflammation of the choroid, either at the time of systemic infection or autoimmune trigger, may lead to the formation of an atrophic scar with disruption of Bruch's membrane. A break in Bruch's membrane may then lead to the formation of a CNV [5].

Table 17.1 Etiology

Inflammatory/infectious
Presumed ocular histoplasmosis syndrome
Toxoplasmosis
Toxocara canis
Rubella retinopathy
Vogt–Koyanagi–Harada syndrome
Chronic uveitis
Sarcoidosis
Inherited retinal disorders
Best's vitelliform macular dystrophy
Stargardt disease
Choroideremia
Disruption of Bruch's membrane
Choroidal rupture
Angioid streaks
Pathologic myopia-lacquer cracks
Optic disc anomalies
Congenital optic pits
Optic nerve head drusen
Optic nerve coloboma
Coats' Disease
Tumors of choroid and RPE
Choroidal osteoma
Combined retinal pigment epithelium: retinal hamartomas
Idiopathic

Ş. Özdek (✉) · H. T. Atalay
Ophthalmology Department, Gazi University Medical School, Ankara, Turkey

J. Chhablani (ed.), *Choroidal Neovascularization*, https://doi.org/10.1007/978-981-15-2213-0_17

Another important cause is ocular toxoplasmosis. Although the frequency of CNV in ocular toxoplasmosis in children is uncertain, most case series of pediatric CNV include this diagnosis [6]. Active inflammation may lead directly to CNV, particularly in cases of sarcoidosis and syphilis [3]. Childhood CNV has also been reported in association with Vogt–Koyanagi–Harada syndrome which is known to have a poor visual prognosis [7].

17.1.2 Inherited Retinal Disorders

CNV has been reported in a number of retinal dystrophies which may be symptomatic in childhood. These are Best disease, Stargardt disease, and Choroideremia [1, 8]. Visual prognosis of Best disease is usually good despite large vitelliform lesions; however, during the disruptive phase, it may be complicated by subretinal hemorrhage and CNV, a major vision-threatening complication [8].

Figure 17.1 shows a case with CNV associated with presumed Stargardt's disease.

Figure 17.2 shows a case as a representative for CNV related to Best disease.

17.1.3 Disruption of Bruch's Membrane

Choroidal ruptures due to blunt trauma may occur directly at the site of injury or, more commonly, at a location distant from the site of injury due to contrecoup injury. The retina is often spared due to its inherent elasticity, whereas the sclera is spared due to its rigidity. CNV has been well recognized as an infrequent but very visually significant complication of choroidal rupture. Longer ruptures and ruptures within the arcades increase the risk of CNV development. It was noted that 81.2% of patients with CNV after choroidal rupture developed it within the first year after the injury, suggesting that follow-up should occur more frequently in the first year after trauma [9, 10].

Angioid streaks result from breaks in a weakened Bruch's membrane, which allows ingrowth of CNV into the subretinal space, can lead to visual impairment. 72–86% of angioid streaks cases present with CNV, the spontaneous evolution is rare and frequently results in legal blindness [11].

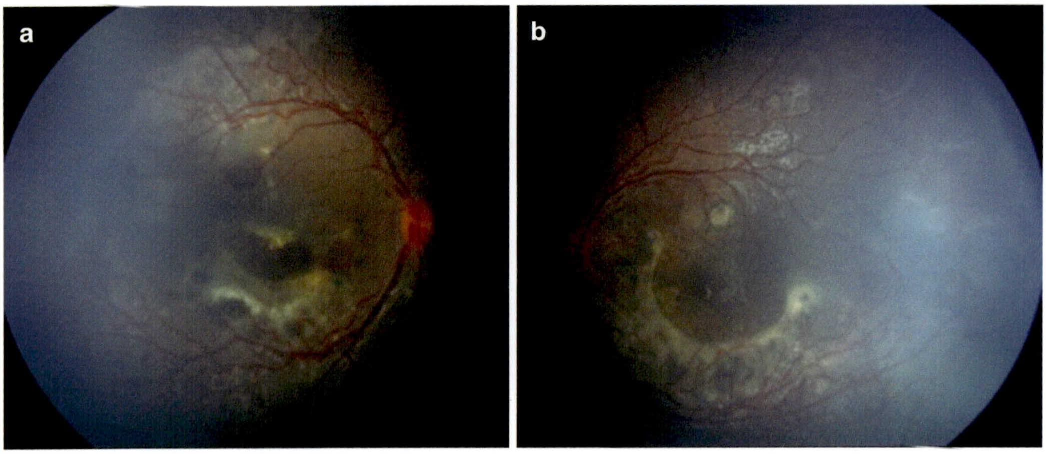

Fig. 17.1 A 2-year-old girl who presented with low vision and esotropia OU (**a**) Fundus picture (OD), subretinal hemorrhage associated with presumed Stargardt's disease with subretinal fibrosis in the macular area of the right eye. (**b**) Fundus picture (OS), perifoveal subretinal fibrosis in the left eye. (**c**) Late-phase fluorescein angiography of the right eye shows late leakage of CNV in the superotemporal and inferonasal areas associated with blocked fluorescence caused by hemorrhage, and staining of subretinal fibrosis in both eyes (**c**, **d**). (**e**, **f**) Color fundus picture of both eyes after monthly injections of ranibizumab (3X1) OD. Note the complete resolution of subretinal hemorrhage OD. (**g**, **h**) FA 6 months of follow-up. Note that there is no late leakage anymore in the RE after anti-VEGF injections

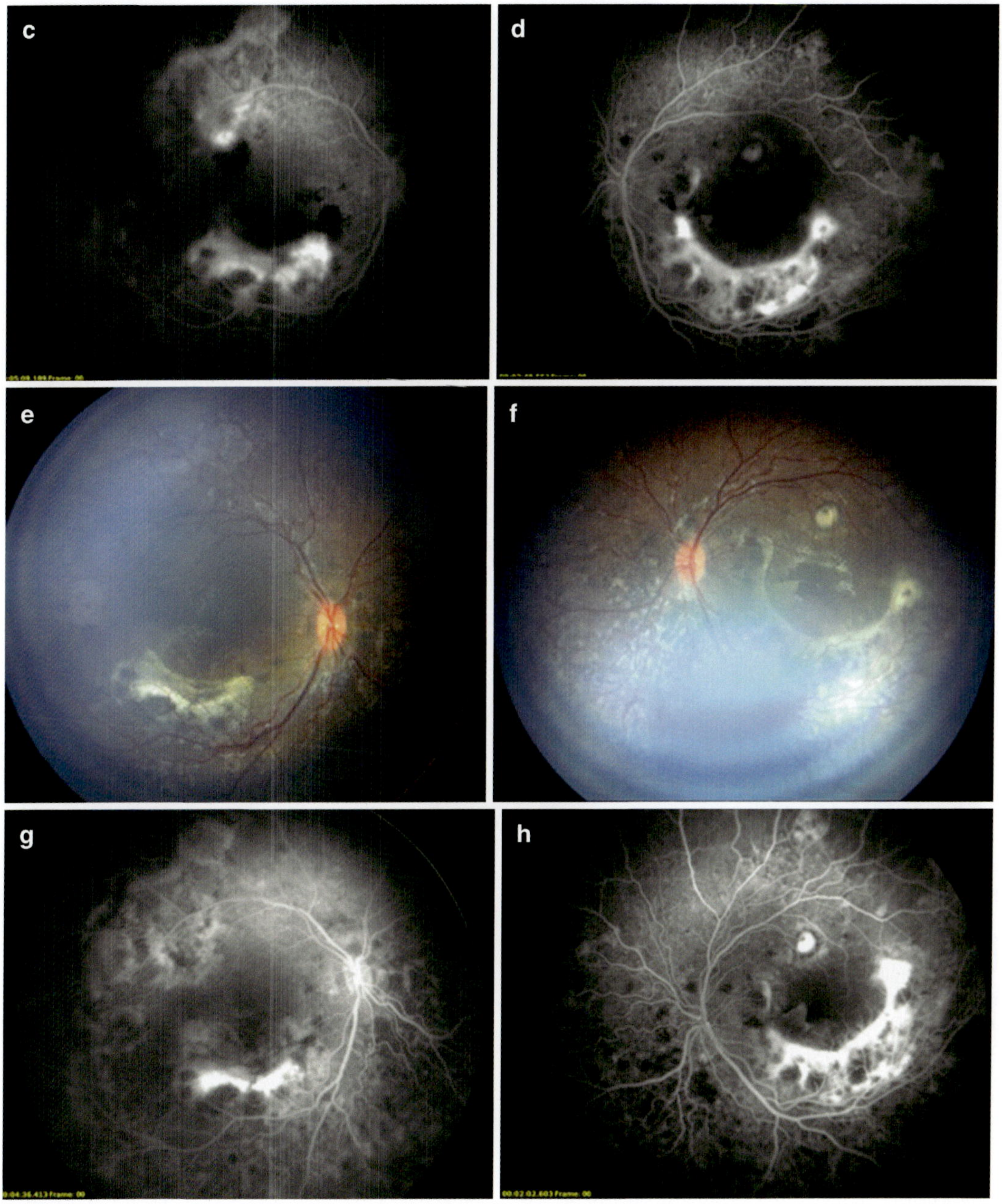

Fig. 17.1 (continued)

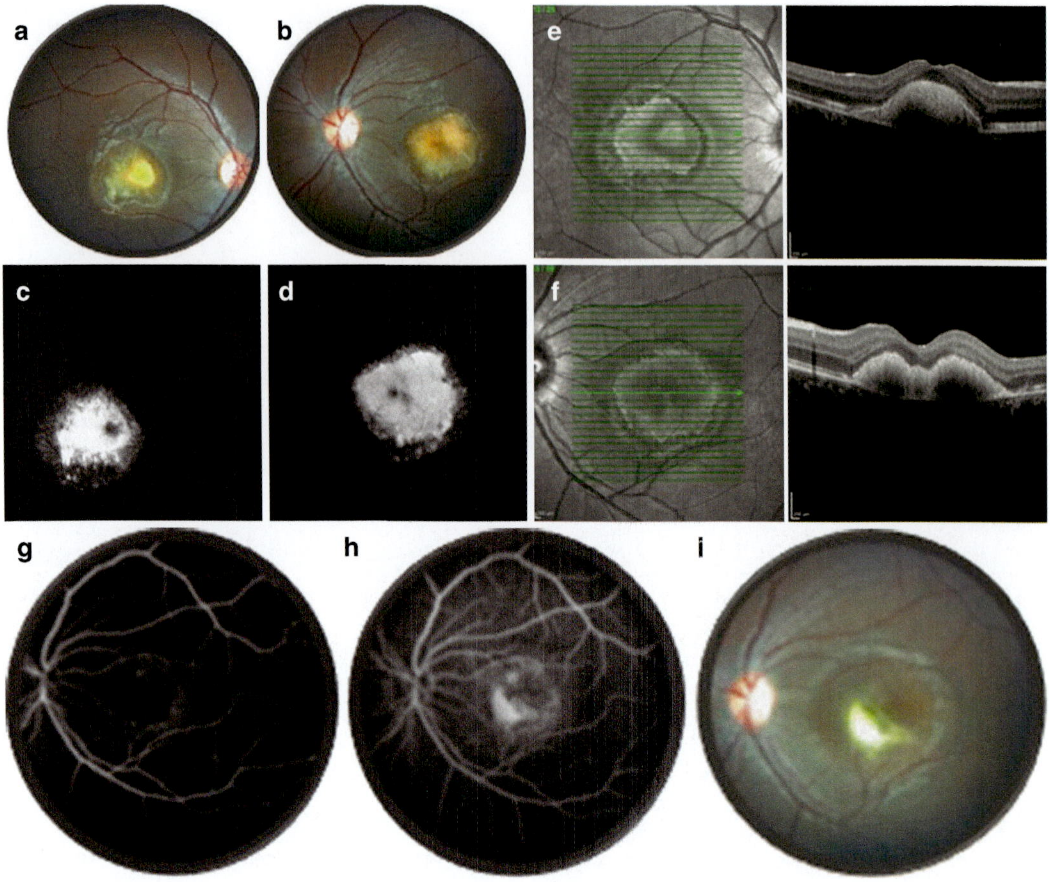

Fig. 17.2 An 8-year-old boy presented with decreased visual acuity OU that was recognized by his teacher in school. Family history was unremarkable. At presentation, BCVA was 0.7 in the right eye and 0.6 in the left eye. (**a**, **b**) Fundus examination of the right and left eyes showed yellow vitelliform lesions in the submacular area that is typical for Best Disease. (**c**, **d**) Fundus autofluorescence images showing macular hyperautofluorescence in both eyes. (**e**, **f**) OCT of the right and left eyes revealed the typical subfoveal hyperreflective material representing the vitelliform material. VA of the LE dropped to 0.1 within 6 months. It was difficult to be sure that there is an associated CNV by looking at the FA since the staining in late stages may be secondary to vitelliruptive stage (**g**, **h**). The amount of the vitelliform material was less, but there was no hemorrhage associated with the lesion in the color picture (**i**). OCT revealed an increase in subfoveal fluid and new intraretinal cyst formation, which is also in favor of CNV (**j**). OCTA, on the other hand, shows the CNV very clearly. OCTA is a very valuable tool for the diagnosis of CNV associated with Best disease. It is possible to see the CNV vessels directly which may not be so clear in fluorescein angiography (**k**). OS underwent intravitreal ranibizumab injections 2 times 1 month apart and vision improved to 0.5 and was stabile afterward for a year (**l**). Color fundus photo of the left eye 1 year after treatment showing a further decrease in the amount of vitelliform material. (**m**) OCT shows subfoveal fluid and persistent intraretinal cysts. (**n**) Vessels of CNV in OCTA were much less than before and represented the inactive lesion

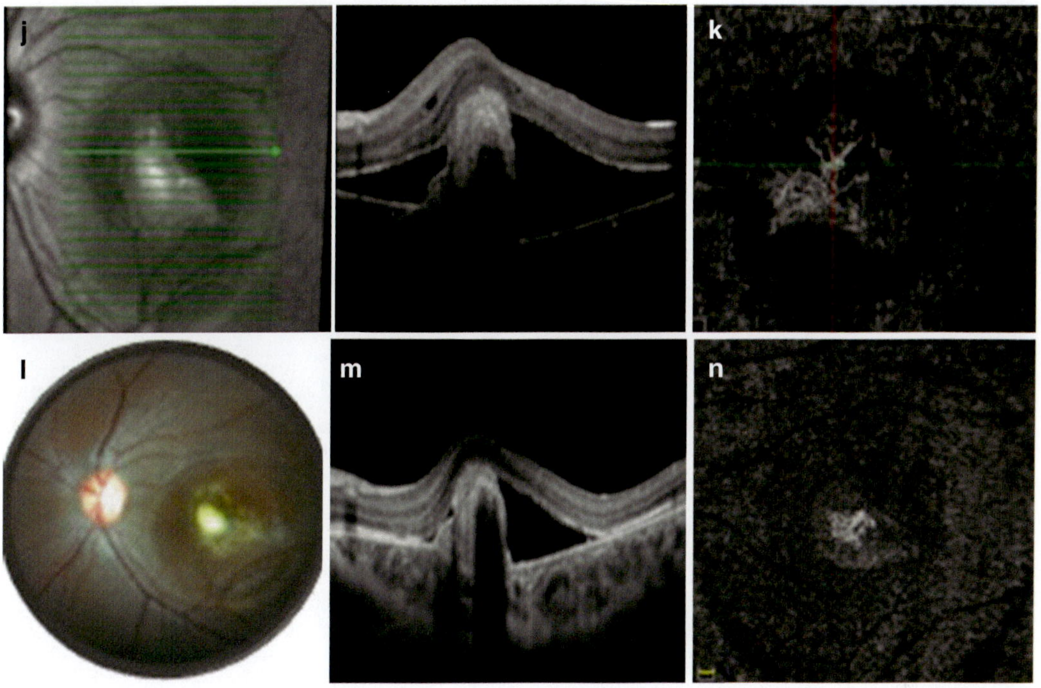

Fig. 17.2 (continued)

Pathologic myopia can induce CNV, commonly in older patients, being rare in children. This may be because of aging which might be important for the development of predisposing factors such as retinal pigment epithelium (RPE) atrophy and lacquer cracks [12]. However, myopic CNV has been reported in children [13]. Secretan et al. performed a retrospective study of 50 treated and 50 untreated eyes with pathologic myopia and CNV. The investigators found that the eyes had a poor prognosis, but treated eyes seemed to do better than untreated eyes at 2 years of follow-up [14]. Patients with pathologic myopia appear to have a very high recurrence rate.

17.1.4 Optic Disc Anomalies

Optic nerve head drusen (ONHD) are a common, benign congenital anomaly of the optic nerve. They have a reported prevalence of 0.4% in children [15]. ONHD has been reported to cause peripapillary CNV which can cause central vision loss by subfoveal progression of the CNV, serous macular detachment, or hemorrhage [16].

Optic nerve coloboma, optic nerve pit, and morning glory syndrome are optic nerve anomalies that are associated with CNV in children [1].

Figure 17.3 shows a case of CNV associated with optic disc coloboma.

17.1.5 Coats' Disease

Daruich et al. reported their series of 40 Coats' patients and found that a subfoveal nodule was detected in 21 patients (52.5%) [17]. Of 18 patients with subfoveal nodules who underwent FA, neovascularization was detected in 2 eyes (11.1%).

Figure 17.4 shows a case of subfoveal nodule with CNV associated with Coats' Disease.

17.1.6 Tumors of Choroid and Retinal Pigment Epithelium

Choroidal osteoma can lead to important vision-threatening problems. Tumor growth, tumor decalcification, and related CNV can contribute

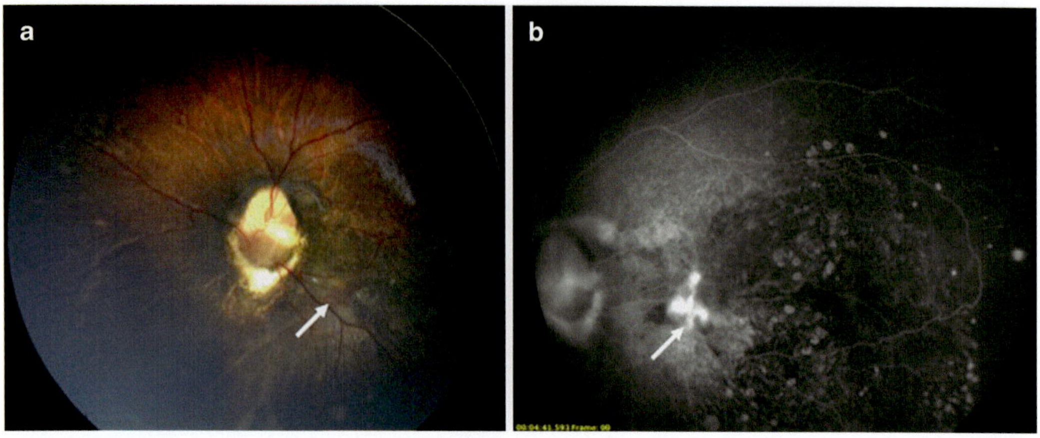

Fig. 17.3 (**a**) Color fundus photo of a 2.5-year-old patient with optic disc coloboma associated with a small subretinal hemorrhage caused by CNV in the inferior part of papillomacular bundle area. (**b**) FA shows frank late leakage indicative of active CNV: arrows indicate CNV

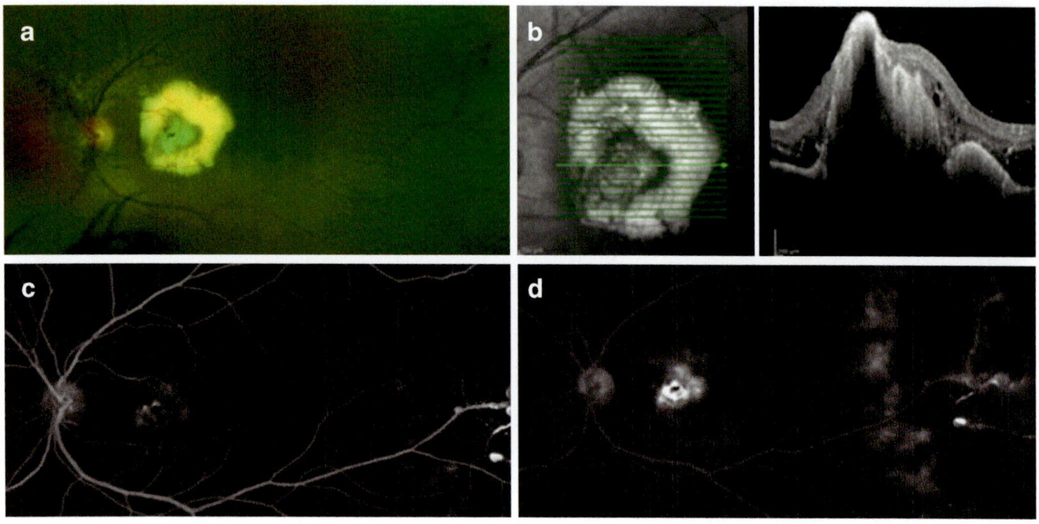

Fig. 17.4 A 10-year-old boy with Coats disease. (**a**) Color picture shows the submacular exudation and central fibrosis together with temporal peripheral telangiectatic vessels. (**b**) OCT shows the subfoveal fibrotic nodule with a CNV lesion. (**c**, **d**) Early and late frames of FA showing late leakage associated with subfoveal CNV and typical telangiectatic vessels associated with capillary dropout areas in the temporal periphery

to substantial visual loss and poor visual acuity. Tumors with overlying hemorrhage and irregular surfaces were at the greatest risk for development of CNV. Disruption of the RPE and thinning or loss of the Bruch membrane and choriocapillaris might contribute to the development of CNV [18].

17.2 Symptoms

Children may complain of metamorphopsia and blurred vision, but often they do not inform their caretakers of any trouble. Fundus findings may include a dark gray membrane, subretinal or intraretinal hemorrhage, hard exudates, and pigmentary changes, most commonly in the macula or peripapillary region [19].

17.3 Diagnostic Tests

Fluorescein angiography (FA) has always been considered the gold standard for the diagnosis, classification, localization, and activity monitoring of CNVs. Indocyanine green angiography (ICGA) is crucial for the diagnosis of neovascular AMD, due to its ability to image sub-RPE structures and to identify the presence and extension of the neovascular lesions. The spectral domain OCT (SD-OCT), has radically changed the diagnostic approach to macular diseases by offering a noninvasive imaging method, highly sensitive in identifying retinal and subretinal abnormalities associated with both neovascular or dry AMD.

Optical coherence tomography angiography (OCTA) enables a depth-resolved assessment of the retinal and choroidal blood flow, far exceeding the levels of detail commonly obtained with dye angiographies. One of the first applications of OCTA was in detecting the presence of CNV and establishing its position in relation to the retinal pigmented epithelium and Bruch's membrane, and thereby classifying the CNV as type 1, type 2, type 3, or mixed lesions. OCTAs, due to the longer wavelength used by OCT, showed a more distinct CNV vascular pattern than FA, since there is less suffering from light scattering or is less obscured by overlying subretinal hemorrhages or exudation [20].

OCTA is a very invaluable tool for the diagnosis of CNV associated with Best disease. Since there is already a hyperfluorescence in FA and subfoveal fluid in OCT associated with vitelliruptive stage of Best disease, it may be difficult to diagnose a CNV lesion without OCTA. However, CNV lesions are very apparent and easily detected with OCTA (Figs. 17.2 and 17.6). On the other hand, there may be no intra/subretinal fluid in OCT and there may be very subtle changes in FA in eyes with degenerative myopia associated CNV where OCTA is again very informative.

17.4 Treatment

CNV in the pediatric population is uncommon. Thus, little has been written in the ophthalmic literature concerning the management of CNV in pediatric patients.

17.4.1 Observation

Pediatric CNV is a rare but sight-threatening retinal disease. CNV in children has a more favorable prognosis than in adults with age-related macular degeneration. Goshorn et al. reported spontaneous involution of CNV in 11 of 19 (58%) untreated eyes in children; nine patients achieved visual acuity better than or equal to 20/50 [2]. Rishi et al. reported spontaneous regression of CNV in 15 of 17 untreated eyes in their pediatric patients [12]. Observation of CNVs in children might seem a reasonable approach; but, it is difficult to predict which CNV will regress or progress. Rishi et al. noted that visual outcome in eyes with treated CNV was better than in eyes with spontaneously regressed CNV [12].

17.4.2 Laser Photocoagulation

Laser photocoagulation of extrafoveal and juxtafoveal CNV can be utilized in cooperative children in a similar fashion used in adults, but it is more challenging in younger children [1]. Wilson and Mazur reported 5 cases of CNV of various causes in children aged 18 years or younger. Of these patients, 3 with extrafoveal CNV had laser photocoagulation, and visual acuity improved in 2 patients [4].

17.4.3 Photodynamic Therapy

Photodynamic therapy (PDT) with verteporfin can be considered in the pediatric population. Sodi et al. reported long-term results of PDT in young patients affected by Best vitelliform macular dystrophy (BVMD) complicated by CNV. PDT was a safe procedure in their series, and it was followed by a CNV regression and a

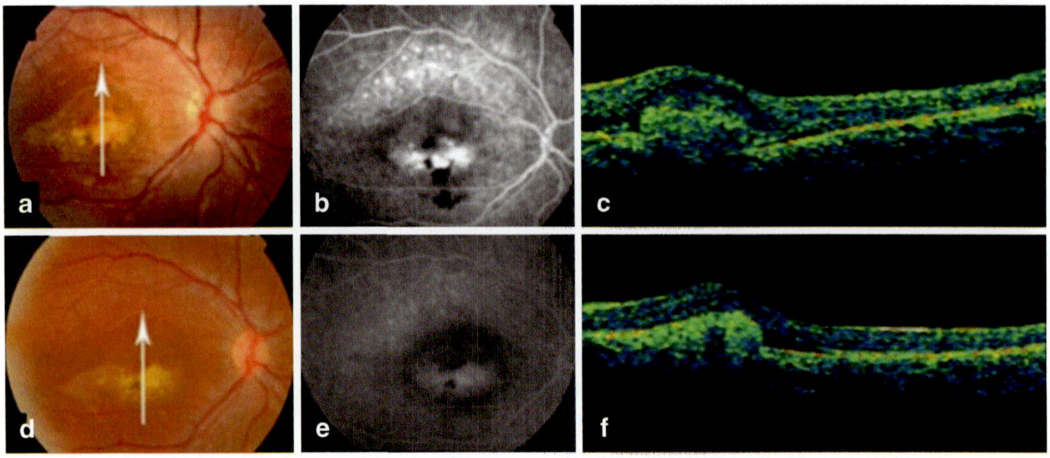

Fig. 17.5 An 8-year-old girl presented with decreased visual acuity. Family history was remarkable with similar complaints in her brother, mother, maternal uncle, and grandfather. At presentation, BCVA was 20/400 in the right eye and 20/32 in the left eye. Fundus examination of the right eye revealed a submacular grayish vitelliform lesion with subretinal hemorrhage at its inferior margin (**a**). The left eye showed a vitelliform lesion in the atrophic phase at the macular region. There were some subretinal fleck-like lesions in the macular areas in both eyes. FA demonstrated subfoveal classic CNV pattern and blocked hypofluorescence due to the subretinal hemorrhage in her right eye (**b**), and hyperfluorescence associated with pigment epithelial window defect in her left eye. OCT of the right eye revealed a subfoveal elevated hyperreflective nodular lesion at the level of the retinal pigment epithelium (RPE) bulging through subretinal space. The apex of this nodular lesion looked in apposition with the neurosensory retina without any intraretinal fluid in the right eye (**c**) and splitting of the RPE with an optically empty space was shown in the OCT of both eyes. The Arden ratio was abnormal (1.12) in both eyes. One session of PDT with verteporfin was performed in the right eye according to the standard treatment protocol. BCVA increased to 20/100 in the first month with clearing of the subretinal hemorrhage and only minimal staining of the lesion in FA, which was maintained throughout the 26-month follow-up period (**d**, **e**). OCT revealed that the lesion got smaller with only splitting of the RPE and some optically empty space (**f**). (Photodynamic therapy for best disease complicated by choroidal neovascularization in children. J Pediatr Ophthalmol Strabismus. 2012;49 (4):216–21. Permission is obtained to use the figures)

consequent improvement in visual acuity that continued to progress even several years after the treatment [21].

We have reported five eyes of four children diagnosed as having BVMD. All eyes responded well to one session of PDT with significant increases in visual acuity in four of the five eyes. Increase or stabilization of visual acuity was reported during a mean follow-up period of 25 months (Fig. 17.5) [8].

17.4.4 Submacular Surgery

Submacular surgery for the treatment of CNV had been popular for a short time in the pre anti-vascular endothelial growth factor (Anti-VEGF) era. Sears et al. reported 12 eyes of 12 consecutive children with subfoveal CNV treated by vitrectomy and excision of the choroidal neovascular complex. 10 of 12 eyes improved from immediate preoperative visual acuity, and four eyes developed recurrence of CNV over a mean follow-up of 18 months. They concluded that selected eyes of children with subfoveal CNV and no evidence of membrane regression may benefit from submacular surgery [22].

In a case series of 17 eyes undergoing surgical removal of CNV of various causes in patients aged 18 years and younger, Uemura et al. reported that 10 (72%) had improvement of 2 or more Snellen lines after surgery, and 6 eyes (43%) had final visual acuity of 20/40 or better. They have noted that removal of these membranes may be a viable alternative to laser photocoagulation in pediatric patients [23]. Nevertheless, in these series in 25–35% of children had a recurrence of CNV. As a conclusion, the role of submacular surgery for the treatment of CNV is very limited in the anti-VEGF era.

17.4.5 Anti-Vascular Endothelial Growth Factor Therapy

Case studies have shown that intravitreal bevacizumab (IVB) and intravitreal ranibizumab (IVR) are effective in the treatment of CNV associated with Best disease, toxoplasmosis, noninfectious uveitis, optic nerve head drusen, optic disc coloboma, choroidal rupture, and other etiologies in children [24–29]. In a study by Henry et al., IVB was found to be efficient in the management of children with CNV due to different underlying conditions. The majority of these patients were successfully treated with a single dose of bevacizumab. Generally, few injections (mean, 3.6 per eye; median, 2) were needed in these patients [30].

Kozak and colleagues retrospectively analyzed the results of 45 eyes of 39 children treated with IVB or IVR for CNV over a mean follow-up period of 12.8 months. A mean of 2.2 injections per eye was required for treatment. An improvement in visual acuity of 3 lines was seen in 22 eyes (49%), and only 1 eye had worsened vision after treatment [31].

Figures 17.1, 17.2, and 17.6 show a case with CNV related to Best Disease and treated successfully with anti-VEGF injection.

Laser photocoagulation, photodynamic therapy with verteporfin, and submacular surgery have been employed successfully for the treatment of pediatric CNVs. However, anti-VEGF therapy and PDT remains the preferred treatment options. The need for retreatments is definitely much less than adults usually between 1 and 3. But still, the long-term effects of suppressing VEGF in children is uncertain.

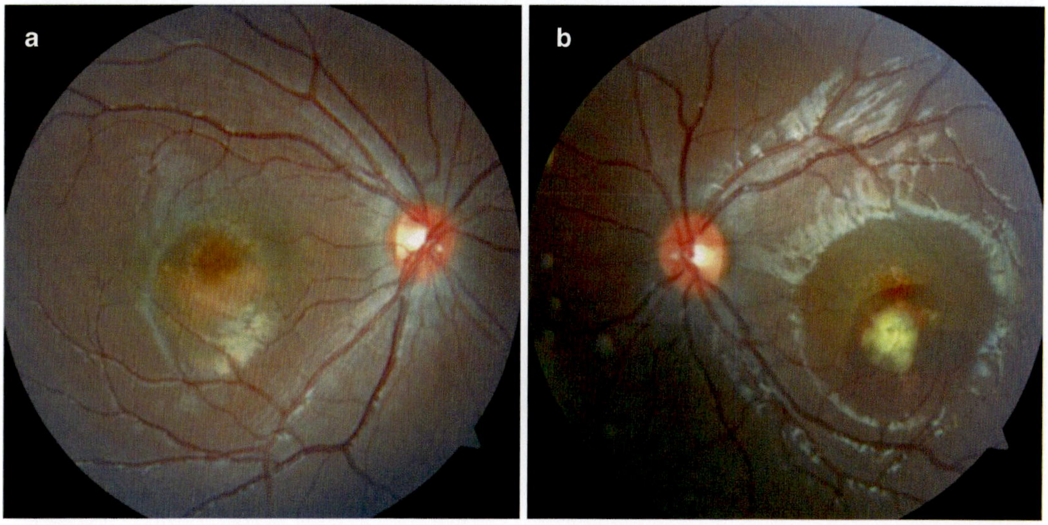

Fig. 17.6 A 5-year-old girl presented with decreased visual acuity during a routine eye examination. At presentation, BCVA was 20/20 OD, 20/200 OS. (**a**) Fundus examination of the right eye revealed a vitelliform lesion at the macula indicating Best Disease. (**b**) The left eye showed a submacular yellow vitelliform lesion associated with subretinal hemorrhage around the vitelliform material. (**c**, **d**) FAF images show splitted hyperautofluorescence of macula more in the RE. (**e**, **f**) FA demonstrated a mild hyperfluorescence in the macular area secondary to vitelliruptive stage of Best disease in the RE and a frank hyperfluorescent leakage consistent with subfoveal CNV and blocked fluorescence around it due to hemorrhage in the LE. (**g**, **h**) OCT revealed subfoveal fluid and some hyperreflective material OD and a subfoveal elevated highly reflective nodular lesion at the level of the RPE protruding through the subretinal space associated with subretinal fluid OS. This young girl was diagnosed as Best Disease in vitelliruptive stage bilaterally, which is complicated with CNV OS. (**i**) Fundus picture of the LE 7 months after intravitreal ranibizumab injections (3×). Her BCVA in the LE improved to 20/60, the hemorrhage resolved totally. (**j**) OCTA revealed inactive CNV and (k) OCT showed contraction of the lesion and a decrease in the subretinal fluid

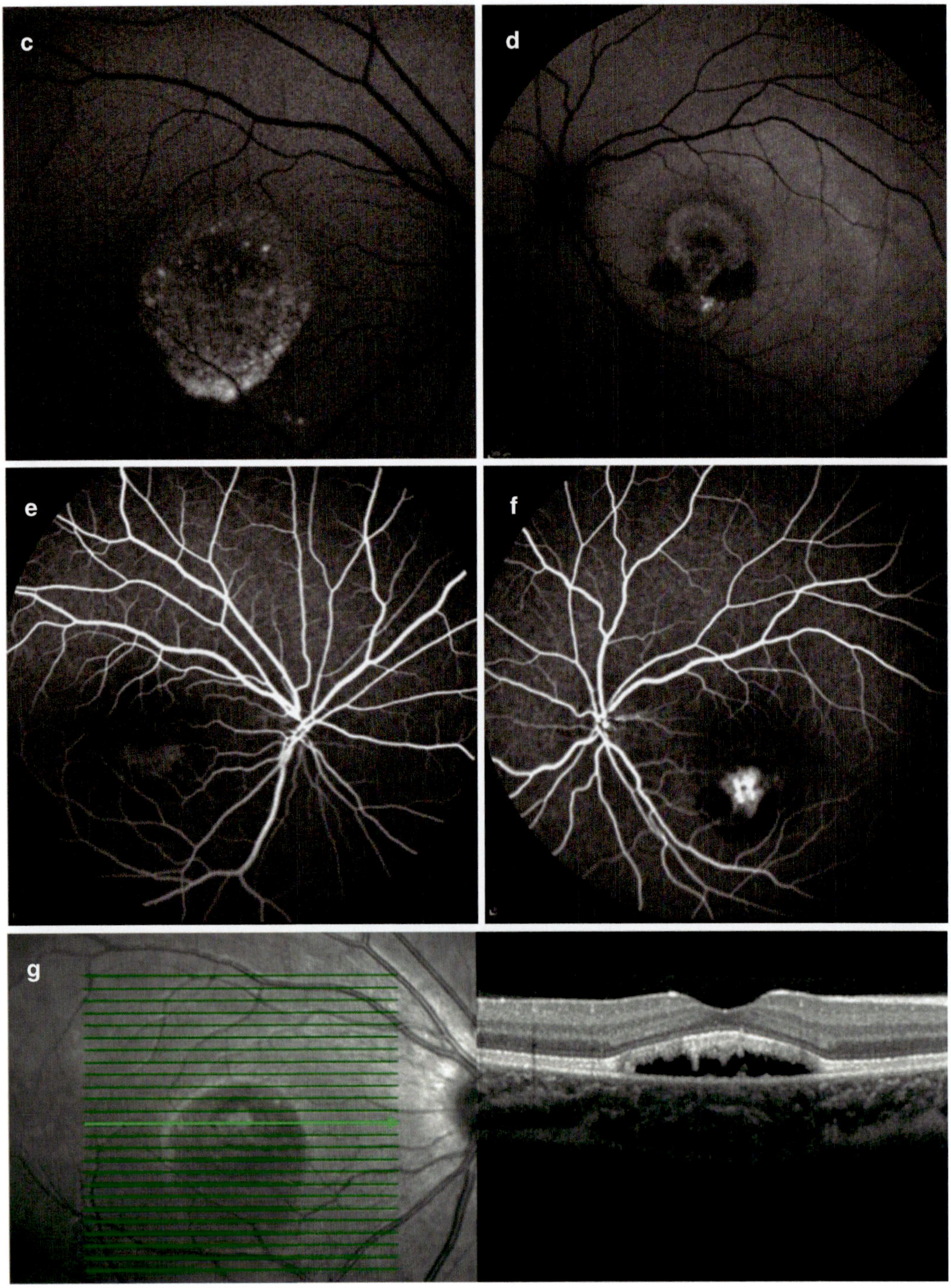

Fig. 17.6 (continued)

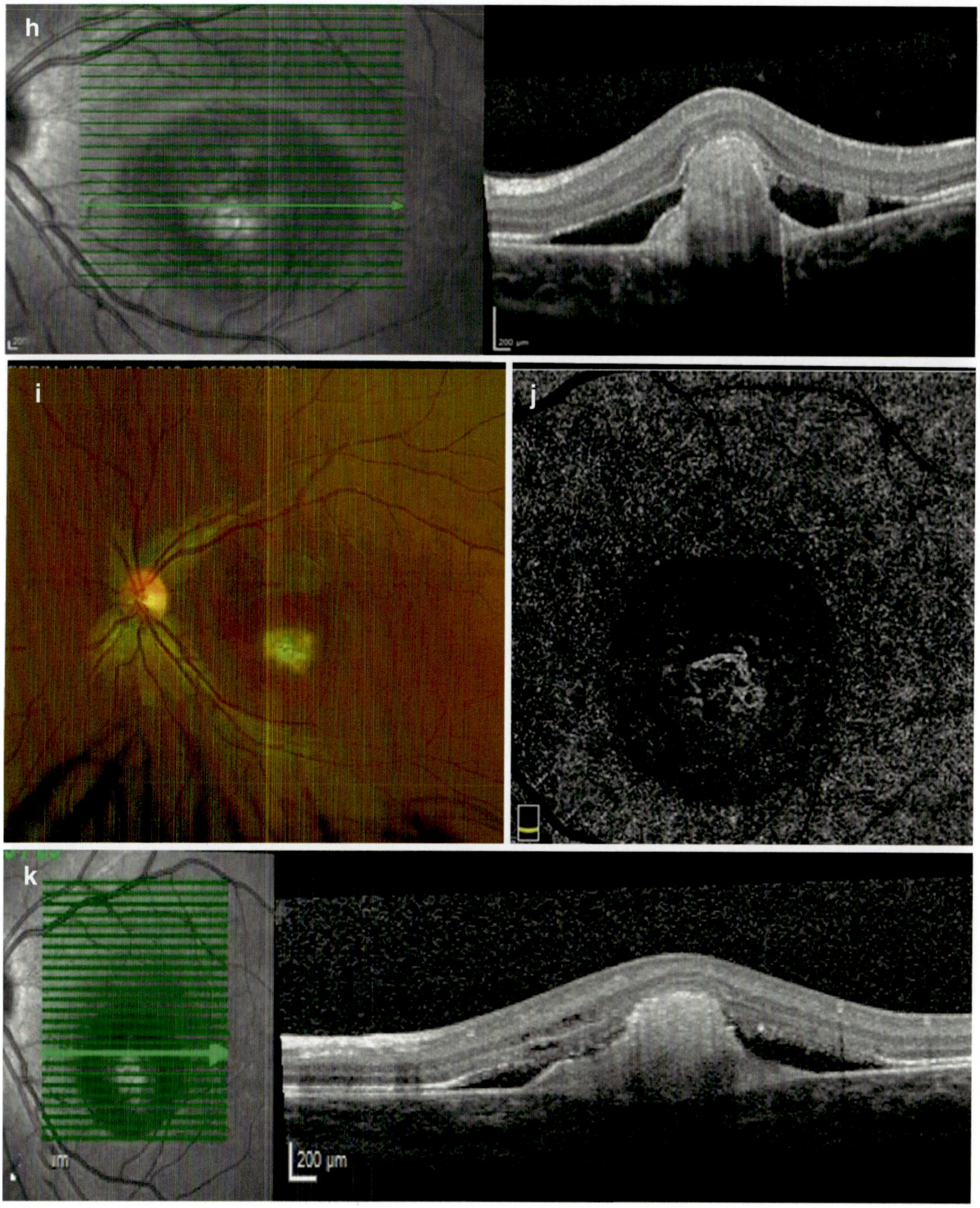

Fig. 17.6 (continued)

Key Points

1. Choroidal neovascularization (CNV) is quite rare in children and adolescents.
2. CNV has been reported in association with infection, inflammation, optic disc anomalies, and retinal dystrophies.
3. Often, no cause is found and the CNV is said to be idiopathic.
4. FA, OCT, recently OCTA are ancillary diagnostic tests.
5. CNV in children has a more favorable prognosis than in adults with age-related macular degeneration.
6. Anti-VEGF therapy and PDT remains the preferred treatment options.

References

1. Sivaprasad S, Moore AT. Choroidal neovascularisation in children. Br J Ophthalmol. 2008;92(4):451–4.
2. Goshorn EB, Hoover DL, Eller AW, Friberg TR, Jarrett WH, Sorr EM. Subretinal neovascularization in children and adolescents. J Pediatr Ophthalmol Strabismus. 1995;32(3):178–82.
3. Spaide RF. Choroidal neovascularization in younger patients. Curr Opin Ophthalmol. 1999;10:177–81.
4. Wilson ME, Mazur DO. Choroidal neovascularization in children: report of five cases and literature review. J Pediatr Ophthalmol Strabismus. 1988;25(1):23–9.
5. Prasad AG, Van Gelder RN. Presumed ocular histoplasmosis syndrome. Curr Opin Ophthalmol. 2005;16(6):364–8.
6. Mavrikakis E, Levin AV, Lam WC. Choroidal neovascularization secondary to congenital toxoplasmosis in an infant. Can J Ophthalmol. 2010;45(6):e11–2.
7. Ketata A, Ben Zina Z, Hajji D, Sellami D, Abdelkefi A, Kharrat W, et al. Two cases of subretinal neovascular membrane in Vogt-Koyanagi-Harada syndrome. J Fr Ophtalmol. 2006;29(3):302–6.
8. Ozdek S, Ozmen MC, Tufan HA, Gurelik G, Hasanreisoglu B. Photodynamic therapy for best disease complicated by choroidal neovascularization in children. J Pediatr Ophthalmol Strabismus. 2012;49(4):216–21.
9. Secretan M, Sickenberg M, Zografos L, Piguet B. Morphometric characteristics of traumatic choroidal ruptures associated with neovascularization. Retina. 1998;18:62–6.
10. Patel MM, Chee YE, Eliott D. Choroidal rupture: a review. Int Ophthalmol Clin. 2013;53(4):69–78.
11. Tilleul J, Mimoun G, Querques G, Puche N, Zerbib J, Lalloum F, et al. Intravitreal ranibizumab for choroidal neovascularization in angioid streaks: four year follow-up. Retina. 2016;36(3):483–91.
12. Rishi P, Gupta A, Rishi E, Shah BJ. Choroidal neovascularization in 36 eyes of children and adolescents. Eye (Lond). 2013;27(10):1158–68.
13. Potter MJ, Szabo SM, Ho T. Combined photodynamic therapy and intravitreal triamcinolone for the treatment of myopic choroidal neovascularization in a 13-year-old girl. Graefes Arch Clin Exp Ophthalmol. 2006;244(5):639–41.
14. Secretan M, Kuhn D, Soubrane G, Coscas G. Long-term visual outcome of choroidal neovascularization in pathologic myopia: natural history and laser treatment. Eur J Ophthalmol. 1997;7:307–16.
15. Erkkilä H. Clinical appearance of optic disc drusen in childhood. Albrecht Von Graefes Arch Klin Exp Ophthalmol. 1975;193(1):1–18.
16. Basdekidou C, Caputo G. Optic nerve abnormalities in pediatric ocular diseases. In: Hartnett ME, Trese M, Capone A, BJB K, Steidl SM, editors. Pediatric retina. 2nd ed. Philadelphia: Wolters Kluver, Lippincott Williams & Wilkins; 2014. p. 148–72.
17. Daruich AL, Moulin AP, Tran HV, Matet A, Munier FL. Subfoveal nodule in Coats' disease: toward an updated classification predicting visual prognosis. Retina. 2017;37(8):1591–8.
18. Shields CL, Sun H, Demirci H, Shields JA. Factors predictive of tumor growth, tumor decalcification, choroidal neovascularization, and visual outcome in 74 eyes with choroidal osteoma. Arch Ophthalmol. 2005;123(12):1658–66.
19. Hollander DA, Stewart JM. Acquired and other retinal diseases. In: Lambert SR, Lyons CJ, editors. Taylor & Hoyt's pediatric ophthalmology and strabismus. 4th ed. Philadelphia: Elsevier; 2013. p. 522–9.
20. Lupidi M, Cerquaglia A, Chhablani J, Fiore T, Singh SR, Cardillo Piccolino F, et al. Optical coherence tomography angiography in age-related macular degeneration: the game changer. Eur J Ophthalmol. 2018;28(4):349–57.
21. Sodi A, Murro V, Caporossi O, Passerini I, Bacci GM, Caputo R, et al. Long-term results of photodynamic therapy for choroidal neovascularization in pediatric patients with best Vitelliform Macular Dystrophy. Ophthalmic Genet. 2015;36(2):168–74.
22. Sears J, Capone A Jr, Aaberg T Sr, Lewis H, Grossniklaus H, Sternberg P Jr, et al. Surgical management of subfoveal neovascularization in children. Ophthalmology. 1999;106(5):920–4.
23. Uemura A, Thomas MA. Visual outcome after surgical removal of choroidal neovascularization in pediatric patients. Arch Ophthalmol. 2000;118(10):1373–8.
24. Kohly RD, Muni RH, Kertes PJ, Lam WC. Management of pediatric choroidal neovascular membranes with intravitreal anti-VEGF agents: a retrospective consecutive case series. Can J Ophthalmol. 2011;46:46–50.
25. Rich R, Vanderveldt S, Berrocal AM, Mavrofrides EC, Murray TG, Gregori N. Treatment of choroidal neovascularization associated with Best's dis-

ease in children. J Pediatr Ophthalmol Strabismus. 2009;46:306–11.

26. Baillif S, Nguyen E, Colleville-El Hayek A, Betis F. Long term follow-up after single intravitreal ranibizumab injection for choroidal neovascularization secondary to optic nerve head drusen in a 5-year old child. Graefes Arch Clin Exp Ophthalmol. 2013;251:1657–9.
27. Vayalambrone D, Misra A. Paediatric choroidal osteoma treated with ranibizumab. BMJ Case Rep. 2012; https://doi.org/10.1136/bcr-2012-007446.
28. Benevento J, Jager RD, Noble AG, Latkany P, Mieler WF, Sautter M, et al. Toxoplasmosis-associated neovascular lesions treated successfully with ranibizumab and antiparasitic therapy. Arch Ophthalmol. 2008;126:1152–6.
29. Piermarocchi S, Benetti E, Fracasso G. Intravitreal bevacizumab for posttraumatic choroidal neovascularization in a child. J AAPOS. 2011;15:314–6.
30. Henry CR, Sisk RA, Tzu JH, Albini TA, Davis JL, Murray TG, et al. Long-term follow-up of intravitreal bevacizumab for the treatment of pediatric retinal and choroidal diseases. J AAPOS. 2015;19(6):541–8.
31. Kozak I, Mansour A, Diaz RI, Calzada JI, Pichi F, Cruz-Villegas V, et al. Outcomes of treatment of pediatric choroidal neovascularization with intravitreal antiangiogenic agents. Retina. 2014;34:2044–52.

18 Polypoidal Choroidal Vasculopathy: Diagnostic and Therapeutic Considerations

Adrian H. C. Koh

18.1 Background

Age-related macular degeneration (AMD) is the leading cause of blindness in elderly people globally and it is estimated that 288 million people will be affected by the year 2040 [1]. Early-stage AMD is characterized by drusen and retinal pigment epithelial (RPE) changes and typically does not cause vision loss. Late-stage AMD, generally classified as geographic atrophy ("dry") AMD or neovascular ("wet") AMD, accounts for 90% of vision loss in AMD.

There is increasing evidence that wet AMD is not a homogeneous entity and that a significant proportion of patients (8–13% of white Caucasians and 20–54% of Asians) have a subtype known as polypoidal choroidal vasculopathy (PCV) [2–5].

Clinically, PCV appears to affect younger individuals than typical wet AMD and frequently presents with large subretinal or intraretinal hemorrhage, but often with minimal scarring. Definitive diagnosis is based on the use of indocyanine green angiography (ICGA), which shows characteristic polyp-like hyperfluorescent lesions, possibly associated with a branching vascular network (BVN). However, other features of PCV are not well defined, thus complicating the interpretation of the epidemiological data. Importantly, although PCV appears to be somewhat more refractory to monotherapy with anti-vascular endothelial growth factor (VEGF) agents than typical wet AMD (i.e., polyps may remain), clinical trials do not always distinguish between these cases; thus, the efficacy of treatments for PCV remains the subject of debate. The disparities in epidemiology, clinical presentation, and treatment response suggest that there may be differences in the underlying pathophysiology of PCV and typical wet AMD.

18.2 Definition and Diagnosis

PCV appears to be a subtype of wet AMD, presenting differently to typical wet AMD. The current understanding that PCV is not a separate disease entity is based on several lines of evidence [6]. First, almost 30% of AMD cases develop polypoidal lesions over time; second, in many cases, ICGA identifies polyps in lesions classified as wet AMD; third, some risk factors for PCV (e.g., smoking) appear to be similar to those for wet AMD [7]; fourth, histopathological analyses have located the vascular network and polyp between Bruch's membrane and the RPE; and finally, there are emerging data that show that the two conditions have largely similar genetic profiles [8].

Clinically, PCV is more likely than typical AMD to present with recurrent serous or

A. H. C. Koh (✉)
Eye & Retina Surgeons, Camden Medical Centre, Singapore, Singapore

J. Chhablani (ed.), *Choroidal Neovascularization*, https://doi.org/10.1007/978-981-15-2213-0_18

hemorrhagic detachments of the RPE and/or vitreous hemorrhage, but less likely to present with fibrous scarring. In wet AMD, the classic appearance of the choroidal neovascularization (CNV) is a dark gray lesion on clinical examination and a "sea fan-like network" seen in the early phases of fundus fluorescein angiography (FA). In contrast, PCV appears as orange-red, bulging polyp-like dilations with submacular hemorrhage in the fundus, and with an FA pattern more likely to be that of occult than classic CNV. While PCV was originally believed to arise from the inner choroidal vascular network, spectral-domain and en-face optical coherence tomography (OCT) imaging has confirmed that the entire complex (consisting of the BVN as well as the polypoidal nodules) arises above the Bruch's membrane and below the basement membrane of the RPE, consistent with type 1 or "occult" CNV [9]. This accounts for why the most common fluorescein angiographic pattern is as "occult" lesions, with granular hyperfluorescence in the early phase and multiple indistinct leakage spots in the later phase. As FA is unable to distinguish between CNV and PCV, the gold-standard diagnosis of PCV is based on the use of ICGA, which shows polyp-like hyperfluorescent lesions possibly with a BVN and other less-well-defined supporting features (see the section on Imaging).

18.2.1 Diagnostic Criteria for PCV

Unfortunately, there is no consensus on ICGA diagnostic criteria, although there are currently two widely used systems: the Japanese Study Group guidelines and the criteria from the EVEREST trial [10, 11]. The Japanese Study Group guidelines propose that a diagnosis of "definite" PCV should be made when the classic features of elevated orange-red lesions on fundus examination and/or polypoidal lesions on ICGA are seen; a diagnosis of "probable" PCV should be made if only the abnormal BVN is seen on ICGA or if there are recurrent hemorrhagic and/or serous RPE detachments without the features of "definite" PCV.

A more elaborate set of criteria was used by the central reading center in the EVEREST clinical trial [11], where a diagnosis of PCV was made if focal hyperfluorescent lesions were observed on confocal scanning laser ophthalmoscope (cSLO)-based ICGA and at least one of the following angiographic or clinical criteria was present: BVN; "pulsatility"; nodular appearance when viewed stereoscopically; hypofluorescent halo; orange subretinal nodule on color photograph; or associated massive submacular hemorrhage. Initial studies suggest that the two systems are largely similar, with the EVEREST study criteria having slightly higher specificity than the use of subretinal focal hyperfluorescence alone [12]. This is a critical area for future research.

18.2.2 Indocyanine Green Angiography (ICGA)

ICGA, either flash-based or cSLO-based, is considered the gold standard for the diagnosis of PCV because it provides imaging of PCV-specific features that are predominantly sub-RPE and therefore poorly visualized using FA. Detailed choroidal vessel morphology can be visualized, as indocyanine green binds plasma protein and so remains within the vascular compartment instead of leaking from the choriocapillaris, hence providing later images with higher definition than FA [13, 14]. Moreover, indocyanine green is imaged using infrared light, which can effectively penetrate the RPE and, to some extent, hemorrhage; this is advantageous because PCV primarily involves the sub-RPE space just above the Bruch's membrane [13]. Although the emitted light is of lower intensity than with fluorescein, the use of the cSLO for ICGA yields images of high resolution [15]. Studies comparing digital fundus photography with cSLO showed both to be similarly effective at detecting PCV [16, 17]. A recent study comparing the individual ICGA features reported that both fundus photography and cSLO-based systems could detect PCV in the presence of typical nodular lesions (seen in over 80% of cases); however, cSLO is superior for detecting additional features, particularly the BVN [16]. Furthermore, other diagnostic features, such as pulsatility of nodules, can only be visualized using the dynamic cSLO videoangiography mode.

PCV exhibits several distinctive angiographic features on ICGA. Polyps exhibit nodularity when viewed stereoscopically and appear early in the ICGA (within the first 6 min) [13]; however, focal hyperfluorescence may also indicate "pseudo-polyp" lesions (such as macroaneurysms or a retinal pigment epithelium defect associated with choroidal vascular knuckle). To add to the specificity for polyps, several additional features have been used under the EVEREST criteria [18]. A distinctive hypofluorescent halo around the polypoidal lesions can be seen in about 45–70% of cases [11, 16]. In many cases, polyps are associated with a BVN with vascular dilation at the borders, which appears as a hyperfluorescent dilated complex of sub-RPE vessels that leaks in the latter stages of the angiogram [13]. However, visualization of the BVN may not always be possible, especially using flash-based ICGA [16].

The Japanese Study Group of PCV describes masses of grape-like clusters on ICGA that start as small nodules in the early phases and gradually expand into the late phase [10]. However, this feature is less common than the typical nodular presentation (only 19% of PCV cases) [16]. In the late ICGA phases, the core of the lesion may become hypofluorescent owing to the washout of the dye, staining the polyps in a ring-like appearance. Polyps that are leaking will be visible as a ring of hyperfluorescence, whereas polyps that are not leaking will appear hypofluorescent [13]. Pulsation of blood flow in polyps may be visualized with dynamic cSLO ICGA; this is thought to be a unique feature of PCV.

Choroidal vascular hyperpermeability is a commonly noted feature in PCV [19] and is visualized during the middle and late phases of ICGA as multifocal hyperfluorescence with blurred margins, distant from the main PCV lesion [19, 20]. In the very late stages of ICGA (45–60 min), one may observe "ghost vessels," where dye has emptied out of the larger choroidal vessels into the surrounding choroidal interstitial tissue causing choroidal vessel silhouetting. Late geographic hyperfluorescence is another characteristic finding in PCV, distinct from choroidal vascular hyperpermeability. This represents the staining of the entire lesion complex, comprising the BVN as well as the polypoidal lesions [19].

18.2.3 Fluorescein Angiography (FA)

Eyes with PCV generally do not display any specific features on FA; therefore, FA alone is not usually adequate to confirm or exclude the diagnosis of PCV. Most eyes with PCV display an occult leakage pattern, or avascularized and hemorrhagic large pigment epithelial detachments (PEDs) on FA [21, 22], which is to be expected because most of the vascular network is located under the RPE. Erosion of the overlying RPE may lead to a variable degree of window defect. Occasionally, a "classic CNV" may coexist with PCV [3, 22]. While FA is not diagnostic of PCV, it is still useful for evaluating treated and recurrent cases, where fluorescein leakage may come from the BVN, either alone or together with residual polypoidal lesions. This distinction between BVN and polyp leakage has important therapeutic implications (see Sect. 18.7.5).

18.2.4 Spectral Domain OCT, Enhanced-Depth OCT, and Swept Source OCT Imaging

The most distinctive OCT feature of the polypoidal nodules in PCV is a sharply angulated inverted V-shaped elevation of the RPE, separating the RPE from the underlying relatively intact Bruch's membrane; this sign has also been dubbed "thumb-like protrusion" in literature. The BVN appears as irregular in the space between the RPE and Bruch's membrane, giving rise to the "double-layer" sign. Kim et al. observed both geographic hyperfluorescence and the double-layer sign in approximately 80% of PCV eyes, indicating that these features are sensitive markers for the diagnosis of PCV [19, 23]. Visualization of the cross-section of the choroid by OCT and enhanced-depth imaging (EDI) suggests that the subfoveal choroid may be thicker in PCV than in typical wet AMD, potentially because of the greater incidence of choroidal vascular hyperpermeability; furthermore, Maruko et al. reported that PCV eyes with ICGA choroidal hyperpermeability tend to have a greater subfoveal choroid thickness than those without [24]. It is now widely accepted that PCV is part of the pachychoroid spectrum of diseases. Therefore, EDI-OCT may be a useful noninvasive tool to help differentiate between PCV and typical AMD subtypes. Recently, swept-source OCT has also shown value in demonstrating the polypoidal lesion and BVN, using both cross-sectional cuts and en-face imaging [25].

18.2.5 Use of ICGA for Differential Diagnosis

ICGA is important, not only to confirm a diagnosis of PCV but also to distinguish it from other lesions such as vascularized PED, central serous chorioretinopathy (CSC), and retinal angiomatous proliferation (RAP). The sensitivity and specificity for PCV is further increased by gathering all data from multimodal imaging, including FA and OCT (see Box 18.1).

Vascularized PED appears on ICGA as late, non-nodular hyperfluorescence (also called "hot spots" or "plaques") within a notch in the margin of a serous PED. There is typically no associated BVN, and the lesion is never pulsatile.

Distinguishing between PCV and CSC can be difficult in atypical cases. Typically, CSC patients present with exudative retinal detachment, multiple small serous PEDs, and patches or tracks of pigment epithelial atrophy. An FA showing pinpoint leaks at the level of the RPE can confirm the diagnosis of CSC. However, in some instances persistent retinal detachment may lead to secondary effects and fluorescein leakage will become more diffuse, resembling PCV and making differential diagnosis difficult [26]. Some atypical cases of PCV may also appear very similar to CSC, presenting with serous detachment of the retina and polypoidal lesions that resemble small PEDs on evaluation by FA [26]. In these cases ICGA is useful to confirm the presence or absence of multifocal areas of choroidal hyperpermeability, which cannot be viewed using FA alone. These areas are known to be indicative of CSC but absent in PCV [26].

Box 18.1 Features Highly Suggestive of PCV

Features highly suggestive of PCV
• Orange-red polyp-like dilations (viewed by routine ophthalmoscopy and contact lens slit-lamp biomicroscopy)
• Large (>2000 μm in diameter) hemorrhagic and exudative PED
• Chronic CSC

CSC central serous chorioretinopathy, *PCV* polypoidal choroidal vasculopathy, *PED* pigment epithelial detachment.

High-speed video ICGA with a cSLO is useful for distinguishing between PCV and RAPs. RAP lesions can be distinguished by the presence of intraretinal small dilated blood vessels within the macula, which are seen to turn sharply from the inner retina to the choroidal interface when stereo pairs of images are viewed; these lesions are often associated with large PEDs and prominent intraretinal cystic fluid [15].

18.3 Epidemiology

Over the past three decades there have been significant advances in our understanding of the epidemiology of AMD, both in white populations and other races [1]. However, epidemiological data on PCV remain limited and those that exist are complicated by inconsistent classification and diagnosis of the disease between populations. As PCV can only be definitively diagnosed using ICGA, most studies have not distinguished it from typical wet AMD [27–29]. Moreover, the prevalence of PCV is likely to be significantly underestimated because ICGA is often not used for routine assessment [30, 31].

PCV was first described more than two decades ago predominantly in black females [32–37]. Although more common in those of African or Asian descent, PCV is now known to affect individuals of all races [3, 6, 38, 39]. Studies of Japanese, Korean, and Chinese patients report a prevalence of 20–54% among patients with wet

AMD [3–5, 40, 41], while the corresponding figure in Caucasian populations is about 8–13% [21, 42, 43]; the prevalence may be higher in patients presenting with large hemorrhagic and exudative neurosensory detachments [37, 44, 45].

Very few studies have examined the incidence and prevalence of PCV in the general, seemingly healthy, population. In a study based on health check-ups in 10,890 participants in Korea, only nine patients with exudative AMD received fluorescein angiography or ICGA; of these, two eyes (22%) were found to have PCV [46].

18.3.1 Demographics

In addition to differences in prevalence, the demographics of PCV in different races also show notable variability [6, 38, 39]. In African and Caucasian patients, a female preponderance has been reported [33, 38], whereas in Asian populations, PCV patients are more likely to be male [2–5, 40, 47, 48]. There are studies which suggest that PCV might affect younger people compared to those with wet AMD [3, 6].

18.3.2 Lesion Location

In African and Caucasian patients, polypoidal lesions appear to have a predilection for the peripapillary area [21, 33, 34, 37, 42, 43]. In Asian patients, however, macular PCV is more prevalent, being found in more than 63% [2, 40, 49].

18.3.3 Laterality

Bilateral involvement is common in wet AMD (over 42% of patients by 5 years after presentation with unilateral disease) [50–53]. However, the frequency of bilateral PCV is less well-studied and reports so far have been inconsistent, giving figures ranging from 7 to 80% [2–5, 21, 32–34, 37, 40, 47–49]. The incidence of bilateral PCV appears to be higher in Caucasian patients than Asian patients [39]. Few prospective studies have examined the incidence of second-eye involvement in PCV or the associated risk factors. Ueta et al. followed up 125 Japanese patients with PCV, while Kim et al. evaluated 47 Korean patients; the cumulative incidence of second-eye involvement was 11% at 3 years and 19% at 2 years, respectively [54, 55].

18.3.4 Risk Factors

18.3.4.1 Ocular

While the presence of drusen is a significant risk factor for wet AMD [53, 56], they appear to be less common in Asians and in patients with PCV (27–33%) [43, 57]. Thus, the role of drusen in the pathogenesis of PCV is unclear.

Other ocular risk factors for PCV include a history of CSC, presence of PED [45], and choroidal hyperpermeability [26, 58]. Ahuja et al. proposed that PCV might develop as a consequence of chronic CSC [58], a theory supported by advances in choroidal imaging [20, 59, 60] and the finding that patients with PCV are more likely to have a history of CSC than those with typical AMD (15 vs. 3% of patients) [61].

18.3.4.2 Systemic

Hypertension has long been regarded as a potential risk factor for PCV [47, 62]; there have been case reports of hypertensive retinopathy and macroaneurysms with coexisting PCV lesions [63], and histopathological studies reporting hyalinization of choroidal vessels similar to that seen in arteriosclerosis [64]. However, not all studies have shown an association [2].

Cigarette smoking, a significant risk factor for wet AMD, has also been shown to increase the risk of PCV with a similar effect size (odds ratio 4.4 for PCV and 4.9 for AMD) [7].

18.4 Pathology and Genetics

18.4.1 Histopathology

In the mid-1990s, several clinicopathological studies of suspected PCV in enucleated eyes described extensive fibrovascular proliferation within the subretinal space and Bruch's membrane [65, 66]. These studies were probably describing the end-stage of PCV. Okubo and colleagues noted a hyaline-like appearance of the vessel walls in a surgically excised specimen while it was still active [67]. This finding was confirmed by Kuroiwa and colleagues [68].

Nakashizuka and colleagues [64] further characterized these lesions in surgical specimens that met the diagnosis criteria of PCV based on ICGA, and documented extensive exudative change and hyalinization of vessels. Hyalinized vessels were characterized by extravasation of plasma protein and deposition of basement membrane-like material, and the smooth muscle component was replaced by amorphous pseudo-collagenous tissue of a poorly defined nature. The authors suggested that these histopathological lesions were similar to retinal arterial macroaneurysms and thus hypertension may be a common risk factor (see Sect. 18.3.4.2).

In a case that included both CNV and PCV portions in the same specimen, the CNV portion showed granulation tissue proliferation, supporting the concept that CNV represents a stereotypic, nonspecific wound-repair response. In contrast, little (if any) fibrosis or granulation tissue proliferation was observed in the PCV portion. Hyalinized vessels in the CNV portion contained pericytes that were immunoreactive for alpha-smooth muscle actin (SMA), while vessels in the PCV portion were negative for alpha-SMA expression, suggesting that the smooth muscle cells of the choroidal vessels had disappeared in the PCV portion. Furthermore, immunoreactive expressions of CD34 revealed discontinuity in the vascular endothelium in the PCV portion. Both of these findings were indicative of vascular damage similar to that seen in hypertension. The hyalinized vessels represented the choroidal vasculature with arteriosclerotic changes, similar to the hyalinization seen in other parts of the body. As such, the authors concluded that these vessels did not represent neovascularization [64].

The relative role of VEGF in the pathogenesis of PCV is variable: while Nakashizuka et al. [64] observed no VEGF expression in vascular endothelial cells of PCV specimens, Matsuoka et al. [69] found strong VEGF positivity. Potential explanations for the disparity include possible differences in the amount of scarring, age-related atherosclerotic changes, or type of PCV (see Sect. 18.5.2). Tong et al. (2006) found higher levels of aqueous VEGF in eyes with PCV compared with normal controls, albeit at lower levels than in wet AMD [70].

18.4.2 Genetics

The underlying genetics of AMD and PCV are largely similar, although some discrepancies have been reported. For example, the strongest association of AMD in the *CFH* gene was through single nucleotide polymorphism (SNP) rs1061170 (Y402H); however, its role in PCV is rather unclear. This discrepancy could be due to ethnic differences in the frequency of the *CFH* risk allele, which is uncommon in Asian populations [71]. A recent meta-analysis found that another variant on *CFH*, rs800292 (I62V), was strongly associated with PCV in Asian patients [72].

A separate comprehensive meta-analysis found that variants at *ARMS2/HTRA1* (rs10490924/rs11200638), *CFH* (rs1061170, rs3753394, rs1329428, rs1410996, and rs800292) and the complement pathway (*C2*; rs547154) were significantly associated with PCV, with the highest odds ratio observed at variants in *ARMS2/HTRA1*. When comparing PCV and wet AMD, only variant rs10490924 of *ARMS2/HTRA1* potentially implicated a genetic and biological difference between these two disease entities. The risk genotypes of rs10490924 were associated with larger lesion size, a greater chance of vitreous hemorrhage, and worse therapeutic response in PCV [73].

The non-synonymous SNPs rs10490924 (A69S) within *ARMS2*, and rs11200638 within *HTRA1*, at 10q26 have been tested for disease susceptibility for both AMD and PCV. Due to a strong linkage disequilibrium across this region, it is difficult to genetically distinguish these two susceptible candidates and prioritize their importance toward disease pathogenesis [6].

Other studies have also examined the association of a number of genetic polymorphisms with PCV in different ethnicities, but a recent meta-analysis of these associations gave inconclusive results [74].

18.5 Classification

At present, there is no generally recognized classification scheme in which PCV is defined. The lack of a clear classification for PCV—either within or outside the wet AMD spectrum—confounds available epidemiological data, and complicates diagnosis and management.

18.5.1 Classification Within CNV

Current opinion, based on published evidence and clinical experience, is that rather than being a discrete clinical entity, PCV is a subtype of wet AMD. However, it is difficult to place PCV within the current classification for CNV, in which disease is categorized according to lesion location (extrafoveal, juxtafoveal, or subfoveal) and subfoveal leakage pattern (occult or classic) based on FA findings. This issue must be viewed alongside the wider limitations of the current classification for CNV. While the present scheme is practical when considering laser photocoagulation—where one needs to be able to direct therapy accurately—it is of questionable value in the era of anti-VEGF therapy, where lesion location is not important for treatment decisions. Accordingly, updating the CNV classification system to improve its value for modern treatment modalities would be a worthwhile undertaking. In doing so, it would be pertinent to account for all possible variants of CNV, including PCV.

One option for a new CNV classification system would be to define neovascularization as sub-RPE (e.g., occult type 1 CNV or PCV), subretinal (e.g., classic type 2 CNV), or intraretinal (e.g., RAP), factors that have implications for prognosis and response to anti-VEGF treatment. Using this classification system, PCV would represent a polyp-exhibiting form of sub-RPE CNV.

18.5.2 Classification of PCV Subtypes

Just as the classification of PCV itself is challenging, so too is the lack of a universally accepted system of classification for PCV subtypes.

One commonly proposed subtyping of PCV is by the presence or absence of a BVN. Type 1 PCV describes the disease in which ICGA shows the polypoidal lesions to be fed and drained by an overt BVN and is characterized by CNV rapidly expanding beneath the RPE with terminal dilatations at the end of the branching vascular network. The BVN typically displays one of two distinct patterns, either an "umbrella" pattern where vessels radiate from the feeder vessel in all directions, or a "rake" pattern in which the vessels extend from the feeder vessel in one direction. In contrast, the type 2 PCV variant shows either a faint BVN or none at all [75–77].

Type 1 PCV, thought to be the less common type, has been shown to be associated with the *ARMS2* A69S genetic polymorphism, which correlates with a larger lesion size and more limited effect of photodynamic therapy (PDT) [75, 76]. Type 1 PCV is associated with a smaller mean subfoveal thickness than type 2 PCV [78].

The type 1/2 classification system described above is not widely used, as interpretation can be subjective and interobserver agreement has not been tested. Other groups have suggested classifying PCV lesions by polyp size (largest diameter of polyp), location (peripapillary, subfoveal, juxtafoveal, or extrafoveal), formation (single, cluster, or string), and a number of discrete polyp areas (single or multiple) [49]. It is also possible to classify PCV based on its primary features, i.e., quiescent, exudative, or hemorrhagic [13, 79].

However, despite the interest in PCV subtypes, evidence relating to the prognostic value of these schemes, and their value in guiding treatment, remain limited.

Recent guidelines for the diagnosis and treatment of PCV described a more pragmatic approach that could be applied in the clinic. In an algorithm for the diagnosis of PCV, the disease was classified as either active or inactive, with active disease defined by a list of features reflecting a likely symptomatic impact and/or possible need for treatment (see Sect. 18.7.3) [13].

As PDT and focal laser remain possible treatment options in addition to anti-VEGF therapy (see Sect. 18.7), lesion location (extrafoveal, juxtafoveal, or subfoveal) also remains an important consideration.

18.6 Natural History and Prognosis

18.6.1 Natural History

In contrast to wet AMD, the natural history of PCV is highly variable and poorly understood [50, 51].

Yannuzzi et al. described a prolonged, relapsing, and remitting course including multiple serosanguinous detachments of the RPE [33]. Long-term vision may be preserved, and fibrous proliferation and scarring are uncommon compared with wet AMD; however, significant vision loss can occur through the development of chronic atrophy or vitreous hemorrhage [33, 35].

Other studies have described PCV as a relatively benign condition [47, 80–82], remaining stable in 50% of eyes for 2 or more years without treatment [83]. In a study by Yamaoka et al., despite persistent serous retinal detachment in 11% of eyes with PCV but no coexisting classic CNV, 89 and 83% had stable or improved vision without treatment at 3 and 12 months, respectively [47]. Furthermore, although patients with PCV have been reported to present later than those with wet AMD (average 21.2 vs. 14.8 months from onset of symptoms to first evaluation), they generally have better visual acuity [2]. Spontaneous involution of polyps may occur [33, 83, 84].

18.6.2 Predictive Factors

18.6.2.1 Clinical and Angiographic Features

As discussed in the Sect. 18.5.2, many investigators have broadly divided PCV by its predominant presenting pattern, either exudative or hemorrhagic. In the exudative pattern, serous RPE or retinal detachment and lipid deposits may continue for a long time in a stable condition, followed by eventual degeneration and atrophy of the RPE and deterioration in vision [83]. In the hemorrhagic pattern, hemorrhagic detachments of the RPE and/or submacular hemorrhage (sometimes acute) can occur, leading to sudden visual deterioration. In these cases, massive retinal hemorrhage may even lead to breakthrough vitreous hemorrhage, which may resolve spontaneously but can recur. Although these patterns may change over the course of follow-up, ultimately, recurrent hemorrhage leads to degeneration of the RPE and outer retina, and loss of vision.

Based on ICGA findings, polyps with a "cluster of grapes" configuration (up to two-thirds of PCV cases) are usually associated with an aggressive disease course, with or without treatment [2, 49, 80, 83, 85]. Bessho et al. followed up 42 eyes with PCV over 12 months and reported that eyes with "clustered" PCV experienced significant deterioration in mean visual acuity, while in those showing "nonclustered" PCV, vision was largely maintained [80]. Polyps that show pulsations (viewed by video ICGA) may also exhibit high disease activity, potentially being associated with extensive hemorrhage [86–88].

Reports have suggested that eyes with better initial vision (≥20/40) tend to maintain this vision at 1 year [47] and 2 years after diagnosis [83]. In a retrospective review of 110 eyes by Okubo et al., smaller lesions and a shorter duration of disturbed vision were associated with a lower rate of decline in visual acuity than larger lesions and a longer history of disturbed vision [89]. In another study of 88 eyes, those with larger PCV complex size (≥1 disc area; n = 66) showed significant progression in the mean area of the lesion, with marked deterioration of vision during follow-up, whereas eyes with smaller PCV complex size (<1 disc area; n = 22) often showed minimal progression with limited exudative change and tended to maintain their initially good vision [90]. Furthermore, severe vision-threatening complications, such as suprachoroidal hemorrhage, vitreous hemorrhage, and RPE tears, were only seen in eyes with larger PCV complexes [90].

Coexisting type 2 CNV has been described in a small proportion of patients with PCV, and is associated with a worse prognosis than PCV alone [3, 22, 47, 91].

18.7 Management

18.7.1 Goals of Treatment

The primary goal of treatment in PCV, as in other forms of wet AMD, is the improvement and subsequent maintenance of vision. This can be achieved through the reduction and resolution of exudation from the two components of PCV: the polyps themselves and/or the BVN [92]. Due to the relapsing and remitting course, which is common in eyes with PCV, an important goal of PCV management that is different from typical wet AMD is the complete closure of polyps, confirmed on ICGA. This secondary objective is especially important in cases with recurrent or persistent fluid at the macula despite multiple repeated anti-VEGF treatments for active polyps [93, 94]. Persistent polyps are associated with a high risk of massive submacular hemorrhage, disciform fibrosis, and RPE atrophy of the macula, leading to severe and irreversible visual loss. Breakthrough vitreous hemorrhage in eyes with PCV may have devastating complications, including secondary glaucoma and phthisis bulbi [95].

18.7.2 Imaging Requirements for Management

In addition to diagnosis (see Sect. 18.2), OCT (and to a lesser extent angiography) are invaluable for guiding the management of PCV. It is important to emphasize that FA alone is insufficient and inaccurate in diagnosing PCV and in guiding its management. However, when ICGA reveals leakage in the absence of visible polyps, the FA is essential in confirming that the source of leakage is the BVN, essentially behaving as typical occult CNV [96]. Lesion location should be based on ICGA findings, and the location of the polypoidal lesions and the BVN should be determined separately. FA and ICGA also serve to delineate the different components of the PCV lesion: FA provides better information on leakage from the BVN, while ICGA is required to visualize the polypoidal lesions themselves. This has a significant bearing on the selection of treatment modality in recurrent and persistent cases (see Sect. 18.7.5).

18.7.3 When to Treat

All active PCV should be treated as soon as possible. PCV may be considered active if there is clinical, OCT, FA, or ICGA evidence of any of the following [13]:

- Symptoms of visual loss and metamorphopsia
- Subretinal fluid and/or intraretinal fluid (with or without PED)
- Subretinal hemorrhage
- Fluorescein leakage on FA
- Polyps and other features on ICGA

The fellow eye should also be monitored carefully for PCV because a significant proportion of patients may have bilateral disease, even though bilaterality has been reported to be lower than in wet AMD. If polyps are present in the fellow eye, the decision to treat should be based on disease activity and presence or absence of symptoms [13].

18.7.4 Treatment Options

Visual morbidity from PCV arises from the activity of polyps and the BVN (bi-component disease), and as such there are several management options to be considered, each of which is discussed below. A summary of the recommended treatment approach is provided in Box 18.2. Representative cases are shown in Figs. 18.1, 18.2, and 18.3.

Box 18.2 Summary of PCV Management

Summary of PCV management
• Visual morbidity from PCV arises from the activity of polyps and the BVN (bi-component disease).
• Polyp closure is more effectively achieved by PDT than with ranibizumab or bevacizumab, while reduction in fluid, visual gains, and control of leakage from BVN are best achieved by anti-VEGF treatment. Intravitreal aflibercept monotherapy may offer polyp closure rates similar to PDT.
• In cases with good initial visual acuity (e.g., 20/40 or better), anti-VEGF monotherapy may be initiated, with PDT added only if there is a persistent activity from active polyps; otherwise, the current treatment of choice is PDT–anti-VEGF combination treatment to the entire lesion, as delineated by ICGA in the first instance.
• Recurrences should be treated based on the primary source of leakage: if polyps are still present, further PDT applied selectively to only the polyps may be administered; if no polyps are present, and leakage is ascertained to be originating only from the BVN, anti-VEGF monotherapy is the treatment of choice.
• Modified PDT protocols may reduce the potential complications of PDT such as submacular hemorrhage and RPE atrophy.
• Ongoing research will demonstrate whether anti-VEGF monotherapy is adequate to achieve and maintain visual acuity gains and polyp closure.

BVN branching vascular network, *ICGA* indocyanine green angiography, *OCT* optical coherence tomography, *PCV* polypoidal choroidal vasculopathy, *PDT* photodynamic therapy, *RPE* retinal pigment epithelial, *VEGF* vascular endothelial growth factor.

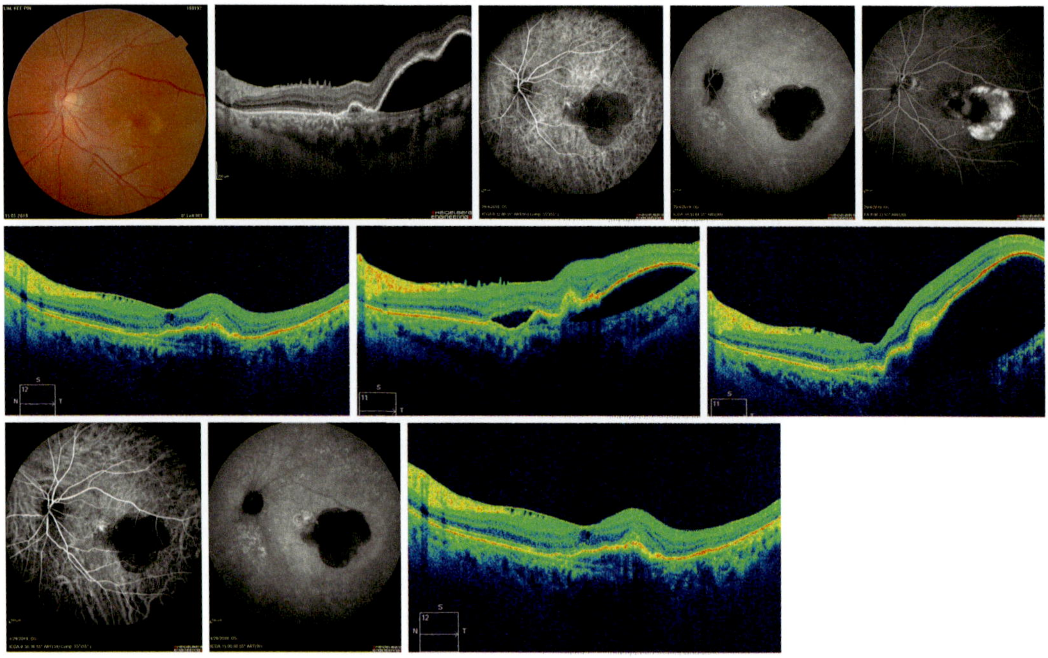

Fig. 18.1 Case 1: A 70-year-old Chinese male presented with reduced central vision with metamorphopsia for 2 months. He had a history of three intravitreal aflibercept injections at monthly intervals in the same eye; however, he did not notice any significant improvement in vision. On examination, fundus examination showed pigment epithelial detachment (PED). Angiography and OCT imaging confirmed the presence of polypoidal choroidal vasculopathy (upper row). The patient underwent combination therapy (PDT and ranibizumab) and responded well (middle row—left OCT). However, he had a recurrence after 4 months (middle row—middle OCT) and underwent three monthly ranibizumab injections with any improvement (middle row—right OCT). Repeat ICG showed polyps and underwent combination therapy which led to recovery (bottom row)

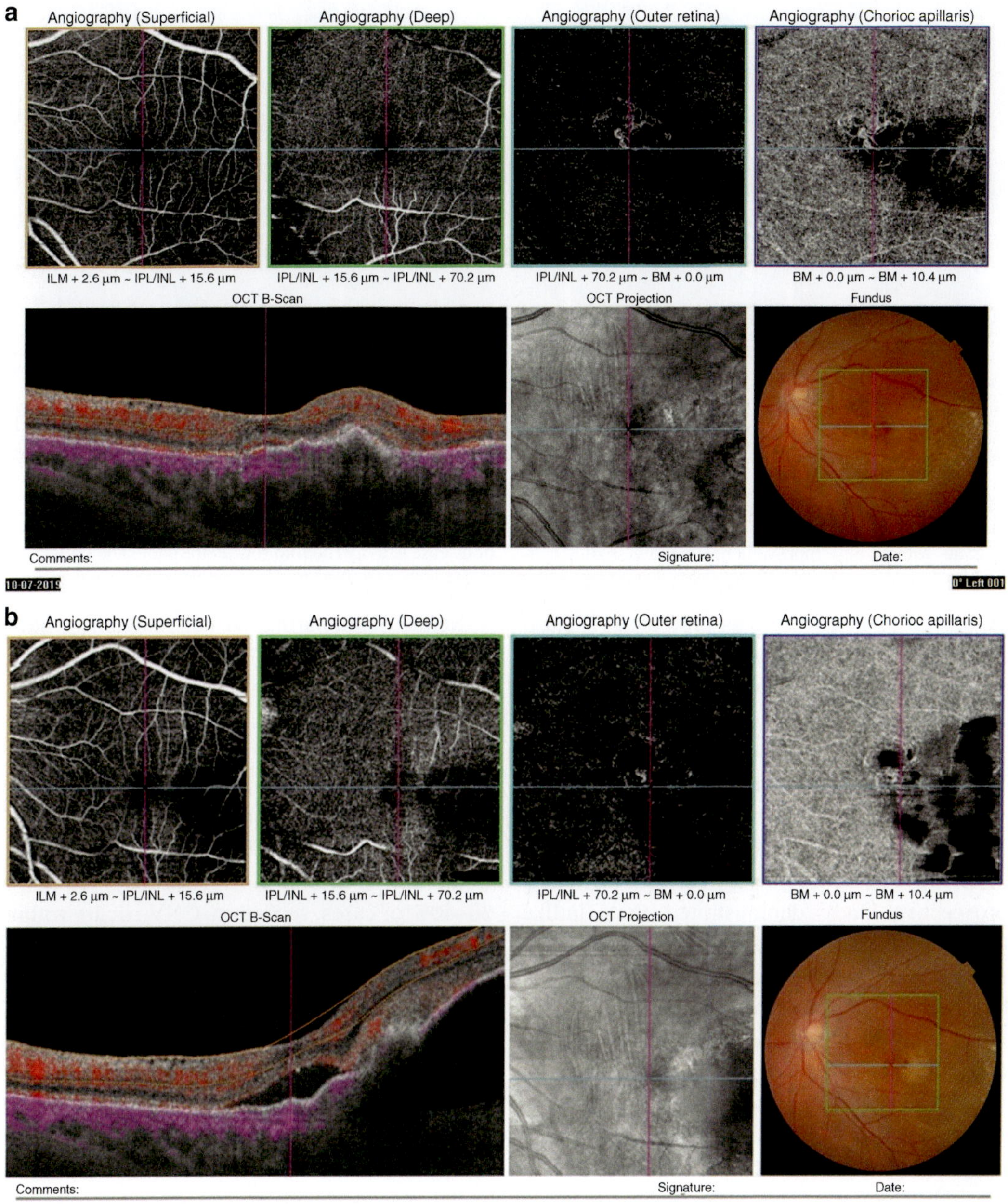

Fig. 18.2 (**a**) OCT angiography of case 1 at presentation shows polyp and BVN. (**b**) OCT angiography of case 1 at the time of recurrence shows polyp and BVN. OCT angiography of case 1 at the last follow-up. Note the persistent and increased flow in BVN; therefore, the patient was asked to continue with aflibercept on treat-and-extend regimen

18.7.4.1 Laser Photocoagulation

Laser photocoagulation only has a role in ablating extrafoveal (preferably extramacular) polyps [97]. Rarely, it may be effective in treating the entire complex of extrafoveal polyps and BVN. The limitations of laser photocoagulation include a high rate of recurrence, formation of new lesions, enlargement of photocoagulation scars, tear or rip of the RPE, as well as iatrogenic CNV. Accordingly, rates of visual loss

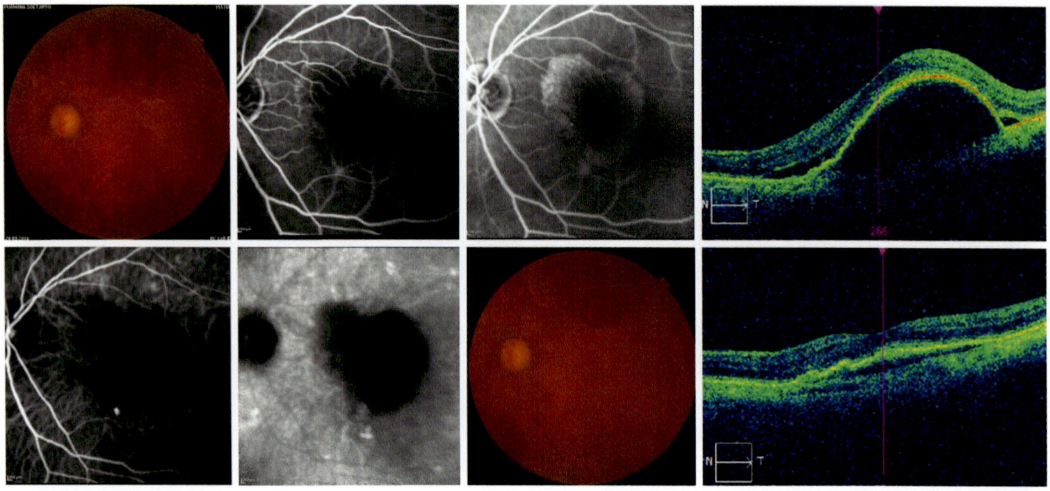

Fig. 18.3 Case 2: A 74-year-old female had a history of intravitreal 3 aflibercept then 3 ranibizumab at monthly intervals without any improvement. Imaging studies confirmed the presence of polyps and she underwent combination therapy and improved from 6/60 to 6/24 with resolution of disease activity (bottom row: color photo and OCT)

have been reported to be as high as 54% [98]. Adjunct anti-VEGF in addition to focal laser has been shown to improve the outcome in extrafoveal PCV [99].

18.7.4.2 Verteporfin (Visudyne™) Photodynamic Therapy

Treatment of PCV with PDT has been shown to be effective in the closure of polyps in PCV. One prospective study demonstrated that, unlike CNV, treatment of PCV with PDT resulted in a mean improvement in visual acuity of 8 letters at 12 months, with 25% of patients experiencing significant gains in vision of at least 3 Snellen lines; only 8% of patients lost 3 or more Snellen lines of vision [100]. In addition, the vast majority of patients (86%) had cessation of fluorescein leakage at 1 year [100, 101]. Similarly, in the EVEREST trial, the mean change in visual acuity in the PDT-treated group was +7.5 letters at 6 months. The rate of complete closure of polyps was 71%, and that of partial but incomplete closure was 86% [11]. The treatment-free period in patients receiving PDT for PCV may also be significantly longer than in those receiving the same treatment for CNV in AMD [101]. However, PDT is relatively ineffective in resolving activity arising from the BVN, with the majority of cases remaining unchanged despite repeated treatment [102, 103].

Studies comparing visual outcomes have shown that anti-VEGF therapy gives better results than PDT [104]. Potential complications of PDT include acute vision decrease, increased subretinal hemorrhage, and RPE tears [105, 106]. Longer-term limitations of PDT monotherapy include reduction of vision, recurrence of polyps, persistence of BVN activity, secondary CNV, and progressive RPE atrophy [107]. In 20–40% of cases, secondary CNV occurs within 2 years [108–110]. Repeated full-fluence PDT may lead to persistent choroidal ischemia, upregulation of VEGF, and RPE atrophy, all of which contribute to unsatisfactory long-term visual outcomes [111]. A recent systematic review and meta-analysis reported stable visual outcomes for up to 2 years of PCV, but worsening by 3 years, particularly in eyes that experienced recurrence [112].

18.7.4.3 Anti-VEGF Monotherapy

Anti-VEGF therapy such as intravitreal aflibercept (EYLEA®), ranibizumab (Lucentis®), and off-label bevacizumab (Avastin®), is currently the gold-standard treatment for wet AMD, with over 95% of patients avoiding moderate visual loss, and about 30% showing a doubling of the visual angle [113–115]; this effect can be maintained over many years with adequate monitoring and retreatment [116]. Ranibizumab monotherapy has been associated with similar visual outcomes in PCV [11, 117, 118]. One indication for anti-VEGF therapy in PCV is for patients with good presenting visual acuity [119]; indeed, current Japanese guidelines recommend anti-VEGF monotherapy for patients presenting with relatively good visual acuity of 20/32 or better [120].

Despite providing improvements in visual acuity, the polyp closure rate with bevacizumab and ranibizumab monotherapy remains low. In the EVEREST trial, complete closure of polyps at 6 months with ranibizumab therapy was 28% compared with over 70% with PDT, while the partial polyp closure rates were 43% in the ranibizumab group and over 83% in the PDT-treated arms [11]. In a retrospective study of three initial monthly injections of bevacizumab, only 1 of 11 cases showed closure of polyps on the ICGA [121]. In addition, while bevacizumab was effective in controlling exudation, the size of the BVN remained unchanged. What is undisputed, however, is that bevacizumab therapy is effective in reducing the activity of the BVN [110, 122].

Intravitreal aflibercept can be used for effective management of PCV, with evidence from VIEW 2 for probable PCV cases suggesting similar VA benefits to "standard" wet AMD [123]. The recently presented results of the PLANET study ($n = 318$) of intravitreal aflibercept in PCV demonstrate that intravitreal aflibercept monotherapy achieves significant visual acuity gains over 1 year and resolves polyp activity in the majority of patients when treated with the approved regimen for wet AMD [124]. Very few patients met the criteria for rescue PDT, suggesting intravitreal aflibercept monotherapy is a safe and efficacious treatment in the vast majority of PCV cases. Furthermore, several case series have reported superior polyp closure with intravitreal aflibercept than is reported for ranibizumab, and intravitreal aflibercept has also been used successfully to treat ranibizumab tachyphylaxis in patients with PCV [125–130].

18.7.4.4 Combination Therapy: PDT with Anti-VEGF Agents

There are sound biologic and scientific rationales for combining PDT with anti-VEGF therapy, as both therapies employ different mechanisms of action that may be synergistic. While PDT may be effective for polyp regression, anti-VEGF therapy improves vision by reducing both exudation from polyps and BVN activity. Anti-VEGF therapy also mitigates the post-PDT upregulation of VEGF that is caused by choroidal ischemia, thereby reducing the risk of the acute vision decrease sometimes observed with PDT monotherapy; it might also minimize the risk of post-PDT subretinal hemorrhage [131, 132]. The EVEREST study demonstrated that the PDT–ranibizumab combination was superior to ranibizumab monotherapy in terms of polyp closure rate while achieving comparable short-term (6-month) visual outcomes [11]. Similar results have been observed in patients receiving PDT with bevacizumab [133]. Moderate vision gains were achieved in the monotherapy arm of the recently presented EVEREST II study ($n = 322$) [134]. The ranibizumab and PDT combination arm of EVEREST II achieved greater vision gains and a rate of polyp regression twice that of the ranibizumab monotherapy arm. However, in studies and real-life evidence generated to date, intravitreal aflibercept as monotherapy has shown similar vision gains and polyp regression rates to the ranibizumab and PDT combination arm of EVEREST II [125, 135, 136]. In the recently presented PLANET study of intravitreal aflibercept in PCV, similar results were achieved using both aflibercept monotherapy and combination therapy (aflibercept + rescue PDT). The majority of patients achieved good vision gains when treated with the approved regimen for wet AMD, with very few patients requiring PDT rescue therapy [124]. Therefore, the use of intravitreal aflibercept has the potential to negate the need for PDT and associated costs and side effects.

The long-term visual results of combination therapy are yet to be established. Some studies indicate that while visual outcomes are good in the first 6–12 months, there is a significant drop-off into the second and third years [137, 138]. A meta-analysis reported greater visual improvement in eyes treated with a combination of PDT and anti-VEGF (ranibizumab or bevacizumab) than in those treated with PDT monotherapy, although the beneficial effect may be lost with longer (2-year) follow-up [112]. Two-year results from the ongoing EVEREST II and PLANET studies will provide more data on the long-term effects of PDT combination therapy in conjunction with a treat-and-extend regimen. Another potential advantage of combination with PDT is that the number of anti-VEGF injections may be reduced without compromising visual acuity gains [139].

Owing to concerns regarding potential complications of PDT, several authors have used modified PDT protocols (e.g., reduced-fluence PDT) alongside anti-VEGF agents, with the aim of reducing the potential complications associated with PDT [140–143]. These protocols are yet to be tested against conventional full-fluence PDT–anti-VEGF combination regimens. However, in recurrent cases, it seems pertinent to minimize the laser treatment size by targeting only polyps (guided by ICGA), rather than the entire lesion complex [144–146].

18.7.5 Treatment in Cases of Persistent Activity and/or Recurrence

Retreatment criteria should be based on disease activity as indicated by reduced visual acuity, macular thickening from fluid, and leakage from polyps and/or the BVN [13]. The treatment modality will then depend on the predominant cause. It is generally agreed that persistent polyps should be selectively treated with PDT in combination with anti-VEGF therapy, while activity from the BVN alone should be managed using anti-VEGF monotherapy, since PDT has little effect on the activity or size of the BVN and might accelerate RPE atrophy and photoreceptor cell loss. However, it is worth considering potential differences in anti-VEGF agents, as intravitreal aflibercept may be associated with a greater likelihood of polyp regression than ranibizumab; indeed, intravitreal aflibercept monotherapy has recently been reported to induce polyp regression in cases that are refractory to ranibizumab treatment. A key objective in retreatment is to minimize complications from PDT by reducing the frequency, spot size, and possibly fluence [146]. A systematic review reported recurrence rates after PDT with or without anti-VEGF (any agent) of 6–50% after 1 year, 9–83% after 2 years, and 40–79% after 3 years of follow-up [112].

18.8 Research Questions

It is evident from the review of the current literature that there remain numerous important questions surrounding PCV and its management.

18.8.1 Questions Regarding Epidemiology and Pathophysiology

- What is the absolute definition of PCV and what are the key features for diagnosis?
- What is the true prevalence and incidence of PCV?
- What are the risk factors associated with PCV, and how do they compare with those for wet AMD?
- What are the underlying genetics in PCV and how they relate to phenotypic presentation, type of PCV, and response to treatment?
- How should PCV be classified in order to predict prognosis and inform management decisions?

18.8.2 Questions Regarding Treatment

- What is the role of combination therapy in PCV and should the different treatment modalities be administered simultaneously or sequentially?
- Is it sufficient to initiate therapy with anti-VEGF monotherapy or would first-line combination with PDT be better?
- Will combination therapy with PDT help improve outcomes in patients whose vision is not improving with anti-VEGF monotherapy?
- Are there significant differences in polyp closure rates by the different anti-VEGF agents?

- Does reducing fluence, especially in repeat treatment, reduce long-term complications of PDT (especially RPE atrophy, macular hemorrhage, and RPE rips)?
- Should treatment-naive and recurrent cases be approached differently?
- Does recurrence indicate undertreatment?

18.8.3 Questions Regarding Outcome

- Can we identify distinct types of PCV that are associated with better or worse outcomes, and should treatment be tailored to the prognosis (e.g., if the risk of persistent BVN activity is high, perhaps these patients should receive proactive rather than reactive therapy)?
- What is the expected long-term visual outcome for PCV patients?
- How does angiographic polyp closure correlate with visual outcome?

18.9 Summary

PCV is increasingly recognized as a major subtype of AMD, estimated to affect nearly 1 million people in China alone, and common elsewhere in Asian populations [147]. While it is historically considered to be a concern only in Asian populations, the condition is now thought to be prevalent globally and may be grossly underestimated in non-Asian populations. The current lack of disease understanding limits optimal diagnosis and treatment.

This chapter brings together the current evidence for PCV and provides expert comment on the available data. Moreover, the paper identifies gaps in our knowledge, which further research is required to address.

Because PCV is considered to be a subtype of wet AMD it should be managed using the currently approved therapies; however, optimal treatment regimens have yet to be determined.

Further research is necessary to improve our understanding of PCV and inform management decisions.

References

1. Wong WL, Su X, Li X, et al. Global prevalence of age-related macular degeneration and disease burden projection for 2020 and 2040: a systematic review and meta-analysis. Lancet Glob Health. 2014;2(2):e106–16.
2. Sho K, Takahashi K, Yamada H, et al. Polypoidal choroidal vasculopathy: incidence, demographic features, and clinical characteristics. Arch Ophthalmol. 2003;121(10):1392–6.
3. Maruko I, Iida T, Saito M, et al. Clinical characteristics of exudative age-related macular degeneration in Japanese patients. Am J Ophthalmol. 2007;144:15–22.
4. Liu Y, Wen F, Huang S, et al. Subtype lesions of neovascular age-related macular degeneration in Chinese patients. Graefes Arch Clin Exp Ophthalmol. 2007;245(10):1441–5.
5. Byeon SH, Lee SC, Oh HS, et al. Incidence and clinical patterns of polypoidal choroidal vasculopathy in Korean patients. Jpn J Ophthalmol. 2008;52(1):57–62.
6. Laude A, Cackett PD, Vithana EN, et al. Polypoidal choroidal vasculopathy and neovascular age-related macular degeneration: same or different disease? Prog Retin Eye Res. 2010;29(1):19–29.
7. Cackett P, Yeo I, Cheung CM, et al. Relationship of smoking and cardiovascular risk factors with polypoidal choroidal vasculopathy and age-related macular degeneration in Chinese persons. Ophthalmology. 2011;118(5):846–52.
8. Cheng CY, Yamashiro K, Jia Chen L, et al. New loci and coding variants confer risk for age-related macular degeneration in East Asians. Nat Commun. 2015;6:6063.
9. Miura M, Makita S, Iwasaki T, et al. Three-dimensional visualization of ocular vascular pathology by optical coherence angiography in vivo. Invest Ophthalmol Vis Sci. 2011;52(5):2689–95.
10. Japanese Study Group of PCV. Criteria for diagnosis of polypoidal choroidal vasculopathy. Nippon Ganka Gakkai Zasshi. 2005;109(7):417–27.
11. Koh A, Lee WK, Chen LJ, et al. EVEREST study: efficacy and safety of verteporfin photodynamic therapy in combination with ranibizumab or alone versus ranibizumab monotherapy in patients with symptomatic macular polypoidal choroidal vasculopathy. Retina. 2012;32(8):1453–64.
12. Cheung GCM, Laude A, Wong W, et al. Improved specificity of polypoidal choroidal vasculopathy diagnosis using a modified EVEREST criteria. Retina. 2015;35(7):1375–80.
13. Koh AH, Chen LJ, Chen SJ, et al. Polypoidal choroidal vasculopathy: evidence-based guidelines for clinical diagnosis and treatment. Retina. 2013;33(4):686–716.
14. Desmettre T, Devoisselle JM, Mordon S. Fluorescence properties and metabolic features of indocyanine green (ICG) as related to angiography. Surv Ophthalmol. 2000;45(1):15–27.

15. Royal College of Ophthalmologists. Age-related macular degeneration: guidelines for management. London: Royal College of Ophthalmologists; 2013.
16. Cheung CM, Lai TY, Chen SJ, et al. Understanding indocyanine green angiography in polypoidal choroidal vasculopathy: the group experience with digital fundus photography and confocal scanning laser ophthalmoscopy. Retina. 2014;34:2397–406.
17. Gomi F, Sawa M, Mitarai K, et al. Angiographic lesion of polypoidal choroidal vasculopathy on indocyanine green and fluorescein angiography. Graefes Arch Clin Exp Ophthalmol. 2007;245(10):1421–7.
18. Lim TH, Laude A, Tan CS. Polypoidal choroidal vasculopathy: an angiographic discussion. Eye (Lond). 2010;24(3):483–90.
19. Kim JH, Kang SW, Kim TH, et al. Structure of polypoidal choroidal vasculopathy studied by colocalization between tomographic and angiographic lesions. Am J Ophthalmol. 2013;156(5):974–80.e972.
20. Koizumi H, Yamagishi T, Yamazaki T, et al. Relationship between clinical characteristics of polypoidal choroidal vasculopathy and choroidal vascular hyperpermeability. Am J Ophthalmol. 2013;155(2):305–13.e301.
21. Lafaut BA, Leys AM, Snyers B, et al. Polypoidal choroidal vasculopathy in Caucasians. Graefes Arch Clin Exp Ophthalmol. 2000;238(9):752–9.
22. Maruko I, Iida T, Saito M, et al. Combined cases of polypoidal choroidal vasculopathy and typical age-related macular degeneration. Graefes Arch Clin Exp Ophthalmol. 2010;248:361–8.
23. De Salvo G, Vaz-Pereira S, Keane PA, et al. Sensitivity and specificity of spectral-domain optical coherence tomography in detecting idiopathic polypoidal choroidal vasculopathy. Am J Ophthalmol. 2014;158:1228–38.e1221.
24. Maruko I, Iida T, Sugano Y, et al. Subfoveal retinal and choroidal thickness after verteporfin photodynamic therapy for polypoidal choroidal vasculopathy. Am J Ophthalmol. 2011;151(4):594–603.e591.
25. Sayanagi K, Gomi F, Akiba M, et al. En-face high-penetration optical coherence tomography imaging in polypoidal choroidal vasculopathy. Br J Ophthalmol. 2015;99(1):29–35.
26. Yannuzzi LA, Freund KB, Goldbaum M, et al. Polypoidal choroidal vasculopathy masquerading as central serous chorioretinopathy. Ophthalmology. 2000;107(4):767–77.
27. Cheung CM, Wong TY. Treatment of age-related macular degeneration. Lancet. 2013;382(9900):1230–2.
28. Cheung CM, Bhargava M, Laude A, et al. Asian age-related macular degeneration phenotyping study: rationale, design and protocol of a prospective cohort study. Clin Exp Ophthalmol. 2012;40:727–35.
29. Jonas JB. Global prevalence of age-related macular degeneration. Lancet Glob Health. 2014;2:e65–6.
30. Kokame GT. Polypoidal choroidal vasculopathy—an important diagnositic tool with therapeutic implications. Retina. 2012;32(8):1446–8.
31. Coscas G, Yamashiro K, Coscas F, et al. Comparison of exudative age-related macular degeneration subtypes in Japanese and French patients: multicenter diagnosis with multimodal imaging. Am J Ophthalmol. 2014;158:309–18.e302.
32. Yannuzzi LA, Wong DW, Sforzolini BS, et al. Polypoidal choroidal vasculopathy and neovascularized age-related macular degeneration. Arch Ophthalmol. 1999;117(11):1503–10.
33. Yannuzzi LA, Ciardella A, Spaide RF, et al. The expanding clinical spectrum of idiopathic polypoidal choroidal vasculopathy. Arch Ophthalmol. 1997;115:478–85.
34. Spaide RF, Yannuzzi LA, Slakter JS, et al. Indocyanine green videoangiography of idiopathic polypoidal choroidal vasculopathy. Retina. 1995;15:100–10.
35. Perkovich BT, Zakov ZN, Berlin LA, et al. An update on multiple recurrent serosanguineous retinal pigment epithelial detachments in black women. Retina. 1990;10:18–26.
36. Stern RM, Zakov ZN, Zegarra H, et al. Multiple recurrent serosanguineous retinal pigment epithelial detachments in black women. Am J Ophthalmol. 1985;100:560–9.
37. Ahuja RM, Stanga PE, Vingerling JR, et al. Polypoidal choroidal vasculopathy in exudative and haemorrhagic pigment epithelial detachments. Br J Ophthalmol. 2000;84(5):479–84.
38. Ciardella AP, Donsoff IM, Huang SJ, et al. Polypoidal choroidal vasculopathy. Surv Ophthalmol. 2004;49(1):25–37.
39. Imamura Y, Engelbert M, Iida T, et al. Polypoidal choroidal vasculopathy: a review. Surv Ophthalmol. 2010;55(6):501–15.
40. Kwok AK, Lai TY, Chan CW, et al. Polypoidal choroidal vasculopathy in Chinese patients. Br J Ophthalmol. 2002;86:892–7.
41. Wen F, Chen C, Wu D, et al. Polypoidal choroidal vasculopathy in elderly Chinese patients. Graefes Arch Clin Exp Ophthalmol. 2004;242(8):625–9.
42. Ladas ID, Rouvas AA, Moschos MM, et al. Polypoidal choroidal vasculopathy and exudative age-related macular degeneration in Greek population. Eye (Lond). 2004;18(5):455–9.
43. Scassellati-Sforzolini B, Mariotti C, Bryan R, et al. Polypoidal choroidal vasculopathy in Italy. Retina. 2001;21(2):121–5.
44. Cackett P, Htoon H, Wong D, et al. Hemorrhagic pigment epithelial detachment as a predictive feature of polypoidal choroidal vasculopathy in a Chinese population. Eye. 2009;24:789–92.
45. Hikichi T, Ohtsuka H, Higuchi M, et al. Causes of macular serous retinal detachments in Japanese patients 40 years and older. Retina. 2009;29(3):395–404.
46. Song SJ, Youm DJ, Chang Y, et al. Age-related macular degeneration in a screened south Korean population: prevalence, risk factors, and subtypes. Ophthalmic Epidemiol. 2009;16:304–410.
47. Yamaoka S, Okada AA, Sugahara M, et al. Clinical features of polypoidal choroidal vasculopathy and visual outcomes in the absence of classic choroidal neovascularization. Ophthalmologica. 2010;224:147–52.

48. Uyama M, Matsubara T, Fukushima I, et al. Idiopathic polypoidal choroidal vasculopathy in Japanese patients. Arch Ophthalmol. 1999;117:1035–42.
49. Cackett P, Wong D, Yeo I. A classification system for polypoidal choroidal vasculopathy. Retina. 2009;29(2):187–91.
50. Chakravarthy U, Evans J, Rosenfeld PJ. Age related macular degeneration. BMJ. 2010;340:c981.
51. Wong TY, Chakravarthy U, Klein R, et al. The natural history and prognosis of neovascular age-related macular degeneration: a systematic review of the literature and meta-analysis. Ophthalmology. 2008;115:116–26.
52. Kawasaki R, Wang JJ, Amirul FM, et al. Is bilateral age-related macular degeneration less common in Asians than Caucasians? Ophthalmic Epidemiol. 2011;18(6):253–8.
53. Age-Related Eye Disease Study Research Group. Risk factors associated with age-related macular degeneration. A case-control study in the age-related eye disease study: Age-Related Eye Disease Study Report Number 3. Ophthalmology. 2000;107(12):2224–32.
54. Kim YT, Kang SW, Chung SE, et al. Development of polypoidal choroidal vasculopathy in unaffected fellow eyes. Br J Ophthalmol. 2012;96:1217–21.
55. Ueta T, Iriyama A, Francis J, et al. Development of typical age-related macular degeneration and polypoidal choroidal vasculopathy in fellow eyes of Japanese patients with exudative age-related macular degeneration. Am J Ophthalmol. 2008;146:96–101.
56. Pauleikhoff D, Barondes MJ, Minassian D, et al. Drusen as risk factors in age-related macular disease. Am J Ophthalmol. 1990;109:38–43.
57. Iwama D, Tsujikawa A, Sasahara M, et al. Polypoidal choroidal vasculopathy with drusen. Jpn J Ophthalmol. 2008;52(2):116–21.
58. Ahuja RM, Downes SM, Stanga PE, et al. Polypoidal choroidal vasculopathy and central serous chorioretinopathy. Ophthalmology. 2001;6:1009–10.
59. Fung AT, Yannuzzi LA, Freund KB. Type 1 (subretinal pigment epithelial) neovascularization in central serous chorioretinopathy masquerading as neovascular age-related macular degeneration. Retina. 2012;32:1829–37.
60. Koizumi H, Yamagishi T, Yamazaki T, et al. Subfoveal choroidal thickness in typical age-related macular degeneration and polypoidal choroidal vasculopathy. Graefes Arch Clin Exp Ophthalmol. 2011;249(8):1123–8.
61. Ueta T, Obata R, Inoue Y, et al. Background comparison of typical age-related macular degeneration and polypoidal choroidal vasculopathy in Japanese patients. Ophthalmology. 2009;116:2400–6.
62. Kikuchi M, Nakamura M, Ishikawa K, et al. Elevated C-reactive protein levels in patients with polypoidal choroidal vasculopathy and patients with neovascular age-related macular degeneration. Ophthalmology. 2007;114:1722–7.
63. Ross RD, Gitter KA, Cohen G, et al. Idiopathic polypoidal choroidal vasculopathy associated with retinal arterial macroaneurysm and hypertensive retinopathy. Retina. 1996;16(2):105–11.
64. Nakashizuka H, Mitsumata M, Okisaka S, et al. Clinicopathologic findings in polypoidal choroidal vasculopathy. Invest Ophthalmol Vis Sci. 2008;49(11):4729–37.
65. MacCumber MW, Dastgheib K, Bressler NM, et al. Clinicopathologic correlation of the multiple recurrent serosanguineous retinal pigment epithelial detachments syndrome. Retina. 1994;14(2):143–52.
66. Spraul CW, Grossniklaus HE, Lang GK. Idiopathic polypoid choroid vasculopathy. Klin Monatsbl Augenheilkd. 1997;210(6):405–6.
67. Okubo A, Sameshima M, Uemura A, et al. Clinicopathological correlation of polypoidal choroidal vasculopathy revealed by ultrastructural study. Br J Ophthalmol. 2002;86(10):1093–8.
68. Kuroiwa S, Tateiwa H, Hisatomi T, et al. Pathological features of surgically excised polypoidal choroidal vasculopathy membranes. Clin Exp Ophthalmol. 2004;32(3):297–302.
69. Matsuoka M, Ogata N, Otsuji T, et al. Expression of pigment epithelium derived factor and vascular endothelial growth factor in choroidal neovascular membranes and polypoidal choroidal vasculopathy. Br J Ophthalmol. 2004;88(6):809–15.
70. Tong JP, Chan WM, Liu DT, et al. Aqueous humor levels of vascular endothelial growth factor and pigment epithelium-derived factor in polypoidal choroidal vasculopathy and choroidal neovascularization. Am J Ophthalmol. 2006;141(3):456–62.
71. Grassi MA, Fingert JH, Scheetz TE, et al. Ethnic variation in AMD-associated complement factor H polymorphism p.Tyr402His. Hum Mutat. 2006;27(9):921–5.
72. Wang D, Zhou J, Hou X, et al. CETP gene may be associated with advanced age-related macular degeneration in the Chinese population. Ophthalmic Genet. 2014;36(4):303–8.
73. Chen H, Liu K, Chen LJ, et al. Genetic associations in polypoidal choroidal vasculopathy: a systematic review and meta-analysis. Mol Vis. 2012;18:816–29.
74. Kuo JZ, Wong TY, Ong FS. Genetic risk, ethnic variations and pharmacogenetic biomarkers in age-related macular degeneration and polypoidal choroidal vasculopathy. Expert Rev Ophthalmol. 2013;8(2):127–40.
75. Miki A, Honda S, Kondo N, et al. The association of age-related maculopathy susceptibility 2 (ARMS2) and complement factor H (CFH) variants with two angiographic subtypes of polypoidal choroidal vasculopathy. Ophthalmic Genet. 2013;34(3):146–50.
76. Tanaka K, Nakayama T, Mori R, et al. Associations of complement factor H (CFH) and age-related maculopathy susceptibility 2 (ARMS2) genotypes with subtypes of polypoidal choroidal vasculopathy. Invest Ophthalmol Vis Sci. 2011;52(10):7441–4.
77. Kawamura A, Yuzawa M, Mori R, et al. Indocyanine green angiographic and optical coherence tomographic findings support classification of polypoidal choroidal vasculopathy into two types. Acta Ophthalmol. 2013;91(6):e474–81.

78. Chung SE, Kang SW, Lee JH, et al. Choroidal thickness in polypoidal choroidal vasculopathy and exudative age-related macular degeneration. Ophthalmology. 2011;118(5):840–5.
79. Chan WM, Lam DS, Lai TY, et al. Photodynamic therapy with verteporfin for symptomatic polypoidal choroidal vasculopathy: one-year results of a prospective case series. Ophthalmology. 2004;111(8):1576–84.
80. Bessho H, Honda S, Imai H, et al. Natural course and funduscopic findings of polypoidal choroidal vasculopathy in a Japanese population over 1 year of follow-up. Retina. 2011;31(8):501–15.
81. Moorthy RS, Lyon AT, Rabb MF, et al. Idiopathic polypoidal choroidal vasculopathy of the macula. Ophthalmology. 1998;105:1380–5.
82. Okubo A, Arimura N, Abematsu N, et al. Predictive signs of benign course of polypoidal choroidal vasculopathy: based upon the long-term observation of non-treated eyes. Acta Ophthalmol. 2010;88(4):e107–14.
83. Uyama M, Wada M, Nagai Y, et al. Polypoidal choroidal vasculopathy: natural history. Am J Ophthalmol. 2002;133(5):639–48.
84. Okubo A, Sameshima M, Sakamoto T. Plasticity of polypoidal lesions in polypoidal choroidal vasculopathy. Graefes Arch Clin Exp Ophthalmol. 2004;242(11):962–5.
85. Lee WK, Kim KS, Kim W, et al. Responses to photodynamic therapy in patients with polypoidal choroidal vasculopathy consisting of polyps resembling grape clusters. Am J Ophthalmol. 2012;154:355–65.
86. Byeon SH, Lew YJ, Lee SC, et al. Clinical features and follow-up results of pulsating polypoidal choroidal vasculopathy treated with photodynamic therapy. Acta Ophthalmol. 2010;88:660–8.
87. Okubo A, Ito M, Sameshima M, et al. Pulsatile blood flow in the polypoidal choroidal vasculopathy. Ophthalmology. 2005;112(8):1436–41.
88. Yuzawa M, Mori R, Kawamura A. The origins of polypoidal choroidal vasculopathy. Br J Ophthalmol. 2005;89:602–7.
89. Okubo A, Hirakawa M, Ito M, et al. Clinical features of early and late stage polypoidal choroidal vasculopathy characterized by lesion size and disease duration. Graefes Arch Clin Exp Ophthalmol. 2008;246:491–9.
90. Tsujikawa A, Ojima Y, Yamashiro K, et al. Association of lesion size and visual prognosis to polypoidal choroidal vasculopathy. Am J Ophthalmol. 2011;151(6):961–72.
91. Tamura H, Tsujikawa A, Otani A, et al. Polypoidal choroidal vasculopathy appearing as classic choroidal neovascularization on fluorescein angiography. Br J Ophthalmol. 2007;91:1152–9.
92. Yannuzzi LA, Sorenson J, Spaide RF, et al. Idiopathic polypoidal choroidal vasculopathy (IPCV). 1990. Retina. 2012;32(Suppl):1–8.
93. Cho M, Barbazetto IA, Freund KB. Refractory neovascular age-related macular degeneration secondary to polypoidal choroidal vasculopathy. Am J Ophthalmol. 2009;148(1):70–8.e71.
94. Hatz K, Prunte C. Polypoidal choroidal vasculopathy in Caucasian patients with presumed neovascular age-related macular degeneration and poor ranibizumab response. Br J Ophthalmol. 2014;98(2):188–94.
95. Matsushita S, Naito T, Takebayashi M, et al. The prognosis of cases with massive subretinal hemorrhage after photodynamic therapy. J Med Investig. 2008;55(3–4):231–5.
96. Windisch R, Windisch BK, Cruess AF. Use of fluorescein and indocyanine green angiography in polypoidal choroidal vasculopathy patients following photodynamic therapy. Can J Ophthalmol. 2008;43(6):678–82.
97. Lee MY, Lee WK, Baek J, et al. Photodynamic therapy versus combination therapy in polypoidal choroidal vasculopathy: changes of aqueous vascular endothelial growth factor. Am J Ophthalmol. 2013;156(2):343–8.
98. Yuzawa M, Mori R, Haruyama M. A study of laser photocoagulation for polypoidal choroidal vasculopathy. Jpn J Ophthalmol. 2003;47(4):379–84.
99. Cheung CM, Yeo I, Li X, et al. Argon laser with and without anti-vascular endothelial growth factor therapy for extrafoveal polypoidal choroidal vasculopathy. Am J Ophthalmol. 2013;155(2):295–304.e291.
100. Gomi F, Ohji M, Sayanagi K, et al. One-year outcomes of photodynamic therapy in age-related macular degeneration and polypoidal choroidal vasculopathy in Japanese patients. Ophthalmology. 2008;115(1):141–6.
101. Honda S, Imai H, Yamashiro K, et al. Comparative assessment of photodynamic therapy for typical age-related macular degeneration and polypoidal choroidal vasculopathy: a multicenter study in Hyogo prefecture, Japan. Ophthalmologica. 2009;223(5):333–8.
102. Akaza E, Mori R, Yuzawa M. Long-term results of photodynamic therapy of polypoidal choroidal vasculopathy. Retina. 2008;28(5):717–22.
103. Akaza E, Yuzawa M, Mori R. Three-year follow-up results of photodynamic therapy for polypoidal choroidal vasculopathy. Jpn J Ophthalmol. 2011;55(1):39–44.
104. Oishi A, Kojima H, Mandai M, et al. Comparison of the effect of ranibizumab and verteporfin for polypoidal choroidal vasculopathy: 12-month LAPTOP study results. Am J Ophthalmol. 2013;156(4):644–51.
105. Hirami Y, Tsujikawa A, Otani A, et al. Hemorrhagic complications after photodynamic therapy for polypoidal choroidal vasculopathy. Retina. 2007;27(3):335–41.
106. Ojima Y, Tsujikawa A, Otani A, et al. Recurrent bleeding after photodynamic therapy in polypoidal choroidal vasculopathy. Am J Ophthalmol. 2006;141(5):958–60.
107. Tsuchihashi T, Mori K, Ueyama K, et al. Five-year results of photodynamic therapy with verteporfin for Japanese patients with neovascular age-

related macular degeneration. Clin Ophthalmol. 2013;7:615–20.
108. Lee WK, Lee PY, Lee SK. Photodynamic therapy for polypoidal choroidal vasculopathy: vaso-occlusive effect on the branching vascular network and origin of recurrence. Jpn J Ophthalmol. 2008;52(2):108–15.
109. Saito M, Iida T, Nagayama D. Photodynamic therapy with verteporfin for age-related macular degeneration or polypoidal choroidal vasculopathy: comparison of the presence of serous retinal pigment epithelial detachment. Br J Ophthalmol. 2008;92(12):1642–7.
110. Wakabayashi T, Gomi F, Sawa M, et al. Marked vascular changes of polypoidal choroidal vasculopathy after photodynamic therapy. Br J Ophthalmol. 2008;92(7):936–40.
111. Dewi NA, Yuzawa M, Tochigi K, et al. Effects of photodynamic therapy on the choriocapillaris and retinal pigment epithelium in the irradiated area. Jpn J Ophthalmol. 2008;52(4):277–81.
112. Wong CW, Cheung CM, Mathur R, et al. Three year results of polypoidal choroidal vasculopathy treated with photodynamic therapy:retrospective study and systematic review. Retina. 2015;35(8):1577–93.
113. Heier JS, Brown DM, Chong V, et al. Intravitreal aflibercept (VEGF trap-eye) in wet age-related macular degeneration. Ophthalmology. 2012;119(12):2537–48.
114. Rosenfeld PJ, Brown DM, Heier JS, et al. Ranibizumab for neovascular age-related macular degeneration. N Engl J Med. 2006;355(14):1419–31.
115. Brown DM, Kaiser PK, Michels M, et al. Ranibizumab versus verteporfin for neovascular age-related macular degeneration. N Engl J Med. 2006;355(14):1432–44.
116. Schmidt-Erfurth U, Kaiser PK, Korobelnik JF, et al. Intravitreal aflibercept injection for neovascular age-related macular degeneration: ninety-six-week results of the VIEW studies. Ophthalmology. 2014;121(1):193–201.
117. Hikichi T, Higuchi M, Matsushita T, et al. Results of 2 years of treatment with as-needed ranibizumab reinjection for polypoidal choroidal vasculopathy. Br J Ophthalmol. 2013;97(5):617–21.
118. Kokame GT, Yeung L, Teramoto K, et al. Polypoidal choroidal vasculopathy exudation and hemorrhage: results of monthly ranibizumab therapy at one year. Ophthalmologica. 2014;231(2):94–102.
119. Mori R, Yuzawa M, Akaza E, et al. Treatment results at 1 year of ranibizumab therapy for polypoidal choroidal vasculopathy in eyes with good visual acuity. Jpn J Ophthalmol. 2013;57(4):365–71.
120. Takahashi K, Ogura Y, Ishibashi T, et al. Treatment guidelines for age-related macular degeneration. Nippon Ganka Gakkai Zasshi. 2012;116(12):1150–5.
121. Gomi F, Sawa M, Sakaguchi H, et al. Efficacy of intravitreal bevacizumab for polypoidal choroidal vasculopathy. Br J Ophthalmol. 2008;92(1):70–3.
122. Wakabayashi T, Gomi F, Sawa M, et al. Intravitreal bevacizumab for exudative branching vascular networks in polypoidal choroidal vasculopathy. Br J Ophthalmol. 2012;96(3):394–9.
123. Ogura Y, VIEW 2 Study Group. Effect of aflibercept on polypoidal choroidal vasculopathy. The results of re-analysis of Japanese patients. Oral presentation at The 53rd Annual Meeting of Japanese Retina and Vitreous Society; 2014 Nov 28–30; Osaka, Japan.
124. Iida T. Efficacy and safety of intravitreal aflibercept in polypoidal choroidal vasculopathy: the PLANET study. Presentation at the 10th Congress of the Asia-Pacific Vitreo-retina Society (APVRS); 2016 Dec 8–10; Bangkok, Thailand.
125. Inoue M, Arakawa A, Yamane S, et al. Short-term efficacy of intravitreal aflibercept in treatment-naive patients with polypoidal choroidal vasculopathy. Retina. 2014;34(11):2178–84.
126. Ijiri S, Sugiyama K. Short-term efficacy of intravitreal aflibercept for patients with treatment-naïve polypoidal choroidal vasculopathy. Graefes Arch Clin Exp Ophthalmol. 2014;253(3):351–7.
127. Yonekawa Y. Aflibercept for the treatment of refractory polypoidal choroidal vasculopathy. Can J Ophthalmol. 2013;48(3):e59–60.
128. Miura M, Iwasaki T, Goto H. Intravitreal aflibercept for polypoidal choroidal vasculopathy after developing ranibizumab tachyphylaxis. Clin Ophthalmol. 2013;7:1591–5.
129. Saito M, Kano M, Itagaki K, et al. Switching to intravitreal aflibercept injection for polypoidal choroidal vasculopathy refractory to ranibizumab. Retina. 2014;34(11):2192–201.
130. Kawashima Y, Oishi A, Tsujikawa A, et al. Effects of aflibercept for ranibizumab-resistant neovascular age-related macular degeneration and polypoidal choroidal vasculopathy. Graefes Arch Clin Exp Ophthalmol. 2015;253(9):1471–7.
131. Gomi F, Sawa M, Wakabayashi T, et al. Efficacy of intravitreal bevacizumab combined with photodynamic therapy for polypoidal choroidal vasculopathy. Am J Ophthalmol. 2010;150(1):48–54.e41.
132. Saito M, Iida T, Kano M, et al. Two-year results of combined intravitreal ranibizumab and photodynamic therapy for polypoidal choroidal vasculopathy. Graefes Arch Clin Exp Ophthalmol. 2013;251(9):2099–110.
133. Kang HM, Koh HJ, Lee CS, et al. Combined photodynamic therapy with intravitreal bevacizumab injections for polypoidal choroidal vasculopathy: long-term visual outcome. Am J Ophthalmol. 2014;157(3):598–606.e591.
134. Koh A. Ranibizumab and vPDT combination therapy versus ranibizumab monotherapy for macular PCV: 12-month results from the EVEREST II study. Presentation at the American Academy of Ophthalmology (AAO) 2016 Annual Meeting; 2016 Oct 14; Chicago, IL, USA; 2016.
135. Hosokawa M, Shiraga F, Yamashita A, et al. Six-month results of intravitreal aflibercept injections for patients with polypoidal choroidal vasculopathy. Br J Ophthalmol. 2015;99(8):1087–91.

136. Oishi A, Tsujikawa A, Yamashiro K, et al. One-year result of aflibercept treatment on age-related macular degeneration and predictive factors for visual outcome. Am J Ophthalmol 2015;159(5):853–60.e851.
137. Kim M, Kim K, Kim DG, et al. Two-year results of photodynamic therapy combined with intravitreal anti-vascular endothelial growth factor for polypoidal choroidal vasculopathy. Ophthalmologica. 2011;226(4):205–13.
138. Nemoto R, Miura M, Iwasaki T, et al. Two-year follow-up of ranibizumab combined with photodynamic therapy for polypoidal choroidal vasculopathy. Clin Ophthalmol. 2012;6:1633–8.
139. Kang HM, Koh HJ. Two-year outcome after combination therapy for polypoidal choroidal vasculopathy: comparison with photodynamic monotherapy and anti-vascular endothelial growth factor monotherapy. Ophthalmologica. 2014;231(2):86–93.
140. Sagong M, Lim S, Chang W. Reduced-fluence photodynamic therapy combined with intravitreal bevacizumab for polypoidal choroidal vasculopathy. Am J Ophthalmol. 2012;153(5):873–82.e872.
141. Sakurai M, Baba T, Kitahashi M, et al. One-year results of intravitreal ranibizumab combined with reduced-fluence photodynamic therapy for polypoidal choroidal vasculopathy. Clin Ophthalmol. 2014;8:235–41.
142. Yamashita A, Shiraga F, Shiragami C, et al. Two-year results of reduced-fluence photodynamic therapy for polypoidal choroidal vasculopathy. Am J Ophthalmol. 2013;155(1):96–102.e101.
143. Yoshida Y, Kohno T, Yamamoto M, et al. Two-year results of reduced-fluence photodynamic therapy combined with intravitreal ranibizumab for typical age-related macular degeneration and polypoidal choroidal vasculopathy. Jpn J Ophthalmol. 2013;57(3):283–93.
144. Eandi CM, Ober MD, Freund KB, et al. Selective photodynamic therapy for neovascular age-related macular degeneration with polypoidal choroidal neovascularization. Retina. 2007;27(7):825–31.
145. Hikichi T, Ohtsuka H, Higuchi M, et al. Factors predictive of visual acuity outcomes 1 year after photodynamic therapy in Japanese patients with polypoidal choroidal vasculopathy. Retina. 2011;31(5):857–65.
146. Jeon S, Lee WK, Kim KS. Adjusted retreatment of polypoidal choroidal vasculopathy after combination therapy: results at 3 years. Retina. 2013;33(6):1193–200.
147. Cheung CM, Wong TY. Ranibizumab and bevacizumab for AMD. N Engl J Med. 2011;365(23):2237, author reply 2237.

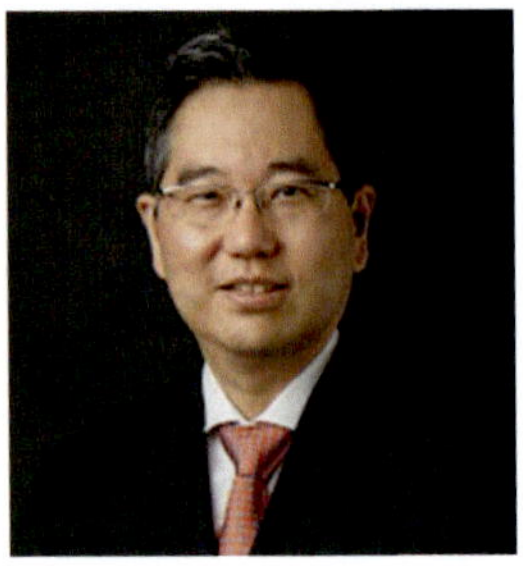

Professor Koh is the Founding Partner and Senior Consultant at the Eye & Retina Surgeons, Camden Medical Centre and Associate Professor at the National University of Singapore. He is the visiting consultant to Singapore National Eye Centre and Tan Tock Seng Hospital. He is the past President of the Singapore Society of Ophthalmology, and a member of the Executive Council of the College of Ophthalmologists. He is the Executive Director of ESASO (European School of Advanced Studies in Ophthalmology) Asia. He was the Secretary-General and Vice President of the 2006 APAO Congress in Singapore and Congress President of the 5th APVRS in 2010. He is an active member of the Macula Society and Club Jules Gonin. He serves on the Executive Council of the Asia Pacific Vitreo Retina Society (APVRS) and was Regional Secretary of the Asia Pacific Academy of Ophthalmology (APAO). He is an active member of EURETINA, American Academy of Ophthalmology, Asia Pacific Academy of Ophthalmology, Vision Academy, and Asia Pacific Vitreoretina Society.

Prof Koh completed Fellowships in Medical Retina at Moorfields Eye Hospital and the Jules Stein Eye Institute. He trained under Professors Alan Bird, Susan Downer, Graham Holder, Bradley Straatsma, and John Heckenlively.

His areas of expertise include degenerative macular disease such as polypoidal choroidal vasculopathy (PCV), choroidal neovascularization, retinal dystrophy, visual electrophysiology, and retinal vascular disease. He is one of the key international opinion leaders in Retina. He was the principal investigator of the EVEREST-1 and EVEREST-2 trials and Chairman of the PCV Roundtable of Experts. He sits on several international advisory boards and steering committees, including Vision Academy Steering Committee and Brolucizumab Global Steering Committee. Prof Koh has published extensively in peer-reviewed journals and ophthalmology textbooks, and lectures in numerous national and international meetings each year.

Choroidal Neovascularization Associated with Rare Entities

19

Pasha Anvari, Masood Naseripour, and Khalil Ghasemi Falavarjani

19.1 Choroidal Nevus

Choroidal nevi are usually found incidentally during routine ophthalmoscopic examination. The prevalence ranges from 4 to 8% in general white population [1, 2] making it the most common benign melanocytic intraocular tumor in adults [3]. Clinically, choroidal nevi appear as flat or slightly elevated, round or oval pigmented gray-brown (and sometimes amelanotic) lesions with well-defined margins. They are located deep to the retina, evenly distributed in all four quadrants of fundus and more common in post-equatorial region [4].

Although mostly asymptomatic, choroidal nevi should be observed for possible malignant transformation [5]. They may result in decreased visual acuity by inducing secondary changes in overlying retinal pigment epithelium (RPE) and retina including RPE atrophy or secondary fibrous metaplasia, pigment epithelial detachments, drusen, and photoreceptor degenerations [4, 6].

Rarely, choroidal nevi may lead to choroidal neovascularization (CNV) with subsequent visual loss, particularly if the fovea is involved. Gass in 1967 [7] was the first to describe the association between choroidal nevus and CNV. In early reports, there was uncertainty regarding this association [8]. Nonetheless, growing evidence suggested that chronic mechanical, inflammatory, or degenerative effects of nevus cells on overlying RPE–Bruch's membrane is presumably responsible for CNV development. The nevus-associated CNV prevalence is estimated to be less than 1% in all choroidal nevi [9]. CNV-complicated choroidal nevi are located in the posterior pole and frequently in the macular area [1, 10, 11]. The reason for this macular predilection remains unclear.

The patients are typically in their sixth decade of life, presenting with blurry vision or metamorphopsia. On examination, subretinal fluid (SRF), lipid exudates, or subretinal hemorrhage, suggestive of presumed CNV is evident at the epicenter or edge of preexisting choroidal nevus. Signs of nevus chronicity including drusen or RPE changes are practically always present. Relatively common age-related macular changes in the same or contralateral eye may lead to an incorrect diagnosis of neovascular age-related macular degeneration (AMD) on cursory examination [12]. In addition, in the case of prominent exuda-

P. Anvari · M. Naseripour
Eye Research Center and Eye Department, Rassoul Akram Hospital, Iran University of Medical Sciences, Tehran, Iran

K. G. Falavarjani (✉)
Eye Research Center and Eye Department, Rassoul Akram Hospital, Iran University of Medical Sciences, Tehran, Iran

Eye Research Center, Rassoul Akram Hospital, Sattarkhan-Niaiesh St, Tehran, Iran

J. Chhablani (ed.), *Choroidal Neovascularization*, https://doi.org/10.1007/978-981-15-2213-0_19

tion from CNV, the underlying choroidal nevus may be overlooked, making the correct diagnosis challenging [13].

Owing to macular predilection of most CNVs complicating nevi, prompt diagnosis of CNV and differentiating from simple nevus, and appropriate treatment is imperative to preserve vision. More to the point is, the onset of symptoms; SRF or increased height of preexisting choroidal nevus may give the wrong impression of malignant transformation to the clinician. In case series of nevus associated CNV by Zografos et al. [10] and Pellegrini et al. [14] suspected choroidal melanoma and choroidal metastasis were the most common initial diagnosis of referred patients. Therefore, an accurate diagnosis may obviate the need for unnecessary work-up or inappropriate treatments.

The diagnosis of choroidal nevus-associated CNV relies on clinical examination and appropriate multimodal imaging. Type 1 CNV, Type 2 CNV, and polypoidal choroidal neovascularization (PCV) [15] have all been described in the context of choroidal nevus with varying incidence. Typical ophthalmoscopic signs of CNV including subretinal hemorrhage, SRF, and exudation may be seen. Fluorescein angiography (FA) and indocyanine green angiography (ICGA) are the standard imaging modalities to demonstrate dye leakage from new vessels. Spectral domain-optical coherence tomography (SD-OCT) is useful by revealing SRF, intraretinal fluid, and PED. In the case of PCV, SD-OCT may show typical features including sharp PED peak, multiple PEDs, and hypo-reflective lumen within hyper-reflective materials [16]. In recent years, optical coherence tomography angiography (OCTA) has gained popularity among ophthalmologists to detect CNV in various ocular pathologies. In a study by Pellegrini et al., OCTA was able to visualize CNV in all 11 cases of nevus associated CNV with "sea fan" or "long filamentous linear vessel" patterns [14]. Major advantages of OCTA to conventional dye-based angiography include its noninvasive nature, rapid acquisition time, and depth-resolved images [17]. Nevertheless, the main drawbacks of this technique are high rates of artifacts [18] and inability to show activity and thus the necessity for treatment.

Generally, the presence of CNV associated with a pigmented choroidal lesion points out to the benign nature of the lesion [19]. Reports describing melanoma-associated CNV are exceedingly rare [20]. However, the wise approach would be to follow these nevi for signs of growth by serial follow-up examinations.

It should be emphasized that choroidal nevus may be associated with overlying subretinal fluid without the evidence of CNV in multimodal imaging evaluation. In the largest analysis of 3422 eyes with choroidal nevus, in 345 (10%) eyes, nevi showed evidence of subretinal fluid. However, these findings indicated the CNV presence only in 20 (0.6%) eyes [9].

Because of the lack of randomized clinical trials, treatment decisions for nevus-associated CNV are mainly guided by small, retrospective case series or reports, and should be tailored to the patient based on clinical findings. Although there are reports of successful management of extrafoveal CNV by conventional argon laser photocoagulation, scar expansion into fovea is a major concern [8].

For subfoveal or juxtafoveal CNV, transpupillary thermotherapy [21] and photodynamic therapy (PDT) [22] have been used with variable results. Some patients may require multiple PDT sessions with subsequent collateral damage to RPE and choriocapillaris [22, 23]. In recent years, with the advent of anti-vascular endothelial growth factors (VEGF), some authors have used intravitreal anti-VEGF injections successfully for the treatment of subfoveal nevus-associated CNV [11, 24, 25]. In a recent report, 73% of eyes with CNV associated with choroidal nevus responded properly to intravitreal bevacizumab injection and a combination of PDT, and bevacizumab led to further regression in unresponsive eyes [26].

In our institution, we manage nevus associated CNV lesions according to the CNV location and patient's symptoms. For the small asymptomatic, extra-macular CNV, we follow the patients closely. If edema or hard exudates are increasing and threatening the fovea, we consider intravitreal injection of anti-VEGF agents, with or without argon laser photocoagulation treatment based on FA findings. For subfoveal or juxtafoveal CNV, we treat the patients by intravitreal anti-VEGF injection. We may consider adjunctive PDT to reduce the frequency of intravitreal injections in selected patients with anti-VEGF resistance or in case of recurrent CNV. An absence of response to anti-VEGF injection should raise a suspicion of malignant lesions [27].

In conclusion, CNV may rarely complicate choroidal nevi in the posterior pole of the fundus. It is recommended to perform appropriate imaging in subjects with choroidal nevi and recent onset of SRF, exudate, or hemorrhage to consider this entity. It is not a harbinger of malignant transformation and could be treated successfully by intravitreal injection of anti-VEGF agents.

19.2 Choroidal Osteoma

Choroidal osteoma (CO) is a rare, benign, intraocular tumor that typically occurs in otherwise healthy young females in their second or third decades of life [28]. Clinically, it appears as a slightly elevated (<2.5 mm) yellow-orange subretinal mass. The tumor is unilateral in 80% of cases and is usually located in the peripapillary or macular area with well-defined, geographic, or scalloped borders [29]. The exact etiology of tumor remained still unclear; however, trauma, congenital, inflammatory, or hormonal theories have been postulated [30–32]. Although patients may initially be asymptomatic or have good visual acuity, the long-term visual prognosis is poor as nearly half of the patients will experience severe vision loss (visual acuity less than 20/200) after 10 years of follow-up [33].

Over the years, the tumor may grow slowly or undergo decalcification. The decalcified portion is characterized by a lighter color (yellow-white) due to retinal pigment epithelium (RPE) depigmentation and increased visibility of underlying choroidal vessels. The tumor decalcification that can occur spontaneously, or following laser treatment is associated with overlying RPE and photoreceptor loss and subsequently can lead to profound vision loss if occurs subfoveally [34].

CNV can complicate CO and is considered a major cause of visual impairment in subjects with CO. In a study by Shields et al. [35] 31% of patients with CO developed CNV by 10 years. Similarly, Aylward et al. [33] reported that 10-year probability for CNV development was 47%.

There is no identified current treatment to induce regression of CO and therapy mainly targets complications. Because the majority of the patients with CO and CNV are relatively young, the burden of visual impairment on quality of life is deemed to be high. This highlights the importance of prompt diagnosis and treatment of CNV.

The pathogenesis of CNV arising from CO is yet to be determined. It has been speculated that thin and degenerated RPE–Bruch's membrane overlying tumor allows growth of abnormal choroidal vessel [35]. The presence of osteoclasts in the surgical specimen obtained from a subject with CO and CNV [36] has raised the possibility that CNV is an extension of tumor vessels. Moreover, inadequate transmural blood supply, high metabolic demand of tumor, and chronic inflammation may result in retinal ischemia and overexpression of VEGF that may contribute to the pathogenesis of CO-associated CNV. Recent reports of choroidal excavation and CNV associated with CO in decalcified cases speculated a common pathogenic pathway for the development of FCE and CNV in choroidal osteoma [37].

Patients commonly present with sudden onset of decreased visual acuity or metamorphopsia. On examination, the tumor along with subretinal hemorrhage (SRH) or subretinal fluid (SRF) is evident. CNV may occur over or at the edge of the tumor and is frequently associated with tumor decalcification and secondary RPE abnormalities. Subretinal pigmentation is usually found around CNV [38]. Cases with CO and CNV occurring at the bottom or slope of choroidal excavation have also been reported [37, 39].

The diagnosis of CO-associated CNV is quite challenging. SRH and tumor surface irregularity are the two strongest predictors of CNV development [35]. However, in subjects with CO, SRH and SRF can occur in the absence of detectable

CNV. Aylward et al. [33] reported that only 22.7% of eyes with CO and serous retinal detachment had concurrent CNV. Similarly, SRH can occur spontaneously or secondary to Valsalva maneuvers rather than from CNV.

FA has been the gold standard for the diagnosis of CNV. Both classic and occult subtypes have been reported, with the predominance of classic components [40]. However, inherent patchy hyperfluorescence of the tumor and RPE abnormalities may either masquerade or obscure leakage from CNV.

OCT is useful in demonstrating SRF, intraretinal fluid (IRF), and subretinal hyper-reflective material. The characteristics of tumor including sponge-like or lattice-like pattern, multiple intralesional horizontal lamellar lines, and intrinsic transparency in addition to a wide range of tumor reflectivity from hypo-to hyperreflectivity are evident, particularly on EDI-OCT. [41]

OCT-angiography is helpful by revealing the neovascular network in the outer retina or choriocapillaris slabs (Fig. 19.1) [42–44]. However, the use of OCT-angiography to diagnose CNV arising from CO has several challenges. First, because of morphologic alterations secondary to tumor, including elevation of the choroidal surface, choriocapillaris compression, RPE, and outer retinal disorganization, automated segmentation will likely result in artifacts; therefore, manual correction of segmentation lines is essential to correctly diagnose CNV in most cases. Second, the distinction of the neovascular network from intrinsic tumor vascularity is crucial. The CNV may appear as a sea fan or tangled network surrounded by a dark halo, in contrast to the fine and thin vascular network of the tumor [44]. Third, the presence of CNV in OCTA images does not necessarily indicate activity and the need for treatment. Despite these limitations, OCTA may be very helpful in differentiating neovascular components from tumor vessels [44].

Various treatment modalities including laser photocoagulation, photodynamic therapy (PDT), transpupillary thermotherapy (TTT) [45], surgical resection [36], and intravitreal injection of anti-VEGF agents have been attempted to manage CNV in patients with CO.

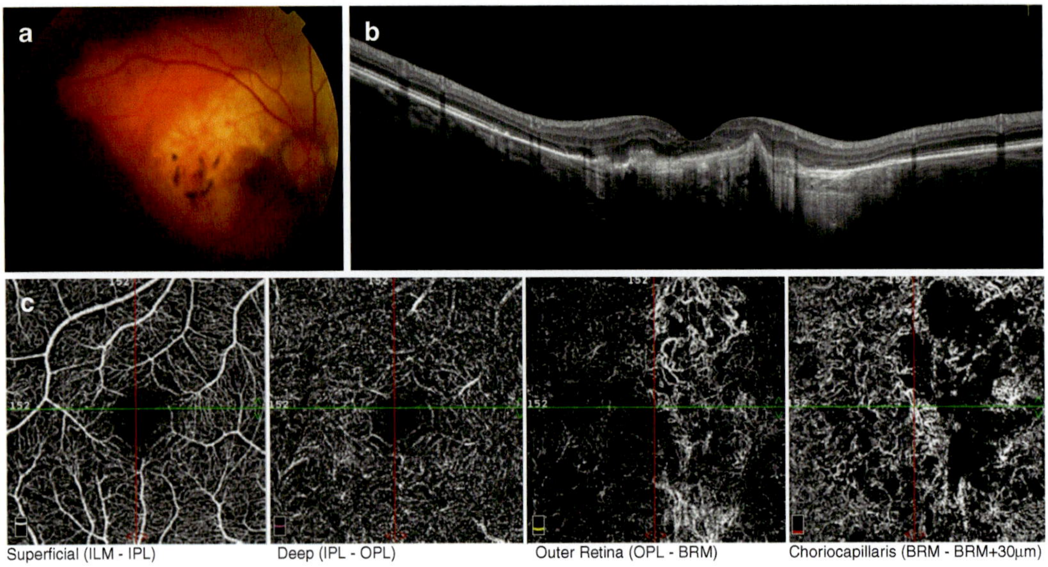

Fig. 19.1 A 33-year-old female with a best-corrected visual acuity of 4/10 OD. (**a**) Color fundus photography showed a large peripapillary choroidal osteoma with macular extension. An area of decalcification and secondary pigmentary alterations was noted. (**b**) OCT revealed subretinal mass with spongy-like appearance and hyper-reflective horizontal lines compatible with choroidal osteoma. No subretinal or intraretinal fluid was evident. (**c**) En-face OCT-angiography demonstrated neovascular tuft in choriocapillaris slab. Given the non-exudative nature of CNV, no treatment was initiated

The results of laser photocoagulation of CNV in CO are disappointing [46]. Insufficient melanin pigmentation of tumor will limit laser absorption. Multiple sessions may be required and the risk of complications including hemorrhage, disciform scar, and decalcification is high. Similarly, surgical resection of CNV in an eye with CO resulted in no significant functional improvement [36].

PDT has been used to successfully treat extrafoveal CNV. However, because of the risk of triggering decalcification or subretinal hemorrhage, it should be used with caution in subfoveal CNV [47]. Half-fluence PDT in combination with intravitreal anti-VEGF injection has also been used (Fig. 19.2) [48]. The rationale of combination therapy is to blunt post-PDT VEGF spike and reduce the number of injections. However, in the absence of a randomized clinical trial, this theoretical benefit is difficult to ascertain.

Several studies have reported the efficacy of intravitreal injection of bevacizumab and ranibizumab in the treatment of CO-associated CNV [49, 50]. In one study, switching to aflibercept was successful in the management of CNV, nonresponder to bevacizumab and ranibizumab [51]. Some authors suggested that the high efficiency of anti-VEGF agents is due to their enhanced penetrance through thin, degenerated RPE–Bruch's membrane complex [52]. The patients may require multiple injections. There might be an increased risk of RPE tear following intravitreal anti-VEGF injections in eyes with CO, as their RPE–Bruch's membrane complex might be brittle [53].

As mentioned earlier, some patients with CO may develop serous retinal detachment in the absence of CNV. The cause of this condition is thought to be chronic RPE decompensation [54]. In most cases, subretinal fluid will resolve spontaneously [55]. The role of anti-VEGF agents in this condition is unclear. However, successful treatment by the use of intravitreal anti-VEGF agents [56, 57] or TTT [58] has been reported.

In summary, CNV is a common, late complication of CO. Multimodal imaging including FA, OCT, and OCTA aids the diagnosis and intravitreal injection of anti-VEGF leads to anatomic improvement in the majority of cases.

19.3 Idiopathic Intracranial Hypertension

Idiopathic intracranial hypertension (IIH), formerly known as pseudotumor cerebri or benign intracranial hypertension, is a syndrome characterized by elevated intracranial pressure (ICP) in the absence of clinical, laboratory, or radiological evidence of intracranial pathology [59]. The typical patient is a young obese woman presenting with headache and transitory blurred vision, commonly lasting less than a minute. Some patients may experience decreased visual acuity at presentation or during the course of the disease. The causes of reduced visual acuity in subjects with IIH can be categorized as optic neuropathy, macular changes, or a combination of both. Optic neuropathy can be progressive and leads to permanent visual loss while macular changes including hard exudate, subretinal fluid, and chorioretinal folds are largely reversible by reducing ICP [60]. Rarely, peripapillary CNV can cause blurred vision.

CNVs complicating IIH are rare. Less than 30 cases have been reported in the literature. The prevalence of CNV in IIH has been estimated to be 0.53% [61]. Although the exact pathogenesis remained unclear, Morse et al. [62] speculated that the pressure deformity of Bruch's membrane's border caused by severe disc edema leads to discontinuity of chorioretinal layers. This anatomical dehiscence coupled with local hypoxia induced by axonal swelling may result in CNV development.

In some cases, IIH-associated CNV was the presenting feature of IIH [63]. Although bilateral cases have been reported, classically, the patient presents with sudden onset of blurry vision in one eye. Previous history of headaches might exist. On examination, features of papilledema including bilateral blurred disc margin and hyperemia are evident. On the affected side, subretinal hemorrhage, hard exudates, and edema suggestive of CNV are present. The peripapillary CNV membrane itself might be obscured by severe disc edema and becomes more clinically visible after the decrease of edema following ICP reduction.

The clinical diagnosis of IIH-associated CNV is usually straightforward and is confirmed by appropriate retinal imaging. FA reveals hyperfluorescence secondary to CNV leakage, dispro-

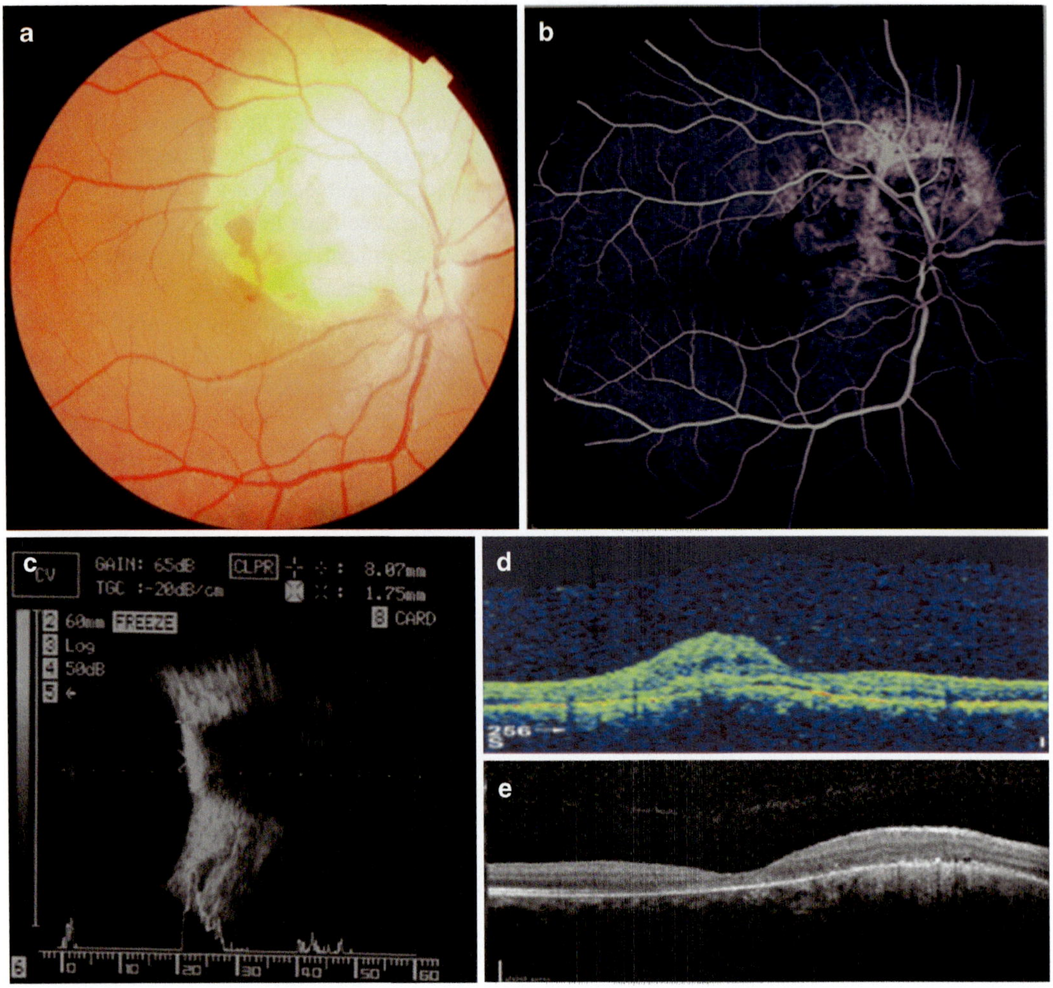

Fig. 19.2 A 25-year-old woman presented with sudden onset of blurry vision in her right eye (OD). Best-corrected visual acuity (BCVA) was 3/10 OD. (**a**) Color fundus photography showed a large yellow-orange peripapillary lesion, deep to retina with extension to macula. Subretinal hemorrhage is visible. (**b**) Fluorescein angiography revealed hypofluorescent area due to blockage of subretinal hemorrhage; diffuse patchy hyperfluorescence secondary to tumor and focal hyperfluorescence due to leakage of choroidal neovascularization. (**c**) B-scan demonstrated hyper-echoic lesion with posterior shadowing, compatible with choroidal osteoma (CO). (**d**) OCT shows subretinal and intraretinal fluid. (**e**) Three months post PDT, and IVB OCT depicted complete regression of fluid and BCVA improved to 8/10

portionate to the disc edema. In addition, disc leakage due to papilledema is evident in the contralateral eye. OCT is useful in demonstrating SRF and intraretinal cystoid edema. Moreover, OCT is an invaluable tool to evaluate the extent of foveal involvement and to monitor treatment response in serial examination. It is noteworthy to mention that, although hard exudates, SRF, and retinal hemorrhages can be found in cases of severe papilledema, subretinal hemorrhage is highly suggestive for CNV.

Differential diagnosis of peripapillary CNV includes neovascular age-related macular degeneration, angioid streaks, excavated disc anomalies, choroidal osteoma, and inflammatory retinochoroidopathies [64]. These conditions can be differentiated by careful examination of the fellow eye and features specific to each entity.

Neurology consults for neuroimaging, measuring CSF opening pressure and composition are warranted in newly diagnosed subjects.

The course of IIH-associated CNV is highly variable. Although some authors reported spontaneous resolution following ICP reduction [65], others described stable or progressive course [66].

Various treatment modalities including surgical resection [67], argon laser photocoagulation [61], photodynamic therapy [61], and intravitreal injection of anti-VEGFs have been used. Surgical resection of the CNV membrane has been disappointing and resulted in choriocapillaris atrophy [67]. Argon laser photocoagulation poses the risk of damage to papillomacular bundle [68]. Recently, several case reports of successful management of IIH-associated CNV by intravitreal anti-VEGFs have been published [69–72]. Some patients may require multiple injections to achieve complete resolution of macular edema; however, the long-term outcomes are promising.

In conclusion, peripapillary CNV may rarely occur in subjects with IIH. It should be considered in any patient with bilateral disc swelling and in the presence of subretinal hemorrhage. Measures to reduce ICP (medically or surgically) and intravitreal injection of anti-VEGF are recommended.

19.4 Laser-Induced CNV

Optical radiations in the visible and near-infrared spectrum of light (380–1400 nm) can pass through ocular media and focus on the retina [73]. Lasers are monochromatic, coherent, unidirectional sources of light with wide applications in medicine, industry, science, and military.

The photochemical, thermal, and mechanical effects of laser may lead to retinal damages. The energy level, pulse duration, and the target location of the beam incidence are among the laser-related factors that determine the severity of retinal injury [73].

19.4.1 Choroidal Neovascularization Secondary to Accidental Laser Exposure

19.4.1.1 Handheld Laser Pointers

Laser pointers are ubiquitous devices used in classrooms and lecture halls to facilitate presentations. Laser pointers are typically red (670 nm wavelength) or green (532 nm wavelength) diode lasers with maximum power output less than 5 mw (class 2 or 3a, according to American National Standard for Safe Use of Lasers classification [74]), and thus generally considered safe during an accidental momentarily eye exposure [75]. However, the incidence of eye injuries secondary to laser pointers appears to be increasing [76]. The reasons behind this rise are considered to be public availability of high-powered lasers (class 3b or 4) with a very similar appearance to low-powered lasers [77] and mislabeling of the actual maximum power of lasers. These devices are perceived as fascinating toys by children that are especially at risk for accidental laser pointer injuries. The normal defensive reaction of adults to laser beam (i.e., blinking and aversion) that limits the exposure to less than 0.25 seconds is probably less prominent in children as they may not fully appreciate the serious hazards of laser eye injuries.

Various retinal pathologies including macular hole, subhyaloid hemorrhage, sub-internal limiting membrane (sub-ILM) hemorrhage and outer retinal disruption following laser pointer injury have been described [78, 79]. However, reports of laser pointer induced CNV are sporadic [80]. Fujinami et al. [81] reported on an intellectually disabled child who suffered from CNV following presumably frequent and repeated exposure to a laser pointer as a toy. Xu et al. [82] described CNV development in a 12-year-old boy after staring into a laser pointer beam for about 15 seconds. His condition was successfully managed by a single injection of intravitreal bevacizumab.

The beneficial role of corticosteroids in the acute stage of laser-induced maculopathy is not well-established. As there is specific treatment for CNV, the correct diagnosis of this rare complication is important. In this regard, utilizing FA and OCT-angiography can be advantageous by demonstrating leakage and neovascular network, respectively. Clear visualization of neovascular membrane by OCT-angiography may obviate the need for performing invasive, time-consuming FA that is particularly a challenge among pediatric age populations. Figure 19.3 shows the utility of the OCTA imaging for

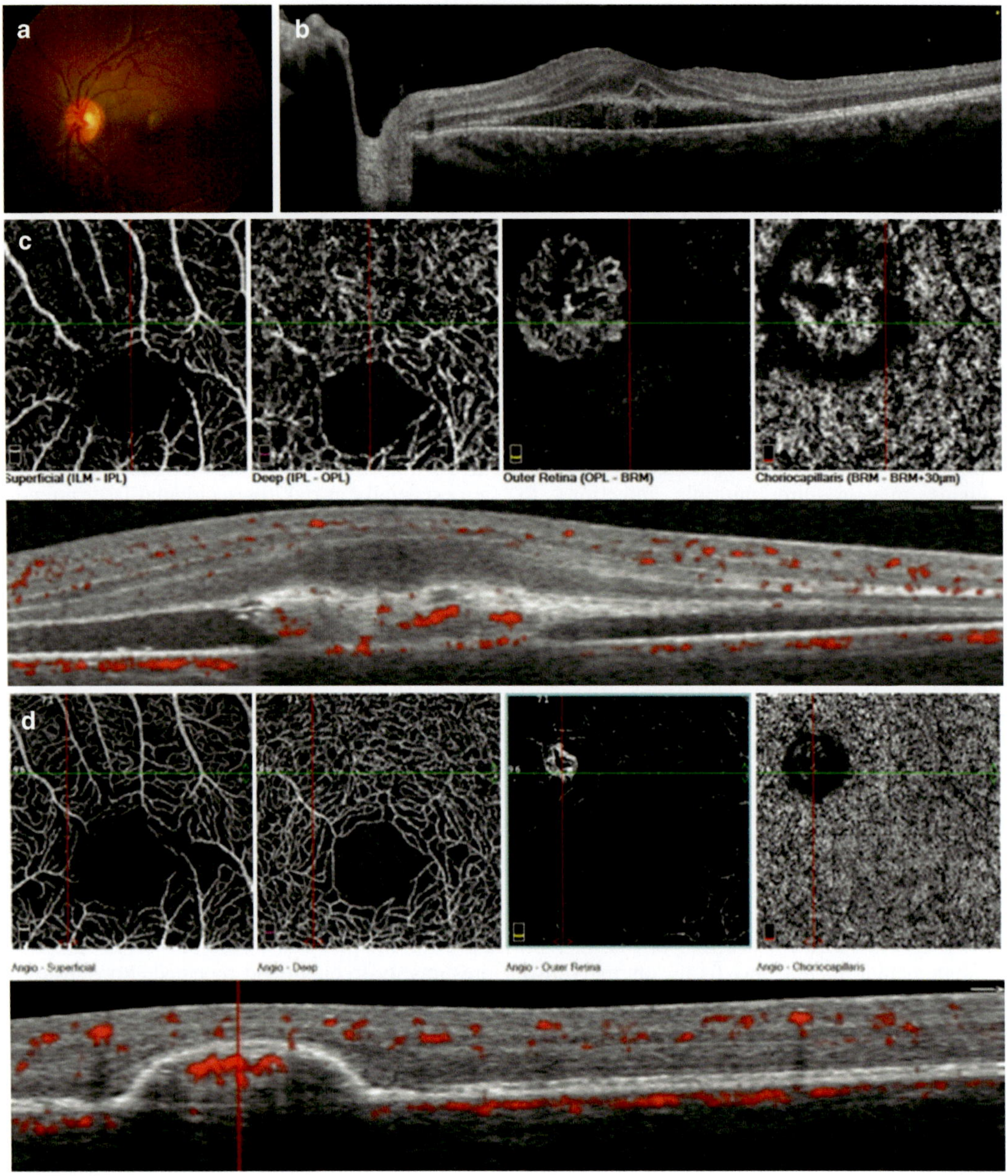

Fig. 19.3 An 8-year-old girl presented with blurry vision in her left eye. Three weeks earlier, she had starred into a green laser pointer for few seconds at a distance of about 1 meter. The laser pointer notification on the device showed a Class III laser production with a maximum output power of less than 1000 mW and a wavelength of 523 nm (Changchun Realpoo Photoelectric CO., Ltd., China). Her best-corrected visual acuity (BCVA) was 20/20 OD and counting fingers OS. (**a**) On funduscopic examination of the left eye, an elevated yellowish lesion in fovea with subretinal hemorrhage and surrounding subretinal fluid was detected. (**b**) Spectral-domain OCT revealed increased retinal thickness, subretinal hyperreflective material (SHRM), and subretinal fluid (SRF) (**c**) Macular OCTA (XR Avanti, Optovue Inc., Fremont CA, USA) demonstrated a neovascular tuft in the outer retinal slab. (**d**) She was treated with a single intravitreal injection of bevacizumab. The size of the neovascular membrane reduced significantly and SRF and SHRM resolved in OCT at 1-month follow-up. Her vision improved to 20/20 and no recurrence was detected until last visit, 5 months after injection

detecting CNV in a patient with accidental laser injury. The prognosis after intravitreal anti-VEGF therapy is generally favorable if patients are treated properly.

19.4.1.2 Other Laser Types

Neodymium:yttrium–aluminum–garnet (Nd:YAG) laser has been associated with CNV development in a physicist from an accidental exposure at work [83]. In addition, CNV development has been reported in a civilian person who unintentionally looked into the laser beam of military range finder [84, 85] and in a dermatologist who suffered CNV following the use of Q-switched Nd:YAG laser while treating a depressed skin scar [86].

Using Alexandrite laser (750 nm) for hair removal has been reported to cause CNV following momentarily accidental exposure in an aesthetician [87].

19.4.2 Choroidal Neovascularization Secondary to Therapeutic Lasers

19.4.2.1 Central Serous Chorioretinopathy

Central serous chorioretinopathy (CSCR) is a major cause of vision loss that affects young and middle-aged men characterized by idiopathic serous neurosensory detachment [88]. CNV can develop during the natural course of the disease or rarely as a complication of laser therapy. The incidence of CSCR-associated CNV varies from 2 to 9% depending on the age and length of follow-up [89, 90].

CNV development has been observed following focal laser photocoagulation [91] or PDT [92–94] in CSCR patients. The underlying RPE and choroidal circulation abnormality may predispose CSCR patients to laser-induced CNV. Thermal laser photocoagulation may lead to Bruch's membrane (BM) defect; however, clinically evident BM defect is usually absent. It is suggested that even the weakening of BM in susceptible individuals might contribute to CNV occurrence [95]. PDT may induce choriocapillaris occlusion, choroidal ischemia, and thus VEGF overexpression. Noteworthy, all reported cases of CNV secondary to PDT occurred after full-fluence PDT rather than half-fluence PDT. Reduced-setting PDT seems to be a safer alternative to conventional PDT.

The time interval between laser and CNV development ranges from 3 weeks to 10 years [95]. Careful assessment of pretreatment images is essential, as preexisting CNV may confound the diagnosis of laser-associated CNV in CSCR patients [96].

The visual prognosis of CNV secondary to focal laser photocoagulation in CSCR is generally favorable because focal laser is usually used to treat extrafoveal RPE leaks, away from the central fovea.

Various treatment modalities including observation, surgical resection, additional laser photocoagulation, and additional PDT have been undertaken to manage laser-induced CNV in CSCR. Recently, Chhablani et al. [95] showed the efficacy and safety of intravitreal injections of anti-VEGF agents for the treatment of laser-associated CNV in CSCR. Notably, PDT-associated CNVs were more resistant to anti-VEGF injections compared to those secondary to thermal laser photocoagulations.

19.4.2.2 Diabetic Macular Edema

Intravitreal injections of anti-VEGF agents have largely supplanted focal/grid laser as the standard of care for patients with center-involving DME, due to their superior anatomical and functional outcome. However, focal/grid laser still holds its role in certain clinical situations including adjunctive treatment, focal DME associated with microaneurysms, or in patients with good visual acuity.

There are several reports of CNV development following macular photocoagulation in DME [97–99]. Intense laser burns, repeated application of laser over the same spot, and smaller spot size appear to be associated with CNV development by damaging to

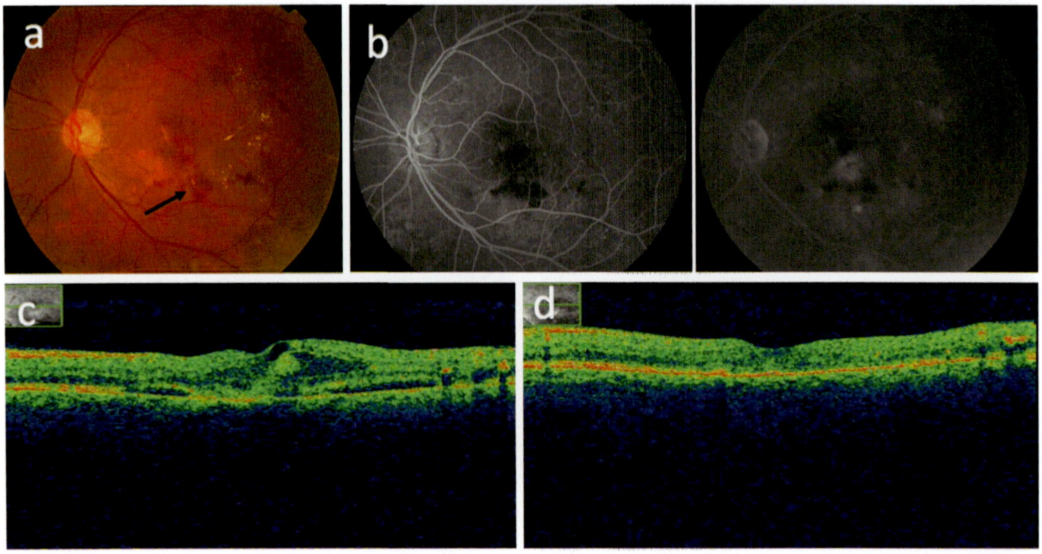

Fig. 19.4 A 54-year-old man with type 2 diabetes presented with acute visual loss in the left eye (OS). There was a history of previous macular photocoagulation a few years ago. Best-corrected visual acuity (BCVA) was counting fingers at 3 meters in OS. (**a**) Hard exudates, microaneurysms, and intraretinal hemorrhages corresponding to non-proliferative diabetic retinopathy along with an area of subretinal hemorrhage (arrow) were evident. (**b**) Fluorescein angiography revealed hypofluorescence due to blockage, compatible to subretinal hemorrhage and an area of hyperfluorescence related to choroidal neovascularization. (**c**) Optical coherence tomography (OCT) demonstrated increased macular thickness, intraretinal fluid, subretinal fluid, and subretinal hyperreflective material. (**d**) OCT showed complete resolution of subretinal and intraretinal fluids after intravitreal injections of bevacizumab. BCVA improved to 2/10

BM. Additionally, underlying ischemia and elevated VEGF levels in diabetic patients may contribute to the pathogenesis of laser-associated CNV [100]. Furthermore, older subjects with associated alterations in RPE and BM are particularly at risk for this complication [101].

The median interval between macular photocoagulation and CNV occurrence is 8 weeks [97, 98]. Thus, timely follow-up examination is essential for prompt diagnosis and treatment of this rare complication to preserve vision. Intravitreal injection of anti-VEGF agents leads to resolution of fluid and improvement in vision (Fig. 19.4).

19.4.2.3 Other Retinal Disorders

CNV may also occur as a complication of laser therapy in various retinal disorders including retinal vein occlusion [102], sickle cell retinopathy [103], Eales disease [104], and age-related macular degeneration [105].

19.5 Trauma

Ocular trauma can lead to temporary or permanent visual impairment through several mechanisms. The main causes of visual decline are hyphema, dislocated lens, vitreous or retinal hemorrhage, commotio retinae, and optic neuropathy. Other causes of decreased vision following trauma include retinal detachment, glaucoma secondary to angle recession, or infrequently CNV. Blunt trauma is the main cause of posttraumatic CNV; however, CNV has been reported after penetrating trauma and alkali burn [106]. In addition, CNV associated with accidental laser burns was discussed in a separate section.

Following blunt trauma, choroidal rupture can occur at the site of impact, known as direct choroidal rupture, or more frequently at the opposite site (counter-coup), which is classified as indirect choroidal rupture (ICR) [107].

Direct choroidal rupture typically occurs anteriorly, parallel to the limbus, and is associated with retinal detachment rather than CNV.

Bruch's membrane (BM) has a lower tensile strength, compared to the elastic retina or rigid sclera. Thus, during blunt trauma, anteroposterior compression and equatorial expansion of the globe creates a shearing force that may cause a break in BM, RPE, and choriocapillaris, resulting in ICR [108].

ICR can be present in 5% of eyes with blunt ocular injuries [109, 110]. Clinically, they appear as yellow-white crescentic or curvilinear streaks, concentric to optic disc. ICRs are commonly located temporal to disc. In acute stage, intraretinal or subretinal hemorrhage can be found alongside them. Over weeks, with resolution of hemorrhage and edema, the white streak with hyperpigmented edges (due to RPE hyperplasia) remains [111].

The incidence of choroidal rupture-associated CNV after blunt injury varies greatly according to different studies [110, 112, 113]. Less than 5% to up to 30% incidence rates have been reported. Eyes with angioid streaks are at special risk for developing CNV after minor trauma. Choroidal ruptures are essential but insufficient for CNV development following ocular injury. It is not clear why some choroidal ruptures are complicated by CNV whereas others remain stable. Older age, macular locations of ruptures, and long ruptures have been identified as predisposing factors for CNV development [114, 115]. A diverse set of interrelated factors contributes to pathogenesis of CNV secondary to choroidal ruptures. Loss of barrier function of BM, loss of RPE and its inhibitory actions against neovascularization, VEGF overexpression caused by trauma-related inflammation, or release of elastin-derived peptides from disrupted BM [116] have been proposed as mechanistic links between trauma and CNV.

Patients usually present with sudden onset of decreased vision following a period of stable visual acuity. The time interval between trauma and CNV development varies from few weeks to several years [110]. However, the majority of patients (nearly 80%) present within 1 year of ocular injury with a median of 5–6 months [117].

The diagnosis of rupture associated with CNV is quite straightforward. On examination, subretinal hemorrhage or subretinal fluid is evident along choroidal rupture. Subretinal hemorrhage may also be present early in the course of trauma, without evidence of neovascularization. FA is useful by showing leakage from CNV network. OCT reveals SRF, IRF, and hyper-reflective subretinal material. Recently, OCT-angiography has been found useful in demonstrating neovascular tuft within choroidal rupture [118, 119]. Care should be taken not to mistake projection artifacts from normal retinal or choroidal vessels with neovascularization.

Various treatment modalities including observation, laser photocoagulation [120], surgical resection [121], and PDT [122] have been attempted to manage CNV complicating choroidal rupture. Recently, several studies [113, 117, 123–126] have reported the efficacy of intravitreal anti-VEGF injection in the treatment of choroidal rupture-associated CNV in adults and children. Remarkably, most patients required only one or few injections and no case of recurrence has been reported. This good prognosis is attributed to the local nature of the disease entity and the young age of patients with remaining healthy RPE.

Penetrating Injury

Reports describing CNV development after penetrating injury are rare. Chen et al. [127] illustrated a case with CNV, developed within months following primary repair and vitrectomy for open globe injury and intraocular foreign body. In another report [128], CNV occurred at the site of retinal perforation, 2 months after globe penetration during retrobulbar anesthesia. Both cases were managed successfully by the use of anti-VEGF intravitreal injections.

In conclusion, CNV secondary to trauma is a major cause of delayed onset visual loss in subjects with a history of trauma and choroidal ruptures. Patients with older age, choroidal rupture in macula, and long ruptures are particularly at risk and should be followed regularly, especially within the first year of trauma. Considering the efficacy and safety of intravitreal anti-VEGF injection, it appears to be the best therapeutic approach.

19.6 Coloboma

Abnormal closure of embryonic fissure during 5–7 weeks of gestation may lead to coloboma of optic nerve, retina, choroid, ciliary body, and iris. These ocular anomalies may occur in isolation or together, depending on the extent of abnormality [129]. Moreover, coloboma may be a part of systemic diseases such as CHARGE syndrome [130] (Coloboma, Heart defects, Atresia of nasal choanae, Retardation of growth, Genitourinary abnormalities, and Ear abnormalities).

Visual acuity varies and is primarily affected by the extent of foveal and papillomacular bundle involvement. Apart from amblyopia management in the affected children, there is no current therapy for coloboma. However, several complications including early cataract [131], retinal detachment [132], and choroidal neovascularization may arise in the course of the disease that needs to be identified and treated promptly to preserve vision.

CNVs complicating optic nerve coloboma (ONC) or retinochoroidal coloboma (RCC) are rare and our knowledge is limited to the case reports and small case series.

As practically all coloboma associated CNVs develop at the margin of coloboma [133], the pathogenesis of this entity is probably related to anatomical alterations at the margin. Histopathologic study of choroidal coloboma has demonstrated discontinuity or disruption of Bruch's membrane (BM) and RPE at the edge of coloboma [131]. Loss of barrier function of BM at the margin of coloboma may permit the invasion of choroidal vessels into the subretinal space and CNV development. In addition, the occurrence of CNVs at the temporal edge of coloboma, in close relation to the fovea, has led some authors to hypothesize the possible role of foveal angiogenic signaling in the pathogenesis of coloboma-associated CNV [134].

CNV can complicate coloboma at any age. A wide range from 10.5 months to 70 years old has been reported [133, 135]. Preverbal children may present with strabismus. Older patients commonly present with recent-onset metamorphopsia or reduced visual acuity.

On examination, the coloboma may involve the optic nerve head, macula, or iris. RCC typically occurs inferonasally. Subretinal grayish-green mass, subretinal hemorrhage, SRF, and lipid exudates at the margin of coloboma are suggestive of CNV development. Care must be taken to differentiate CNV membrane from choroidal thickening and RPE hyperplasia that typically develops at the coloboma margin [134]. The diagnosis can be confirmed by FA that shows leakage from the neovascular membrane. OCT is useful by demonstrating SRF, intraretinal fluid, and subretinal hyper-reflective material, and in monitoring treatment response. It is noteworthy to mention that retinoschisis and serous retinal detachment can occur in subjects with optic nerve coloboma in the absence of CNV [136].

Several treatment modalities including observation [135, 137–139], laser photocoagulation [130, 140–144], PDT alone [145] or in combination with intravitreal anti-VEGF injection, [146] intravitreal anti-VEGF injection monotherapy [147, 148] and surgical resection [149] have been used in coloboma-associated CNV. In the absence of a randomized controlled trial (which may not be feasible, given the rarity of this entity), it is not possible to recommend the best treatment option with certainty. However, intravitreal anti-VEGF injections are thought to be the first treatment option, especially in subfoveal or juxtafoveal CNVs where laser photocoagulation will likely result in permanent collateral damage.

Prophylactic barrier laser around the margin of coloboma might reduce the risk of retinal detachment [150]. Gupta and colleagues [137] suggested that chorioretinal adhesion induced by laser photocoagulation at the margin of coloboma might prevent the growth of choroidal vessels and CNV development; however, the efficacy of this approach is not clear.

In summary, CNV can rarely complicate optic nerve or retinochoroidal coloboma. Regular examination, particularly in children might be helpful in the timely diagnosis and treatment of this entity.

Subjects with coloboma should be instructed to seek ophthalmologic examination upon occurrence of sudden onset metamorphopsia, decreased visual acuity, floaters, or flashing. Intravitreal anti-VEGF injections appear to be safe and efficient in the treatment of coloboma-associated CNV.

Key Learning Points

- Nevus-associated CNV should be included in the differential diagnosis of any pigmented choroidal lesion with associated subretinal fluid, subretinal hemorrhage, or exudates.
- CNV is a common, late complication of choroidal osteoma and is a major cause of visual impairment.
- CNV may rarely complicate idiopathic intracranial hypertension.
- To reduce the risk of MPC-induced CNV, do not strive to intensely blanch microaneurysms, and avoid repeated laser application over the same spot.
- High-powered handheld laser pointers are not playthings as they may result in retinal injuries including CNV.
- Subjects with traumatic choroidal rupture in macula should be followed regularly, particularly during the first year after trauma to detect early signs of CNV development.
- Patients with retinochoroidal coloboma should be instructed to seek ophthalmologic examination upon the occurrence of sudden onset of metamorphopsia, and decreased visual acuity, to detect possible CNV.

Competing Interest Statement None of the authors has any financial interest in the subject matter of this chapter.

References

1. Callanan DG, Lewis ML, Byrne SF, Gass JD. Choroidal neovascularization associated with choroidal nevi. Arch Ophthalmol (Chicago, Ill 1960) [Internet]. 1993 Jun;111(6):789–94. Available from: http://www.ncbi.nlm.nih.gov/pubmed/7685589.
2. Sumich P, Mitchell P, Wang JJ. Choroidal nevi in a white population: the Blue Mountains Eye Study. Arch Ophthalmol (Chicago, Ill 1960) [Internet]. 1998 May;116(5):645–50. Available from: http://www.ncbi.nlm.nih.gov/pubmed/9596501.
3. Shields JA, Shields CL. Intraocular tumors: a text and atlas. Philadelphia: W.B. Saunders Company; 1992. p. 85–100.
4. Shields CL, Furuta M, Mashayekhi A, Berman EL, Zahler JD, Hoberman DM, et al. Clinical spectrum of choroidal nevi based on age at presentation in 3422 consecutive eyes. Ophthalmology [Internet]. 2008 Mar;115(3):546–552.e2. Available from: http://www.ncbi.nlm.nih.gov/pubmed/18067966.
5. Shields CL, Furuta M, Berman EL, Zahler JD, Hoberman DM, Dinh DH, et al. Choroidal nevus transformation into melanoma: analysis of 2514 consecutive cases. Arch Ophthalmol (Chicago, Ill 1960) [Internet]. 2009 Aug;127(8):981–7. Available from: http://www.ncbi.nlm.nih.gov/pubmed/19667334.
6. Gonder JR, Augsburger JJ, McCarthy EF, Shields JA. Visual loss associated with choroidal nevi. Ophthalmology [Internet]. 1982 Aug;89(8):961–5. Available from: http://www.ncbi.nlm.nih.gov/pubmed/6182515.
7. Gass JD. Pathogenesis of disciform detachment of the neuroepithelium. Am J Ophthalmol [Internet]. 1967 Mar;63(3):Suppl:1–139. Available from: http://www.ncbi.nlm.nih.gov/pubmed/6019308.
8. Waltman DD, Gitter KA, Yannuzzi L, Schatz H. Choroidal neovascularization associated with choroidal nevi. Am J Ophthalmol [Internet]. 1978 May;85(5 Pt 1):704–10. Available from: http://www.ncbi.nlm.nih.gov/pubmed/566035.
9. Shields CL, Furuta M, Mashayekhi A, Berman EL, Zahler JD, Hoberman DM, et al. Visual acuity in 3422 consecutive eyes with choroidal nevus. Arch Ophthalmol (Chicago, Ill 1960) [Internet]. 2007 Nov;125(11):1501–7. Available from: http://www.ncbi.nlm.nih.gov/pubmed/17998511.
10. Zografos L, Mantel I, Schalenbourg A. Subretinal choroidal neovascularization associated with choroidal nevus. Eur J Ophthalmol [Internet]. 14(2):123–31. Available from: http://www.ncbi.nlm.nih.gov/pubmed/15134109.
11. Chiang A, Bianciotto C, Maguire JI, Park CH, Baker PS, Shields JA, et al. Intravitreal bevacizumab for choroidal neovascularization associated with choroidal nevus. Retina [Internet]. 2012 Jan;32(1):60–7. Available from: http://www.ncbi.nlm.nih.gov/pubmed/21886019.
12. Namavari A, Zheng F, Motulsky EH, de Oliveira Dias JR, Gregori G, Rosenfeld PJ. Swept-Source OCT Angiography identifies Choroidal neovascularization arising from a Choroidal nevus. Ophthalmic Surg lasers imaging Retina [Internet]. 2018;49(5):360–3. Available from: http://www.ncbi.nlm.nih.gov/pubmed/29772047.
13. Tuncer S, Tugal-Tutkun I. Choroidal neovascularization secondary to choroidal nevus simulating an inflammatory lesion. Indian J Ophthalmol [Internet]. 2013 Jun;61(6):305–6. Available from: http://www.ncbi.nlm.nih.gov/pubmed/23571241.
14. Pellegrini M, Corvi F, Say EAT, Shields CL, Staurenghi G. Optical coherence tomography angi-

ography features of choroidal neovascularization associated with choroidal nevus. Retina [Internet]. 2018;38(7):1338–46. Available from: http://www.ncbi.nlm.nih.gov/pubmed/28570484.
15. Pascual-Camps I, López-Corell PM, Andreu-Fenoll M, Gallego-Pinazo R. Polypoidal choroidopathy associated with choroidal nevus. Indian J Ophthalmol [Internet]. 2017;65(11):1213–4. Available from: http://www.ncbi.nlm.nih.gov/pubmed/29133655.
16. De Salvo G, Vaz-Pereira S, Sehmi KS, Andrews RM, Sagoo MS. Spectral-domain optical coherence tomography of Polypoidal Choroidal vasculopathy associated with benign Choroidal nevus. Ophthalmic Surg lasers imaging Retina [Internet]. 46(10):1062–4. Available from: http://www.ncbi.nlm.nih.gov/pubmed/26599253.
17. Falavarjani KG, Sarraf D. Optical coherence tomography angiography of the retina and choroid; current applications and future directions. J Curr Ophthalmol. 2017;29(1):1–4.
18. Ghasemi Falavarjani K, Al-Sheikh M, Akil H, Sadda SR. Image artefacts in swept-source optical coherence tomography angiography. Br J Ophthalmol [Internet]. 2017 May [cited 2017 Jul 13];101(5):564–8. Available from: http://www.ncbi.nlm.nih.gov/pubmed/27439739.
19. Gass JD. Problems in the differential diagnosis of choroidal nevi and malignant melanomas. The XXXIII Edward Jackson Memorial Lecture. Am J Ophthalmol [Internet]. 1977 Mar;83(3):299–323. Available from: http://www.ncbi.nlm.nih.gov/pubmed/848534.
20. Lubin JR, Gragoudas ES, Albert DM. Choroidal neovascularization associated with malignant melanoma: a case report. Acta Ophthalmol [Internet]. 1982 Jun;60(3):412–8. Available from: http://www.ncbi.nlm.nih.gov/pubmed/6182734.
21. Parodi MB. Transpupillary thermotherapy for subfoveal choroidal neovascularization associated with choroidal nevus. Am J Ophthalmol [Internet]. 2004 Dec;138(6):1074–5. Available from: http://www.ncbi.nlm.nih.gov/pubmed/15629316.
22. Parodi MB, Boscia F, Piermarocchi S, Ferrari TM, Furino C, Sborgia C. Variable outcome of photodynamic therapy for choroidal neovascularization associated with choroidal nevus. Retina [Internet]. 2005 Jun;25(4):438–42. Available from: http://www.ncbi.nlm.nih.gov/pubmed/15933589.
23. Stanescu D, Wattenberg S, Cohen SY. Photodynamic therapy for choroidal neovascularization secondary to choroidal nevus. Am J Ophthalmol [Internet]. 2003 Sep;136(3):575–6. Available from: https://linkinghub.elsevier.com/retrieve/pii/S0002939403003210.
24. Cavalcante ML, Villegas VM, Gold AS, Cavalcante LL, Lonngi M, Shah N V, et al. Treatment of vascular activity secondary to atypical choroidal nevus using intravitreal bevacizumab. Clin Ophthalmol [Internet]. 2014;8:1377–82. Available from: http://www.ncbi.nlm.nih.gov/pubmed/25092961.
25. Papastefanou VP, Nogueira V, Hay G, Andrews RM, Harris M, Cohen VML, et al. Choroidal naevi complicated by choroidal neovascular membrane and outer retinal tubulation. Br J Ophthalmol [Internet]. 2013 Aug;97(8):1014–9. Available from: http://www.ncbi.nlm.nih.gov/pubmed/23686326.
26. Munie MT, Demirci H. Management of Choroidal Neovascular Membranes Associated with Choroidal Nevi. Ophthalmol Retin [Internet]. 2018 Jan;2(1):53–8. Available from: http://www.ncbi.nlm.nih.gov/pubmed/31047303.
27. Lee J, Kwon HJ, Kim M, Lee CS, Lee SC. Treatment response to intravitreal bevacizumab in small pigmented choroidal lesions with subretinal fluid. BMC Ophthalmol [Internet]. 2019 May 3;19(1):103. Available from: http://www.ncbi.nlm.nih.gov/pubmed/31053116.
28. Gass JDM, Guerry RK, Jack RL, Harris G. Choroidal Osteoma. Arch Ophthalmol [Internet]. 1978 Mar 1;96(3):428–35. Available from: http://archopht.jamanetwork.com/article.aspx?articleid=632514
29. Shields CL, Shields JA, Augsburger JJ. Choroidal osteoma. Surv Ophthalmol [Internet] 1988 Jul;33(1):17–27. Available from: https://linkinghub.elsevier.com/retrieve/pii/0039625788900690
30. Trimble SN, Schatz H. Choroidal Osteoma after intraocular inflammation. Am J Ophthalmol [Internet]. 1983 Dec;96(6):759–64. Available from: https://linkinghub.elsevier.com/retrieve/pii/S000293941471921X
31. Gass JD. New observations concerning choroidal osteomas. Int Ophthalmol [Internet]. 1979 Feb;1(2):71–84. Available from: http://www.ncbi.nlm.nih.gov/pubmed/553048.
32. McLeod BK. Choroidal osteoma presenting in pregnancy. Br J Ophthalmol [Internet] 1988 Aug 1;72(8):612–4. Available from: http://bjo.bmj.com/cgi/doi/10.1136/bjo.72.8.612
33. Aylward GW. A long-term follow-up of choroidal osteoma. Arch Ophthalmol [Internet]. 1998 Oct 1;116(10):1337. Available from: http://archopht.jamanetwork.com/article.aspx?doi=10.1001/archopht.116.10.1337
34. Shields CL, Perez B, Materin MA, Mehta S, Shields JA. Optical coherence tomography of Choroidal Osteoma in 22 cases. Ophthalmology [Internet]. 2007 Dec;114(12):e53–8. Available from: https://linkinghub.elsevier.com/retrieve/pii/S0161642007008536
35. Shields CL, Sun H, Demirci H, Shields JA. Factors predictive of tumor growth, tumor decalcification, choroidal neovascularization, and visual outcome in 74 eyes with choroidal osteoma. Arch Ophthalmol. 2005;123(12):1658–66.
36. Foster BS. Surgical Removal and Histopathologic Findings of a Subfoveal Neovascular Membrane Associated With Choroidal Osteoma. Arch Ophthalmol [Internet]. 2003 Feb 1;121(2):273. Available from: http://archopht.jamanetwork.com/article.aspx?doi=10.1001/archopht.121.2.273
37. Pierro L, Marchese A, Gagliardi M, Introini U, Battaglia Parodi M, Casalino G, et al. Choroidal excavation in choroidal osteoma complicated by

choroidal neovascularization. Eye [Internet] 2017 Dec 21;31(12):1740–3. Available from: http://www.nature.com/doifinder/10.1038/eye.2017.136
38. Yoshikawa T, Takahashi K. Long-term outcomes of intravitreal injection of bevacizumab for choroidal neovascularization associated with choroidal osteoma. Clin Ophthalmol [Internet]. 2015 Mar;429. Available from: http://www.dovepress.com/long-term-outcomes-of-intravitreal-injection-ofnbspbevacizumab-for-cho-peer-reviewed-article-OPTH
39. Chawla R, Azad SV, Takkar B, Sharma A, Kashyap B. Nonconforming Deep Focal Choroidal Excavation in a Patient With Choroidal Osteoma: A Diagnostic Dilemma. Ophthalmic Surgery, Lasers Imaging Retin [Internet]. 2017 Nov 1;48(11):944–7. Available from: http://www.healio.com/doiresolver?doi=10.3928/23258160-20171030-12
40. Papastefanou VP, Pefkianaki M, Al Harby L, Arora AK, Cohen VML, Andrews RM, et al. Intravitreal bevacizumab monotherapy for choroidal neovascularisation secondary to choroidal osteoma. Eye (Lond) [Internet]. 2016 Jun;30(6):843–9. Available from: http://www.ncbi.nlm.nih.gov/pubmed/27034203.
41. Mello PC de, Berensztejn P, Brasil OFM. Enhanced depth imaging optical coherence tomography of choroidal osteoma with secondary neovascular membranes: report of two cases. Arq Bras Oftalmol [Internet] 2016;79(3):197–9. Available from: http://www.gnresearch.org/doi/10.5935/0004-2749.20160057
42. Shen C, Yan S, Du M, Zhao H, Shao L, Hu Y. Assessment of choroidal osteoma complicating choroidal neovascularization by optical coherence tomography angiography. Int Ophthalmol [Internet]. 2018 Apr;38(2):787–92. Available from: http://link.springer.com/10.1007/s10792-017-0503-9
43. Olguin-Manríquez F, Enríquez AB, Crim N, Meraz-Gutierrez M, Soberón-Ventura V, Ávila I, et al. Multimodal imaging in choroidal osteoma. Int J Retin Vitr [Internet]. 2018;4:30. Available from: http://www.ncbi.nlm.nih.gov/pubmed/30128167.
44. Furino C, Di Antonio L, Grassi MO, Rispoli M, Reibaldi M, Niro A, et al. Choroidal neovascularization due to choroidal osteoma treated with anti–vascular endothelial growth factor therapy: An optical coherence tomography angiography study. Eur J Ophthalmol [Internet]. 2018 Aug 13;112067211879218. Available from: http://journals.sagepub.com/doi/10.1177/1120672118792187
45. Sharma S, Sribhargava N, Shanmugam MP. Choroidal neovascular membrane associated with choroidal osteoma (CO) treated with trans-pupillary thermo therapy. Indian J Ophthalmol [Internet]. 2004 Dec;52(4):329–30. Available from: http://www.ncbi.nlm.nih.gov/pubmed/15693329.
46. Aylward GW, Chang TS, Pautler SE, Gass JD. A long-term follow-up of choroidal osteoma. Arch Ophthalmol (Chicago, Ill 1960) [Internet]. 1998 Oct;116(10):1337–41. Available from: http://www.ncbi.nlm.nih.gov/pubmed/9790633.
47. Palamar M, Uretmen O, Gündüz K. Transient subretinal hemorrhage after photodynamic therapy of subfoveal choroidal osteoma. Retin cases brief rep [Internet]. 2012;6(2):166–8. Available from: http://www.ncbi.nlm.nih.gov/pubmed/25390953.
48. Morris R, Shah P, Prabhu V, Narendran V. Combination therapy of low-fluence photodynamic therapy and intravitreal ranibizumab for choroidal neovascular membrane in choroidal osteoma. Indian J Ophthalmol [Internet]. 2011;59(5):394. Available from: http://www.ijo.in/text.asp?2011/59/5/394/83622
49. Mansour AM, Arevalo JF, Al Kahtani E, Zegarra H, Abboud E, Anand R, et al. Role of Intravitreal Antivascular endothelial growth factor injections for Choroidal neovascularization due to Choroidal Osteoma. J Ophthalmol [Internet] 2014;2014:1–8. Available from: http://www.hindawi.com/journals/joph/2014/210458/
50. Khan MA, DeCroos FC, Storey PP, Shields JA, Garg SJ, Shields CL. Outcomes of anti-vascular endothelial growth factor therapy in the management of choroidal neovascularization associated with choroidal osteoma. Retina [Internet]. 2014 Sep;34(9):1750–6. Available from: http://www.ncbi.nlm.nih.gov/pubmed/24936941.
51. Saitta A, Nicolai M, Neri P, Reibaldi M, Giovannini A, Mariotti C. Rescue therapy with intravitreal aflibercept for choroidal neovascularization secondary to choroidal osteoma non-responder to intravitreal bevacizumab and ranibizumab. Int Ophthalmol [Internet]. 2015 Jun 12;35(3):441–4. Available from: http://link.springer.com/10.1007/s10792-015-0059-5
52. Ahmadieh H, Vafi N. Dramatic response of choroidal neovascularization associated with choroidal osteoma to the intravitreal injection of bevacizumab (Avastin). Graefe's Arch Clin Exp Ophthalmol [Internet]. 2007 Sep 24;245(11):1731–3. Available from: http://link.springer.com/10.1007/s00417-007-0636-z
53. Erol MK, Coban DT, Ceran BB, Bulut M. Retinal pigment epithelium tear formation following intravitreal ranibizumab injection in choroidal neovascularization secondary to choroidal osteoma. Cutan Ocul Toxicol [Internet] 2014 Sep 11;33(3):259–63. Available from: http://www.tandfonline.com/doi/full/10.3109/15569527.2013.844702
54. Chen J, Lee L, Gass JDM. Choroidal osteoma: evidence of progression and decalcification over 20 years. Clin Exp Optom [Internet] 2006 Mar;89(2):90–4. Available from: http://doi.wiley.com/10.1111/j.1444-0938.2006.00012.x
55. Mansour A, Alameddine R, Kahtani E. Review of choroidal osteomas. Middle East Afr J Ophthalmol [Internet]. 2014;21(3):244. Available from: http://www.meajo.org/text.asp?2014/21/3/244/134686
56. Song JH, Bae JH, Rho MI, Lee SC. Intravitreal bevacizumab in the management of subretinal fluid associated with choroidal osteoma. Retina [Internet] 2010 Jun;30(6):945–51. Available from: https://insights.ovid.com/crossref?an=00006982-201006000-00015

57. Najafabadi F, Hendimarjan S, Zarrin Y, Najafabadi M. Intravitreal bevacizumab for management of choroidal osteoma without choroidal neovascularization. J Ophthalmic Vis Res [Internet]. 2015;10(4):484. Available from: http://www.jovr.org/text.asp?2015/10/4/484/176905
58. Ben Yahia S, Zaouali S, Attia S, Messaoud R, Ladjimi A, Khairallah M. Serous retinal detachment secondary to choroidal osteoma successfully treated with transpupillary thermotherapy. Retin Cases Brief Rep [Internet]. 2008;2(2):126–7. Available from: https://insights.ovid.com/crossref?an=01271216-200800220-00014
59. Skau M, Brennum J, Gjerris F, Jensen R. What is new about idiopathic intracranial hypertension? An updated review of mechanism and treatment. Cephalalgia [Internet]. 2006 Apr;26(4):384–99. Available from: http://www.ncbi.nlm.nih.gov/pubmed/16556239.
60. Chen JJ, Thurtell MJ, Longmuir RA, Garvin MK, Wang J-K, Wall M, et al. Causes and Prognosis of Visual Acuity Loss at the Time of Initial Presentation in Idiopathic Intracranial Hypertension. Invest Ophthalmol Vis Sci [Internet]. 2015 Jun;56(6):3850–9. Available from: http://www.ncbi.nlm.nih.gov/pubmed/26070058.
61. Wendel L, Lee AG, Boldt HC, Kardon RH, Wall M. Subretinal neovascular membrane in idiopathic intracranial hypertension. Am J Ophthalmol [Internet]. 2006 Mar;141(3):573–4. Available from: http://www.ncbi.nlm.nih.gov/pubmed/16490514.
62. Morse PH, Leveille AS, Antel JP, Burch J V. Bilateral juxtapapillary subretinal neovascularization associated with pseudotumor cerebri. Am J Ophthalmol [Internet]. 1981 Mar;91(3):312–7. Available from: http://www.ncbi.nlm.nih.gov/pubmed/6163360.
63. Belliveau MJ, Xing L, Almeida DRP, Gale JS, ten Hove MW. Peripapillary choroidal neovascular membrane in a teenage boy. J Neuro-Ophthalmology [Internet] 2013 Mar;33(1):48–50. Available from: https://insights.ovid.com/crossref?an=00041327-201303000-00012
64. Browning D, Fraser C. Ocular Conditions associated with peripapillary subretinal neovascularization, their relative frequencies, and associated outcomes. Ophthalmology [Internet]. 2005 Jun;112(6):1054–1061.e2. Available from: https://linkinghub.elsevier.com/retrieve/pii/S016164200500117X
65. Kaeser P-F, Borruat F-X. Peripapillary neovascular membrane: a rare cause of acute vision loss in pediatric idiopathic intracranial hypertension. J Am Assoc Pediatr Ophthalmol Strabismus [Internet] 2011 Feb;15(1):83–6. Available from: https://linkinghub.elsevier.com/retrieve/pii/S1091853110005422
66. Sathornsumetee B, Webb A, Hill DL, Newman NJ, Biousse V. Subretinal hemorrhage from a peripapillary choroidal neovascular membrane in papilledema caused by idiopathic intracranial hypertension. J Neuro-Ophthalmology [Internet]. 2006 Sep;26(3):197–9. Available from: https://insights.ovid.com/crossref?an=00041327-200609000-00011
67. Castellarin AA, Sugino IK, Nasir M'a., Zarbin MA. Clinicopathological correlation of an excised choroidal neovascular membrane in pseudotumour cerebri. Br J Ophthalmol [Internet]. 1997 Nov 1;81(11):994–1000. Available from: http://bjo.bmj.com/cgi/doi/10.1136/bjo.81.11.994
68. Jamison RR. Subretinal neovascularization and papilledema associated with pseudotumor cerebri. Am J Ophthalmol [Internet] 1978 Jan;85(1):78–81. Available from: https://linkinghub.elsevier.com/retrieve/pii/S0002939414766693
69. Jamerson SC, Arunagiri G, Ellis BD, Leys MJ. Intravitreal bevacizumab for the treatment of choroidal neovascularization secondary to pseudotumor cerebri. Int Ophthalmol [Internet] 2009 Jun 15;29(3):183–5. Available from: http://link.springer.com/10.1007/s10792-007-9186-y
70. Más-Ramírez AM, Villegas VM, Garcia JM, Acevedo S, Serrano L. Intravitreal bevacizumab for peripapillary subretinal neovascular membrane associated to papilledema: a case report. P R Health Sci J. 2012;31(3):148–150.
71. Lee I-J, Maccheron LJ, Kwan AS. Intravitreal Bevacizumab in the treatment of Peripapillary Choroidal Neovascular membrane secondary to idiopathic intracranial hypertension. J Neuro-Ophthalmology [Internet]. 2013 Jun;33(2):155–7. Available from: http://content.wkhealth.com/linkback/openurl?sid=WKPTLP:landingpage&an=00041327-201306000-00014
72. Kumar N, Tigari B, Dogra M, Singh R. Successful management of peripapillary choroidal neovascular membrane secondary to idiopathic intracranial hypertension with intravitreal ranibizumab. Indian J Ophthalmol [Internet]. 2018;66(9):1358. Available from: http://www.ijo.in/text.asp?2018/66/9/1358/239359
73. Barkana Y, Belkin M. Laser eye injuries. Surv Ophthalmol [Internet]. 2000 May;44(6):459–78. Available from: http://linkinghub.elsevier.com/retrieve/pii/S0039625700001120
74. Laser Institute of America LIA. ANSI Z136.1: American national standard for safe use of lasers. SPIE Med Imaging. 2007;
75. Ajudua S, Mello MJ. Shedding some light on laser pointer eye injuries. Pediatr Emerg Care. 2007;23(9):669–72.
76. Torp-Pedersen T, Welinder L, Justesen B, Christensen UC, Solborg Bjerrum S, La Cour M, et al. Laser pointer maculopathy – on the rise? Acta Ophthalmol. 2018;96(7):749–54.
77. Wyrsch S, Baenninger PB, Schmid MK. Retinal injuries from a handheld laser pointer. N Engl J Med [Internet] 2010;363(11):1089–91. Available from: http://www.nejm.org/doi/abs/10.1056/NEJMc1005818
78. Alsulaiman SM, Alrushood AA, Almasaud J, Alzaaidi S, Alzahrani Y, Arevalo JF, et al. High-power handheld blue laser-induced maculopathy: the results of the king khaled eye specialist hospital collaborative retina study group. Ophthalmology [Internet] 2014;121(2):566–72. Available from: https://doi.org/10.1016/j.ophtha.2013.09.006

79. Turaka K, Bryan JS, Gordon AJ, Reddy R, Kwong HM, Sell CH. Laser pointer induced macular damage: case report and mini review. Int Ophthalmol. 2012;32(3):293–7.
80. Ghasemi Falavarjani K, Au A, Anvari P, Mollaei S, Ghasemizadeh S, Verma A, et al. En face OCT of type 2 neovascularization: a reappraisal of the pitchfork sign. Ophthalmic Surg Lasers Imaging Retin. 2019;50(11):719–25.
81. Fujinami K, Yokoi T, Hiraoka M, Nishina S, Azuma N. Choroidal neovascularization in a child following laser pointer-induced macular injury. Jpn J Ophthalmol [Internet] 2010 Nov 28;54(6):631–3. Available from: http://link.springer.com/10.1007/s10384-010-0871-4
82. Xu K, Chin EK, Quiram PA, Davies JB, Parke DW, DRP A. Retinal injury secondary to laser pointers in pediatric patients. Pediatrics. 2016;138(4):e20161188.
83. Ying HS, Symons RCA, Lin KL, Solomon SD, Gehlbach PL. Accidental Nd:YAG laser-induced choroidal neovascularization. Lasers Surg Med. 2008;40(4):240–2.
84. Roider J, Buesgen P, Hoerauf H, Schmidt-Erfurth U, Laqua H, Birngruber R. Macular injury by a military range finder. Retina. 1999;19:531–5.
85. Modarres-Zadeh M, Parvaresh MM, Pourbabak S, Peyman GA. Accidental parafoveal laser burn from a standard military ruby range finder. Retina. 1995;15(4):356–8.
86. Lee YH, Kim YC. Foveal choroidal neovascularization secondary to accidental laser exposure in a dermatologist. Medicine (Baltimore) [Internet]. 2019 May;98(18):e15429. Available from: http://insights.ovid.com/crossref?an=00005792-201905030-00049
87. Wang R, Wykoff CC, Christie L, Croft DE, Major JC, Fish RH, et al. Choroidal neovascularization secondary to alexandrite laser exposure. Retin Cases Br Rep. 2016;10(3):244–8.
88. Daruich A, Matet A, Dirani A, Bousquet E, Zhao M, Farman N, et al. Central serous chorioretinopathy: recent findings and new physiopathology hypothesis. Prog Retin Eye Res. 2015;48:82–118.
89. Loo RH, Scott IU, Flynn HW, JDM G, Murray TG, Lou LM, et al. Factors associated with reduced visual acuity during long-term follow-up of patients with idiopathic central serous chorioretinopathy. Retina. 2002;22(1):19–2.
90. Spaide RF, Campeas L, Haas A, Yannuzzi LA, Fisher YL, Guyer DR, et al. Central serous chorioretinopathy in younger and older adults. Ophthalmology. 1996;103(12):2070–9.
91. Çakir M, Çekiç O, Yilmaz ÖF. Photodynamic therapy for iatrogenic CNV due to laser photocoagulation in central serous Chorioretinopathy. Ophthalmic Surg Lasers Imaging. 2009;40(4):405–8.
92. Yaman A, Arikan G, Saatci AO, Cingil G. Choroidal neovascularization following photodynamic therapy in a patient with chronic central serous chorioretinopathy. Bull Soc Belge Ophtalmol. 2007;303:69–73.
93. Colucciello M. Choroidal neovascularization complicating photodynamic therapy for central serous retinopathy. Retina. 2006;26(2):239–4.
94. Chan WM, Lam DSC, Lai TYY, Tam BSM, Liu DTL, Chan CKM. Choroidal vascular remodelling in central serous chorioretinopathy after indocyanine green guided photodynamic therapy with verteporfin: a novel treatment at the primary disease level. Br J Ophthalmol. 2003;87(12):1453–8.
95. Chhablani J, Pichi F, Silva R, Casella AM, Murthy H, Banker A, et al. Antiangiogenics in Choroidal Neovascularization associated with laser in central serous Chorioretinopathy. Retina. 2016;36(5):901–8.
96. Matsunaga H, Nangoh K, Uyama M, Nanbu H, Fujiseki Y, Takahashi K. Occurrence of choroidal neovascularization following photocoagulation treatment for central serous retinopathy. Nihon Ganka Gakkai Zasshi [Internet]. 1995 Apr;99(4):460–8. Available from: http://www.ncbi.nlm.nih.gov/pubmed/7537938.
97. Varley MP, Frank E, Purnell EW. Subretinal neovascularization after focal argon laser for diabetic macular edema. Ophthalmology. 1988;95(5):567–73.
98. Lewis H, Schachat AP, Haimann MH, Haller JA, Quinlan P, von Fricken MA, et al. Choroidal neovascularization after laser photocoagulation for diabetic macular edema. Ophthalmology [Internet]. 1990 Apr;97(4):503–10; discussion 510–1. Available from: http://www.ncbi.nlm.nih.gov/pubmed/1691477.
99. Shah GK. Photodynamic therapy for choroidal neovascularization after thermal laser photocoagulation for diabetic macular edema. Am J Ophthalmol [Internet]. 2003 Jan;135(1):114–6. Available from: http://www.ncbi.nlm.nih.gov/pubmed/12504717.
100. Deschler EK, Sun JK, Silva PS. Side-effects and complications of laser treatment in diabetic retinal disease. Semin Ophthalmol. 2014;29(5–6):290–300.
101. Berger AR, Boniuk I. Bilateral subretinal neovascularization after focal argon laser photocoagulation for diabetic macular edema. Am J Ophthalmol. 1989;108(1):88–90.
102. Yarng SS, Hsieh CL. Choriovitreal neovascularization following laser-induced chorioretinal venous anastomosis. Ophthalmology. 1996;103(suppl):136.
103. Jacobson MS, Gagliano DA, Cohen SB, Rabb MF, Jampol LM, Farber MD, et al. A randomized clinical trial of feeder vessel photocoagulation of sickle cell retinopathy. A long-term follow-up. Ophthalmology [Internet]. 1991 May;98(5):581–5. Available from: http://www.ncbi.nlm.nih.gov/pubmed/2062489.
104. Theodossiadis G, Velissaropoulos P. Choroidal vascular involvement in Eales' disease. Ophthalmologica. 1973;166(1):1–9.
105. Choroidal Neovascularization Prevention Trial Research Group. Laser treatment in eyes with large drusen. Ophthalmology [Internet]. 1998 Jan;105(1):11–23. Available from: http://www.ncbi.nlm.nih.gov/pubmed/9442774.
106. Al-Husainy S, Stavrou P, Hope-Ross MW. Alkali injury complicated by choroidal neovascularisation.

Eye (Lond) [Internet]. 2000 Dec;14(Pt 6):904–5. Available from: http://www.ncbi.nlm.nih.gov/pubmed/11584853.

107. Aguilar JP, Green WR. Choroidal rupture. A histopathologic study of 47 cases. Retina [Internet]. 4(4):269–75. Available from: http://www.ncbi.nlm.nih.gov/pubmed/6531524.
108. Pujari A, Chawla R, Agarwal D, Gagrani M, Kapoor S, Kumar A. Pathomechanism of traumatic indirect choroidal rupture. Med Hypotheses [Internet]. 2019 Mar;124:64–6. Available from: https://linkinghub.elsevier.com/retrieve/pii/S0306987718311617
109. Bellows JG. Observations on 300 consecutive cases of ocular war injuries. Am J Ophthalmol [Internet]. 1947 Mar;30(3):309–23. Available from: http://www.ncbi.nlm.nih.gov/pubmed/20288592.
110. Wood CM, Richardson J. Chorioretinal neovascular membranes complicating contusional eye injuries with indirect choroidal ruptures. Br J Ophthalmol [Internet]. 1990 Feb;74(2):93–6. Available from: http://www.ncbi.nlm.nih.gov/pubmed/1690025.
111. Pierro L, Giuffrè C, Rabiolo A, Gagliardi M, Arrigo A, Bandello F. Multimodal imaging in a patient with traumatic Choroidal ruptures. Eur J Ophthalmol [Internet] 2017 Nov 8;27(6):e175–8. Available from: http://journals.sagepub.com/doi/10.5301/ejo.5001005
112. Secrétan M, Sickenberg M, Zografos L, Piguet B. Morphometric characteristics of traumatic choroidal ruptures associated with neovascularization. Retina [Internet]. 1998;18(1):62–6. Available from: http://www.ncbi.nlm.nih.gov/pubmed/9502283.
113. Chanana B, Azad R V, Kumar N. Intravitreal bevacizumab for subfoveal choroidal neovascularization secondary to traumatic choroidal rupture. Eye [Internet]. 2009 Nov 23;23(11):2125–6. Available from: http://www.nature.com/articles/eye2008434
114. Ament CS. Predictors of visual outcome and choroidal neovascular membrane formation after traumatic choroidal rupture. Arch Ophthalmol [Internet]. 2006 Jul 1;124(7):957. Available from: http://archopht.jamanetwork.com/article.aspx?doi=10.1001/archopht.124.7.957
115. Secrétan M, Sickenberg M, Zografos L, Piguet B. Morphometric characteristics of traumatic choroidal ruptures associated with neovascularization. Retina [Internet]. 1998;18(1):62–6. Available from: http://www.ncbi.nlm.nih.gov/pubmed/9502283.
116. Wang H, Ninomiya Y, Sugino IK, Zarbin MA. Retinal pigment epithelium wound healing in human Bruch's membrane explants. Invest Ophthalmol Vis Sci [Internet]. 2003 May;44(5):2199–210. Available from: http://www.ncbi.nlm.nih.gov/pubmed/12714662.
117. Joo K, Um T, Park SJ, Cho JH, Ahn J, Kim JT, et al. Efficacy of bevacizumab for posttraumatic choroidal neovascularization. Acta Ophthalmol [Internet] 2019 Mar;97(2):e324–6. Available from: http://doi.wiley.com/10.1111/aos.13896
118. Preziosa C, Corvi F, Pellegrini M, Bochicchio S, Rosar AP, Staurenghi G. Optical coherence tomography angiography findings in a case of choroidal neovascularization secondary to traumatic choroidal rupture. Retin Cases Brief Rep [Internet]. 2018 Mar;1. Available from: http://insights.ovid.com/crossref?an=01271216-900000000-98840
119. Lorusso M, Micelli Ferrari L, Nikolopoulou E, Micelli Ferrari T. Optical coherence tomography angiography evolution of choroidal neovascular membrane in choroidal rupture managed by intravitreal bevacizumab. Case Rep Ophthalmol Med [Internet]. 2019 Jan 6;2019:1–4. Available from: https://www.hindawi.com/journals/criopm/2019/5241573/
120. Smith RE, Kelley JS, Harbin TS. Late macular complications of Choroidal ruptures. Am J Ophthalmol [Internet]. 1974 May;77(5):650–8. Available from: https://linkinghub.elsevier.com/retrieve/pii/0002939474905261
121. Abri A, Binder S, Pavelka M, Tittl M, Neumuller J. Choroidal neovascularization in a child with traumatic choroidal rupture: clinical and ultrastructural findings. Clin Exp Ophthalmol [Internet] 2006 Jul;34(5):460–3. Available from: http://doi.wiley.com/10.1111/j.1442-9071.2006.01248.x
122. Harissi-Dagher M, Sebag M, Gauthier D, Marcil G, Labelle P, Arbour JD. Photodynamic therapy in young patients with choroidal neovascularization following traumatic choroidal rupture. Am J Ophthalmol [Internet]. 2005 Apr;139(4):726–8. Available from: https://linkinghub.elsevier.com/retrieve/pii/S0002939404012498
123. Liang F, Puche N, Soubrane G, Souied EH. Intravitreal ranibizumab for choroidal neovascularization related to traumatic Bruch's membrane rupture. Graefe's Arch Clin Exp Ophthalmol [Internet] 2009 Sep 26;247(9):1285–8. Available from: http://link.springer.com/10.1007/s00417-009-1098-2
124. De Benedetto U, Battaglia Parodi M, Knutsson KA, Librando A, Bandello F, Lanzetta P, et al. Intravitreal bevacizumab for extrafoveal choroidal neovascularization after ocular trauma. J Ocul Pharmacol Ther [Internet] 2012 Oct;28(5):550–2. Available from: http://www.liebertpub.com/doi/10.1089/jop.2012.0022
125. Artunay O, Rasier R, Yuzbasioglu E, Sengül A, Bahcecioglu H. Intravitreal bevacizumab injection in patients with choroidal neovascularization due to choroid rupture after blunt-head trauma. Int Ophthalmol [Internet]. 2009 Aug 30;29(4):289–91. Available from: http://link.springer.com/10.1007/s10792-008-9226-2
126. Prasad A, Patel CC, Puklin JE. Intravitreal bevacizumab in the treatment of choroidal neovascularization from a traumatic choroidal rupture in a 9-year-old child. Retin Cases Brief Rep [Internet] 2009;3(2):125–7. Available from: https://insights.ovid.com/crossref?an=01271216-200900320-00006
127. Chen T-L, Sun M-H, Lin K-K, Lai C-C, Chen K-J. Intravitreal Bevacizumab With Regression of Subretinal Neovascularization After Intraocular Foreign Body Trauma. J Trauma Inj Infect Crit Care [Internet]. 2010 Mar;68(3):747. Available from: https://insights.ovid.com/crossref?an=00005373-201003000-00046

128. Dikci S, Yılmaz T, Gök Z, Demirel S, Genç O. Choroidal neovascularization secondary to ocular penetration during retrobulbar anesthesia and its treatment. Oman J Ophthalmol [Internet]. 2017;10(1):44. Available from: http://www.ojoonline.org/text.asp?2017/10/1/44/200695
129. Maumenee IH, Mitchell TN. Colobomatous malformations of the eye. Trans Am Ophthalmol Soc [Internet]. 1990;88:123–32; discussion 133-5. Available from: http://www.ncbi.nlm.nih.gov/pubmed/2095017.
130. Guirgis MF, Lueder GT. Choroidal neovascular membrane associated with optic nerve coloboma in a patient with CHARGE association. Am J Ophthalmol [Internet]. 2003 Jun;135(6):919–20. Available from: http://www.ncbi.nlm.nih.gov/pubmed/12788148.
131. Onwochei BC, Simon JW, Bateman JB, Couture KC, Mir E. Ocular colobomata. Surv Ophthalmol [Internet]. 45(3):175–94. Available from: http://www.ncbi.nlm.nih.gov/pubmed/11094243.
132. Jesberg DO, Schepens CL. Retinal detachment associated with Coloboma of the choroid. Arch Ophthalmol [Internet] 1961 Feb 1;65(2):163–73. Available from: http://archopht.jamanetwork.com/article.aspx?articleid=626425
133. Hussain RM, Abbey AM, Shah AR, Drenser KA, Trese MT, Capone A. Chorioretinal Coloboma complications: retinal detachment and choroidal neovascular membrane. J Ophthalmic Vis Res [Internet]. 12(1):3–10. Available from: http://www.ncbi.nlm.nih.gov/pubmed/28299000.
134. Grewal DS, Tran-Viet D, Vajzovic L, Mruthyunjaya P, Toth CA. Association of pediatric choroidal neovascular membranes at the temporal edge of optic nerve and retinochoroidal Coloboma. Am J Ophthalmol [Internet]. 2017 Feb;174:104–12. Available from: https://linkinghub.elsevier.com/retrieve/pii/S0002939416305220
135. Leff SR, Britton WA, Brown GC, Lucier AC, Brown JF. Retinochoroidal coloboma associated with subretinal neovascularization. Retina [Internet]. 5(3):154–6. Available from: http://www.ncbi.nlm.nih.gov/pubmed/2416022.
136. Jeng-Miller KW, Cestari DM, Gaier ED. Congenital anomalies of the optic disc: insights from optical coherence tomography imaging. Curr Opin Ophthalmol [Internet]. 2017 Nov;28(6):579–86. Available from: http://www.ncbi.nlm.nih.gov/pubmed/28817389.
137. Gupta V, Gupta A, Dogra MR. Subretinal neovascularization associated with retinochoroidal coloboma. Indian J Ophthalmol [Internet]. 1997 Jun;45(2):116–7. Available from: http://www.ncbi.nlm.nih.gov/pubmed/9475031.
138. Rouland JF, Constantinides G. Retinochoroidal coloboma and subretinal neovascularization. Ann Ophthalmol [Internet]. 1991 Feb;23(2):61–2. Available from: http://www.ncbi.nlm.nih.gov/pubmed/2029115.
139. Takenaka J, Yamane K, Minamoto A, Mishima HK, Hayashida H. Subretinal neovascularization associated with retinochoroidal coloboma. Eur J Ophthalmol [Internet]. 15(6):815–7. Available from: http://www.ncbi.nlm.nih.gov/pubmed/16329073.
140. Maberley AL, Gottner MJ, Antworth M V. Subretinal neovascularization associated with retinochoroidal colobomas. Can J Ophthalmol [Internet]. 1989 Jun;24(4):172–4. Available from: http://www.ncbi.nlm.nih.gov/pubmed/2472858.
141. Brodsky MC, Ford RE, Bradford JD. Subretinal neovascular membrane in an infant with a retinochoroidal coloboma. Arch Ophthalmol (Chicago, Ill 1960) [Internet]. 1991 Dec;109(12):1650–1. Available from: http://www.ncbi.nlm.nih.gov/pubmed/1726773.
142. Steahly LP. Laser treatment of a subretinal neovascular membrane associated with retinochoroidal coloboma. Retina [Internet]. 6(3):154–6. Available from: http://www.ncbi.nlm.nih.gov/pubmed/2432636.
143. Dailey JR, Cantore WA, Gardner TW. Peripapillary choroidal neovascular membrane associated with an optic nerve coloboma. Arch Ophthalmol (Chicago, Ill 1960) [Internet]. 1993 Apr;111(4):441–2. Available from: http://www.ncbi.nlm.nih.gov/pubmed/7682407.
144. Spitzer M, Grisanti S, Bartz-Schmidt KU, Gelisken F. Choroidal neovascularization in retinochoroidal coloboma: thermal laser treatment achieves long-term stabilization of visual acuity. Eye (Lond) [Internet]. 2006 Aug;20(8):969–72. Available from: http://www.ncbi.nlm.nih.gov/pubmed/16151482.
145. von Eicken J, Höh H, Rehfeldt K. [Photodynamic therapy for choroidal neovascularisation due to choroidal coloboma in a 5 1/2-year-old child]. Klin Monbl Augenheilkd [Internet]. 2007 Feb;224(2):140–5. Available from: http://www.ncbi.nlm.nih.gov/pubmed/17309012.
146. Bhende M, Suganeswari G, Gopal L, Bhende PS, Gopal L, Rao C. Choroidal neovascularization associated with coloboma of the choroid: a series of three cases. Indian J Ophthalmol [Internet]. 59(2):148–51. Available from: http://www.ncbi.nlm.nih.gov/pubmed/21350286.
147. Rajendran A, Gupta SR, Brahadeesh S, Ramasamy K. Intravitreal bevacizumab for choroidal neovascularization associated with a retinochoroidal coloboma. Eye (Lond) [Internet]. 2010 May;24(5):933–4. Available from: http://www.ncbi.nlm.nih.gov/pubmed/19713977.
148. Naithani P, Vashisht N, Mandal S, Sankaran P, Garg S. Intravitreal bevacizumab in choroidal neovascularization associated with congenital choroidal and optic nerve coloboma in children: long-term improvement in visual acuity. J AAPOS Off Publ Am Assoc Pediatr Ophthalmol Strabismus [Internet]. 2010 Jun;14(3):288–90. Available from: http://www.ncbi.nlm.nih.gov/pubmed/20603066.
149. Uemura A. Visual outcome after surgical removal of choroidal neovascularization in pediatric patients. Arch Ophthalmol [Internet]. 2000 Oct 1;118(10):1373. Available from: http://archopht.jamanetwork.com/article.aspx?doi=10.1001/archopht.118.10.1373
150. Uhumwangho OM, Jalali S. Chorioretinal coloboma in a paediatric population. Eye (Lond) [Internet]. 2014 Jun;28(6):728–33. Available from: http://www.ncbi.nlm.nih.gov/pubmed/24675580.

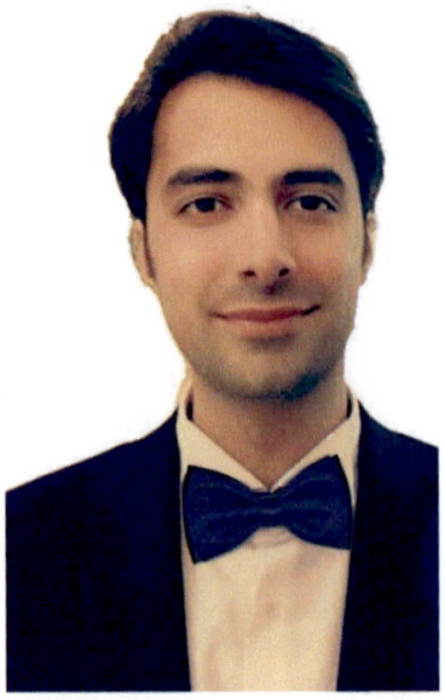

Pasha Anvari, MD MPH is an Assistant Professor of Ophthalmology at the Rassoul Akram Hospital, Iran University of Medical Sciences. He received his medical degree and Master of Public Health from the Tehran University of Medical Sciences and completed his ophthalmology residency at the Farabi Eye Hospital, Tehran University of Medical Sciences, and his retina fellowship at the Rassoul Akram Hospital, Iran University of Medical Sciences.

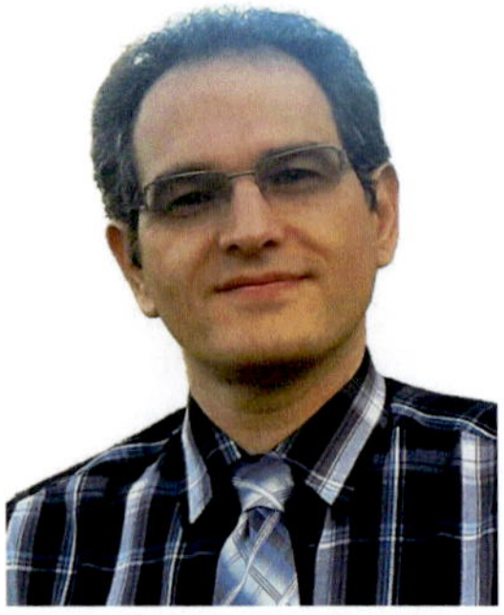

Khalil Ghasemi Falavarjani MD graduated in Ophthalmology from Iran University of Medical Sciences, Tehran, Iran. He was trained in Surgical and Medical Fellowship in Retina in the same institution. He completed a Clinical and Research Fellowship in Retina at the University of California, Los Angeles (UCLA). Currently, he is the Chair of the Department of the Ophthalmology, Iran University of Medical Sciences. He has been elected as the Editor in Chief of the Journal of Current Ophthalmology since 2015. In addition, he is a member of the Editorial Board of Middle East African Journal of Ophthalmology (MEAJO) and Journal of Ophthalmic and Vision Research.

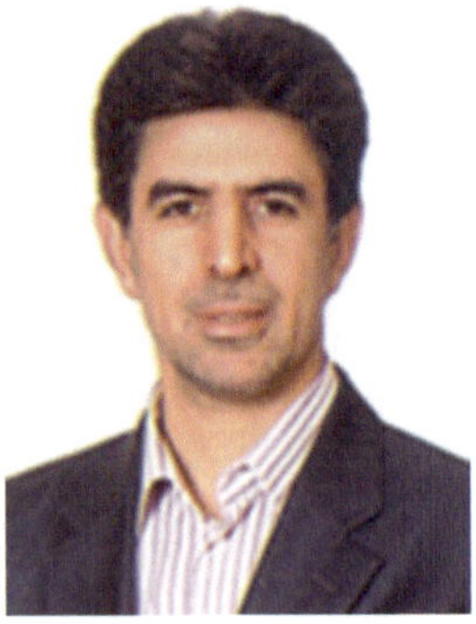

Masood Naseripour MD is a Professor of Ophthalmology and head of Eye Research Center, and Ocular Oncology Unit at the Rassoul Akram Hospital, affiliated with the Iran University of Medical Sciences, Tehran, Iran. He is also the Head of the Iranian Board of Ophthalmology. He finished his Ophthalmology training at the Tabriz University of Medical Sciences in 1993 and obtained his fellowship in Vitreoretinal Surgery in 1995. He completed his fellowship in Ocular Oncology at the Wills Eye Hospital, Philadelphia, USA in 2001.

Part III

Clinical Trials

Clinical Trials Related to Choroidal Neovascularization Secondary to Age-Related Macular Degeneration

20

Paisan Ruamviboonsuk, Peranut Chotcomwonse, Variya Nganthavee, Warissara Pattanapongpaiboon, and Kornwipa Hemarat

Acronyms and Titles of Selected Clinical Trials of CNV-AMD

ABC	Avastin (bevacizumab) for choroidal neovascular age-related macular degeneration
ANCHOR	Anti-VEGF antibody for the treatment of predominantly classic choroidal neovascularization in age-related macular degeneration
BRAMD	Comparing the effectiveness of bevacizumab to ranibizumab in patients with exudative age-related macular degeneration
CATT	The comparison of age-related macular degeneration treatments trials
DAWN	Dorzolamide-timolol in combination with anti-vascular endothelial growth factor injections for wet age-related macular degeneration
DENALI	Verteporfin plus ranibizumab for choroidal neovascularization in age-related macular degeneration
EXCITE	Efficacy and safety of monthly versus quarterly ranibizumab treatment in neovascular age-related macular degeneration
FOCUS	RhuFab V2 ocular treatment combining the use of Visudyne to evaluate safety
GEFAL	The Groupe d'Etude Français Avastin versus Lucentis dans la DMLA néovasculaire
HARBOR	The pHase III, double-masked, multicenter, randomized, active treatment-controlled study of the efficacy and safety of 0.5 mg and 2.0 mg Ranibizumab administered monthly or on an as-needed basis (PRN) in patients with subfoveal neOvasculaR age-related macular degeneration
HAWK and HARRIER	Phase 3, multicenter, randomized, double-masked trials of brolucizumab for neovascular age-related macular degeneration

P. Ruamviboonsuk (✉) · P. Chotcomwongse
V. Nganthavee · W. Pattanapongpaiboon
Department of Ophthalmology, Rajavithi Hospital, Bangkok, Thailand

K. Hemarat
Department of Ophthalmology, Faculty of Medicine, Vajira Hospital, Navamindradhiraj University, Bangkok, Thailand

J. Chhablani (ed.), *Choroidal Neovascularization*, https://doi.org/10.1007/978-981-15-2213-0_20

HORIZON	Open-label extension trial of Ranibizumab for Choroidal neovascularization secondary to age-related macular degeneration
IVAN	The inhibition of VEGF in age-related choroidal neovascularization trial
LUCAS	The Lucentis compared to Avastin study
MANTA	A randomised double-masked trial comparing the visual outcome after treatment with ranibizumab or bevacizumab in patients with neovascular age-related macular degeneration
MARINA	Minimally classic/occult trial of the anti-VEGF antibody Ranibizumab in the treatment of Neovascular age-related macular degeneration
MONT BLANC	Verteporfin plus ranibizumab for choroidal neovascularization in age-related macular degeneration
PIER	A phase IIIb, multicenter, randomized, double masked, sham injection controlled study of the efficacy and safety of Ranibizumab in subjects with Subfoveal Choroidal neovascularization [CNV] with or without classic CNV secondary to age-related macular degeneration
PrONTO	Prospective optical coherence tomography (OCT) imaging of patients with Neovascular age-related macular degeneration (AMD) treated with intraOcular Ranibizumab
PROSPERO	Conbercept for patients with age-related macular degeneration: a systematic review
REACH	Evaluation of AGN-150998 in exudative age-related macular degeneration
RIVAL	The comparison of Ranibizumab and Aflibercept for the development of geographic atrophy in (wet) AMD patients
SALUTE	A randomized trial to compare the safety and efficacy of two ranibizumab dosing regimens in a Turkish cohort of patients with choroidal neovascularization secondary to AMD
SUSTAIN	Safety and efficacy of a flexible dosing regimen of Ranibizumab in Neovascular age-related macular degeneration
TAP	Photodynamic therapy of subfoveal choroidal neovascularization in age-related macular degeneration with verteporfin
TREND	TReat and extend study
TREX-AMD	Treat-and-extend versus monthly dosing for Neovascular age-related macular degeneration
VIEW	The VEGF trap-eye: Investigation of efficacy and safety in wet AMD
VIP	Verteporfin therapy of subfoveal choroidal neovascularization in age-related macular degeneration

The number of clinical trials for age-related macular degeneration (AMD) increases dramatically in the past decades. There were at least 200 published papers on the subject in the 1990s, 700 in the 2000s, and 1000 in the 2010s until mid-2019. The results from many phase III clinical trials of treatment for choroidal neovascularization (CNV) secondary to AMD have shifted the treatment paradigm in favor of anti-vascular endothelial growth factor (anti-VEGF) as the gold standard treatment [1]. The clinical trials for neovascular AMD (nAMD) or CNV secondary to AMD (CNV-AMD) were reviewed extensively in both systematic [2–4] and non-systematic methods [5, 6]. This chapter aims to explore into the design, analysis, and interpretation [7, 8] of the results of the clinical trials of CNV-AMD.

20.1 Superiority Versus Non-inferiority Trials

Every clinical trial should start with a research question [9]. A well-designed clinical trial is conducted to answer that particular question with the primary outcome. If the question is whether an intervention is better than another, the trial is usually designed as prospective randomized controlled trial (RCT) in which an intervention is designated as a comparator or control, with the outcome is the difference between two interventions [9]. An RCT should have enough power to make sure that the statistical significance of the outcome is actual by having enough samples [10].

In the era when laser photocoagulation was becoming the gold standard treatment of subfoveal CNV-AMD, since there was no other treatment or comparator, the laser treatment was compared with observation in the Macular Photocoagulation Study (MPS) [11]. Although the laser treatment caused immediate vision loss after treatment, the MPS concluded that the final vision was significantly superior to observation ($p = 0.002$) in the long-term follow-up [8]. In the era when the treatment was shifted to photodynamic therapy (PDT) with verteporfin, major clinical trials, such as TAP [12] and VIP [13], demonstrated that PDT was superior to sham treatment for preventing visual loss. These studies used sham instead of laser photocoagulation as control. The results from TAP and VIP showed that only predominantly classic CNV identified by fluorescein angiography (FA) had benefit from PDT based on the secondary outcome that 59% of PDT-treated patients compared with 31% of placebo-treated patients lost fewer than 15 letters at the month 24 examination ($p < 0.001$) [14].

PDT was then used as control in clinical trials for assessing an anti-VEGF agent, ranibizumab, as a treatment for CNV-AMD. The trials for ranibizumab were therefore split into a trial for predominantly classic CNV or ANCHOR [15] using PDT as control against ranibizumab and another trial for minimally classic and occult with no classic CNV or MARINA [16] using sham as control since PDT did not provide visual benefits in this group of patients. Ranibizumab was found to be superior to sham by 18 letters ($p < 0.001$) and to PDT by 20 letters ($p < 0.001$) with 95% power in both trials. It was the first time that we could document with strong evidence from clinical trials that a modality for treatment of CNV-AMD could improve vision. Intravitreal injection of ranibizumab since then has become the gold standard for treatment of CNV-AMD [17]. Newer anti-VEGF agents or newer kinds of treatments are investigated against ranibizumab for their efficacy including safety.

The clinical trials designed to compare the other anti-VEGFs, such as bevacizumab and aflibercept, with ranibizumab, however, were not aimed to prove that these two medications were superior to ranibizumab but aimed to prove that they were not inferior to ranibizumab for improving vision, i.e., CATT [18] and VIEW [19] studies. Proving that bevacizumab was not inferior to ranibizumab in terms of efficacy and safety was the aim of CATT because treatment by the former was economical [20] but off-label. It would be justified for clinical use if non-inferiority in efficacy and safety between the two agents were found. Proving that aflibercept was not inferior to ranibizumab would also be justified because treatment with aflibercept might be less burden.

Generally, when a published RCT did not have a statement clarifying that it was designed as non-inferiority trial, we might assume that it was superiority trial. This is always true to RCT comparing between a drug and a placebo, such as TAP, VIP, and MARINA. Superiority and non-inferiority trials are different in terms of design, data analysis, and interpretation of results [21]. It is plausible to switch from interpretation of inferiority outcome to superiority [22], however, this should be done under certain circumstances and a predesign of the trial allowing the switch should be made.

On statistical point of view, the null hypothesis of non-inferiority trial would be easier to be

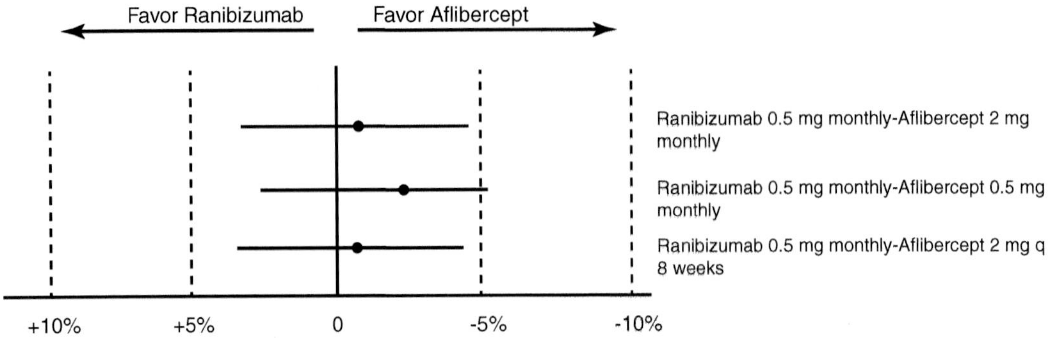

Fig. 20.1 Primary endpoint of VIEW studies. Difference in proportion of patients with best-corrected visual acuity (BCVA) losing <15 letters. The horizontal lines indicated 95% confidence interval (95% CI) of each treatment arm of the studies without actual value shown. The 95% CI for each arm was within +5% margin to −5% margin. This chart shows non-inferiority of aflibercept comparing to ranibizumab in all treatment arms. (Reproduced from the published VIEW studies)

rejected than superiority trial [21, 23]. Its sample size is generally smaller. It is important to specify the difference margin of the efficacy between interventions that were investigated in both superiority and non-inferiority trials [21]. The margin is used primarily for sample size estimation in a superiority trial whereas it is used for both sample size estimation and interpretation of trial results in a non-inferiority trial [24].

In ANCHOR [15], for example, a superiority trial comparing ranibizumab and PDT for treatment of CNV-AMD at 52 weeks, the margin of difference of 17% was pre-specified in the sample size estimation. The results from ANCHOR showed that, with respect to the primary efficacy endpoint (the proportion of patients who lost fewer than 15 letters from baseline best-corrected visual acuity [BCVA]), 94.3% of patients in the 0.3-mg group and 96.4% in the 0.5-mg group of ranibizumab injection reached the primary endpoint compared with 64.3% in PDT group ($p < 0.001$ for each comparison). This was both statistical significance and clinical importance at the time when this study was conducted. The P-value was important to show that the superiority of approximately 30% from ranibizumab had a small chance to be false positive and 95% power made sure that this was actual. The pre-specified margin of difference, 17%, was not as important on the trial analysis and interpretation.

In VIEW 1 and VIEW 2 [19], for example, which were designed as non-inferiority trials comparing between aflibercept and ranibizumab for CNV-AMD at 52 weeks, the primary endpoint was similar to ANCHOR: the proportion of patients who lost fewer than 15 letters from baseline BCVA. The difference margin between these two agents for measuring this endpoint was pre-specified at 10% for assessing non-inferiority and the U.S. Food and Drug Administration recommended a 5% margin for assessing clinical equivalence. In addition, the investigators stated that the non-inferiority margin of 7% was also set according to the European Medicines Agency/ Committee for Medicinal Products for Human Use for analysis of the integrated data from VIEW 1 and VIEW 2. The investigators were able to claim non-inferiority in all arms of aflibercept in VIEW 1 and VIEW 2 because the 95% Confidence Interval (95% CI) of the difference between each of the six aflibercept arms and ranibizumab for the primary endpoint had the lower margin of the CI above the pre-specified difference margin of 10%. This occurred when the mean difference was also in favor of aflibercept. In addition, the 95% CI for each arm was within +5% margin to −5% margin for claiming clinical equivalence between aflibercept and ranibizumab (Fig. 20.1).

The investigators found further in VIEW 1 that only the group of aflibercept 2 mg every 4 weeks showed statistically superior to the group of ranibizumab with a gain of mean of +10.9 letters from baseline compared to +8.1 letters. It was shown in the published table of this study (reproduced as Fig. 20.2) that only 95% CI of the

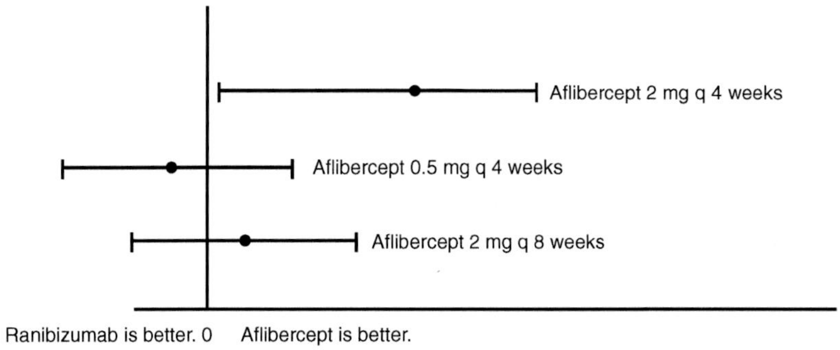

Fig. 20.2 Secondary endpoint of VIEW 1. Mean best-corrected visual acuity (BCVA) difference between each of the three aflibercept treatment arms and ranibizumab at 52 weeks. The horizontal lines indicate 95% confidence interval (95% CI) of least square mean difference of BCVA between aflibercept and ranibizumab of each treatment arm. Only the arm of 2 mg aflibercept every 4 weeks shows superiority over ranibizumab interpreted by the lower limit of the 95% CI greater than zero. No superiority was shown in the other 2 arms. (Recreated from VIEW studies, only values without graph shown in the published manuscript of VIEW)

least square mean difference between aflibercept and ranibizumab in this arm of the VIEW 1 had the lower margin above zero. This is the interpretation of a non-inferiority trial when the claim for superiority is to be made [22]. However, this mean difference of BCVA in letters was not the primary endpoint in these studies.

For superiority trial, analysis of data from all patients in each randomized arm, i.e., the full analysis set, is recommended [23]. This is because it is more conservative to claim superiority when those with missing data, drop out, or nonresponsive to treatment after randomization are included for analysis. For non-inferiority trial, however, an even more conservative approach may be recommended. To decrease bias, both analyses on full dataset or "intention-to-treat" analysis, and "per-protocol" analysis, which is an analysis of data from patients who only completed the treatment at the end excluding those with missing, dropout, nonresponsive, are recommended [25, 26]. The LUCAS Study [27] that was a non-inferiority randomized controlled clinical trial for ranibizumab vs. bevacizumab in treat and extended dosing regimen is a good example. This study showed a clear figure of study groups with intention-to-treat (ITT) and per-protocol (PP) analyses in each arm. Both ITT and PP analyses in LUCAS shown non-inferiority between the two agents for achieving the primary outcome. In addition, the investigators claimed equivalence efficacy in achieving the endpoint by demonstrating that the 95% CI of the difference between the two agents fell within the pre-specified equivalence margin, both sides.

20.2 Assessment of Primary Outcomes in Clinical Trials of CNV-AMD

20.2.1 Clinical Trials on Different Agents

20.2.1.1 Comparison Between Bevacizumab and Ranibizumab: CATT and IVAN

IVAN was another major non-inferiority RCT comparing between bevacizumab and ranibizumab conducted in the United Kingdom whereas CATT was in the United States. The other smaller RCTs, included GEFAL, MANTA, BRAMD, and LUCAS, were conducted in other countries with a similar aim to show that bevacizumab was non-inferior to ranibizumab for visual improvement in CNV-AMD.

One-Year Results of CATT

There were 1185 patients from 44 clinical centers randomized into 4 groups defined by drugs, ranibizumab or bevacizumab, and dosing regimens, monthly or as-needed, without initial loading injections [18]. This study was pre-designed with the ability to test for superiority if a treatment was found to be non-inferior. The non-inferiority margin for the difference between study groups in the mean change of BCVA at 1 year was 5 letters.

At one year, among the six comparisons in the trial, only the comparisons of visual gain between bevacizumab PRN and bevacizumab monthly and between bevacizumab PRN and ranibizumab monthly could not reach the non-inferiority margin. The lower margins of the 95% CIs of both comparisons fell below the pre-specified −5.0 letters. The favor of ranibizumab over bevacizumab was found in each arm of the comparisons, except that bevacizumab monthly was favorable to ranibizumab PRN. BCVA gain from baseline was 8.5 in the ranibizumab-monthly group, 8.0 in the bevacizumab-monthly group, 6.8 in the ranibizumab-as-needed group, and 5.9 in the bevacizumab as-needed group, respectively. This BCVA gain between 5 and 10 letters found in CATT is a benchmark for BCVA gain from treatment of CNV-AMD with a new anti-VEGF agent or a new kind of treatment in later clinical trials.

Two-Year Results of CATT

A total of 93.4% of participants from year 1 continued in CATT year 2 [28]. During the second year, approximately half of patients in monthly groups were randomized to switch to PRN regimen. This created 6 groups of treatments, instead of four groups as in the first year. This re-randomization reduced the sample size of groups originally treated monthly but yielded larger sample sizes, greater precision, and increased power to assess the actual effects of PRN treatment. This approach provided an accurate description of the results when there was no interaction between drug and dosing regimen [28].

On analysis, the investigators pooled data from all arms to compare the differences between the two drugs: ranibizumab and bevacizumab and between the two treatment regimens: monthly and PRN. At the end of year 2, bevacizumab was non-inferior to ranibizumab for visual gain, 95% CI was −3.7–0.8, the mean BCVA change was −1.4 letters in favor of ranibizumab ($p = 0.21$). This held true as an overview assessment between the two drugs at the end of the second year. There was non-inferiority for a comparison between PRN and monthly when both medications were pooled together within each dosing regimen. The results were in favor of monthly regimen and non-inferiority could be claimed with the mean change of −2.4 letters, 95% CI between −4.8 and −0.1 ($p = 0.046$) at the end of the second year. The results were still similar after applying alternative methods for handling missing visual acuity data at 2 years (ITT analysis).

Two-Year Results of IVAN

IVAN randomized 628 patients into four treatment groups similar to CATT year 1 but 3 monthly loading injections were applied in the PRN regimens [29]. The investigators of IVAN used more conservative approach than CATT for designing this trial. They specified a non-inferiority margin of 3.5 letters, instead of 5 letters; the retreatment regimen of IVAN required 3 monthly injections instead of one injection as CATT.

At 2 years, 84% of patients from the first year were still in the study. A total of 271 eyes received ranibizumab and 254 eyes received bevacizumab whereas 261 received monthly and 264 PRN regimens. The analysis on these 2-year data showed inconclusive evidence that the mean change in BCVA from baseline between both drugs (bevacizumab vs. ranibizumab difference, −1.37 letters; $p = 0.26$, 95% CI −3.75 to 1.01) and the mean change between both treating regimens (monthly vs. PRN difference, −1.63 letters; $p = 0.18$, 95% CI −4.01 to 0.75) could reach non-inferiority. The lower margin of both 95% CIs fell below −3.5 letters prespecified margin. Although it seemed that the non-inferiority in IVAN could have been reached if the non-inferiority margin of 5 letters was pre-specified as in CATT; however, the sample size would be re-estimated and the results would be uncertain.

20.2.1.2 Comparisons Between Bevacizumab and Ranibizumab Other than CATT and IVAN

In MANTA [30], the RCT in Austria, patients in each arm of ranibizumab and bevacizumab received three initial monthly injections followed by monthly evaluation of BCVA and lesion activity for re-treatment (PRN regimen). At month 12, the mean gain of BCVA of bevacizumab and ranibizumab group was 4.9 and 4.1 letters, respectively ($p = 0.78$) from intention-to-treat analysis. The investigators interpreted that this mean change in BCVA of bevacizumab was equivalent to ranibizumab because the 95% CI was within −7 to +7 letters (the pre-specified margin of 7 letters of non-inferiority) without showing the actual value of the 95% CI in the article. The 7 letters margin may be too wide to claim non-inferiority in real clinical practice since this is a change of more than a line on ETDRS visual acuity chart.

GEFAL [31], the RCT in France, had similar study design as MANTA comparing ranibizumab and bevacizumab in PRN regimen. The margin of clinical non-inferiority was pre-specified at 5 letters. At 1 year, bevacizumab was non-inferior to ranibizumab (bevacizumab vs. ranibizumab +2.36 letters; 95% CI −0.72 to 5.44, $p < 0.0001$, from intention-to-treat analysis) and the mean number of injections was not significantly different between the two drugs (bevacizumab 6.8, ranibizumab 6.5, $p = 0.39$). The main difference between GEFAL and other well-designed non-inferiority trials like IVAN and CATT might lay on the aspect of conducting the trial. The investigators stated that the effective double-masking was remained throughout the entire study of GEFAL, unlike CATT and IVAN in which the masking differed between centers.

BRAMD [32] was the RCT to compare between monthly regimen of both ranibizumab and bevacizumab in the Netherlands. The non-inferiority margin was pre-specified at 4 letters. AT 1 year, the mean gain in BCVA was 5.1 letters in the bevacizumab group and 6.4 letters in the ranibizumab group ($p = 0.37$) in intention-to-treat analysis. The lower limit of 95% CI of the difference in BCVA gain between the two groups was 3.72 which allowed the investigators to claim non-inferiority.

LUCAS [27] was the RCT to compare bevacizumab and ranibizumab in the Treat-and-Extend (T&E) regimen in Norway. At 1 year, there was no difference between both drugs in mean BCVA improvement (bevacizumab 7.9, ranibizumab 8.2, $p = 0.845$, 95% CI −2.4 to 2.9 according to per-protocol analysis; bevacizumab 7.8, ranibizumab 8.0, $p = 0.550$, 95% CI −2.2 to 2.5 according to intention-to-treat analysis). The non-inferiority could also be claimed.

20.2.1.3 Systematic Review of Comparisons Between Bevacizumab and Ranibizumab

In a systematic review from Cochrane Group that included 16 randomized controlled trials that enrolled 6347 patients with CNV-AMD (the number of patients per trial ranged from 23 to 1208) for assessment of the efficacy and safety of three anti-VEGF agents, ranibizumab, bevacizumab, and pegatanib [2]. The overall certainty of the evidence among the included trials was moderate to high, and most trials had an overall low risk of bias. There were 10 trials compared between bevacizumab and ranibizumab.

According to this review, at 1 year, patients who received intravitreal injections of any of the three anti-VEGF agents had a significantly higher chance of gaining 15 letters or more (risk ratio [RR] 4.19, 95% CI 2.32 to 7.55; the evidence was moderate-certainty), lost fewer than 15 letters (RR 1.40, 95% CI 1.27 to 1.55; the evidence was high-certainty), and showed better mean improvement in visual acuity (mean difference [MD] 6.7 letters, 95% CI 4.4 to 9.0 in one pegaptanib trial; MD 17.8 letters, 95% CI 16.0 to 19.7 in three ranibizumab trials; the evidence was moderate-certainty), compared to controls. Patients treated with anti-VEGF agents also showed improvement in central retinal thickness (CRT) and size of CNV and other morphologic outcomes (the evidence was moderate-certainty).

Also in this review, at 1 year when bevacizumab was compared with ranibizumab, visual acuity outcomes were similar in terms of gaining 15 letters or more (RR 0.95, 95% CI 0.81 to 1.12) and loss of fewer than 15 letters (RR 1.00, 95% CI 0.98 to 1.02). The mean improvement in visual acuity in those received ranibizumab were from 3 to 8 letters whereas those with bevacizumab improved 0.5 letters or fewer in average (95% CI −1.5 to 0.5). The mean reduction in CRT in those received ranibizumab were from 30 to 182 μm whereas those with bevacizumab were 13.97 μm in average (95% CI −26.52 to −1.41). All of these evidence were in high certainty [2].

20.2.1.4 Comparisons Between Aflibercept and Ranibizumab

The first RCT that compared aflibercept with ranibizumab was VIEW study, in which two parallel phase III studies were conducted in different countries as VIEW 1 and VIEW 2. A total of 1217 patients were included in VIEW 1 and 1240 patients were included in VIEW2. Patients enrolled were classified into four groups: (1) 0.5 mg aflibercept monthly injection for 3 doses then every 4 weeks (A0.5q4); (2) 2 mg aflibercept monthly injection for 3 doses then every 4 weeks (A2q4); (3) 2 mg aflibercept monthly injection for 3 doses then every 8 weeks (A2q8); and (4) 0.5 mg ranibizumab every 4 weeks (R0.5q4). The results of the primary endpoint were stated previously [19].

20.2.1.5 Clinical Trials of Ziv-Aflibercept

Ziv-aflibercept is a drug containing a fusion protein, aflibercept, and approved by U.S. Food and Drug Administration as a systemic chemotherapeutic agent for treatment of colorectal cancer [33]. For treatment of CNV-AMD, ziv-aflibercept was used off-label similar to bevacizumab. Ziv-aflibercept, however, could potentially be more harmful than bevacizumab due to the higher osmolality of the drug, approximately 1000 mOsm/kg, compared with the vitreous. On the other hand, aflibercept itself has undergone a different purification process and contained different buffer solutions resulting in a lower osmolality of 286 mOsm/kg [34]. Despite this safety concern of ziv-aflibercept, in vitro studies showed safety of ziv-aflibercept for cellular viability of cultured retinal pigment epithelium cells (ARPE-19 [35]) as well as the rabbit retina with intravitreal injection [36]. Many clinical studies of intravitreal injection of ziv-aflibercept showed no particular safety concern. This included a 26-week case series on visual outcome and electroretinographic findings of treatment of CNV-AMD with ziv-aflibercept [37]. There were two clinical studies reported on relatively long-term outcomes. One had a follow-up of 52 weeks [38] and another of 30 months [39].

In the 52-week study, ziv-aflibercept was given initially for three monthly injections of 1.25 mg/0.05 ml (regular dose of aflibercept is 2 mg/0.05 ml), followed by PRN, BCVA was improved from 0.95 ± 0.41 (20/200) at baseline to 0.75 ± 0.51 (20/125) logMAR units ($p = 0.0066$); the central retinal thickness decreased from 478.21 ± 153.48 mm at baseline to 304.43 ± 98.59 mm ($p = 0.0004$). Full-field electroretinography parameters were used to assess retinal toxicity after the injections (rod response and oscillatory potentials). It was found that both parameters remained unchanged during the follow-up. The average multifocal electroretinography macular response in 5° showed increased N1-P1 amplitude and decreased P1 implicit time from baseline ($p < 0.05$). The investigators discussed that these significant changes could be from disease processes rather than from the drug.

In the 30-month study, the investigators prospectively treated consecutive cases of macular diseases with ziv-aflibercept using the Treat and Extend (T&E) regimen. Of a total of 53 eyes in the study, 35 were CNV-AMD. Central macular thickness of these patients decreased by 107.8 μm ($p = 0.012$) with BCVA gain of 0.52 ($p = 0.001$). Initiation of T&E in CNV-AMD occurred after a mean of 8.0 injections (range 4–16) at 9.9 months (range 5–18 months). No eye with CNV-AMD had initiation of T&E after three injections. One eye in this case series developed a single episode of transient iritis, which recovered well to topical treatment. No systemic complications were noted. The high visual gain from T&E of ziv-aflibercept in this study, compared with T&E of aflibercept in another study [40], might come from selection bias of recruiting patients with poorer vision at baseline.

There has not yet been a published RCT of ziv-aflibercept for CNV-AMD. The only publication of RCT of ziv-aflibercept to date was a comparison between ziv-aflibercept and bevacizumab for diabetic macular edema in T&E regimen [41].

20.2.1.6 Clinical Trials of Conbercept

Conbercept (KH902) is another anti-VEGF agent, which was designed as a recombinant fusion protein with high affinity to all VEGF isoforms and placental growth factor (PIGF) similar to aflibercept, developed in China. Currently, it is still approved only in China. Almost all trials of conbercept were also conducted in China and most of them were written in Chinese.

The only prospective RCT on conbercept published in English is the PHOENIX study [42] which was phase III trial. Patients with CNV-AMD and PCV were included, but the definite diagnosis of PCV was not clear in some cases due to the unavailability of indocyanine green angiography in some periods of the study. A total of 124 patients were randomized into conbercept or sham. Conbercept 0.5 mg was injected monthly with three loading doses then fixed at every 3 months until month 12. Sham injection was performed monthly for the first 3 months followed by conbercept 0.5 mg monthly injection for three doses, then every 3 months until month 12. This study design was not defined as superiority or non-inferiority. The primary endpoint was mean BCVA change at 3 months.

At 3 months, BCVA improvement in conbercept group was statistically better than sham. This was +9.2 letters compared to +2.02 (mean difference + 7.27 letters, 95% CI 3.36–11.18; $p < 0.001$). At 12 months, the mean changes from baseline BCVA were + 9.98 letters in the conbercept group and + 8.81 letters in the sham group (95% CI 4.47–13.15; $p = 0.64$). The statistical significance was only shown when the data were analyzed with per-protocol analysis (mean difference + 7.27 letters: 95% CI 3.27–11.26; $p < 0.001$), not intention-to-treat analysis (mean difference + 1.24 letters: 95% CI −4.01 to 6.50; $p < 0.64$).

There was a systematic review on conbercept entitled "PROSPERO" [43]. Of the 18 RCTs selected from 780 trials of conbercept, there were three trials with the longest follow up of 12 months. One compared with ranibizumab whereas the other two compared with triamcinolone. The primary outcome of these trials was central retinal thickness (CRT), not BCVA. Nine trials had a follow-up of three months or less. According to this review, conbercept might improve BCVA slightly compared to triamcinolone acetonide (mean difference = 0.11, 95% CI 0.08–0.15), and reduce CRT compared to the other four therapies (conservative treatment, ranibizumab, transpupillary thermotherapy, and triamcinolone acetonide).

20.2.1.7 Clinical Trials of Brolucizumab

Brolucizumab is a new small (26 kDa), humanized, single-chain antibody fragment, which is another potent anti-VEGF. Preclinical data demonstrated a 2.2- and 1.7-fold higher exposure in the retina and in the retinal pigment epithelium and choroid, respectively, compared with ranibizumab [44].

HAWK and HARRIER studies were conducted to assess the efficacy and safety between brolucizumab and aflibercept at the dosing regimens of three-monthly injections followed by every 12 weeks (q12w) for the former and every 8 weeks (q8w) for the latter. Any patients in brolucizumab arm who met the criteria defining disease activity at the assessment visits, assessed by masked investigators, would be changed dosing to q8w. The selection of q12w and q8w dosing was based on the results of the OSPREY study [45], in which a head-to-head comparison of the q8w treatment regimen between brolucizumab 6 mg and aflibercept 2 mg showed anatomical advantages with brolucizumab while reaching non-inferiority in BCVA. In the same study, brolucizumab-treated patients were subsequently challenged with q12w dosing interval, with an outcome suggesting that half of the patients were adequately treated.

Non-inferiority of mean BCVA change from baseline at week 48 was set as a primary objective in both HAWK (6 mg and 3 mg of brolucizumab) and HARRIER (6 mg brolucizumab). At Week 48, each brolucizumab arm demonstrated non-inferiority to aflibercept in BCVA change from baseline as +6.6 letters, +6.1 letters, and + 6.8 letters in brolucizumab 6 mg group, brolucizumab 3 mg group, and aflibercept group, respectively, with 95% CI of −2.5 to 1.3 and −2.7 to 1.3 in HAWK study; as +6.9 letters and + 7.6 letters in brolucizumab 6 mg and aflibercept, respectively, with 95% CI of −2.1 to 1.2 in HARRIER. Greater than 50% of brolucizumab

6 mg-treated eyes were maintained on q12w dosing through Week 48 (56% in HAWK and 51% in HARRIER).

20.2.2 Clinical Trials on Different Dosing Regimens of Anti-VEGF Agents

20.2.2.1 Case Series on PRN of Ranibizumab

PrONTO [46] was a small study without control arm to evaluate the potential benefit of using findings from Optical Coherence Tomography (OCT) to adjust treatment regimen of ranibizumab. It was one of the first studies assessing ranibizumab in PRN treatment. A total of 40 patients were enrolled to receive three monthly loadings of 0.5 mg ranibizumab then followed monthly for a year. At each monthly visit, the patients would have re-treatment if they had the following criteria: (1) persistent subretinal fluid after a 1-month period post injection, (2) increase in CRT on OCT of at least 100 μm, (3) new macular hemorrhage or new classic CNV, and (4) loss of 5 letters on BCVA with OCT evidence of fluid in the macula. The investigators did not have the option "not to treat" in case of good visual acuity, a flat retina, or futility of treatment.

At month 12, the mean visual acuity improved by 9.3 letters compared with baseline ($p < 0.001$) and the mean CRT on OCT decreased by 178 μm compared with baseline ($p < 0.001$). The average number of injections was 5.6 over 12 months. The mean injection-free interval was 4.5 months.

During the second year, the re-treatment criteria were amended to include re-treatment if any qualitative increase in the amount of macular fluid was detected using OCT. At month 24, the mean visual acuity improved by 11.1 letters ($p < 0.001$) and the CRT decreased by 212 μm ($p < 0.001$). Visual acuity improved by 15 letters or more in 43% of patients. These vision and OCT outcomes were achieved with an average of 9.9 injections over 24 months. The potential of using OCT-based PRN regimen for treatment of CNV-AMD found in PrONTO was carried over to be investigated in many studies.

SUSTAIN [47] was also a case series to investigate ranibizumab given in PRN regimen similar to PrONTO but with much larger population: 513 treatment-naive patients. The re-treatment criteria were focused on both visual acuity and OCT change as equally important whereas PrONTO focused mainly on OCT findings. All included patients received three initial monthly injections of ranibizumab (0.3 mg) then followed up monthly for one year. The pre-specified re-treatment criteria during the follow-up were BCVA better than 79 letters or the CRT was lower than 225 μm together with either one or two of (1) a decrease of BCVA by more than 5 letters or (2) an increase in CRT by more than 100 μm compared with best value at any prior visit.

The best mean BCVA was achieved at month 3 at +5.8 letters. The mean final BCVA was +3.6 at month 12. The mean number of injections was 5.6 which was unexpectedly a similar number as PrONTO at one year. However, the primary outcome of SUSTAIN was assessment of adverse events, not visual efficacy.

20.2.2.2 Fixed Monthly Versus PRN of Ranibizumab Other than CATT

HARBOR [48] was conducted to evaluate ranibizumab in the higher than usual dose, 2.0 mg, in superiority comparison with the usual dose, 0.5 mg. This study also evaluated whether PRN dosing were non-inferiority to monthly dosing. The HARBOR was different from CATT for the non-inferiority comparison in the way that HARBOR have initial three loading doses in the PRN arm; the non-inferiority margin, 4 letters, was smaller than CATT. All four treatment arms in HARBOR demonstrated clinically significant BCVA improvement at months 12 and 24, but the 2.0 mg monthly dose failed to show superiority to the 0.5 mg monthly dose (model-adjusted mean difference, −1.1 letters; 95.1% CI, −3.4 to 1.3; $p = 0.8145$). The mean change in BCVA at month 24 were + 9.1, +7.9, +8.0, and + 7.6 for the 0.5 mg monthly, 0.5 mg PRN, 2 mg monthly and 2 mg PRN, respectively. The non-inferiority comparison between 0.5 mg PRN and 0.5 mg monthly had a model-adjusted mean difference of −2.0 letters (97.5% CI, −4.5 to 0.6) and inconclusive results. The comparison between 2.0 mg PRN and 0.5 mg monthly had a model-adjusted mean difference of −1.6 letters (98.4% CI, −4.4 to 1.1) and also showed inconclusive results for non-inferiority.

20.2.2.3 Monthly Versus "Treat & Extend" (T&E) Regimen of Ranibizumab

The T&E regimen was introduced to decrease the treatment burden from PRN regimen by decreasing patient visits and providing the potential to treat patients proactively before disease activity recurred.

TREX-AMD [49] was a relatively small prospective, multicenter, randomized, controlled clinical trial with 60 naive patients randomized to ranibizumab monthly or T&E in the proportion of 1:2. The T&E protocol in this study had a requirement that the injections were no more frequently than every 4 weeks and no less frequently than every 12 weeks which was similar to other studies on T&E. However, the protocol for extension of visiting intervals in this study was relatively more conservative than the others.

At each visit, the enrolled eyes were treated monthly until a dry macula was achieved. The dry macula was defined as either resolution of subretinal and intraretinal hemorrhage related to CNV or resolution of intraretinal and subretinal fluid on Spectral Domain-OCT. The dry macula also included cases with a pigment epithelial detachment without intraretinal or subretinal fluid.

When the dry macula was found, the interval between treatment visits was extended by the increments of 2 weeks. If recurrent disease activity was found, the interval was reduced by the increments of 2 weeks until the dry macula was achieved. At this point, the interval then was extended by the increments of only 1 week until the disease was recurred. If this recurrence was again found, the interval then was reduced by the increments of 1 week until the macular was dry. At this point, the most recent interval between treatment visits was maintained for an additional visit; if the macula remained dry, the interval was extended by the increments of 1 week once again. If an eye showed recurrent disease activity three times at any given intervals, treatment was continued at the next shorter interval for three consecutive visits.

TREX-AMD found that the mean maximum extension interval in the T&E cohort was 8.4 weeks; 22% of patients still required monthly dosing and visit. At month 12, it was found that 37% required treatment at 9-week intervals or longer. These proportions are coincidentally similar to the respective 19 and 34% reported in another study [50], which was from patients treated with T&E regimen of ranibizumab in the real world. TREX-AMD also showed comparable BCVA change from baseline between the two treatment groups, +9.2 letters in monthly and + 10.5 letters in T&E group ($p = 0.60$) and significantly lower number of injections in the T&E group (13 vs. 10.1, $p < 0.001$). However, there was still a limitation in the study design of TREX-AMD in a way that we may not be able to strongly confirm non-inferiority of the T&E to monthly protocol.

A larger and recently published trial assessing ranibizumab in T&E regimen was TREND study [51]. TREND was designed as non-inferiority trial comparing 323 eyes with T&E and 327 eyes with monthly ranibizumab. The T&E arm was treated with two initial monthly doses, not three as in TREX-AMD or other studies. The primary outcome was mean change of BCVA from baseline until one year and the non-inferiority margin was pre-specified at 5 letters.

The T&E regimen in TREND was slightly different from TREX-AMD in the way that the treatment interval between visits, no matter extended or reduced interval, would be 2 weeks. There was no 1-week interval as in TREX-AMD. The regimen in TREND is commonly used in real-world practice. T&E in TREND was shown to be non-inferior to monthly regimen. The least-square mean difference between the two treatments was −1.9 letters (95% CI −3.83 to 0.07; $p < 0.001$ for non-inferiority). The mean change in BCVA was + 7.6 and + 6.6 letters and mean change in CST were −169.2 μm and −173.3 μm for the monthly and T&E, respectively. The average duration between the visits was 40.1 days in T&E and 28.5 days in monthly group. In the T&E group, 51.7% of the patients received 6–9 injections.

Despite the differences in T&E protocols, TREX-AMD and TREND had a comparable proportion of patients who required monthly dosing (22.6% in TREND and 22% in TREX-AMD) and proportion of patients who required treatment at 9-week intervals or longer at month 12 (41.8% in TREND and 37% in TREX-AMD).

20.3 Interpretation of Secondary Outcome, Ad Hoc, and Post Hoc Analyses

Only on some occasions when clinical trials are powered to cover secondary outcomes or variables other than the primary outcome [52]. It may not be justified to increase the sample size large enough to cover other outcomes since more resources and time are needed. Ad hoc or post hoc analysis (by definition, the former is usually conducted additionally when the trial has not yet been completed whereas the latter is conducted after the trial has been completed) [53], on the other hand, usually conducts on data already available in well-designed, prospective, RCTs to determine variables that are not accounted for during the design of a clinical trial. These analyses can be conducted because of the availability of plenty of data in the trials. The data may be used to explore some additional research questions. The results of ad hoc, and post hoc analyses, including the results of the secondary outcomes, should be interpreted carefully [52]. They may better be used for pointing out the direction for future research.

20.3.1 Post Hoc Study from ANCHOR and MARINA

Following the ANCHOR and MARINA, an extension study called HORIZON [54] was conducted to further evaluate the safety of ranibizumab in patients who had already completed one of the three RCTs, ANCHOR, MARINA, or FOCUS [55] for 2 years. They were classified into three groups in the following two more years: (1) patients treated with ranibizumab ($n = 600$), (2) patients randomized to control who crossed over to receive ranibizumab ($n = 253$), and (3) ranibizumab-naïve patients ($n = 253$). Ranibizumab was administered at the investigator's discretion without pre-specified re-treatment criteria in this extension period. Systemic and ocular side effects, which were primary outcomes in HORIZON, were uncommon and consistent with other previous studies (one mild endophthalmitis in 3552 injections in all ranibizumab-treated patients).

This study had limitations as post hoc analysis and the assessment of safety might suffer from inadequate sample size. The investigators also found that the mean change in BCVA from the initial study baseline (the secondary outcome) was only +2.0 letters in the ranibizumab-treated initial group vs. −11.8 in the other two groups. These results might be difficult to interpret since many confounders might not be controlled.

20.3.2 Additional Analyses from CATT and IVAN

Analysis of pooled data [29] between CATT and IVAN could be considered as another post hoc analysis since the data from both trials, albeit were from relatively similar inclusion and exclusion criteria, should not be combined together as a group for analysis. These pooled data, however, might demonstrate some trends. Pooled bevacizumab ($n = 629$) was shown to be non-inferior to pooled ranibizumab ($n = 666$) with the mean difference of BCVA of −1.15 letters (95% CI −2.82 to 0.51). In addition, the pooled PRN regimen ($n = 775$) was found to be inferior to the pooled monthly regimen ($n = 522$) with the mean difference of −2.23 letters (95% CI −3.93 to −0.53).

Based on data from CATT alone, there are at least 40 published papers on additional post hoc analyses. Among these are analyses of baseline characteristics, newly defined associated features, such as subretinal hyperreflective material (SHRM) [56] and hyperreflective foci on OCT [57], angiographic cystoid macular edema

(CME) [58], retinal angiomatous proliferation (RAP) [56], or genetic risk factors [59].

20.3.2.1 Development of Geographic Atrophy (GA) in CATT and IVAN

Among the 1011 participants who did not have GA at baseline and had follow-up images gradable for GA in CATT, the cumulative incidence was 12% at 1 year, 17% at 2 years, and 38% at 5 years. Older age, hypercholesterolemia, worse initial visual acuity, larger CNV area, retinal angiomatous proliferation (RAP) lesion, GA in the fellow eye, and intraretinal fluid were associated with a higher risk of incidence of GA. GA in the fellow eye, subretinal hemorrhage, and absence of subretinal pigment epithelium fluid at baseline were associated with a higher growth rate. Thicker subretinal tissue complex and presence of subretinal fluid were associated with less GA development. Eyes treated with ranibizumab in the first 2 years had a higher growth rate than bevacizumab (adjusted growth rate, 0.38 vs. 0.28 mm/year; $p = 0.009$) [60].

Both the use of ranibizumab and bevacizumab monthly treatment was associated with an increased rate of development of GA. At the end of year 2, eyes treated with ranibizumab had a higher incidence of GA (21% vs. 17%; $p = 0.02$) [61]. on contrary, post hoc of IVAN showed the incidence was similar to both agents (28% vs. 31%; $p = 0.46$) [29]. This seemed to decrease the likelihood of ranibizumab on development of GA more often than bevacizumab. The association of monthly treatment with an increased rate of development of GA might be more consistent. At the end of year 2 of CATT and IVAN, eyes that received monthly treatment were more likely to demonstrate GA than those receiving PRN (24% vs. 15%; $p = 0.003$ in CATT and 34% vs. 26%; $p = 0.03$ in IVAN). In HARBOR, eyes received monthly ranibizumab also showed a higher incidence of GA compared with PRN (hazard ratio, 1.3; 95% CI 1.0–1.7) [62]. The association between GA and the number of anti-VEGF injections raised initially by CATT and IVAN post hoc analyses prompted many investigators to investigate this relationship which has not yet been concluded with strong evidence.

20.3.2.2 Macular Morphology and Visual Acuity in CATT

In another study on macular morphology and visual acuity in CATT which were published sequentially based on the data in year one, two, and five, it was found that associations between VA and morphologic features previously identified in year 1 were maintained or strengthened at year 5 [63]. New foveal scar, CNV, intraretinal fluid, SHRM and retinal thinning, development or worsening of foveal GA, and increased lesion size are important contributors to VA decline from years 2 to 5.

20.3.2.3 Five-Year CATT

Another pivotal post hoc analysis from CATT was a report on 5-year results [64]. This report included 647 of 914 (70.8%) living patients with an average follow-up of 5.5 years (the interval of 4.3–85 months) who were still in the trial until year 5. However, if we include patients who did not participate for 5-year follow-up ($n = 203$) and patients who died after the CATT trials ended ($n = 203$), 57.9% of patients from the original trial participated and most of them (91.3%) continued to have eye care at a CATT center after release from the trial.

Despite the limitation of high patient dropout, which is common in long-term research, the investigators could report the overall results of both ranibizumab and bevacizumab together, without comparison between drugs and dosing regimens. It was found that BCVA of the follow-up patients decreased 3 letters from baseline and 11 letters from year 2. On the other hand, 50% of these patients had VA 20/40 or better, whereas only 20% had VA of 20/200 or worse and almost 10% had VA of 20/20. The investigators found further that these patients were 2 years younger, had VA that was 3 letters better at baseline, and had VA that was 5 letters better at 2 years compared with patients who did not return. The decrease vision was found to be accompanied by expansion of the size of the total neovascular complex comprising neovascularization, scarring, and atrophy and by persistence of fluid on OCT.

20.3.3 Additional Analyses from VIEW 1 and VIEW 2 Studies

20.3.3.1 Secondary Outcome of Year 1 VIEW Studies: NEI VFQ-25

The assessment of vision-related quality of life using the 25-item National Eye Institute Visual Function Questionnaire (NEI VFQ-25) is common in clinical trials of CNV-AMD. This assessment is a descriptive study and interpretation of scores from NEI VFQ-25 is straightforward.

In VIEW 1 and 2, the NEI VFQ-25 assessments [65] were conducted by trained interviewers who were masked to treatment arm at the screening visit, and at weeks 12, 24, 36, and 52. Among the four arms of treatment in VIEW 1 and 2, the investigators chose to compare the NEI VFQ-25 subscale scores between aflibercept A2q8 and ranibizumab R0.5q4 as primary outcome.

Baseline NEI VFQ-25 scores were similar in both VIEW studies although the questionnaire was administered by phone in VIEW 1 and face to face in VIEW 2. Mean change from baseline to 52 weeks was similar for ranibizumab R0.5q4 and aflibercept A2q8 across all 12 subscales. Improvement of 4 points or more was observed in both treatments, and in both studies for subscales near vision, distance vision, role difficulties, and dependency.

20.3.3.2 Post Hoc Analysis of Year 1 VIEW Studies: Persistent Fluid at 3 Months

A total of 1815 eyes (75% of the original studies) were analyzed to find an association between early persistent retinal fluid after 3 initial injections and the effect of aflibercept or ranibizumab on visual outcomes [66]. The analysis included patients with known retinal fluid status at baseline and weeks 4, 8, and 12 in the three treatment arms: ranibizumab R0.5q4 ($n = 595$), aflibercept A2q4 ($n = 613$), and A2q8 ($n = 607$) after 3 monthly injections. The proportion of eyes with persistent fluid was approximately 20% in each arm. In these eyes, mean BCVA gain from baseline to week 52 was greater in A2q4 compared with Rq4 ($p < 0.01$) and A2q8 ($p < 0.05$), whereas the statistical difference was not found between Rq4 and A2q8 ($p = 0.294$). In eyes without persistent fluid, BCVA changes were similar across treatment groups.

20.3.3.3 Visual Outcome of Year 2 VIEW Studies

During year 2, the dosing intervals in all treatment arms were changed to a common regimen of modified quarterly dosing with respect to their originally randomized dose and drug (all patients were monitored monthly and received a minimum of dosing every 12 weeks with interim PRN monthly injections) [67]. The results of the second-year data revealed 81.6–85.7% patient retention in all groups. This retention rate might be high enough to uphold enough power to identify statistical significance of these second-year data. Comparable visual acuity maintenance (91–92%) was found in each arm at week 96. The total number of active injections (from baseline to week 96) was 16.0–16.2 in the two original monthly aflibercept groups, 16.5 in the original R0.5q4, and 11.2 in the original A2q8 arm. The finding showed that visual acuity maintenance could be achieved for up to 96 weeks in the A2q8 arm with similar gains in BCVA compared with ranibizumab despite more than five fewer injections.

20.3.3.4 Subgroup Analysis on Final Visual Outcomes of Year 2 VIEW Studies

The investigators classified the patients who completed week 96 follow-up into four groups [68]. They were (1) patients who lost more than 5 letters from week 52 to week 96, (2) patients who at week 96 lost more than 5 letters from the previous best BCVA time point, (3) patients who received the scheduled treatment of 3 injections during week 52–96, and (4) patients who lost 5 letters or more at two consecutive visits from week 52 to 96 and received active treatment at that second visit.

It was found that the patterns of response to treatment of these four groups during the first year were indistinguishable. At week 96, patients in Group 1 had the worst final BCVA, fell to be lower than baseline, among the four groups. Patients in Group 3 had the best final BCVA, which was maintained from week 52 despite having the least number of injections. Patients in Group 4, despite having the greatest number of treatments among the four groups, did not regain final BCVA up to the level at week 52 as Group 3. This post hoc showed that switching from monthly to PRN during weeks 52–96 might have created the different patterns of response among patients. Data from VIEW 1 and 2 themselves might not explain these patterns. These post hoc analyses revealed certain groups of patients that warranted future studies.

20.3.4 Interim Analysis of Secondary Outcome of Ranibizumab Versus Aflibercept in T&E: RIVAL Study

RIVAL study [69] was a recent RCT designed to compare treatment with ranibizumab and aflibercept for the development of geographic atrophy (GA) in nAMD patients. The primary objective was the mean change in area of macular atrophy from baseline to month 24 and safety results. The recently published paper showed interim analysis at 12 months for the secondary endpoints as BCVA gain and number of injections.

The head-to-head comparison between ranibizumab and aflibercept in RIVAL was in T&E regimen. The criteria to determine treatment interval were a loss of visual acuity of 5 or more letters from the baseline, a new retinal hemorrhage, and retinal fluid. Injection interval was every 4 weeks and it was extended by 2 weeks until maximum 12 weeks if there was no disease activity defined to determine treatment interval as above. The interval was reduced for 2 weeks with any sign of disease activity. If two or more disease activities were found during the T&E period, the interval was reset to 4 weeks. At month 12, the change of BCVA from baseline was statistically significant in either ranibizumab or aflibercept, but no difference of BCVA change from baseline between both groups (letter score difference 2.3; 95% CI −0.1 to 4.7; $p = 0.06$) and no difference in the number of injection (rate ratio = 1.00; 95% CI 1.0–1.1; $p = 0.86$) at month 12.

20.4 Safety Data

According to CATT 2-year data, the rates of death were 5.3% in ranibizumab and 6.1% in bevacizumab ($p = 0.60$). The proportion of patients with one or more systemic serious adverse events was higher with bevacizumab than ranibizumab (39.9% vs. 31.7%; adjusted risk ratio, 1.30; 95% CI 1.07–1.57; $p = 0.009$) [28]. According to IVAN 2-year data, the atherothrombotic events were not different among all treatment arms. The mortality rate was found to be lower with monthly than as-needed treatment (OR 0.47, 95% CI 0.22–1.03; $p = 0.05$) with no difference between drug groups (OR 0.96, 95% CI 0.46–2.02; $p = 0.91$) [29]. Pooled estimates from both IVAN and CATT of safety outcomes showed no difference by drugs for deaths and atherothrombotic events. However, bevacizumab treatment might increase the risk of any systemic adverse events ($p = 0.008$) [29].

With longer follow-up at 5 years, data from CATT showed that 7.6% of patients who completed the follow-up and originally assigned to ranibizumab had an atherothrombotic event compared with 4.5% of bevacizumab ($p = 0.04$) [64]. There was no new safety concern reported in clinical trials of newer anti-VEGF agents, such as aflibercept [7] and brolucizumab [44].

Based on the systematic review, available information on the adverse effects of each medication, ranibizumab, aflibercept, did not suggest a higher incidence of potentially vision-threatening complications compared with controls; however, clinical trial sample sizes were not sufficient to estimate differences in rare safety outcomes [2]. The systematic review of conbercept showed the incidence of adverse events in patients receiving conbercept was significantly lower than those receiving triamcinolone acetonide (RR = 0.25, 95% CI 0.09–0.72), but was similar to the other therapies [43]. There were a few recent case reports on brolucizumab-associated retinal vasculitis.

20.5 Failed Clinical Trials of CNV-AMD

We may judge the word "failed clinical trials" in at least two ways. On a statistical standpoint, some trials may fail because they cannot reject the null hypothesis. On clinical standpoint, some trials may fail, even though they can reject the null hypothesis and the alternate hypothesis can be accepted, because the statistical significance is not clinically meaningful.

20.5.1 Combination Therapy

FOCUS [55] was conducted to assess the combination of PDT with ranibizumab monthly injections in CNV-AMD compared with PDT alone. At month 24, 25% of patients in combined treatment group had gained >15 letters (vs 7% for PDT alone; $p = 0.006$), and the two treatment groups differed by 12.4 letters in mean VA change ($p < 0.001$). Furthermore, the combined group exhibited less lesion growth, greater reduction of CNV leakage, reduction of subretinal fluid accumulation, and required fewer PDT re-treatments. It was clear from FOCUS that the combination therapy was superior to PDT alone.

MONT BLANC [70] assessed whether combination of PDT and ranibizumab in PRN regimen was non-inferior to ranibizumab PRN monotherapy. At 12 months, the mean change in BCVA from baseline was +2.5 and + 4.4 letters in the combination arm and monotherapy arm respectively with 95% CI, −5.76 to 1.86; the lower limit was greater than the present −7 letters of non-inferiority margin. This study achieved the primary endpoint. However, it was the secondary endpoint, the number of ranibizumab injections, which failed the combination therapy to be applied for CNV-AMD in the real world. It was shown that the combination might not decrease treatment burden from the monotherapy. Patients received 4.8 ranibizumab injections in the combination arm vs. 5.1 injections in the monotherapy arm over 12 months; the mean number of ranibizumab retreatments was 1.9 in the combination arm and 2.2 in the monotherapy arm ($p = 0.1373$).

DENALI study [71] assessed the efficacy and safety of PDT in either standard fluence (SF) or reduced fluence (RF) combined with ranibizumab PRN regimen vs. ranibizumab monotherapy in monthly regimen. Mean BCVA change at month 12 was +5.3 and + 4.4 letters in PDT-SF plus ranibizumab and PDT-RF plus ranibizumab, respectively, compared with +8.1 letters with ranibizumab monotherapy. Non-inferiority of either combination regimen to monthly ranibizumab monotherapy (97.5% CI, 7.90 to infinity; $p = 0.0666$ for PDT-SF plus and 97.5% CI, 8.51 to infinity; $p = 0.1178$ for PDT-RF plus) was not demonstrated.

The lessons learned from these trials of combination therapy was that MONT BLANC could reject the null hypothesis, but analysis of secondary outcome did not provide clinically meaningful data. On the other hand, DELANI could not even reject the null hypothesis. The combination therapy did not gain popularity in real-world treatment of CNV-AMD.

20.5.2 Fixed Quarterly Dosing Regimen

PIER study [72] was a 24-month RCT evaluating ranibizumab with fixed quarterly regimen for patients with CNV-AMD. The two doses, 0.3 and 0.5 mg, were compared with sham injection. Ranibizumab was initially administered monthly for 3 doses, then switched to every 3 months (quarterly dosing). The results from the first 12 months revealed that the treatment effect declined during quarterly dosing.

The protocols were subsequently revised in the following year to have eligible patients in the sham group cross over to 0.5 mg ranibizumab quarterly and all eligible randomized patients cross over to 0.5 mg ranibizumab monthly. At month 24, visual acuity decreased even further at the mean of 2.2, and 2.3 letters from baseline in the original 0.3 mg and 0.5 mg groups and decreased at the mean of

21.4 letters from baseline in the sham group, ($p < 0.0001$ for each ranibizumab group vs sham). BCVA of patients in 0.3 mg and 0.5 mg groups who were crossed over to monthly from quarterly dosing increased at the mean of 2.2 and 4.1 letters, respectively. PIER study showed the fixed quarterly was superior to sham but provided visual loss.

EXCITE study [73] was the RCT assessing whether the fixed quarterly dosing was non-inferior to fixed monthly dosing of ranibizumab. Two quarterly dosing regimens, 0.3 mg and 0.5 mg were compared with 0.3 mg monthly regimen. A non-inferiority limit of −6.8 was predetermined based on the results of MARINA in which the value of 6.8 was approximately half of the minimum estimated difference (13.6 which was the lower limit of a 2-sided 95% CI) of the mean change in BCVA from baseline to month 12 between ranibizumab 0.3 mg and sham injection.

The results of EXCITE showed that in per-protocol analysis, BCVA increased from baseline to month 12 by +4.9, +3.8, and + 8.3 letters in 0.3 mg quarterly, 0.5 mg quarterly and the monthly group with 95% CI −7.1 to −0.2 and −7.9 to −0.7 when both quarterly dosing arms were compared with monthly arm. In the intention-to-treat analysis, mean BCVA improvement were + 4.0, +2.8, and + 8.0 letters and the 95% CIs are −7.7 to −0.9 and −8.6 to −1.7, for the same comparisons in PP analysis, respectively. The non-inferiority of the quarterly dosings was not reached in this study.

PIER and EXCITE have given quarterly dosing the same fate as MONT BLANC and DELANI had given to combination therapy.

20.5.3 Failed Phase III Trials

There were a few clinical trials on new drugs for treatment of CNV-AMD which demonstrated promising results in phase I and II clinical trials but failed to duplicate the results in the larger following phase III RCTs recently.

Of the three recently failed phase III RCTs of new drugs for AMD over the past 2 years, there were two for CNV-AMD: fovista and squalamine eye drop. Fovista is an inhibitor of platelet-derived growth factor (PDGF), which was studied in combination with anti-VEGF for the treatment of CNV-AMD [74, 75]. Another failed phase III trial was from the study of lampalizumab for treatment of GA [76].

In the phase II study of fovista, a total of 449 eyes with "classic-containing" CNV-AMD were randomized 1:1:1 among 3 monthly treatment arms: 0.3 mg fovista combined with ranibizumab, 1.5 mg fovista combined with ranibizumab, and ranibizumab alone. The primary outcome, change in visual acuity at 24 weeks, strongly supported a treatment benefit from combination of 1.5 mg fovista and ranibizumab over ranibizumab alone. However, it was found that there was a substantial imbalance in clinical characteristics, such as lesion sizes, between the groups in phase II data. Despite this, instead of adherence to the phase II protocol in phase III trial of fovista, the investigators decided to change the inclusion criteria to include eyes with subretinal hyper-reflective material (SHRM)-containing CNV, instead of classic-containing CNV, in the phase III trial. This decision was based on a subgroup analysis of the phase II trial showing CNV associated with SHRM, regardless of the presence of the classic component, responded best to fovista combined with ranibizumab. It was very likely that this protocol change might not allow the results from the phase II trial to be carried over into the phase III trial. This is a lesson learned for investigators of clinical trial [74].

In the phase II trial of topical squalamine, all types of treatment-naïve CNV-AMD were randomized to receive a ranibizumab injection at baseline followed by topical squalamine twice a day or vehicle drops twice a day. All eyes then received as-needed monthly injections of ranibizumab. After 36 weeks, better visual acuity was found in the arm receiving topical squalamine. However, according to pre-specified subgroup analysis, an even greater visual benefit was found in eyes with classic-containing lesions and eyes with any occult CNV measuring less than 10 mm^2. The protocol in the phase III trial was then changed, according to these positive outcomes, to include eyes with any occult CNV measuring less than 10 mm^2 (ClinicalTrials.gov Identifier: NCT02727881). This phase III trial of topical squalamine followed the same fate as the trial of fovista. It failed to replicate the results of the subgroup analysis of the phase II trial. Another lesson learned [74, 77].

20.6 Real-World Clinical Trials

Clinical trials are almost always conducted in an ideal situation when most variables are controlled to prevent bias and confounding factors. The situation in clinical trials is rarely found in the real world. In fact, it is the real world where we would like to apply the results from clinical trials for treating our patients. A gap between real-world evidence and clinical trial evidence always exists [78]. The gap has increasingly caused one of the frequently asked questions in clinical practice: Can the drugs in clinical trials achieve similar efficacy in the real world? This question may be answered by studies conducted in the real world.

There was a study claimed to be the first real-world study on head-to-head comparison between ranibizumab and aflibercept in fixed dosing regimen for both drugs (three loading monthly injections followed by bimonthly injections) [79]. However, this study was not RCT but a single-center, retrospective, comparative, and nonrandomized study. The retrospective nature of data revealed discrepancy in the number of patients and age between the two groups. The results showed that the aflibercept arm had better BCVA, approximately 1–4 letters, and also better CRT improvement than ranibizumab at every time point. Could this occur because of the suboptimal dosing (bimonthly) of ranibizumab group or because of the older age of the patients in this group? It might be difficult to answer from data in this study in which there were no actual controls.

In another study of real-world evidence, treatment of CNV-AMD by ranibizumab and aflibercept was compared from observational database [69]. This study, however, tried to overcome limitation of retrospective nature of real-world data by matching baseline characteristics, such as VA, lesion size, and lesion type, between the eyes received the two agents. The investigators adapted principles in the design of RCT into this observational data, such as identifying zero time for determination of patient eligibility and baseline features. They also used intention-to-treat analysis as in the RCT.

The investigators found significant BCVA improvement of both treatment groups, +3.7 and + 4.3 letters for ranibizumab and aflibercept respectively at 12 months with a similar number of injections. These results supported data from some observational case series that the efficacy in the real world was somehow lower than the efficacy in RCTs in which improvement of more than 5 letters was relatively common. The investigators found further that there was a low rate of switching treatment between the two agents. However, once it occurred, there was more switching from ranibizumab to aflibercept than vice versa. This might also reflect real-world impression that aflibercept might have higher efficacy than ranibizumab and the switching should be performed from the agent with a lower efficacy.

This latter study, although based on retrospective data as the former study, demonstrated how we could conduct a clinical trial by using real-world data in more reliable ways to yield stronger evidence.

20.7 Future Directions

The ongoing clinical trials of CNV-AMD are investigating on some new anti-VEGF agents [80, 81], port delivery system [82], gene therapy [83, 84], etc. Some of these trials aim to decrease treatment burden by lowering number of treatments, some aim to increase magnitude of visual improvement or to be alternatives to the current anti-VEGF agents. Proving these new modalities effective in real-world practice may be a long way to go. The first steps for achieving this goal, however, still count on well-designed, well-conducted, and well-interpreted clinical trials.

References

1. Özkiris A. Anti-VEGF agents for age-related macular degeneration. Expert Opin Ther Pat. 2010;20(1):103–18.

2. Solomon SD, Lindsley K, Vedula SS, Krzystolik MG, Hawkins BS. Anti-vascular endothelial growth factor for neovascular age-related macular degeneration. Cochrane Database Syst Rev. 2019;3:1–123.
3. Guo MY, Cheng J, Etminan M, Zafari Z, Maberley D. One year effectiveness study of intravitreal aflibercept in neovascular age-related macular degeneration: a meta-analysis. Acta Ophthalmol. 2019;97(1):e1–7.
4. Li J, Xu J, Chen Y, Zhang J, Cao Y, Lu P. Efficacy comparison of intravitreal anti-VEGF therapy for three subtypes of neovascular age-related macular degeneration: a systematic review and meta-analysis. J Ophthalmol. 2018;2018:1–10.
5. Kovach JL, Schwartz SG, Flynn HW, Scott IU. Anti-VEGF treatment strategies for wet AMD. J Ophthalmol. 2012;2012:1–7.
6. Wykoff CC, Clark WL, Nielsen JS, Brill JV, Greene LS, Heggen CL. Optimizing anti-VEGF treatment outcomes for patients with neovascular age-related macular degeneration. J Manag Care Spec Pharm. 2018;24(2-a):S3–15.
7. Schmidt-Erfurth UM, Richard G, Augustin A, Aylward WG, Bandello F, Corcòstegui B, et al. Guidance for the treatment of neovascular age-related macular degeneration. Acta Ophthalmol Scand. 2007;85(5):486–94.
8. Macular Photocoagulation Study Group. Laser photocoagulation of subfoveal neovascular lesions of age-related macular degeneration updated findings from two clinical trials. Arch Ophthalmol. 1993;111:1200–9.
9. Al Jundi A, Sakka S. Protocol writing in clinical research. J Clin Diagn Res. 2016;10(11):ZE10–3.
10. Dawn Teare M, Dimairo M, Shephard N, Hayman A, Whitehead A, Walters SJ. Sample size requirements to estimate key design parameters from external pilot randomised controlled trials: a simulation study. Trials. 2014;15:264.
11. Macular Photocoagulation Study Group. Subfoveal neovascular lesions in age-related macular degeneration. Guidelines for evaluation and treatment in the macular photocoagulation study. Macular photocoagulation study group. Arch Ophthalmol. 1991;109(9):1242–57.
12. TAP study group. Photodynamic therapy of subfoveal choroidal neovascularization in age-related macular degeneration with verteporfin: two-year results of 2 randomized clinical trials-tap report 2. Arch Ophthalmol. 1999;117(10):1329–45.
13. VIP study group. Verteporfin therapy of subfoveal choroidal neovascularization in age-related macular degeneration: two-year results of a randomized clinical trial including lesions with occult with no classic choroidal neovascularization—verteporfin in photodynamic therapy. Am J Ophthalmol. 2001;131:541–60.
14. Brown GC, Landy J. Photodynamic therapy of subfoveal choroidal neovascularization in pathologic myopia with verteporfin. Arch Ophthalmol. 2001;119:198–207.
15. Brown DM, Kaiser PK, Michels M, Soubrane G, Heier JS, Kim RY, et al. Ranibizumab versus verteporfin for neovascular age-related macular degeneration. N Engl J Med. 2006;355(14):1432–44.
16. Rosenfeld PJ, Brown DM, Heier JS, Boyer DS, Kaiser PK, Chung CY, et al. Ranibizumab for neovascular age-related macular degeneration. N Engl J Med. 2006;355(14):1419–31.
17. Triantafylla M, Massa HF, Dardabounis D, Gatzioufas Z, Kozobolis V, Ioannakis K, et al. Ranibizumab for the treatment of degenerative ocular conditions. Clin Ophthalmol. 2014;8:1187–98.
18. The CATT Research Group. Ranibizumab and bevacizumab for neovascular age-related macular degeneration. N Engl J Med. 2011;364(20):1897–908.
19. Heier JS, Brown DM, Chong V, Korobelnik JF, Kaiser PK, Nguyen QD, et al. Intravitreal aflibercept (VEGF trap-eye) in wet age-related macular degeneration. Ophthalmology. 2012;119(12):2537–48.
20. Smiddy WE. Economic implications of current age-related macular degeneration treatments. Ophthalmology. 2009;116(3):481–7.
21. Wang B, Wang H, Tu XM, Feng C. Comparisons of superiority, non-inferiority, and equivalence trials. Shanghai Arch Psychiatry. 2017;29(6):385–8.
22. Murray GD. Switching between superiority and non-inferiority switching between superiority and non-inferiority: an introductory note. Br J Clin Pharmacol. 2001;52(3):219.
23. Christensen E. Methodology of superiority vs. equivalence trials and non-inferiority trials. J Hepatol. 2007;46(5):947–54.
24. Schumi J, Wittes JT. Through the looking glass: understanding non-inferiority. Trials. 2011;12:106.
25. Hahn S. Understanding noninferiority trials. Korean J Pediatr. 2012;55(11):403–7.
26. Ferreira-Gonzalez I. Basis for the interpretation of noninferiority studies: considering the ROCKET–AF, RE-LY, and ARISTOTLE studies. Rev Esp Cardiol (Engl Ed). 2014;67(6):432–5.
27. Berg K, Pedersen TR, Sandvik L, Bragadóttir R. Comparison of ranibizumab and bevacizumab for neovascular age-related macular degeneration according to LUCAS treat-and-extend protocol. Ophthalmology. 2015;122(1):146–52.
28. The CATT Research Group, Martin DF, Maguire MG, Fine SL, Ying GS, Jaffe GJ, et al. Ranibizumab and bevacizumab for treatment of neovascular age-related macular degeneration: two-year results. Ophthalmology. 2012;119(7):1388–98.
29. Chakravarthy U, Harding SP, Rogers CA, Downes SM, Lotery AJ, Culliford LA, et al. Alternative treatments to inhibit VEGF in age-related choroidal neovascularisation: 2-year findings of the IVAN randomised controlled trial. Lancet. 2013;382(9900):1258–67.
30. Krebs I, Schmetterer L, Boltz A, Told R, Vécsei-Marlovits V, Egger S, et al. A randomised double-masked trial comparing the visual outcome after treatment with ranibizumab or bevacizumab in patients with neovascular age-related macular degeneration. Br J Ophthalmol. 2013;97(3):266–71.

31. Kodjikian L, Souied EH, Mimoun G, Mauget-Faÿsse M, Behar-Cohen F, Decullier E, et al. Ranibizumab versus bevacizumab for neovascular age-related macular degeneration: results from the GEFAL noninferiority randomized trial. Ophthalmology. 2013;120(11):2300–9.
32. Schauwvlieghe AME, Dijkman G, Hooymans JM, Verbraak FD, Hoyng CB, Dijkgraaf MGW, et al. Comparing the effectiveness of bevacizumab to ranibizumab in patients with exudative age-related macular degeneration. The BRAMD study. PLoS One. 2016;11(5):1–16.
33. Chung C, Pherwani N. Ziv-aflibercept: a novel angiogenesis inhibitor for the treatment of metastatic colorectal cancer. Am J Heal Pharm. 2013;70(21):1887–96.
34. Cheng YD, Yang H, Chen GQ, Zhang ZC. Molecularly targeted drugs for metastatic colorectal cancer. Drug Des Devel Ther. 2013;7:1315–22.
35. Malik D, Tarek M, Del Carpio JC, Ramirez C, Boyer D, Kenney MC, et al. Safety profiles of anti-VEGF drugs: Bevacizumab, ranibizumab, aflibercept and ziv-aflibercept on human retinal pigment epithelium cells in culture. Br J Ophthalmol. 2014;98:11–6.
36. de Oliveira DJ, Badaró E, Novais E, Colicchio D, Chiarantin G, Matioli M, et al. Preclinical investigations of intravitreal ziv-aflibercept. Ophthalmic Surg Lasers Imaging Retina. 2014;45(6):577–84.
37. de Oliveira DJ, de Andrade G, Kniggendorf V, Novais E, Maia A, Meyer C, et al. Clinical and electrophysiological evaluation after intravitreal ziv-aflibercept for exudative age-related macular degeneration. Ophthalmologica. 2017;37(8):1499–507.
38. de Oliveira D, de Andrade G, Kniggendorf V, Novais E, Takahashi VKL, Maia A, et al. Intravitreal Ziv-aflibercept for neovascular age-related macular degeneration: 52-week results. Retina. 2019;39:648–55.
39. Mansour AM, Charbaji A, Farah ME, Mansour HA, Chhablani J. Long-term outcome of treat and extend intravitreal ziv-aflibercept therapy. Br J Ophthalmol. 2018;103:1–4.
40. Jørstad ØK, Faber RT, Moe MC. Two-year functional and anatomical results after converting treatment resistant eyes with exudative age-related macular degeneration to aflibercept in accordance with a treat and extend protocol. Acta Ophthalmol. 2017;95(5):460–3.
41. Baghi A, Jabbarpoor Bonyadi MH, Ramezani A, Azarmina M, Moradian S, Dehghan MH, et al. Two doses of intravitreal Ziv-Aflibercept versus bevacizumab in treatment of diabetic macular edema: a three-armed. Double-blind randomized trial. Ophthalmol Retina. 2016;1(2):103–10.
42. Liu K, Song Y, Xu G, Ye J, Wu Z, Liu X, et al. Conbercept for treatment of neovascular age-related macular degeneration: results of the randomized phase 3 PHOENIX study. Am J Ophthalmol. 2019;197:156–67.
43. Zhang J, Liang Y, Xie J, Li D, Hu Q, Li X, et al. Conbercept for patients with age-related macular degeneration: a systematic review. BMC Ophthalmol. 2018;18(1):1–12.
44. Dugel PU, Koh A, Ogura Y, Jaffe G, Schmidt-Erfurth U, Brown D, et al. HAWK and HARRIER: phase 3, multicenter, randomized, double-masked trials of brolucizumab for neovascular age-related macular degeneration. Ophthalmology. 2020;127:72–84.
45. Singerman LJ, Weichselberger A, Sallstig P. OSPREY trial: randomized, active-controlled, phase II study to evaluate safety and efficacy of RTH258, a humanized single-chain anti-VEGF antibody fragment, in patients with neovascular AMD. Investig Ophthalmol Vis Sci. 2015;56
46. Csaky KG. A variable-dosing regimen with intravitreal ranibizumab for neovascular age-related macular degeneration: year 2 of the PrONTO study: comment. Evidence-Based Ophthalmol. 2010;11(1):26–7.
47. Holz FG, Amoaku W, Donate J, Guymer RH. Safety and efficacy of a flexible dosing regimen of ranibizumab in neovascular age-related macular degeneration. Ophthalmology. 2010;118(4):663–71.
48. Busbee BG, Ho AC, Brown DM, Heier JS, Suñer IJ, Li Z, et al. Twelve-month efficacy and safety of 0.5 mg or 2.0 mg ranibizumab in patients with subfoveal neovascular age-related macular degeneration. Ophthalmology. 2013;120(5):1046–56.
49. Wykoff CC, Croft DE, Brown DM, Wang R, Payne JF, Clark L, et al. Prospective trial of treat-and-extend versus monthly dosing for neovascular age-related macular degeneration elated macular degeneration TREX-AMD 1-year results. Ophthalmology. 2015;122:2514–22.
50. Gillies MC, Nguyen V, Daien V, Arnold JJ, Morlet N, Barthelmes D. Twelve-month outcomes of ranibizumab vs. aflibercept for neovascular age-related macular degeneration: data from an observational study. Ophthalmology. 2016;123(12):2545–53.
51. Silva R, Berta A, Larsen M, Macfadden W, Feller C, Monés J. Treat-and-extend versus monthly regimen in neovascular age-related macular degeneration: results with ranibizumab from the TREND study. Ophthalmology. 2018;125(1):57–65.
52. Freemantle N. Interpreting the results of secondary end points and subgroup analyses in clinical trials: should we lock the crazy aunt in the attic? Br Med J. 2001;322(7292):989–91.
53. Fridman M, Erder MH. Interpreting the results of a retrospective comparison of test and reference treatments in a randomized clinical trial setting. Clin Drug Investig. 2014;35(2):133–40.
54. Singer MA, Awh CC, Sadda S, Freeman WR. HORIZON: an open-label extension trial of ranibizumab for choroidal neovascularization secondary to age-related macular degeneration. Ophthalmology. 2012;119(6):1175–83.
55. Heier JS, Boyer DS, Ciulla TA, Ferrone PJ, Jumper JM, Gentile RC, et al. Ranibizumab combined with verteporfin photodynamic therapy in neovascular age-related macular degeneration: year 2 results of the FOCUS study. Arch Ophthalmol. 2006;124(11):1532–42.
56. Daniel E, Shaffer J, Ying GS, Grunwald JE, Martin DF, Jaffe GJ, et al. Outcomes in eyes with retinal angiomatous proliferation in the comparison of

age-related macular degeneration treatments trials (CATT). Ophthalmology. 2016;123(3):609–16.
57. Willoughby AS, Ying GS, Toth CA, Maguire MG, Burns RE, Grunwald JE, et al. Subretinal hyperreflective material in the comparison of age-related macular degeneration treatments trials. Ophthalmology. 2015;122(9):1846–1853.e5.
58. Shah N, Maguir MG, Martin DF, Shaffer J, Ying G-S, Grunwald JE, et al. Angiographic cystoid macular edema and outcomes in the comparison of age-related macular degeneration treatments trials (CATT). J Autism Dev Disord. 2017;47(3):549–62.
59. Hagstrom SA, Ying GS, Pauer GJT, Sturgill-Short GM, Huang J, Callanan DG, et al. Pharmacogenetics for genes associated with age-related macular degeneration in the comparison of AMD treatments trials (CATT). Ophthalmology. 2013;120(3):593–9.
60. Grunwald JE, Daniel E, Huang J, Ying GS, Maguire MG, Toth CA, et al. Risk of geographic atrophy in the comparison of age-related macular degeneration treatments trials. Ophthalmology. 2014;121(1):150–61.
61. Grunwald JE, Pistilli M, Daniel E, Ying GS, Pan W, Jaffe GJ, et al. Incidence and growth of geographic atrophy during 5 years of comparison of age-related macular degeneration treatments trials. Ophthalmology. 2017;124(1):97–104.
62. Ho AC, Busbee BG, Regillo CD, Wieland MR, Van Everen SA, Li Z, et al. Twenty-four-month efficacy and safety of 0.5 mg or 2.0 mg ranibizumab in patients with subfoveal neovascular age-related macular degeneration. Ophthalmology. 2014;121(11):2181–92.
63. Sharma S, Toth CA, Daniel E, Grunwald JE, Maguire MG, Ying GS, et al. Macular morphology and visual acuity in the second year of the comparison of age-related macular degeneration treatments trials. Ophthalmology. 2016;123(4):865–75.
64. Maguire MG, Martin DF, Shuang YG, Jaffe GJ, Daniel E, et al. Five-year outcomes with anti–vascular endothelial growth factor treatment of neovascular age-related macular degeneration: the comparison of age-related macular degeneration treatments trials. Ophthalmology. 2016;123(8):1751–61.
65. Yuzawa M, Fujita K, Wittrup-Jensen KU, Norenberg C, Zeitz O, Adachi K, et al. Improvement in vision-related function with intravitreal aflibercept: data from phase 3 studies in wet age-related macular degeneration. Ophthalmology. 2015;122(3):571–8.
66. Jaffe GJ, Kaiser PK, Thompson D, Gibson A, Saroj N, Vitti R, et al. Differential response to anti-VEGF regimens in age-related macular degeneration patients with early persistent retinal fluid. Ophthalmology. 2016;123(9):1856–64.
67. Schmidt-Erfurth U, Kaiser PK, Korobelnik J-F, Brown DM, Chong V, Nguyen QD, et al. Intravitreal aflibercept injection for neovascular age-related macular degeneration: ninety-six-week results of the VIEW studies. Ophthalmology. 2014;121(1):193–201.
68. Richard G, Monés J, Wolf S, Korobelnik JF, Guymer R, Goldstein M, et al. Scheduled versus pro re Nata dosing in the VIEW trials. Ophthalmology. 2015;122(12):2497–503.
69. Gillies MC, Hunyor AP, Arnold JJ, Guymer RH, Wolf S, Ng P, et al. Effect of ranibizumab and aflibercept on best-corrected visual acuity in treat-and-extend for neovascular age-related macular degeneration: a randomized clinical trial. JAMA Ophthalmol. 2019;137(4):372–9.
70. Larsen M, Schmidt-Erfurth U, Lanzetta P, Wolf S, Simader C, Tokaji E, et al. MONT BLANC study group. Verteporfin plus ranibizumab for choroidal neovascularization in age-related macular degeneration: twelve-month MONT BLANC study results. Ophthalmology. 2012;119(5):992–1000.
71. Kaiser PK, Boyer DS, Cruess AF, Slakter JS, Pilz S, Weisberger A, DENALI Study Group. Verteporfin plus ranibizumab for choroidal neovascularization in age-related macular degeneration: twelve-month results of the DENALI study. Ophthalmology. 2012;119(5):1001–10.
72. Abraham P, Yue H, Wilson L. Randomized, double-masked, sham-controlled trial of ranibizumab for neovascular age-related macular degeneration: PIER study year 2. Am J Ophthalmol. 2010;150(3):239–48.
73. Schmidt-Erfurth U, Eldem B, Guymer R, Korobelnik J-F, Schlingemann RO, Axer-Siegel R, et al. Efficacy and safety of monthly versus quarterly ranibizumab treatment in neovascular age-related macular degeneration: the EXCITE study. Ophthalmology. 2010;118(5):831–9.
74. Rosenfeld PJ, Feuer WJ. Lessons from recent phase III trial failures: don't design phase III trials based on retrospective subgroup analyses from phase II trials. Ophthalmology. 2018;125(10):1488–91.
75. Dunn EN, Hariprasad SM, Sheth VS. An overview of the fovista and rinucumab trials and the fate of anti-PDGF medications. Ophthalmic Surg Lasers Imaging Retina. 2017;48(2):100–4.
76. Holz FG, Sadda SR, Busbee B, Chew EY, Mitchell P, Tufail A, et al. Efficacy and safety of lampalizumab for geographic atrophy due to age-related macular degeneration: Chroma and spectri phase 3 randomized clinical trials. JAMA Ophthalmol. 2018;136(6):666–77.
77. Wroblewski JJ, Hu AY. Topical squalamine 0.2% and intravitreal ranibizumab 0.5 mg as combination therapy for macular edema due to branch and central retinal vein occlusion: an open-label, randomized study. Ophthalmic Surg Lasers Imaging Retina. 2016;47(10):914–23.
78. Kim HS, Lee S, Kim JH. Real-world evidence versus randomized controlled trial: clinical research based on electronic medical records. J Korean Med Sci. 2018;33(34):1–7.
79. Providência J, Rodrigues TM, Oliveira M, Bernardes J, Marques JP, Murta J, et al. Real-world results of aflibercept versus ranibizumab for the treatment of exudative AMD using a fixed regimen. Biomed Res Int. 2018;2018:1–7.
80. Callanan D, Kunimoto D, Maturi RK, Patel SS, Staurenghi G, Wolf S, et al. Double-masked, randomized, phase 2 evaluation of abicipar pegol (an anti-VEGF DARPin therapeutic) in neovascular age-related macular degeneration. J Ocul Pharmacol Ther. 2018;34(10):700–9.

81. Graybug Vision I. GB-102 and GB-103 [Internet]. 2019. Available from: https://graybug.com/pipeline/gb-102-gb-103/
82. Campochiaro PA, Marcus DM, Awh CC, Regillo C, Adamis AP, Bantseev V, Chiang Y, Ehrlich JS, Erickson S, Hanley WD, Horvath J, Maass KF, Singh N, Tang F, Barteselli G. The port delivery system with ranibizumab for neovascular age-related macular degeneration: results from the randomized phase 2 ladder clinical trial. Ophthalmology. 2019;126:1141–54.
83. Rockville M. REGENXBIO Reports First Quarter 2019 Financial and Operating Results and Additional Positive Interim Phase I/IIa Trial Update for RGX-314 for the Treatment of Wet AMD [Internet]. 2019. Available from: https://www.pharmiweb.com/press-release/2019-05-07/regenxbio-reports-first-quarter-2019-financial-and-operating-results-and-additional-positive-interim
84. Kirkner RM. Wet AMD gene therapy shows promise Phase I/IIa results of RGX-314 confirm protein uptake over months [Internet]. 2019. Available from: https://www.retina-specialist.com/article/wet-amd-gene-therapy-shows-promise

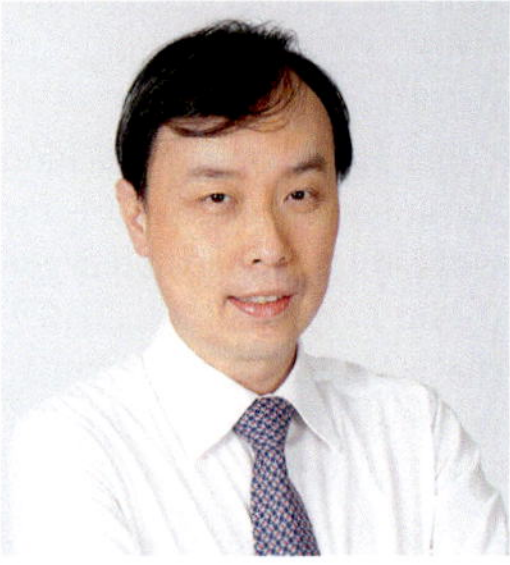

Dr. Paisan Ruamviboonsuk is the Scientific Secretary of Asia-Pacific Vitreo-Retina Society and a council member of the Asia-Pacific Academy of Ophthalmology (APAO). He is the Immediate Past President of the Royal College of Ophthalmologists of Thailand and the Past President of Thai Retina Society. He is well recognized internationally and received many important international awards, including the United Nations Public Service Award for Prevention of Diabetic Blindness Project in Thailand, APAO Arthur Lim Award, American Academy of Ophthalmology Achievement Award.

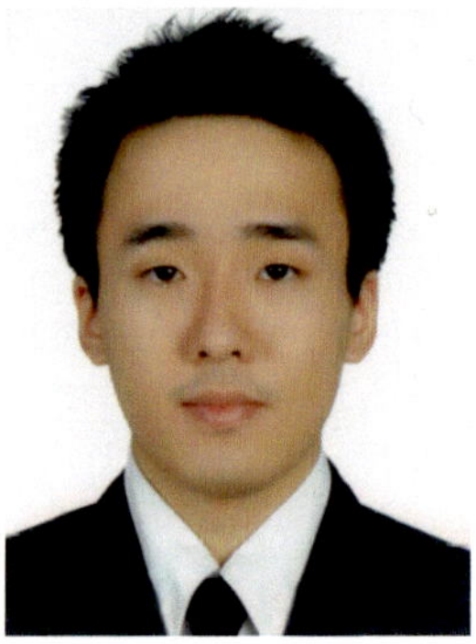

Dr. Peranut Chotcomwongse is currently a resident of ophthalmology at the Department of Ophthalmology, Rajavithi Hospital, Bangkok. He worked in EVEREST Study, a randomized controlled trial for polypoidal choroidal vasculopathy. His published studies are on artificial intelligence for detection of optical coherent tomography-based centered-involved diabetic macular edema from color fundus photography and for classifying diabetic retinopathy severity levels.

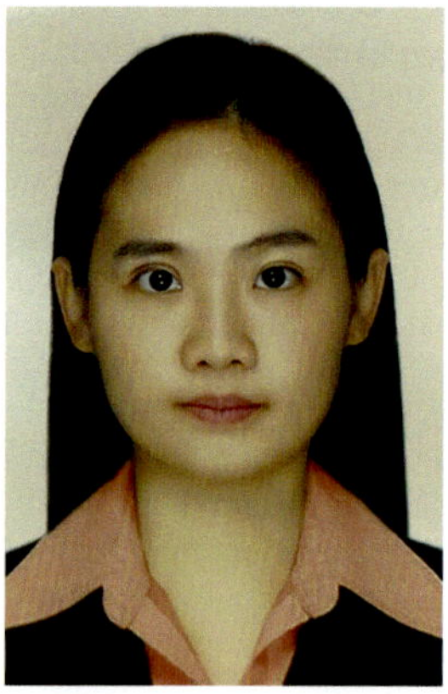

Dr. Variya Nganthavee got her First Class Honor for her bachelor degree from Faculty of Medicine, Siriraj Hospital, Mahidol University, Bangkok. She has been working as a research fellow at the Department of Ophthalmology, Rajavithi Hospital, Bangkok. Her published papers are on artificial intelligence for early detection of diabetic retinopathy and diabetic macular edema; her ongoing works are clinical trials of diabetic macular edema and age-related macular degeneration.

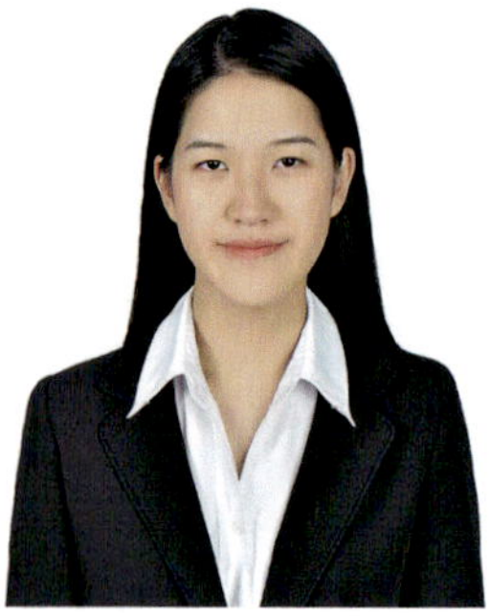

Dr. Warisara Pattanapongpaiboon works as a research fellow at the Departement of Ophthalmology, Rajavithi Hospital, Bangkok. She is currently working on clinical trials for diabetic macular edema, age-related macular degeneration, and deploying artificial intelligence in real-world diabetic retinopathy screening.

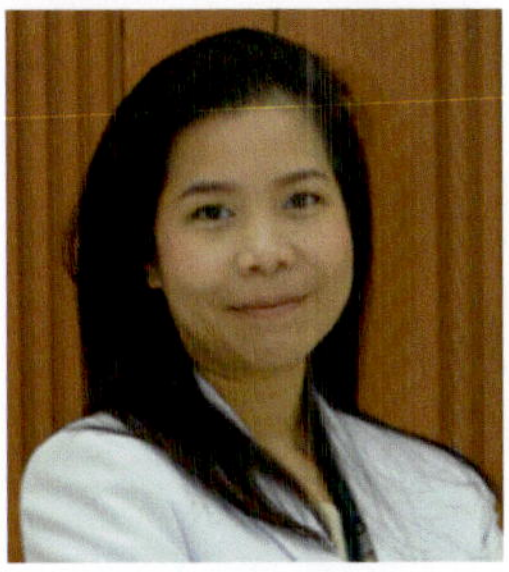

Dr. Kornwipa Hemarat is currently the attending physician at the Ophthalmology department, Navamindradhiraj University. She completed her residency and Vitreoretinal fellowship program from the Faculty of Medicine, Siriraj hospital, Mahidol University. She also completed the post-doctoral research fellowship at the University of California, San Francisco. Her published studies are on artificial intelligence for early detection of diabetic retinopathy and diabetic macular edema, dexamethasone implant for macular edema. She has been working on clinical trials for wet macular degeneration and deploying artificial intelligence in real-world diabetic retinopathy screening.

Clinical Trials Related to Myopic Choroidal Neovascularization

21

Christine P. S. Ho and Timothy Y. Y. Lai

21.1 Introduction and Natural History of Myopic CNV

Pathologic myopia affects up to 3% of the world's population and is a major cause of blindness worldwide. The prevalence of visual impairment resulting from pathologic myopia ranges from 0.1% to 0.5% in European studies and from 0.2% to 1.4% in Asian studies [1]. A number of complications relating to the posterior segment can develop in patients with pathologic myopia, and the development of choroidal neovascularization (CNV) is one of the most serious complications, often leading to sudden onset but later progressive central vision loss [2]. Myopic CNV has been estimated to develop in around 5% to 11% of pathologic myopia patients, [1] with 35% of patients with myopic CNV also developing CNV in the fellow eye within 8 years, which could disturb the patients' binocular visual function [3]. Myopic CNV is also the most common cause of CNV in individuals younger than 50 years of age who are often part of the working population, and thus it has an immense impact on the patients' quality of life [4]. Several factors are associated with worse visual prognosis of myopic CNV, including the age of onset being >40 years, subfoveal location of CNV, larger size of CNV (>400 μm), and lower best-corrected visual acuity (BCVA) at baseline [1].

Various extent of visual loss can develop in the three stages during the natural course of myopic CNV. The initial active phase involves direct photoreceptor damage caused by the CNV, resulting in central vision loss. CNV then regresses with the formation of localized fibrous scars known as Fuchs' spot, and macular chorioretinal atrophy develops around the regressed CNV as a late complication [5]. A long-term follow-up study by Yoshida et al. demonstrated that patients with untreated myopic CNV generally have poor visual outcomes due to development and enlargement of macular chorioretinal atrophy around the regressed CNV. A reduction in visual acuity to <20/200 was seen in 88.9% and 96.3% of patients at 5 and 10 years after the onset of CNV, respectively [6].

Various treatment modalities have been proposed for the treatment of myopic CNV, including thermal focal laser photocoagulation, verteporfin photodynamic therapy (vPDT), surgical excision of CNV, and macular translocation. However, these modalities demonstrated suboptimal long-term visual outcomes due to potential

C. P. S. Ho
Faculty of Medicine, The University of Hong Kong, Pok Fu Lam, Hong Kong

T. Y. Y. Lai (✉)
Department of Ophthalmology and Visual Sciences, The Chinese University of Hong Kong, Hong Kong Eye Hospital, Kowloon, Hong Kong

2010 Retina and Macula Centre, Tsim Sha Tsui, Kowloon, Hong Kong
e-mail: tyylai@cuhk.edu.hk

J. Chhablani (ed.), *Choroidal Neovascularization*, https://doi.org/10.1007/978-981-15-2213-0_21

CNV recurrence or complications such as macular scar, macular atrophy, and postoperative retinal detachment [7]. Vascular endothelial growth factor (VEGF) is an important cytokine involved in angiogenesis and vascular permeability, and has been implicated in the development of myopic CNV. Elevated levels of VEGF have been found in the aqueous humor of eyes with myopic CNV [8]. In recent years, intravitreal anti-VEGF therapies have been introduced for the treatment of patients with myopic CNV. Large randomized controlled clinical trials have demonstrated good efficacy and safety of anti-VEGF therapy, and anti-VEGF therapy has subsequently become the standard of care treatment for myopic CNV. Agents including ranibizumab, aflibercept, and conbercept are currently approved for treatment of myopic CNV in various countries.

This chapter summarizes the design and major results from key clinical trials in the past two decades concerning vPDT and anti-VEGF therapies, demonstrating the efficacies of different therapeutic agents available for the treatment of patients with myopic CNV.

21.2 Verteporfin Photodynamic Therapy Clinical Trial: VIP Study

The Verteporfin in Photodynamic Therapy (VIP) study was a multicenter, double-masked, placebo-controlled, randomized controlled trial evaluating the efficacy of vPDT compared with placebo, in stabilizing or improving vision in patients with subfoveal myopic CNV over a period of 12 months (Table 21.1) [9]. Patients with subfoveal CNV caused by pathologic myopia (defined as less than or equal to −6.0 diopters, or less myopic than −6.0 diopters with retinal abnormalities consistent with pathologic myopia and axial length of ≥26.5 mm), with lesion greatest linear dimension ≤5400 μm and BCVA ≥50 Early Treatment for Diabetic Retinopathy Study (ETDRS) letters were included in the study. Eligible patients ($n = 120$) were randomized in a 2:1 ratio to receive vPDT or placebo at baseline. Patients were followed up every 3 months until month 24, and received retreatment with vPDT or placebo if leakage from CNV was detected on fluorescein angiogram (FA). The primary outcome of the study was the proportion of eyes that lost fewer than 8 letters at month 12 compared with baseline, and the secondary outcome was the proportion of eyes that lost <15 letters or <30 letters at month 12 compared with baseline.

For the primary outcomes of the study, patients treated with vPDT were more likely to maintain stable BCVA compared with the placebo group, with 72% of eyes in the vPDT group lost fewer than 8 letters at month 12 compared with 44% in the placebo group ($P < 0.01$). A smaller proportion of patients in the vPDT group had a loss of BCVA ≥15 letters (moderate visual loss) or 30 letters (severe visual loss) at month 12, with 14% and 7% of eyes in the vPDT group reported to have moderate or severe loss of visual acuity, respectively, compared with 33% and 8% of eyes in the group receiving placebo ($P = 0.01$).

In terms of BCVA gains, a greater proportion of patients who had vPDT experienced improvement in visual acuity. 32% and 6% eyes in the vPDT group reported to have slight (≥5 letters) and large (≥15 letters) improvements in visual acuity at month 12, respectively, compared with 15% and 3% in the placebo group. Moreover, the two treatment groups differed by 10 letters in terms of median change in visual acuity, with a gain of 1 letter in the vPDT group and a loss of 9 letters in the placebo group. The median BCVA remained stable in the vPDT group at month 12, but decreased to 20/80–2 in the placebo group. Patients in the vPDT group also had higher mean contrast sensitivity scores at month 12, with patients in the vPDT and placebo groups experienced a mean gain of 0.1 letters and a mean loss of 2 letters, respectively. Furthermore, patients who received vPDT demonstrated better anatomical outcomes at month 12 compared with patients in the placebo group. Examination at month 12 revealed progression of classic CNV beyond the area of lesion identified at baseline in 36% of patients in the vPDT group and 54% of patients in the placebo group. 35% of patients in the vPDT group also demonstrated resolved classic CNV leakage at month 12, compared with

Table 21.1 Summary of main findings of clinical trials on anti-VEGF agents for treating myopic CNV

Study	Treatment groups	Number of eyes	Mean age (years)	Mean BCVA (ETDRS letters)	Mean axial length (mm)	CNV location	Main visual outcomes
VIP [9, 10]	vPDT	81	51 (median)	62 (median)	N/A	• Subfoveal 62% • Probably subfoveal 19% • Not subfoveal 14% • No CNV or cannot grade 6%	Mean BCVA gain of 1 letter at 12 months
	Sham injection	39	46 (median)	58 (median)	N/A	• Subfoveal 69% • Probably subfoveal 18% • Not subfoveal 8% • No CNV/cannot grade 5%	Mean BCVA loss of 9 letters at 12 months
REPAIR [12, 13]	Ranibizumab 0.5 mg	65	55.5	59.5	N/A	• Subfoveal 66.2% • Juxtafoveal 26.2% • Probably subfoveal/juxtafoveal 7.7%	Mean BCVA gain of 13.8 letters at 12 months
RADIANCE—main study [15]	Ranibizumab 0.5 mg guided by stabilization of BCVA	106	54	55.4	29.3	• Subfoveal 67.0% • Juxtafoveal 24.5% • Extrafoveal 6.6%	Mean BCVA gain of 10.5 letters at 3 months and 13.8 letters at 12 months
	Ranibizumab 0.5 mg guided by disease activity	116	56.1	55.8	28.8	• Subfoveal 69.8% • Juxtafoveal 20.7% • Extrafoveal 2.6%	Mean BCVA gain of 10.6 letters at 3 months and 14.4 letters at 12 months
	vPDT	55	57.4	54.7	29.4	• Subfoveal 69.1% • Juxtafoveal 29.1% • Extrafoveal 1.8%	Mean BCVA gain of 2.2 letters at 3 months and 9.3 letters at 12 months
RADIANCE—Subgroup analysis [16]	Caucasian patients	70	58.0	55.9	28.9	• Subfoveal 65.7% • Juxtafoveal 20.0% • Extrafoveal 4.3%	Mean BCVA gain of 14.1 letters at 12 months
	East-Asian patients	35	54.2	54.2	28.4	• Subfoveal 74.3% • Juxtafoveal 22.9% • Extrafoveal 0%	Mean BCVA gain of 17.0 letters at 12 months

(Continued)

Table 21.1 (Continued)

Study	Treatment groups	Number of eyes	Mean age (years)	Mean BCVA (ETDRS letters)	Mean axial length (mm)	CNV location	Main visual outcomes
RADIANCE—long-term outcomes [17]	Additional anti-VEGF required	7	55.3	59.7	29.7	• Subfoveal 57.1% • Juxtafoveal 42.9% • Extrafoveal 0%	Mean BCVA gain of 19.4 letters at 48 months
	No further treatment required	34	55.0	55.8	28.9	• Subfoveal 67.6% • Juxtafoveal 26.5% • Extrafoveal 2.9% • Cannot grade 2.9%	Mean BCVA gain of 11.0 letters at 48 months
BRILLIANCE [18]	Ranibizumab 0.5 mg guided by stabilization of BCVA	182	52.0	53.6	28.9	• Subfoveal 73.1% • Juxtafoveal 8.8% • Extrafoveal 16.5%	Mean BCVA gain of 9.5 letters at 3 months and 12.0 letters at 12 months
	Ranibizumab 0.5 mg guided by disease activity	184	51.5	54.2	29.0	• Subfoveal 70.1% • Juxtafoveal 12.0% • Extrafoveal 17.4%	Mean BCVA gain of 9.8 letters at 3 months and 13.1 letters at 12 months
	Verteporfin PDT	91	49.1	52.1	28.8	• Subfoveal 68.1% • Juxtafoveal 15.4% • Extrafoveal 13.2%	Mean BCVA gain of 4.5 letters at 3 months and 10.3 letters at 12 months
MYRROR [19]	Aflibercept 2 mg	90	58.5	56.4	28.8	• Subfoveal 60.0% • Juxtafoveal 38.9% • Extrafoveal 1.1%	Mean BCVA gain of 12.1 letters at 6 months and 13.5 letters at 12 months
	Sham/aflibercept 2 mg	31	57.5	56.6	28.6	• Subfoveal 64.5% • Juxtafoveal 35.5% • Extrafoveal 0%	Mean BCVA loss of 2.0 letters at 6 months and gain of 3.9 letters at 12 months
SHINY [20]	Conbercept 0.5 mg	132	49.30	54.05	N/A	N/A	Mean BCVA gain of 12.0 letters at 3 months and 13.3 letters at 9 months
	Sham/conbercept 0.5 mg	44	51.93	49.77	N/A	N/A	Mean BCVA gain of 0.6 letters at 3 months and 11.3 letters at 9 months

28% of patients in the placebo group. For the lesion size at month 12, patients who had vPDT were more likely to have lesions ≤1 disc area in size, while patients who had placebo were more likely to have lesions size of >3 disc areas. Patients in the vPDT group were also reported to have decreased greatest linear dimension of CNV leakage, compared with an increase in the placebo group. No serious ocular or systemic adverse events of vPDT were reported in the study.

The VIP study demonstrated the efficacy of vPDT compared with placebo in stabilizing or improving vision, and improving anatomical outcomes in patients with subfoveal myopic CNV over a period of 12 months. vPDT subsequently became the first therapy approved for the treatment of mCNV. However, in the 2-year follow-up of the study, although vPDT was able to stabilize vision, no significant improvement in BCVA was observed [10].

21.3 Ranibizumab Clinical Trials

Ranibizumab (Lucentis/Accentrix, Novartis, Basel, Switzerland) is a monoclonal anti-VEGF antibody fragment that binds to all VEGF-A isoforms specifically designed for intraocular use. It is currently approved for the treatment of myopic CNV, with a recommended dosing regimen of a single injection of intravitreal ranibizumab 0.5 mg followed by retreatment with as a pro re nata (PRN) approach [11].

21.3.1 REPAIR Study

The REPAIR (Ranibizumab for the treatment of Choroidal Neovascularization secondary to Pathological Myopia: an Individualized Regimen) study was a phase II, prospective, multicenter, open-label study exploring the efficacy of intravitreal ranibizumab 0.5 mg in patients with myopic CNV over a period of 12 months (Table 21.1) [12, 13]. The study included patients aged ≥18 years with myopia less than or equal to −6 diopters, with active subfoveal or juxtafoveal myopic CNV, and BCVA of 24 to 78 ETDRS letters. Patients ($n = 65$) received an initial intravitreal injection of 0.5 mg ranibizumab, with subsequent PRN injections if subretinal or intraretinal fluid was detected on optical coherence tomography (OCT), or CNV leakage was detected on fluorescein angiography during monthly monitoring until month 12. The primary outcome of the study was the mean change in BCVA from baseline to month 12. Following ranibizumab treatment, patients demonstrated a mean BCVA improvement of 12.2 letters at month 6 ($P < 0.001$), and the gain was sustained up to month 12. At month 12, a mean BCVA gain of 13.8 letters was observed, with the greatest mean visual gain of 8.4 letters seen in the first month of treatment. 86% of patients demonstrated improvement in BCVA over 12 months, with 36.9% of patients gaining ≥15 letters and 50.8% of patients gaining ≥10 letters. 1.5% of patients reported to have a loss of ≥15 letters. Prior to receiving treatment, 73.8% of study eyes were the worse-seeing eyes and 14.4% of eyes became the better-seeing eyes upon receiving treatment. Over 12 months, patients were given a median number of 3 injections, with retreatment rates of 21.5%, 18.5%, 16.9%, and 15.5% for 0, 1, 2, and 3 additional injections, respectively. The study demonstrated that a minimal number of retreatments with intravitreal ranibizumab 0.5 mg were required to achieve and maintain visual gains in patients with myopic CNV.

Regarding anatomical outcomes, a substantial mean reduction in OCT central macular thickness (CMT) of 108 and 135 μm was observed from baseline to month 6 and month 12, respectively ($P < 0.001$), with the greatest mean reduction of 109 μm seen in the first month of treatment, which was consistent with the trend observed in BCVA improvement. A mean decrease in lesion size was also observed on FA, with a mean decrease of 0.54 mm^2 by month 6, and a mean decrease of 0.37 mm^2 by month 12 ($P = 0.0287$). Patients were also evaluated with OCT for the presence of subretinal fluid, intraretinal cysts, or edema. At month 12, there were significant reductions in the proportion of patients with subretinal fluid, intraretinal cysts, and edema compared with baseline, with reductions of 60%, 38.5%, and 80%, respectively (all $P < 0.001$). No new safety issues were identified with the use of intravitreal ranibizumab treatment in the study. One ocular and three non-ocular serious adverse events (SAEs) were reported in the study period, which were considered unrelated to intravitreal ranibizumab treatment [12, 13].

The study also evaluated two patient-reported outcomes, including treatment satisfaction measured using the Macular Treatment Satisfaction Questionnaire (MacTSQ), and patient wellbeing measured using the 12-item Wellbeing Questionnaire (W-BQ12). Regarding treatment satisfaction, the mean MacTSQ scores increased from 55.0 at month 1 to 64.9 at month 12 ($P = 0.0001$), with the greatest increase in mean MacTSQ scores observed in patients aged 68 years or older. For the W-BQ12 general wellbeing score, the mean general wellbeing score was 25.6 at baseline. It remained similar at months 1 and 6, and increased significantly at month 12 to 27.3 ($P = 0.03$). Patients aged 40 years or younger had the greatest improvement in general well-being. Overall, no significant correlations were found between patients' changes in BCVA, MacTSQ score and W-BQ12 general well-being score [14].

In conclusion, the REPAIR study demonstrated the efficacy of intravitreal ranibizumab 0.5 mg injection in producing substantial visual and anatomical improvements in patients with myopic CNV. A minimal number of retreatments were required after the initial dose of intravitreal ranibizumab, and good patient satisfaction and maintenance of well-being were reported.

21.3.2 RADIANCE Study

The RADIANCE (Ranibizumab and PDT (verteporfin) evaluation in myopic choroidal neovascularization) study was a 12-month, phase III, randomized, double-masked, multicenter study, which compared the efficacy and safety of intravitreal ranibizumab 0.5 mg, as guided by visual acuity stabilization criteria (group 1) or disease-activity guided criteria (group 2), with vPDT (group 3) in patients with myopic CNV (Table 21.1) [15]. The study included patients aged ≥ 18 years with myopia less than or equal to −6 diopters, active CNV, and BCVA of 24 to 78 ETDRS letters. Eligible patients ($n = 277$) were randomized in a 2:2:1 ratio into three treatment groups. Patients in group 1 received intravitreal ranibizumab 0.5 mg on day 1 and month 1, followed by a PRN regimen, with retreatment determined by visual acuity (VA) stabilization criteria, defined as no change in BCVA compared with the two previous monthly assessments. Patients in group 2 received intravitreal ranibizumab 0.5 mg on day 1 followed by PRN regimen, with retreatment determined by disease-activity guided criteria, which was defined as an impairment of vision due to intraretinal or subretinal fluid, or active CNV leakage. Patients in group 3 were treated with vPDT on day 1, and received vPDT, intravitreal ranibizumab 0.5 mg, or a combination of both, guided by disease activity following a PRN regimen from month 3. All patients also received either sham injections or sham PDT depending on treatment groups they were allocated to. Baseline demographics were similar among the 3 study groups. The primary objective of the study was to demonstrate the superiority of intravitreal ranibizumab treatment over vPDT in mean BCVA gain at month 3, while the secondary objective was to show that ranibizumab retreatment guided by disease activity was non-inferior to ranibizumab retreatment guided by visual acuity stabilization criteria at month 6.

Regarding visual outcomes, patients who received intravitreal ranibizumab 0.5 mg, irrespective of retreatment criteria, demonstrated superiority over vPDT based on mean BCVA changes from baseline to month 3. Patients in groups 1 and 2 showed similar mean BCVA improvements, with a mean gain of 10.5 letters and 10.6 letters, respectively, at month 3, and a mean gain of 13.8 and 14.4 letters, respectively, at month 12 ($P < 0.00001$). Patients who had vPDT demonstrated lower mean BCVA gain of 2.2 letters at month 3. However, upon switching to intravitreal ranibizumab with or without vPDT at month 3, patients showed a significant mean improvement of 9.3 letters at month 12, although the mean visual gain was less prominent than patients who received intravitreal ranibizumab from baseline. Moreover, the two different individualized ranibizumab dosing regimens demonstrated similar efficacies in stabilizing vision. Ranibizumab retreatment guided by disease activity was non-inferior to ranibizumab retreatment guided by VA stability based on mean changes in BCVA at month 6, with a mean gain of 11.7 letters and 11.9 letters, respectively ($P < 0.00001$). The study proposed the use of disease activity as a guide to retreatment, as it could possibly control disease progression with fewer intravitreal ranibizumab injections than using VA stabilization criteria. Furthermore, at month 3, a greater proportion of patients in the ranibizumab groups gained ≥10 letters and ≥15 letters compared to patients in the vPDT group. With intravitreal ranibizumab introduced to patients in the vPDT group, an increased proportion of patients gained ≥10 letters and ≥15 letters at month 12. However, the proportion was still lower than that those who had ranibizumab from baseline. Hence, the study suggested early initiation of ranibizumab treatment in patients diagnosed with myopic CNV.

For anatomical outcomes, a decreased proportion of patients with subretinal fluid, intraretinal edema, and intraretinal cysts were observed in all treatment groups at month 12. Patients in groups 1 and 2 demonstrated a decrease in mean central retinal thickness (CRT) (66.6 and 71.3 μm, respectively) at month 12, which was comparable to the decrease in CRT of 60.8 μm seen in patients in the group receiving vPDT followed by PRN intravitreal ranibizumab treatment. At month 12, resolution of CNV leakage was also observed in 63.8% to 65.7% patients. Moreover, patients in groups 1 and 2 who had intravitreal ranibizumab demonstrated a mean ± standard deviation (SD) decrease in lesion size of 0.31 ± 1.65 mm^2 and 0.57 ± 1.94 mm^2, compared with a mean ± SD increase in lesions size of 0.28 ± 2.96 mm^2 in patients in group 3.

In terms of treatment exposure, a relatively low number of intravitreal ranibizumab injections was required in the study to stabilize vision. Patients in group 1 received a median number of 4.0 intravitreal ranibizumab injections over 12 months, compared with a median of 2.0 injections for group 2. The difference in treatment exposure was attributed to different loading dosage regimens of the two groups as required by the protocol. The number of retreatment was low in the ranibizumab groups, with 62% of patients who did not require additional ranibizumab in groups 1 and 2. From months 6 to 11, 30.9% of patients in group 3 received intravitreal ranibizumab injections, with a median of 2.0 injections. Regarding the safety of treatment, no new safety concerns were identified with ranibizumab and vPDT treatment, with a low incidence of ocular and non-ocular serious adverse effects in the study groups [15].

Additional subgroup analyses of the RADIANCE study were performed to evaluate the influence of age, ethnicity, and various ocular characteristics such as axial length, refractive error, and CNV size on the efficacy of intravitreal ranibizumab in the treatment of myopic CNV [16]. Patients from group 2 of the RADIANCE study who had intravitreal ranibizumab retreatment guided by disease activity were included in this post hoc analysis (n = 116), as this retreatment protocol based on disease activity was used for the approval of ranibizumab in the treatment of myopic CNV. Regarding the impact of ethnicity on visual outcomes, East-Asian and Caucasian patients had similar baseline BCVA. However, East-Asians demonstrated a greater mean BCVA improvement of 17.0 letters compared to a mean gain of 14.1 letters in Caucasians at month 12. Differences in baseline ocular characteristics also influenced patients' mean BCVA gains at month 12. Patients with the highest level of baseline BCVA (≥73 letters) demonstrated the lowest mean gain in BCVA of 8.2 letters, while patients with lowest BCVA at baseline (<45 letters) demonstrated the greatest mean BCVA gain of 20.3 letters. This is likely due to the ceiling effect in patients with good visual acuity as observed in other ophthalmology clinical trials. For treatment exposure, East-Asians required a median number of 2 injections compared with 3 injections in Caucasians over 12 months, with 74.3% East-Asians not requiring reinjections from month 6. Patients in the category with the lowest baseline BCVA had a higher median number of 4 ranibizumab injections, compared with patients in the category with the highest baseline BCVA, which requires only one single injection. A higher median number of injections was also required in patients with larger baseline CNV lesion area. In summary, the subgroup analysis of RADIANCE demonstrated the efficacy of ranibizumab in treating myopic CNV patients with different baseline characteristics, and recommended the use individualized treatment in using ranibizumab as guided by disease activity criteria for treating myopic CNV. In addition, regardless of the baseline characteristics, ranibizumab resulted in good visual acuity improvement across all subgroups [16].

After the completion of the RADIANCE study, a post-RADIANCE retrospective cohort study was also conducted to investigate the long-term efficacy and safety in the use of intravitreal ranibizumab in the treatment of myopic CNV in East-Asian patients from the RADIANCE study [17]. Patients ($n = 41$) were followed for up to 48 months in order to evaluate the mean BCVA changes, recurrence of myopic CNV, and ocular adverse events. During the period, patients with myopic CNV could be treated without restriction on anti-VEGF agents or treatment regimens. Patients were categorized into two groups, with 7 (17.1%) patients received additional anti-VEGF injections, and 34 (82.9%) patients did not require any further treatment during the observation period. Out of the 7 patients who had retreatment, 4 patients were treated with intravitreal ranibizumab, while the other 3 patients were treated with other anti-VEGF agents. A mean number of 5.0 injections were required in patients who had additional treatment; with a mean duration of 29.4 months of follow-up in the post-RADIANCE observation period.

The primary outcome of the study was the long-term efficacy of ranibizumab in terms of mean BCVA change from baseline to each follow-up. During the follow-up, patients had significant improvement in mean ± SD visual acuity from baseline, with +14.3 ± 11.4 letters at month 12 ($P < 0.0001$), +10.4 ± 22.3 letters at month 24 ($P = 0.0143$), +11.0 ± 22.4 letters at month 30 ($P = 0.0134$), +12.9 ± 20.9 letters at month 42 ($P = 0.0051$) and +16.3 ± 18.7 letters at month 48 ($P = 0.0034$). During the post-RADIANCE observation period, a low rate of myopic CNV recurrences was observed, with recurrences reported in 9.8% of patients, and the overall annual rate of myopic CNV recurrence being 0.06 recurrence per patient per year. No serious ocular adverse events related to anti-VEGF treatment was reported during the study period. Overall, patients with myopic CNV demonstrated positive visual outcomes up to 48 months, with low incidence of myopic CNV recurrence, and few reinjections required to maintain or improve BCVA [17].

21.3.3 BRILLIANCE Study

The BRILLIANCE study was a phase III, 12-month, randomized, active-controlled, double-masked study, which compared the efficacy and safety of intravitreal ranibizumab 0.5 mg, as guided by criteria based on visual acuity stabilization or disease activity, with vPDT in patients with myopic CNV (Table 21.1) [18]. The BRILLIANCE study design was identical to the RADIANCE study, except that the BRILLIANCE study involved predominately Asian patients, while the RADIANCE study involved Asians, Caucasians, and other races. A total of 431 patients completed the study, with a majority being female (68.1%) and Chinese (84.0%) patients. Patients were also randomized in a 2:2:1 ratio to receive intravitreal ranibizumab 0.5 mg guided by visual acuity stabilization (group 1), intravitreal ranibizumab 0.5 mg guided by disease activity (group 2), and vPDT (group 3). The baseline demographics were comparable among the 3 study groups. The primary objective of the study was to demonstrate the superiority of intravitreal ranibizumab treatment over vPDT at month 3, while the secondary objective was to show that ranibizumab retreatment guided by disease activity was non-inferior to ranibizumab retreatment guided by visual acuity stabilization criteria at month 6.

Regarding visual outcomes of the study, intravitreal ranibizumab 0.5 mg, irrespective of retreatment criteria, was superior over vPDT treatment based on mean BCVA changes from baseline to month 3, with patients in groups 1, 2, and 3 gained 9.5 letters, 9.8 letters, and 4.5 letters at month 3, respectively ($P < 0.001$). Ranibizumab retreatment guided by disease activity was also non-inferior to ranibizumab retreatment guided by VA stability based on mean changes in BCVA at month 6, with a mean gain of 10.4 letters and 10.7 letters, respectively ($P < 0.001$). At month 12, all three treatment groups demonstrated improvement in BCVA, with patients in groups 1, 2, and 3 gained a mean of 12.0 letters, 13.1 letters, and 10.3 letters, respectively. However, patients in group 3 who received vPDT/intravitreal ranibizumab had reduced visual gains compared with patients who received intravitreal ranibizumab from baseline.

For anatomical outcomes, reduced proportions of patients with subretinal fluid, intraretinal edema, and intraretinal cysts were observed in all treatment groups at month 12. Reductions in mean CNV leakage and lesion areas were also observed. Patients in groups 1 and 2 who received intravitreal ranibizumab demonstrated a decrease in mean CRT up to month 3, with stabilization of CRT up to month 12. Patients in group 3 demonstrated a decrease in mean CRT, with stabilization of CRT up to month 3. With the introduction of intravitreal ranibizumab to patients in the vPDT group at month 3, a further reduction in mean CRT was observed. For treatment exposure, a median number of 4.0 and 3.0 intravitreal ranibizumab injections were required in groups 1 and 2, respectively, up to month 12, while patients in group 3 received a median number of 3.2 intravitreal ranibizumab injections from months 3 to 12. Regarding the safety of treatment, low frequencies of adverse events and serious adverse events (SAE) were recorded, with 3 patients presenting with ocular SAEs and 24 patients with non-ocular SAEs, which were considered to be unrelated to the study drug.

Overall, the results from the BRILLIANCE study were comparable to that of the RADIANCE study, showing the superiority of intravitreal ranibizumab, regardless of retreatment criteria, over vPDT up to 3 months in the treatment of patients with myopic CNV.

In summary, the phase II REPAIR study, the phase III RADIANCE, and BRILLIANCE studies have shown consistent results, demonstrating that intravitreal ranibizumab is efficacious and safe in stabilizing and improving vision in patients with myopic CNV. It has been proposed that the slight differences in BCVA improvement reported in different studies could be due to the differences in baseline demographics of different patient groups [18].

21.4 Aflibercept Clinical Trial

Aflibercept (Eylea, Bayer, Leverkuensen, Germany) is a recombinant protein with activities inhibiting VEGF-A, VEGF-B, and placental growth factor, and has also been approved for the treatment of myopic CNV in various countries.

21.4.1 MYRROR Study

The MYRROR study was an international, phase III, multicenter, randomized controlled trial evaluating the efficacy of intravitreal aflibercept 2.0 mg compared with sham treatment in patients with myopic CNV, with the primary endpoint measured at week 24 (Table 21.1) [19]. Patients aged ≥18 years with high myopia (defined as less than or equal to −6.0 diopters or axial length of ≥26.5 mm), with active subfoveal or juxtafoveal myopic CNV and BCVA of 35 to 73 ETDRS letters were included in the study. Patients ($n = 121$) were randomized in a 3:1 ratio into intravitreal aflibercept group or sham/intravitreal aflibercept treatment group. Patients in the intravitreal aflibercept group received one single injection of 2.0 mg aflibercept at baseline, followed by additional PRN injections in case of CNV persistence or recurrence up to week 44 if the retreatment criteria were met. The retreatment criteria were defined as reduction in ≥5 letters from the previous visit, increase in CRT by >50 μm, presence of cystic retinal changes, subretinal fluid, or pigment epithelial detachment with CNV or hemorrhage. Patients in the sham group received one sham injection at baseline, followed by sham injections every 4 weeks up to week 20. From week 24 onwards, patients in the sham group were eligible to receive intravitreal aflibercept 2.0 mg injection on a PRN basis in case of CNV persistence or recurrence according to the retreatment criteria.

The primary outcome of the study was the mean change in BCVA from baseline to week 24, and the secondary outcome was the proportion of patients in the two treatment groups who gained ≥15 letters at week 24. For treatment exposure, the median number of aflibercept injections in the aflibercept group was 2.0 in the first 12 weeks and 0 in the remaining study period. The median number of aflibercept injections in the sham/intravitreal aflibercept group was 3.0 during the study period, with a median number of 2.0 and 1.0 injections in the third and fourth study quarters, respectively. The study demonstrated that a minimal number of reinjections were required following initial intravitreal aflibercept injection to stop the myopic CNV disease process.

Intravitreal aflibercept demonstrated superior efficacy compared with sham treatment in both primary and secondary endpoints of the study. For the primary endpoint, the mean BCVA change from baseline to week 24 was a gain of 12.1 letters and a loss of 2.0 letters in the intravitreal aflibercept and sham groups, respectively ($P < 0.0001$). For the confirmatory key secondary endpoint, a greater proportion of patients in the intravitreal aflibercept group (38.9%) gained ≥15 letters at week 24 compared to the sham group (9.7%) ($P = 0.0001$). For other visual acuity endpoints, a greater proportion of patients who were treated with aflibercept gained ≥10 letters and ≥5 letters compared to patients in the sham group at both 24 and 48 weeks. The improvement in BCVA in the intravitreal aflibercept group was sustained to week 48, with a mean gain of 13.5 letters and 50% gain in ≥15 letters. Patients in the sham/intravitreal aflibercept group received intravitreal aflibercept at week 24 with a PRN regimen thereafter, and demonstrated a mean improvement of 5.9 letters from week 24 to week 48. Since the visual outcomes in the first 24 weeks of aflibercept treatment were significantly better in patients in the aflibercept group compared with patients in the sham/intravitreal aflibercept group, the study recommended early evaluation of visual change in patients with pathologic myopia for detection of myopic CNV so that anti-VEGF treatment can be initiated as soon as possible.

Regarding the anatomical outcomes, patients who received intravitreal aflibercept injections had a significantly higher mean reduction in CRT from baseline to week 24 compared with patients in the sham group (−80.7 μm vs. −13.9 μm) ($P < 0.0001$). However, the difference between the two groups was not statistically significant at week 48. A difference in mean CNV size was also observed between the two groups at week 24 compared with baseline, with a decrease in 0.24 disc areas (DA) in patients in the aflibercept group, and an increase in 0.31 DA in patients in the sham group ($P < 0.0001$). At week 48, patients in both groups demonstrated a decrease in mean CNV size, with a reduced difference between the two groups. Patients in the aflibercept group also showed a significant reduction in the area of FA leakage at week 24, with a mean decrease of 0.48 DA, compared with an increase of 0.19 DA in patients in the sham group ($P < 0.0001$). At week 48, a greater proportion of patients in the aflibercept group had resolution of CNV leakage compared to the sham/aflibercept group.

In terms of quality of life indicator, patients in the intravitreal aflibercept group demonstrated a better vision-related quality of life than patients in the sham/aflibercept group, as measured by the National Eye Institute Visual Function Questionnaire 25 at weeks 24 and 48. Regarding the safety of treatment, intravitreal aflibercept was generally well tolerated, and no new safety concerns emerged during the study. Patients in the aflibercept and sham/intravitreal aflibercept groups had a similar incidence of ocular treatment–emergent adverse events in the study period, with most being mild intensity events.

In summary, the MYRROR study demonstrated the efficacy of intravitreal aflibercept 2.0 mg compared with sham/intravitreal aflibercept in the treatment of patients with myopic CNV, producing significant visual and anatomical outcomes over a period of 48 weeks, with a limited number of injections required in the early course of treatment [19].

21.5 Conbercept Clinical Trial

Conbercept is a fusion protein that inhibits the activity of VEGF-A, VEGF-B, and placental growth factor, and is currently approved in China for the treatment of myopic CNV.

21.5.1 SHINY Study

The SHINY study was a 9-month, multicentered, double-masked, sham-controlled, randomized controlled trial, which compared the efficacy and safety of intravitreal conbercept 0.5 mg with sham treatment in patients with myopic CNV (Table 21.1) [20]. Patients (n = 176) were randomized in a 3:1 ratio to receive intravitreal conbercept 0.5 mg or sham injection. Patients in the intravitreal conbercept group received monthly intravitreal injections of conbercept 0.5 mg for 3 months, followed by conbercept injections with a PRN regimen up to month 9. Patients in the sham treatment group received monthly sham injections for 3 months, and at 3 months, they were eligible to receive intravitreal conbercept 0.5 mg on a PRN basis.

The baseline demographics were similar between the two study groups. The primary objective of the study was to assess the mean change in BCVA from baseline to month 3. A final assessment of BCVA was then conducted at month 9. At month 3, patients in the conbercept group demonstrated a significant mean BCVA gain of 12.00 letters ($P < 0.001$), while patients who received sham injections showed a mean gain of 0.56 letters ($P = 0.656$). At month 9, patients in both groups demonstrated substantial improvement in BCVA, with patients in the conbercept and sham/intravitreal conbercept groups achieved a mean gain of 13.28 letters and 11.26 letters, respectively.

For anatomical outcomes, at month 3, a mean reduction of 61.97 μm in CRT was observed in patients who had intravitreal conbercept 0.5 mg ($P < 0.001$), while the change in mean CRT was not statistically significant in patients who had sham injections. However, significant reductions in mean CRT were observed in both study groups at month 9, with patients in the conbercept and sham/intravitreal conbercept groups demonstrated a mean reduction of 73.7 and 55.9 μm, respectively ($P < 0.001$).

Regarding treatment exposure, patients who had conbercept injections from baseline received a mean of 4.78 conbercept injections over 9 months, with 27% of patients required no further injections following the initial 3 loading doses. Patients in the sham/intravitreal conbercept group required a mean number of 3.49 conbercept injections from months 3 to 9.

21.6 Conclusions

The above major clinical trials demonstrated the efficacy of vPDT and anti-VEGF therapy in improving vision in patients with myopic CNV, with anti-VEGF therapy being superior over vPDT regardless of the retreatment criteria adopted. The phase 3 randomized controlled trials including RADIANCE, BRILLIACE, MYRROR, and SHINY studies have all demonstrated the efficacy and safety of ranibizumab, aflibercept, and conbercept in improving visual and anatomical outcomes in patients with myopic CNV.

As early diagnosis and initiation of treatment for myopic CNV are crucial, patients with high myopia presenting with blurred vision, central scotoma, and/or metamorphopsia, or signs of CNV should be promptly referred to an ophthalmologist or a retinal specialist with expertise in treating myopic CNV [21]. Licensed anti-VEGF agents are currently the first-line therapy for treating myopic CNV, and the use of initial anti-VEGF injections followed by a PRN regimen is supported by results from the above mentioned pivotal clinical trials. In all these RCTs in the use of anti-VEGF therapy for myopic CNV, patients demonstrated improvement in visual outcomes regardless of the time of initiation of treatment. However, compared with prompt treatment, any delay in applying anti-VEGF therapy resulted in reduced visual gains. Hence, early treatment during the active stage of the disease is critical in limiting the disease activity. Following initial treatment, patients should be monitored regularly for disease activity or visual changes, and receive prompt retreatment if required. The above RCTs also demonstrated that the majority of patients with myopic CNV required much fewer intravitreal anti-VEGF injections to prevent disease progression, compared with CNV due to neovascular age-related macular degeneration. If intravitreal anti-VEGF therapy is contraindicated in patients, vPDT can be still adopted in the treatment of myopic CNV, though the visual gains are likely to be substantially lower than that of using anti-VEGF therapy [11, 21].

Key Learning Points

- Choroidal neovascularization is a major complication in patients with pathologic myopia causing central vision loss.
- The long-term visual outcomes of myopic CNV without treatment are extremely poor.
- The VIP study demonstrated that vPDT was effective in improving vision in patients with myopic CNV in the short-term, but vPDT was unable to result in significant visual improvement at 24 months.
- Anti-VEGF therapy is currently the standard of care treatment for myopic CNV.
- The phase 2 REPAIR study and phase 3 large-scaled randomized controlled trails including RADIANCE, BRILLIANCE, MYRROR, and SHINY studies have demonstrated the favorable efficacy and good safety of anti-VEGF agents including ranibizumab, aflibercept, and conbercept in the treatment of myopic CNV.
- Early diagnosis and prompt treatment of myopic CNV is crucial to prevent severe irreversible vision loss.
- A low number of anti-VEGF injections are required in the treatment of myopic CNV.

References

1. Wong TY, Ferreira A, Hughes R, Carter G, Mitchell P. Epidemiology and disease burden of pathologic myopia and myopic choroidal neovascularization: an evidence-based systematic review. Am J Ophthalmol. 2014;157:9–25.e12.
2. Hotchkiss ML, Fine SL. Pathologic myopia and choroidal neovascularization. Am J Ophthalmol. 1981;91:177–83.
3. Ohno-Matsui K, Yoshida T, Futagami S, Yasuzumi K, Shimada N, Kojima A, et al. Patchy atrophy and lacquer cracks predispose to the development of choroidal neovascularisation in pathological myopia. Br J Ophthalmol. 2003;87:570–3.
4. Cohen SY, Laroche A, Leguen Y, Soubrane G, Coscas GJ. Etiology of choroidal neovascularization in young patients. Ophthalmology. 1996;103:1241–4.
5. Neelam K, Cheung CM, Ohno-Matsui K, Lai TY, Wong TY. Choroidal neovascularization in pathological myopia. Prog Retin Eye Res. 2012 Sep;31:495–525.
6. Yoshida T, Ohno-Matsui K, Yasuzumi K, Kojima A, Shimada N, Futagami S, et al. Myopic choroidal neovascularization: a 10-year follow-up. Ophthalmology. 2003;110:1297–305.
7. Ohno-Matsui K, Ikuno Y, Lai TYY, Gemmy Cheung CM. Diagnosis and treatment guideline for myopic choroidal neovascularization due to pathologic myopia. Prog Retin Eye Res. 2018 Mar;63:92–106.
8. Tong JP, Chan WM, Liu DT, Lai TY, Choy KW, Pang CP, Lam DS. Aqueous humor levels of vascular endothelial growth factor and pigment epithelium derived factor in polypoidal choroidal vasculopathy and choroidal neovascularization. Am J Ophthalmol. 2006;141:456–62.
9. Verteporfin in Photodynamic Therapy Study Group. Photodynamic therapy of subfoveal choroidal neovascularization in pathologic myopia with verteporfin. 1-year results of a randomized clinical trial – VIP report no. 1. Ophthalmology. 2001;108:841–52.
10. Blinder KJ, Blumenkranz MS, Bressler NM, Bressler SB, Donato G, Lewis H, et al. Verteporfin therapy of subfoveal choroidal neovascularization in pathologic myopia: 2-year results of a randomized clinical trial – VIP report no. 3. Ophthalmology. 2003;110:667–73.
11. Cheung CMG, Arnold JJ, Holz FG, Park KH, Lai TYY, Larsen M, et al. Myopic choroidal neovascularization: review, guidance, and consensus statement on management. Ophthalmology. 2017;124:1690–711.
12. Tufail A, Patel PJ, Sivaprasad S, Amoaku W, Browning AC, Cole M, et al. Ranibizumab for the treatment of choroidal neovascularisation secondary to pathological myopia: interim analysis of the REPAIR study. Eye (Lond). 2013;27:709–15.
13. Tufail A, Narendran N, Patel PJ, Sivaprasad S, Amoaku W, Browning AC, et al. Ranibizumab in myopic choroidal neovascularization: the 12-month results from the REPAIR study. Ophthalmology. 2013;120:1944–5.e1.
14. Amoaku WM, Gale RP, Lotery AJ, Menon G, Sivaprasad S, Petrillo J, et al. Treatment satisfaction and Well-being in patients with myopic choroidal neovascularization treated with ranibizumab in the REPAIR study. PLoS One. 2015;10(6):e0128403.
15. Wolf S, Balciuniene VJ, Laganovska G, Menchini U, Ohno-Matsui K, Sharma T, et al. RADIANCE: a randomized controlled study of ranibizumab in patients with choroidal neovascularization secondary to pathologic myopia. Ophthalmology. 2014;121:682–92.e2.
16. Holz FG, Tufail A, Leveziel N, Lai TY, Lanzetta P, Wong TY, et al. Ranibizumab in myopic choroidal neovascularization: a subgroup analysis by ethnicity, age, and ocular characteristics in RADIANCE. Ophthalmologica. 2016;236:19–28.
17. Tan NW, Ohno-Matsui K, Koh HJ, Nagai Y, Pedros M, Freitas RL, et al. Long-term outcomes of ranibizumab treatment of myopic choroidal neovascularization in east-Asian patients from the RADIANCE study. Retina. 2018;38:2228–38.
18. Chen Y, Sharma T, Li X, Song Y, Chang Q, Lin R, et al. Ranibizumab versus verteporfin photodynamic therapy in Asian patients with myopic choroidal neovascularization: BRILLIANCE, a 12-month, randomized, Double-Masked Study. Retina. 2018; https://doi.org/10.1097/IAE.0000000000002292.
19. Ikuno Y, Ohno-Matsui K, Wong TY, Korobelnik JF, Vitti R, Li T, et al. Intravitreal Aflibercept injection

in patients with myopic choroidal neovascularization: the MYRROR Study. Ophthalmology. 2015;122:1220–7.
20. Chen Y. Efficacy and safety of conbercept ophthalmic injection in treatment of choroidal neovascularization secondary to pathological myopia (Shiny trial). Presented in angiogenesis, exudation and degeneration meeting 2016, Miami, FL.
21. Wong TY, Ohno-Matsui K, Leveziel N, Holz FG, Lai TY, Yu HG, et al. Myopic choroidal neovascularisation: current concepts and update on clinical management. Br J Ophthalmol. 2015;99:289–96.

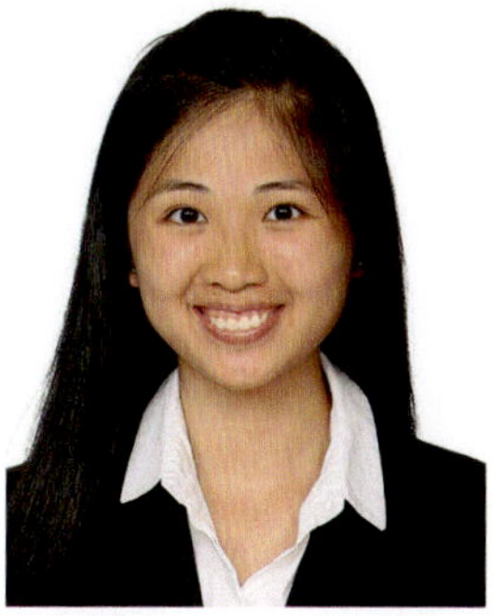

Christine P. S. Ho is a fifth-year medical student currently studying in the Faculty of Medicine at the University of Hong Kong. She has developed a strong interest in ophthalmology and has previously published review articles in macular diseases including polypoidal choroidal vasculopathy and choroidal neovascularization due to uncommon causes. She has been awarded various scholarships including the HKU Entrance Scholarship and the Dean's Scholarship.

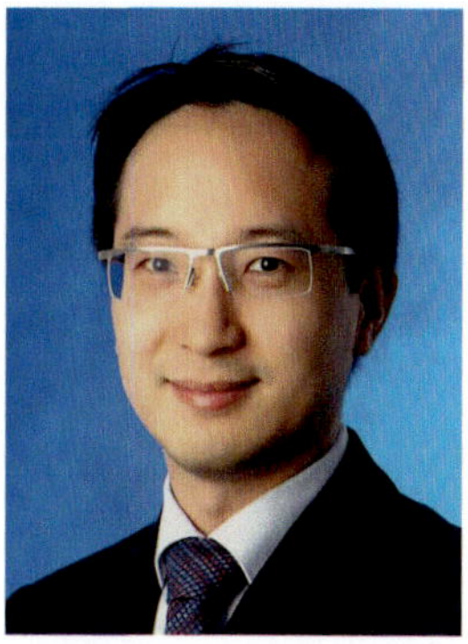

Timothy Y. Y. Lai is currently a Clinical Professor (Honorary) of the Department of Ophthalmology & Visual Sciences, The Chinese University of Hong Kong; and Director of the 2010 Retina and Macula Centre, Hong Kong. His clinical and research interests lie in the medical and surgical management of retinal diseases, particularly polypoidal choroidal vasculopathy, myopic maculopathy, choroidal neovascularization, central serous chorioretinopathy, visual electrophysiology, and genetics of retinal diseases and uveitis. Prof. Lai has published over 230 papers in international peer-reviewed journals and has a Scopus *h*-index of 46. His academic achievements are well-recognized internationally and has received many awards including the Nakajima Award of the Asia-Pacific Academy of Ophthalmology (2008), Achievement Award of the American Academy of Ophthalmology (2010), Achievement Award of the Asia-Pacific Academy of Ophthalmology (2011), Victor Yong Lecture of the NHG Eye Institute in Singapore (2013), Senior Achievement Award of the American Academy of Ophthalmology (2017), Constable Lecture Award of the Asia-Pacific Vitreo-Retina Society (2017), and Senior Achievement Award of the Asia-Pacific Academy of Ophthalmology (2019).

Clinical Trials Related to Non-AMD Choroidal Neovascularization

22

Tariq Alzahem, Nayef Alswaina, and Marwan A. Abouammoh

22.1 Introduction

The condition that most commonly leads to the development of choroidal neovascularization (CNV) in industrialized nations is age-related macular degeneration (AMD) [1–3]. However, especially in younger patients, there are other causes for CNVs. These include high myopia, presumed ocular histoplasmosis syndrome (POHS), hereditary, traumatic, and inflammatory ocular disorders [4]. Polypoidal choroidal vasculopathy (PCV) is another entity in which type 1 CNV has a characteristic abnormal branching network of vessels and aneurysmal dilations [5]. Thus, some believe that PCV is a variant of neovascular AMD. Idiopathic CNV is a term used to describe CNV's with no specific cause.

Before the introduction of intravitreal anti-vascular endothelial growth factor (VEGF) agents to treat CNV, laser photocoagulation, verteporfin with photodynamic therapy (PDT), and surgical intervention were performed to treat CNV. In the last few years, revolutionary advancements in patient outcomes have been observed after the institution of anti-VEGF therapy.

T. Alzahem · M. A. Abouammoh (✉)
Department of Ophthalmology, College of Medicine, King Saud University, Riyadh, Saudi Arabia

N. Alswaina
Department of Ophthalmology, College of Medicine, Qassim University, Buraydah, Saudi Arabia

The objective of this chapter is to summarize the key clinical trials that have made the most noticeable transformations in the management of patients affected with non-AMD causes of CNV. We will focus on clinical trials addressing CNV associated with POHS, angioid streaks, uveitis, central serous chorioretinopathy (CSCR), pattern dystrophy, and idiopathic CNV's.

22.2 Methodology

We conducted a literature review on all clinical trials focusing on non-AMD, non-myopia, and non-PCV related choroidal neovascularizations. We searched MEDLINE and EMBASE for all published phase III clinical trials written in the English language. Search terms used included: "*Choroidal neovascularization*" OR "*Choroidal neovascular membrane*" OR "*CNV*." No limits were placed on the year of publication. We excluded animal studies. The search results, using the previously mentioned terms and filters, returned 653 articles (MEDLINE: 604, EMBASE: 49).

In the initial screening, abstracts were reviewed by a single reviewer for obvious exclusion criteria (AMD, myopia, and PCV trials). Then, the full publications were retrieved for all clinical trials recognized at the initial screening. They were then rescreened by two investigators. This resulted in 48 articles being used to develop this chapter. Then, the articles were categorized

J. Chhablani (ed.), *Choroidal Neovascularization*, https://doi.org/10.1007/978-981-15-2213-0_22

according to the disease entity. The clinical trials categories are CNV's associated with ocular histoplasmosis syndrome (17 articles), idiopathic CNV's (9 articles), angioid streaks (4 articles), inflammatory CNV's (6 articles), CSCR (2 articles), and pattern dystrophy (1 article). Retinal angiomatous proliferation (9 articles) are covered under AMD trials.

22.3 Clinical Trials

We will detail the clinical trials for non-AMD causes of choroidal neovascular membranes in the following order:

22.3.1 Presumed Ocular Histoplasmosis Syndrome (POHS).
22.3.2 Idiopathic choroidal neovascularization.
22.3.3 Angioid streaks.
22.3.4 Inflammatory choroidal neovascularization.
22.3.5 Central serous chorioretinopathy (CSCR).
22.3.6 Pattern dystrophy.

22.3.1 Presumed Ocular Histoplasmosis Syndrome

Various historical treatment modalities were proposed for patients with POHS. They include stress management, discontinuing aspirin, avoiding valsalva maneuvers, use of corticosteroids, and others [6–8]. Those interventions were not proven effective with no known treatment for inactive lesions. In the presence of active chorioretinal lesions and subfoveal CNV, corticosteroids also have been suggested [9]. However, since the advent of laser photocoagulation, PDT, and anti-VEGF agents, the previous modalities are generally of historic interest.

22.3.1.1 Laser Treatment

Light Coagulation in Presumed Histoplasmic Choroiditis [10]

The objective of this trial was to assess the effect of light coagulation (Xenon-arc) on macular hemorrhagic disciform degeneration of the macula as measured by visual acuity and the activity of the chorioretinal scar in patients with POHS. A total of 29 patients were randomized to either treatment (15 patients) or control (14 patients). All patients were followed for a minimum of 1 year. In the treatment group, the final visual acuity improved 1 Snellen line in 33.3%, remained the same in 6.66%, and worsened in 60% of patients. In the control group, the final visual acuity improved 1 Snellen line in 42.8% and worsened in 57.1% of patients. The intervention did not significantly change the activity of the lesions compared to the control group. Thus, short-term improvement was observed in some patients, but the Xenon-arc photocoagulation was not effective in the long-term management of CNV in patients with POHS [10].

Macular Photocoagulation Study in POHS [11–17]

The Macular Photocoagulation Study (MPS) Group conducted a number of randomized, controlled clinical trials to assess the laser treatment of CNV in patients with AMD, POHS, and idiopathic CNV's. The effect of Argon and Krypton laser photocoagulation in the treatment of extrafoveal and juxtafoveal CNV secondary to POHS was reported in the MPS. In all MPS trials, the primary outcome was the change in best-corrected visual acuity from baseline. The clinical trials of Argon laser followed by Krypton laser are described below.

Argon Laser Photocoagulation for Extrafoveal CNV's in POHS [11–13]

In 1983, the MPS Group published the first trial addressing the effect of argon laser photocoagulation in preventing severe visual loss in eyes with extrafoveal CNV's and a clinical evidence of POHS [11]. Severe visual loss was defined as loss of 6 or more lines from the baseline. A baseline best-corrected visual acuity of 20/100 or better was required in the study eye. Eligible patients (no. of eyes = 245) were randomly assigned to either blue-green laser photocoagulation (n = 124) or observation only (n = 121). Supplementary treatment was performed when new vessels recurred 200 μm away from the center of the FAZ. The data were based on 231 eyes (117 treated vs. 114 untreated) followed for at least 6 months with a median follow-up for 18 months. In the most recent follow-up, 39 out of 114 (34.2%) untreated eyes lost 6 lines compared to 11 out of 117 (9.4%) treated eyes. At the same visit, 36% of untreated eyes had visual acuity worse than 20/100 compared to 12.8% in the treated group. Two years after starting the study, half of the untreated eyes and 22% of the treated eyes had lost 6 or more lines of visual acuity. The risk of losing 6 lines was estimated to be 2.3 times greater for untreated eyes compared to treated eyes. The most common complications of laser photocoagulation were hemorrhage and internal limiting membrane wrinkles. This trial has demonstrated that argon laser photocoagulation of CNV related to POHS is superior to no treatment [11]. Additionally, patients' recruitment has been terminated in 1983 because of the short-term treatment benefit described. However, follow-up of all patients continued to establish the long-term outcomes (described below).

The 3 and 5 years' results of argon laser treatment were reported in 1986 and 1991, respectively [12, 13]. At the end of summer, 1985, a minimum of three or more years of planned follow-up examinations had been completed for 203 (77%) of 262 eyes enrolled from the commencement date of the study. The data were based on 194 eyes (104 treated vs. 90 untreated). At the 3-year visit, 47.8% of untreated eyes had a visual acuity worse than 20/100 compared to 14.4% in the treated group. In addition, 47.8% of the untreated eyes and 8.6% of the treated eyes had lost 6 or more lines of visual acuity. The relative risk of experiencing severe loss of vision in the untreated eyes after 3 years was 5.5 (95% CI: 3.9 to 10.8). Two-thirds of the treated eyes had a visual acuity of 20/40 or better in comparison with approximately a third of the untreated group [12]. At 5 years, the data of 232 eyes (116 in each group) were analyzed. Visual acuity of 20/100 or worse was observed in 45% of untreated and 17% of the treated eyes. A loss of 6 or more lines of visual acuity was detected in 44% of the untreated eyes compared to 9% of the treated eyes. In 5 years, the relative risk of losing 6 or more lines of visual acuity among untreated vs. treated eyes was 3.6 ($P < 0.0001$). Similar to the 3-year results, 68% of the treated group had a visual acuity of 20/40. The percentage of having a 20/40 visual acuity or better in the untreated group increased from 38% at 3 years to 43% at 5 years. In the laser-treated group, recurrent CNV had been observed in 26% of eyes by 5 years after the start of the trial. In conclusion, the 5 years' follow-up results emphasized the superiority of argon laser photocoagulation in the treatment of well-defined extrafoveal CNV's secondary to POHS compared to no treatment [13].

Krypton Laser Photocoagulation for Juxtafoveal CNV's in POHS [14–16]

Extrafoveal CNV's represent 46.2% of CNV's occurring in patients with POHS. The remaining CNV's, i.e. 53.7%, are extending under the foveal avascular zone [18]. Those patients were not eligible for the previously mentioned trial because of proximity of the neovascular lesion to the FAZ. Argon laser was not used on those lesions because of the theoretical harm it would induce in the area within 200 μm of the center of the FAZ [19]. Therefore, a second randomized clinical trial using Krypton laser was initiated [14].

In 1987, the results of Krypton laser photocoagulation for juxtafoveal CNV's in patients with POHS were published [14]. This trial differs from the first one described above in 3 points: the location of CNV's, the wavelength of the laser used for photocoagulation, and that treatment was permitted up to the center of the FAZ. The aim of this study is to determine whether krypton laser treatment would be beneficial in halting the progressive visual loss in eyes with POHS and juxtafoveal CNV's. Eligible patients should have an angiographic evidence of CNV located between 1 and 199 μm from the center of the FAZ, or between 200 and 2500 μm from the center if associated with an adjacent blood or pigment ring involving the FAZ. The best-corrected visual acuity should be equal or better than 20/400 in the study eye. A total of 288 eyes were included in the study. 143 and 145 eyes were randomly assigned to treatment and observation groups, respectively. The data were based on 125 eyes completing the 36-month visit. In both groups, an almost even percentage of eyes attained or preserved a visual acuity of 20/20 or better (20.3% in the treatment group, 21.3% in the observation group). However, 26.2% of the observation group had a visual acuity worse than 20/200 compared to 4.7% in the treatment group. Similarly, 15 out of 61 untreated eyes (24.6%) lost 6 lines compared to 3 out of 64 treated eyes (4.7%). A worse baseline visual acuity was associated with a greater proportion of visual improvement. It has been concluded that treatment with Krypton laser photocoagulation was associated with better visual acuity outcomes regardless of baseline variables [14].

The 5 years' results were reported in 1994. A total of 236 eyes, 118 in each group, eyes were evaluated [15]. After 5 years, the median visual acuity was significantly better in the treated group (Snellen visual acuity; 20/40) compared to in observation group (Snellen visual acuity; 20/64). Almost similar to the earlier data described above, 23 treated eyes (19%) and 24 untreated eyes (20%) had visual acuity that is equal or better than 20/20. On the other hand, 0.8% and 13.6% had a visual acuity of 20/400 or worse in the treated and observation groups, respectively. 10 treated eyes (8%) had lost 6 or more lines of visual acuity compared to 33 untreated eyes (28%). Thus, early beneficial effects of Krypton laser photocoagulation continued for at least 5 years in eyes with POHS-related CNV [15].

The occurrence of persistent and recurrent CNV after initial treatment with laser photocoagulation has been published in a separate report [16]. The eyes assigned to krypton red laser photocoagulation (n = 144) were examined. Eyes in which fluorescein angiograms showing fluorescein dye leakage taken during the first 6 weeks after initial treatment were classified as having a persistent CNV. Recurrence of CNV was defined as the observation of leakage on fluorescein after the 6-week posttreatment visit without previous persistence. Persistent CNV's were documented in 23% of treated eyes while recurrent CNV's were detected among an additional 8%. An increased frequency of severe visual loss was seen in those eyes. Persistent CNV was approximately 2.5 times more common in patients with systemic hypertension than in patients without [16].

Laser Photocoagulation for Peripapillary CNV's and CNV's Located Nasal to the Fovea in POHS [17]

There were some concerns regarding the treatment of two types of CNV's: peripapillary CNV's, and large CNV's located nasal to the fovea in which the longest diameter is greater than 750 μm. Laser treatment of CNV's in these two areas was thought to carry the risk of damaging the optic nerve and the papillomacular bundle, respectively. Thus, the specific results of laser treatment of these CNV's in the eyes included in the previous MPS trials were published in a separate report [17]. The objective was to determine whether laser treatment of these CNV's was better than observation. The same protocol for laser treatment described above was applied in which extrafoveal CNV's were treated by argon laser and juxtafoveal CNV's were treated by krypton laser.

The etiologies of CNV's in this report were POHS and idiopathic causes with a total of 113 eyes included. The results published were based on CNV type and not on etiology. However, 51 out of 58 treated eyes (88%) and 46 out of 55 untreated eyes (84%) were diagnosed to have CNV's secondary to POHS. The data were based on 105 eyes (54 treated vs 51 untreated) followed for at least 3 years. Regardless of the lesion type, treated eyes had better visual acuity ($P = 0.03$), with 72% of treated eyes and 56% untreated eyes having a visual acuity of 20/100 or better. Compared to the baseline visual acuity, 11% of the treated eyes vs. 41% of the untreated eyes lost 6 or more lines ($P < 0.001$). In the peripapillary CNV subgroup, treated eyes had a slightly better visual acuity with 64% vs. 60% in the untreated group having a visual acuity of 20/100 or better. Approximately 14% of the treated eyes in this subgroup had lost 6 or more lines of visual acuity compared to 26% of the untreated eyes. In the nasal CNV subgroup, the differences were more marked with 78% treated eyes vs. 50% untreated eyes achieving a visual acuity of 20/100 or better. Among patients in this subgroup, 9% of the treated eyes lost 6 or more lines of visual acuity compared with 54% of the untreated eyes ($P < 0.001$). The study findings confirmed beneficial effects of laser photocoagulation for peripapillary and papillomacular CNV's. It is important to note that the beneficial outcome was less pronounced in the peripapillary CNV's subgroup [17].

Argon Green Versus Krypton Red Laser Photocoagulation for Extrafoveal Choroidal Neovascularization: One-Year Results in Ocular Histoplasmosis—The Canadian Ophthalmology Study Group [20]

The Canadian Ophthalmology Study Group carried out a randomized clinical trial to determine whether krypton laser is superior to argon laser in the treatment of extrafoveal CNV's secondary to POHS in terms of visual acuity at 1 year. Eligible patients should have an angiographic evidence of an active CNV in which the posterior edge is 200 to 2500 μm from the center of the FAZ, a clinical exam suggesting POHS, and best-corrected visual acuity of 20/200 or better in a previously untreated eye.

A total of 127 eyes were eligible (63 in the argon laser group and 64 in the krypton laser group). At 1 year, 6% of the eyes in the argon laser group had lost 6 or more lines of visual acuity compared with 14% of eyes in the krypton red laser group. The difference was not statistically significant between the two groups. In the argon laser group, 21% of eyes required more than one treatment, compared with 39% of the eyes in the krypton red laser group. The Canadian Ophthalmology Study Group concluded that krypton laser photocoagulation treatment is not superior to argon laser photocoagulation therapy for well-defined extrafoveal CNV's in patients with POHS [20].

Laser Treatment for Subfoveal Neovascular Membranes in Ocular Histoplasmosis Syndrome: Results of a Pilot Randomized Clinical Trial [21]

This was a pilot clinical trial published in 1993 to evaluate the effect of laser photocoagulation in patients with POHS and subfoveal CNV's, new and recurrent. New CNV's and recurrent previously treated CNV's were enrolled in the study. The sizes of the new membranes and the recurrent membranes should be equal or less than 3.5 and 4 disc areas, respectively [21].

A total of 25 patients (12 in the treatment group, 13 in the observation group) were evaluated. Among the treatment group, there were 4 new CNV's and 8 recurrent CNV's. Among the observation group, there were 6 new CNV's and 7 recurrent CNV's. The mean visual acuity for both groups at baseline was 20/125. The results were based on 15 patients (7 in the treatment group and 8 in the observation group) at 12 months after treatment. The mean visual acuity at 12 months was 20/200 in both groups. The results were inconclusive and do not suggest any benefit or harm to the eyes receiving laser photocoagulation.

22.3.1.2 Photodynamic Therapy (PDT) in POHS

Verteporfin in Ocular Histoplasmosis Study [22–24]

The Verteporfin in Ocular Histoplasmosis (VOH) study is an open-label, uncontrolled, multicenter clinical trial to evaluate the effect of PDT on subfoveal CNV secondary to POHS. For patients to be eligible, there should be an angiographic evidence of classic or occult CNV involving the center of the FAZ. Best-corrected Snellen visual acuity at baseline ranged from 20/40 to 20/200. The treatment protocol starts with a 10-minute infusion of Verteporfin at a dose of 6 mg/m^2 of body surface area. Then, 15 min after the start of infusion, a light application (689 nm) of 600 mW/cm^2 for 83 s to reach a total of 50 J/cm^2 of energy. Outcomes to be measured were visual acuity changes from baseline and contrast sensitivity scores.

A total of 26 patients were eligible. The mean visual acuity was 20/80 and the mean contrast sensitivity score was 29 letters. At 12 months, 14 patients (56%) had gained 1 or more lines of visual acuity, half of them (7 patients, 28%) gained 3 or more lines. Four patients (16%) lost 1 or more lines of visual acuity from baseline with two patients (8%) losing 3 or more lines. Seven patients (28%) had a stable visual acuity. Only one patient had a visual acuity of 20/200 or worse at the 12-month visit. Contrast sensitivity increased by 3 or more letters in 12 patients (48%) and decreased by 3 or more lines in 3 patients (12%). Ten patients (40%) had stable contrast sensitivity. At the 12-month visit, 43% and 100% of patients did not show fluorescein leakage from classic CNV and occult CNV, respectively. The authors concluded that PDT with verteporfin is safe and well tolerated in patients with subfoveal CNV due to POHS for at least 1 year. Approximately half of the patients experienced some improvement in visual acuity [22].

After 2 years, 22 out of the 26 patients (85%) were followed [23]. At 24 months, there was an improvement of 1 or more lines from baseline in 14 patients, similar to the 12-month results. Eight patients (36%) gained 3 or more lines of visual acuity compared to 7 patients (28%) at the 12-month examination. Visual acuity scores were stable in 4 patients (18%) at the 24-month visit. Similar to the 1-year results visual acuity decreased by 1 or more lines from baseline in 4 patients, with 1 patient having a visual acuity of 20/200 or worse. Fluorescein angiographic leakage was absent in 17 out of 20 (85%) having classic CNV. No leakage was observed in the occult CNV cases. The same conclusion was reached at the 2-year follow-up [23].

Fifteen patients completed the 48-month follow-up examination [24]. A mean of 4.4 treatments was given to the patients during the 48 months. The median visual acuity improvement from the baseline was 15 letters. The median contrast sensitivity improved by 3 letters compared to baseline. Through 48 months of PDT therapy for subfoveal CNV's due to POHS, the visual acuity and contrast sensitivity were maintained or improved in the majority of patients [24].

22.3.1.3 Surgical Management of CNV's in POHS

Management of Subfoveal Choroidal Neovascularization [25]

This interventional case series studied the use of vitreoretinal surgical techniques in subfoveal CNV's secondary to AMD, POHS, and miscellaneous causes. The results of CNV's secondary to POHS will be discussed here. Inclusion criteria included angiographic proof of a CNV beneath the center of the FAZ. In all cases, a small retinotomy (about 200 μm) eccentric to the fovea was made. Then, two variations to remove or manipulate the neovascular complex through the small retinotomy were performed in POHS patients. The first technique involved CNV extraction using an angled subretinal pick or forceps. The second technique involved CNV disconnection without removal.

Out of 58 consecutive patients, 20 eyes of 20 patients had CNV secondary to POHS. In 85% of the cases, the CNV had been present from 6 months to 1 year. Preoperative visual acuities ranged from 20/30 to counting fingers at 2 feet. In eyes where the subfoveal CNV was removed (n = 16), all but one of the eyes had preoperative visual acuities of 20/200 or worse. In eyes where the subfoveal CNV was disconnected without removal (n = 4), the initial visual acuities were 20/100 or better. In eyes where CNV was removed, with a mean follow-up of 4.8 months, the final visual acuity significantly improved in 6 eyes, worsened in one, and remained the same in nine eyes. A visual acuity of 20/70 or better was achieved in 4 eyes. In 37% of eyes, persistent or recurrent neovascularization were observed in which the final visual acuity was negatively affected. In the four eyes where the subfoveal CNV was disconnected without removal, the mean follow-up duration was 3.8 months. All four patients experienced a postoperative significant reduction in visual acuity. Complications include subretinal hemorrhage, rhegmatogenous retinal detachment, and RPE injury. Surgical management of subfoveal CNV's in patients with POHS showed better results in some of the cases. Recurrence of CNV following surgery is an important cause of visual decline and warrants careful follow-ups [25].

Submacular Surgery Trials Research Group: Surgical Removal vs Observation for Subfoveal Choroidal Neovascularization, Either Associated with the Ocular Histoplasmosis Syndrome or Idiopathic [26]

The Submacular Surgery Trials (SST) Research Group conducted randomized trials of surgical removal of subfoveal CNV's secondary to POHS, and idiopathic CNV's. The aim was to assess the effectiveness of this intervention on visual acuity. Eligible patients had a subfoveal CNV that had a classic component. The best-corrected visual acuity scores of eligible patients ranged from 20/50 to 20/800. A retinotomy was made by the surgeon to provide access to the CNV. The fibrovascular complex was disconnected and then removed manually with a micro forceps. The primary outcome was a success if there was an improvement or stabilization of visual acuity at the 2-year visit. Stabilization was defined as no change of vision or a change of no more than 1 line worse than the baseline at 2 years.

Two hundred twenty-five patients (112 in the surgery arm and 113 in the observation arm) were enrolled in the trial. Out of 225 patients, 192 (85%) patients were having CNV secondary to POHS (95 patients in the surgery arm and 97 in the observation arm). The Median visual acuity of study eyes at baseline was 20/100 for both arms [26].

At the 24-month visit, 200 patients (including POHS and idiopathic) were evaluated. The median visual acuity was 20/160 in the surgery arm compared to 20/250 in the observation arm ($P = 0.07$). The median visual acuity changes at the 24-month follow-up were a loss of 1 line in the surgery arm and 2 lines in the observation arm ($P = 0.14$). The SST definition of successful outcomes at 24 months was achieved in 53% of the patients in the surgery arm and 45% in the observation arm ($P = 0.26$). The mean visual acuity improvement was more prominent when the baseline visual acuity was worse than 20/100. For this subgroup of patients ($n = 92$), the mean visual acuity in the surgery group was 20/200 compared to 20/320 in the observation group. At 2 years, the primary successful outcome was achieved in 76% in the surgery group vs. 50% in the observation group. Complications encountered in the surgery group include cataract (39%) and rhegmatogenous retinal detachments (4.5%). The 24-month cumulative incidence of fluorescein leakage from the CNV was 58% in the treated eyes. By the 24-month examination, 38% of operated eyes had 1 or more additional treatments. It was concluded from this trial that submacular surgery was not beneficial in eyes that had best-corrected visual acuity of 20/100 or better. On the other hand, if the best-corrected visual acuity is worse than 20/100, submacular surgery is considered to improve the chances of preserving or improving visual acuity for at least 2 years [26]. An improved vision targeted quality of life was observed more after submacular surgery compared with observation [27].

22.3.1.4 Anti-Vascular Endothelial Growth Factors Agents in POHS

Treatment of CNV Secondary to Presumed Ocular Histoplasmosis with Intravitreal Aflibercept 2.0 mg Injection [28]

This was an open-label, prospective, randomized, phase II/III clinical trial investigating the safety and efficacy of aflibercept 2 mg injections for CNV in patients with POHS. The CNV should be less than 1 year in duration, subfoveal, or juxtafoveal in location, with best-corrected visual acuity ranging between 20/25 and 20/400.

A total of 5 patients were included. The mean baseline visual acuity was 62, measured in Early Treatment Diabetic Retinopathy (ETDRS) letters. The mean baseline central foveal thickness and volume were 293 μm and 10.1 mm^3, respectively. Subretinal fluid was observed in all patients by OCT at baseline. All patients received a total of 7 intravitreal aflibercept injections in 12 months. No adverse systemic or ocular events were reported during the study period. One year following the initiation of therapy, the mean visual acuity improved by 12.4 letters. The mean central subfoveal thickness and OCT volume reduced by 34.6 μm and 0.58 mm^3. Four of 5 patients had resolved fluid on OCT at the 12-month visit. It was concluded that intravitreal aflibercept 2 mg given monthly for 3 months and then every 8 weeks is safe and effective for the treatment of neovascular POHS for at least 1 year. [28].

22.3.2 Idiopathic Choroidal Neovascularization

22.3.2.1 Laser Treatment

Laser Photocoagulation for Idiopathic Neovascularization: Results of a Randomized Clinical Trial [29]
This was the first randomized clinical trial published by the MPS group addressing the effect of argon laser photocoagulation in the treatment of extrafoveal CNV's without an apparent cause, i.e., idiopathic. The aim of this trial was to determine whether laser treatment would be of benefit in preventing severe visual loss.

A total of 67 patients (33 patients in the laser group and 34 in the observation group) were included. At 1 year, 51 patients were evaluated (26 in the treatment group and 25 in the observation group). At the most recent follow-up, 86.7% vs. 63.6% of the patients in the treatment and the observation groups were having a visual acuity of 20/100 or better, respectively. Sixteen percent of patients in the treatment group had lost six or more lines of visual acuity compared to 33.3% in the observation group. The most common complication of treatment was the development of hemorrhage. Although the sample size was not large enough to derive a definitive conclusion, the pattern of treatment benefit is similar to that observed in the POHS patients mentioned above [29].

Fifty-one patients completed the 3-year follow-up (27 in the treatment group and 24 in the observation group). Approximately 85% of patients in the laser group had a visual acuity of 20/100 or better vs. 61% in the observation group. Severe visual loss was seen in 15% of patients in the laser group compared to 35% of patients in the observation group. If left untreated, the relative risk of losing six or more lines after 3 years is 2.3 [12]. Five years after enrollment, 57 patients were evaluated (30 in the treatment group and 27 in the observation group). The mean visual acuities in eyes assigned to treatment were 20/64 vs. 20/80 in the observed eyes. The mean lines of visual acuity lost after 5 years were 3 lines in the treatment group and 4 lines in the observation group ($P = 0.22$). Similar to the three-year results, the relative risk of having a severe visual loss at 5 years in the untreated group was 2.3. Five years after entry, 57% of the treated eyes had a visual acuity of 20/40 or better compared to 41% in the untreated eyes. Thirty-four percent of laser-treated eyes had recurrent CNV throughout the 5 years. The argon laser treatment for idiopathic extrafoveal CNV's had a favorable outcome. However, the beneficial outcome was less pronounced than that in the POHS trial [13].

Laser Photocoagulation for Idiopathic Neovascular Lesions: Results of a Randomized Clinical Trial [30]
The aim of this clinical trial was to evaluate whether krypton laser treatment would be of benefit in preventing visual acuity loss in eyes with idiopathic juxtafoveal CNV's. As mentioned earlier in the POHS study, the posterior edge of the CNV should be located 1 to 199 μm from the center of the FAZ or from 200 to 2500 μm from the center of FAZ if there was associated blood or blockage of fluorescence extending to the central 200-micron circle. There should be no drusen or atrophic scars suggestive of AMD or POHS, respectively.

A total of 49 eyes were enrolled at the start of the study (24 eyes in the laser group and 25 eyes were observed). Ninety-two percent of the eyes in the laser group vs. 76% of eyes in the observation group had a baseline visual acuity of 20/100 or better. At the 36-month visit, 40% of eyes in the laser group vs. 42% of eyes in the observation group had a visual acuity of 20/40 or better. On the other hand, 10% of treated eyes had a visual acuity of 20/200 or worse vs. 40% of untreated eyes. Regarding the change of visual acuity from baseline, 10% of treated eyes sustained severe visual loss compared to 37% of observed eyes. Thus large visual acuity losses in eyes affected with juxtafoveal idiopathic CNV's were seen less frequently after krypton laser treatment at the 3-year visit [30].

Five years following patients' enrollment (20 eyes in the treatment group and 18 eyes in the observation group), the median visual acuity in eyes that received krypton laser was 20/50 compared to 20/80 in the observed eyes ($P = 0.27$). Twenty over forty vision was achieved by 45% of the treated eyes and 39% of the untreated eyes.

The benefit of laser treatment was less defined in the 5-year results. In addition, the number of patients was small for reliable estimation of the treatment benefit [15].

22.3.2.2 Photodynamic Therapy (PDT)

Photodynamic Therapy with Verteporfin for Subfoveal Idiopathic Choroidal Neovascularization: One-Year Results from a Prospective Case Series [31]
That was a prospective, open-label, consecutive, interventional case series that investigated the outcome of PDT with verteporfin on eyes with idiopathic CNV involving the subfoveal zone in Chinese patients. The patients included were aged 50 years or younger. The location of the CNV or any associated blood or blocked fluorescence should involve the foveal center. The best-corrected visual acuity was required to be 20/200 or better. There should be evidence of leakage within the lesion on fluorescein angiography.

A total of 17 patients received PDT with verteporfin according to the standardized protocol described above. The patients were followed-up every 3 months for 1 year. The primary outcome was improved (2 or more lines), stable (within 1 line), or decreased (2 or more lines) visual acuity 1 year after enrollment. The secondary outcomes included a change in the mean and median best-corrected visual acuity following treatment at 1 year. All cases had predominantly classic subfoveal CNV. The median baseline best-corrected visual acuity was 20/70 with a range of 20/50 to 20/200. At the end of 1 year, 10 eyes (58%) showed improvement of visual acuity, 6 eyes (35%) were stable, and one eye (6%) demonstrated worsening. The median visual acuity after treatment was 20/50 with a mean of 2.3 lines of improvement. Fourteen CNV's (82%) converted into fibrotic scars without any leakage in fluorescein angiography. The remaining CNV's (18%) showed mild leakage. A mean of 1.8 PDT treatments was performed per eye within the study period. The retreatments, if required, were given 3 months after the initial treatment. It was concluded that PDT with verteporfin demonstrated a beneficial outcome in the treatment of idiopathic subfoveal CNV's[31].

Photodynamic Treatment Versus Photodynamic Treatment Associated with Systemic Steroids for Idiopathic Choroidal Neovascularization [32]
That was a prospective, open-label, consecutive, and randomized controlled trial. The purpose was to investigate the efficacy of PDT vs. systemic steroids with PDT in patients with idiopathic CNV's. Patients were randomized into two groups. The first group received PDT according to the standard protocol (group 1). The second group received intravenous methylprednisolone 1 gram daily for 3 days, followed by oral prednisone 1 mg/kg daily, and then tapered thereafter (median duration was 5 months), in addition to PDT (group 2). The median time between the start of steroids and PDT was 1.5 months.

A total of 20 patients were included (10 patients in each group). The median follow-up for both groups was 23 months. The baseline mean visual acuity was 0.34 and 0.26 in group 1 and 2, respectively (decimal visual acuity). The mean numbers of PDT treatments were 2.3 for group 1 and 1.5 for group 2. At the last follow-up, the mean best-corrected visual acuity was 0.31 in group 1 compared to 0.41 in group 2. At the last follow-up, 40% of group 1 vs. 90% of group 2 patients had stable/improved visual acuity. With regard to the CNV size at the last follow-up, 40% of group 1 vs. 90% of group 2 patients had stable/reduced lesions. It was concluded from this small trial that PDT preceded by systemic steroids was better than PDT alone in the visual acuity outcome, the number of PDT treatments, and the size of the scar in patients with idiopathic CNV's [32].

Small Laser Spot Versus Standard Laser Spot Photodynamic Therapy for Idiopathic Choroidal Neovascularization: A Randomized Controlled Study [33]
This was a randomized controlled trial designed to compare PDT with small laser spot (spot diameter size is equal to CNV's greatest linear dimension (GLD) + 500 μm) and PDT with standard laser spot (CNV's GLD + 1000 μm) in terms of visual outcome and RPE damage in patients with idiopathic CNV.

A total of 52 patients were randomly assigned to a study group (27 patients, small laser spot) and a control group (25 patients, standard laser spot). Approximately half of the patients completed the 1-year follow-up. All patients received intravenous infusion of verteporfin (6 mg/m^2 of body surface area) over 10 minutes. Then, a 689-nm laser source (spot size is equal to GLD + 500 μm in the study group vs. GLD + 1000 μm in the control group) was used to deliver 50 J/cm^2 over 83 s. The mean baseline best-corrected visual acuity was 52.5 and 55.2 ETDRS letters in the study and control groups, respectively. Subfoveal CNV was present in 44.4% of eyes in the study group and 40% of eyes in the control group. At 6- and 9-months follow-ups, the mean improvement in the best-corrected visual acuity in the study group (25.5 and 27.5 ETDRS letters, respectively) was significantly better than that in the control group (14.7 and 15.5 ETDRS letters, respectively). The ETDRS scores at 12 months were better in the study group compared to the control group. At 3 and 6 months of follow-ups, the study group had 1.5 and 2.5 quadrants involved compared to 3 and 4 quadrants affected in the control group, respectively. At 12 months, the difference was minimized to 3 and 4 quadrants affected in the study and control groups, respectively. There was no statistically significant difference between the two groups in the proportion of cases with decreased or stabilized CNV leakage size and the height of subretinal fluids. Thirty-seven percent of the study group and 32% of the control group had recurrent CNV during the 12-month follow-up. In summary, a trend toward a better visual improvement and a less RPE alteration was noted in the group with small laser spot PDT compared to the standard laser spot PDT over 1 year [33].

22.3.2.3 Transpupillary Thermotherapy (TTT)

Transpupillary Thermotherapy for Idiopathic Subfoveal Choroidal Neovascularization [34]
This was a prospective, noncontrolled case series of patients with idiopathic subfoveal CNV treated with transpupillary thermotherapy (TTT). It is a treatment modality in which the choroid and the overlying retinal pigment epithelium are heated through the use of 810-nm infrared diode laser with subsequent closure of the vascular complex. Patients with idiopathic subfoveal CNV with visual acuity better than 10/200 in previously untreated eyes were included. Laser spot sizes and power settings ranged between 1.2–3 mm in diameter and 300–600 mW, respectively.

A total of 21 patients were treated. Twelve CNV's were predominantly classic and 9 were predominantly occult. The mean follow-up duration was 5.1 months with a minimum follow-up of 3 months. The mean number of treatments given was 1.14. Out of 12 predominantly classic CNV's, 11 CNV's (92%) regressed. Eight out of 9 predominantly occult CNV's (89%) showed regression. Persistence of subretinal fluid was noted in one predominantly classic CNV and 3 predominantly occult CNV's. None of the eyes showed recurrence. Overall, 17 out of 21 eyes (81%) had either a stable or improved visual acuity. Out of 17 eyes, 11 (52%) had improvement of one or more lines of visual acuity and the remaining 6 eyes were stable. Four eyes (19%) showed worsening visual acuity compared to baseline. Three of the 21 eyes (14%) required retreatment with TTT. The study findings suggested that TTT has a potential role in the treatment of idiopathic subfoveal CNV's [34].

22.3.2.4 Anti-Vascular Endothelial Growth Factor Agents

Intravitreal Bevacizumab for Subfoveal Idiopathic Choroidal Neovascularization [35]
This was a prospective, non-comparative, consecutive, interventional case series aimed to evaluate the short-term outcomes and safety of intravitreal bevacizumab in eyes with idiopathic subfoveal CNV. Patients included were ≤50 years with an OCT demonstrating intraretinal edema, subretinal fluid, or pigment epithelial detachment (PED).

Thirty-two consecutive patients were eligible. All patients received a 1.25 mg/0.05 ml of intravitreal bevacizumab. The injection was repeated at a 4-week interval if OCT was still showing intraretinal edema, subretinal fluid, and/or PED. The median best-corrected visual acuity at baseline was 20/200. The means of baseline OCT central macular thickness and volume were 314.37 μm and

6.9 μL, respectively. The mean duration of follow-up was 4.2 months with a minimum of 3 months of follow-up. At 12 weeks, 19 eyes (59%) improved 3 lines or more of visual acuity, 11 eyes (34%) were stable, and 2 eyes (6%) lost 3 or more lines. The median posttreatment best-corrected visual acuity was 20/50 with a mean improvement of 4.9 lines. The means of central macular thickness and macular volume at 12 weeks were 236.84 μm and 6.7 μL, respectively. The mean number of intravitreal injections was 1.7 injections per eye. The short-term results suggested that intravitreal bevacizumab is safe and effective in patients with subfoveal idiopathic CNV [35].

Intravitreal Bevacizumab for Treatment of Subfoveal Idiopathic Choroidal Neovascularization: Results of a 1-Year Prospective Trial [36]

This was a prospective, consecutive, nonrandomized, noncomparative, and interventional case series that investigated the visual, anatomic, and safety outcomes of intravitreal bevacizumab in patients with subfoveal idiopathic CNV.

A total of 40 consecutive Chinese patients with subfoveal idiopathic CNV were included. All patients received an intravitreal injection of bevacizumab (1.25 mg/0.05 mL) at baseline. All patients were followed monthly for 12 months. Reinjection was done for persistent or recurrent activity as indicated by OCT. The median best-corrected visual acuity at baseline was 20/63. The mean OCT central macular thickness at baseline was 321 μm. At 12 months, the median best-corrected visual acuity was 20/32 with the mean of 2.4 lines of improvement. Seventy percent of eyes showed improved visual acuity, 30% were stable, and no eye had deterioration. After 1 year, the mean central macular thickness was 237 μm, and all eyes were in the cicatricial stage with no recurrence during the study period. A mean of 2 injections per eye were given, all retreatments were in the first 3 months. No severe ocular or systemic adverse event was observed. The results of this study demonstrated the beneficial effects of intravitreal bevacizumab in the treatment of subfoveal idiopathic CNV's [36].

Efficacy and Safety of Ranibizumab for the Treatment of Choroidal Neovascularization Due to Uncommon Cause: Twelve-Month Results of the MINERVA Study [37] (Please Refer to the Previous Chapter for More Details)

The MINERVA study was a phase III, prospective, double-masked, controlled, and randomized clinical trial. The objective was to assess the effectiveness and safety of intravitreal ranibizumab 0.5 mg/0.05 ml in patients with CNV due to uncommon causes (idiopathic, angioid streak, post inflammatory, central serous chorioretinopathy, and miscellaneous) over 1 year.

The study enrolled 178 patients who were randomized 2:1 to take either intravitreal ranibizumab injection (119 patients) or sham (59 patients) at baseline, and if required, month one. An open-label tailored ranibizumab injection started from month two until the twelfth month for both arms. Out of 178 patients, 63 patients were having idiopathic CNV (37 patients receiving ranibizumab and 26 patients receiving sham), and 27 patients were having CNV related to angioid streaks (18 patients receiving ranibizumab and 9 patients receiving sham). The mean baseline visual acuity for all subgroups was 62.2 ETDRS letters. At month 2, the ranibizumab group patients gained 9.5 letters vs. loss of 0.4 letters in the sham group. At month 12 (10 months after the open-label individualized ranibizumab injection), the difference was minimized to +11 letters and +9.3 in the ranibizumab and the sham groups, respectively. The least square means demonstrated a treatment effect of 10 letters gained compared to sham in patients with idiopathic CNV, CNV associated with angioid streaks, and CNV in the miscellaneous groups. The underlying etiology of the CNV did not contribute to the generally positive result. Over 1 year, the mean number of ranibizumab injections was 5.8 in the ranibizumab group and 5.4 injections in the sham group. Overall, intravitreal ranibizumab was safe and effective in treating CNV's and improving visual acuity regardless of the etiology [37].

22.3.3 CNV's Associated with Angioid Streaks

22.3.3.1 Photodynamic Therapy

Verteporfin Photodynamic Therapy of Choroidal Neovascularization in Angioid Streaks: One-Year Results of a Prospective Case Series [38]

This was a prospective, open-label, multicenter, interventional case series of patients treated with PDT for subfoveal/juxtafoveal CNV secondary to angioid streaks. PDT was carried out according to the standard protocol (see above). Patients were reassessed every 3 months and retreatment was done if there was evidence of fluorescein leakage on angiography. All patients were followed for 12 months.

A total of 23 eyes of 22 patients were included. Out of 23 eyes, 16 eyes were having subfoveal CNV's and 7 eyes had juxtafoveal CNV's. All CNV's were classic with no occult component at presentation. Over 1 year, 38% of the patients in the subfoveal group gained 8 or more letters and 88% lost fewer than 15 letters. Six eyes (38%) showed fluorescein leakage from the CNV at the 12-month visit. The mean number of PDT performed was 2.9. Two of 7 eyes (29%) gained 8 or more letters and 4 eyes (57%) lost more than 15 letters at 12 months. The mean number of PDT treatments done on eyes in this group was 3.4. This case series suggested that PDT can minimize visual loss patients with CNV's secondary to angioid streaks. Subfoveal CNV's showed better results than juxtafoveal lesions in which PDT did not limit the progression of CNV into the subfoveal area [38].

22.3.3.2 Anti-Vascular Endothelial Growth Factor Agents

Long-Term Control of Choroidal Neovascularization Secondary to Angioid Streaks Treated with Intravitreal Bevacizumab [39]

This study was a prospective, consecutive, open-label, interventional case series to study the efficacy of intravitreal bevacizumab in the long-term management of subfoveal CNV associated with angioid streaks. The study enrolled 11 patients who received an intravitreal injection of bevacizumab 1.25 mg/0.05 ml. The mean duration of follow-up was 23.8 months. The mean best-corrected visual acuity improved from 0.28 (ETDRS letters) at baseline to 0.56 at 20 months. All patients had a stable/improved visual acuity and 90.9% had improved vision at the 20-month visit. In addition, all patients had a stable/reduced CNV size at the same visit. The mean number of injections was 3.5 with no documented systemic or local adverse events. In summary, intravitreal bevacizumab was a safe and effective treatment modality for the long-term management of CNV secondary to angioid streaks [39].

Intravitreal Bevacizumab for Nonsubfoveal Choroidal Neovascularization Associated with Angioid Streaks: 3-Year Follow-Up Study [40]

This was a prospective interventional case series aiming to study the effects of intravitreal bevacizumab for juxtafoveal/extrafoveal CNV secondary to angioid streaks. The CNV's were treatment naïve. Primary end-points were the change in the best-corrected visual acuity and the proportion of eyes gaining 10 letters or more over 3 years. Secondary end-points included the change in the central macular thickness (CMT) and progression of the lesion to the fovea at the conclusion of the study.

Eighteen patients were eligible to be studied with 15 patients completing the 3-year follow-up on which the results were based. Juxtafoveal CNV was present in 8 patients (53.3%) while the remaining 7 patients (46.7%) presented with extrafoveal CNV. The mean best-corrected visual acuity showed a nonsignificant positive change from 77.9 ETDRS letters (20/28 Snellen equivalent) at baseline to 80.1 letters at the 1-year examination. At the 24- and 36-months' examinations, a statistically significant worsening (when compared to the 1-year results) of visual acuities were noted, with the mean visual acuities being 72.8 and 65.8 (20/50 Snellen equivalent) ETDRS letters, respectively. However, the visual acuities were stable between the time points in the second and third year and between the time points at baseline and the third year. On the other hand, 5 patients in the juxtafoveal group and 4 patients in the extrafoveal group lost 10 or more letters at the 3-year visit. The CMT changes were statistically insignificant in both groups.

Six CNV's (3 juxtafoveal and 3 extrafoveal) extended to the subfoveal area at the second-year follow-up with no more eyes observed to progress at the third-year visit. The mean number of intravitreal bevacizumab injections over 3 years was 5.2 (6.2 injections in the juxtafoveal CNV group and 4.1 injections in the extrafoveal CNV group). In conclusion, intravitreal bevacizumab was beneficial for nonsubfoveal CNV's secondary to angioid streaks over a 3-year follow-up and monitoring recurrence/progression was recommended on a monthly basis [40].

Intravitreal Ranibizumab Treatment of Macular Choroidal Neovascularization Secondary to Angioid Streaks: One-Year Results of a Prospective Study [41]
This was a prospective interventional case series that investigated the efficacy of intravitreal ranibizumab in the treatment of macular CNV's associated with angioid streaks.

A total of 15 eyes of 14 consecutive patients were included and observed for 1 year. Five eyes were having a subfoveal CNV, five eyes with juxtafoveal CNV, and 5 eyes with extrafoveal CNV. All eyes were injected with intravitreal ranibizumab 0.5 mg/0.05 ml monthly for 4 months. Then, patients were asked to come back in 6 weeks for re-evaluation. If the CNV was inactive (no hemorrhage, retinal edema, or subretinal fluid), the eye was injected and the patient was evaluated in 8 weeks. The same was done in this 8-week extension visit for inactive lesions except that the patients were requested to come back after 3, 4, and 5 months for injections until completing a total of 24 months. If the CNV was active at any visit after the 4 initial injections, the eye was injected and the patients were followed up at the same time interval as that before the preceding injection. The mean best-corrected visual acuity at baseline was 20/100 which improved to 20/50 at 1 year. The primary outcome (stable or improved visual acuity) was achieved in 93.3% at the end of follow-up. The best-corrected visual acuity improved in 53.3% and stabilized in 40.0% of the eyes. A worse best-corrected visual acuity was observed in 1 eye (6.7%). The mean greatest OCT lesion height was reduced and the lesion size on fluorescein angiography decreased/stabilized in 14 eyes (93.3%). The mean number of injections was 7.1 per eye. It was concluded that repeat intravitreal ranibizumab injections had beneficial visual and anatomical outcomes in patients with CNV's secondary to angioid streaks over 1 year [41].

22.3.4 Inflammatory Choroidal Neovascularization

22.3.4.1 Corticosteroids Therapy for Inflammatory CNV's

The Use of Corticosteroids for Choroidal Neovascularization in Young Patients [42]
The aim of this prospective study was to evaluate the effect of systemic corticosteroids in the treatment of sight-threatening choroidal neovascularization (CNV) in patients with punctate inner choroidopathy (PIC) and multifocal inner choroiditis (MIC). It included all cases where the CNV was not suitable for laser photocoagulation. Systemic oral prednisolone was started with a dose of 1 mg/kg and reduced gradually every 3–5 days over the course of 6–8 weeks. This corticosteroids course was repeated if retreatment deemed necessary. Main outcome measures were best-corrected visual acuity changes, and leakage on FFA during a mean follow-up period of 13 months.

Twelve eyes of 10 patients with symptomatic CNV due to PIC or MIC were identified. Mean initial visual acuity was 20/60 (range: 20/15–3/200). Ten of 12 eyes showed either improvement in Snellen visual acuity or stabilization of vision after the corticosteroids course. Mean final visual acuity was 20/40 (range: 20/20–20/200). Resolution of leakage on FFA was achieved in 9 eyes, and reduction of leakage on FFA was seen in the remaining 3 eyes. Four patients required more than one course of treatment. No systemic complications were observed during the study period. The study concluded that oral corticosteroids course in healthy young patients with subfoveal CNV secondary to PIC or MIC may reduce vascular leakage as seen on FFA, and stabilize vision when no other treatment option is available [42].

22.3.4.2 Photodynamic Therapy

Photodynamic Therapy for Juxtafoveal Choroidal Neovascularization Associated with Multifocal Choroiditis [43]

This study was an open-label, prospective, interventional case series to evaluate the effect of PDT on visual acuity outcomes in patients with juxtafoveal CNV secondary to multifocal choroiditis (MC).

Seven eyes of seven patients were treated in accordance with the treatment of age-related macular degeneration with photodynamic therapy (TAP) study. The median baseline visual acuity score increased from 75 letters (mean: 70 ± 12.5 SD) to 76 letters (mean: 74.5 ± 6.2 SD), and 79 letters (mean: 76.2 ± 7.6 SD) at 12- and 24-month follow-up, respectively. Visual acuity decreased by 1.5 or more lines in only one patient, but three patients (43%) gained at least 1.5 lines of visual acuity, and three patients (43%) maintained their baseline visual acuity at the 24-month follow-up. There were no side effects recorded during follow up. The study concluded that PDT can be considered as a safe and practical treatment option for juxtafoveal CNV secondary to MC [43].

22.3.4.3 Anti-Vascular Endothelial Growth Factor Agents

Intravitreal Bevacizumab for Juxtafoveal Choroidal Neovascularization Secondary to Multifocal Choroiditis [44]

This study was a prospective interventional case series to evaluate the effect of intravitreal bevacizumab injection on juxtafoveal CNV in multifocal choroiditis (MC) patients. The treatment protocol was as follows; intravitreal bevacizumab injection at baseline, then reassess every month for a total of 12 months. Repeat injection was done during the monthly follow-up visits if fluid on optical coherence tomography is seen and/or leakage on fluorescein angiography is detected.

Fourteen eyes of 14 patients were included. Mean BCVA improved from 0.41 ± 0.23 LogMAR at baseline (20/50 Snellen equivalent) to 0.16 ± 0.13 LogMAR at 12-month follow-up (20/28 Snellen equivalent) ($P = 0.002$). Mean central macular thickness decreased to 239 μm at the 12-month examination compared to 318 μm at baseline ($P < 0.001$). Mean number of injections was 2 ± 0.6 (range, 1–3) over the 12-month follow-up. No active CNV or extension of the CNV to the fovea at the 12-month follow-up was noted. No systemic or ocular side effects were observed. The study concluded that intravitreal bevacizumab is a useful treatment for juxtafoveal choroidal neovascularization associated with MC [44].

Choroidal Neovascularization Associated with Multiple Evanescent White Dot Syndrome Treated with Intravitreal Ranibizumab [45]

This prospective, interventional, case series study was conducted to evaluate the outcomes of subfoveal CNV associated with multiple evanescent white dot syndrome (MEWDS) after intravitreal ranibizumab injection. Patients were evaluated monthly for 12 months after the first ranibizumab injection and re-treatment was performed if activity was detected in the form of fluid on optical coherence tomography and/or leakage on fluorescein angiography.

Four eyes of four female patients were included in the study. All eyes (100%) showed functional improvement of at least 15 ETDRS letters. At 12-month examination, mean CMT decreased to 228 ± 14 μm compared to 330 ± 32 μm at baseline. The mean number of ranibizumab injections administered was 2.2 at the end of 12 months. No systemic complications or ocular side-effects were noted during follow-up. The study concluded that intravitreal ranibizumab treatment is a valuable therapeutic option for the management of CNV associated with MEWDS [45].

22.3.4.4 Combined Therapy for Inflammatory CNV's

Photodynamic Therapy Combined with Systemic Corticosteroids for Choroidal Neovascularization Secondary to Punctate Inner Choroidopathy (PIC) [46]
This study was a prospective consecutive case series to evaluate functional and angiographic outcomes of subfoveal CNV secondary to PIC after a combined PDT/systemic corticosteroid treatment regimen. All patients received oral prednisolone (1 mg/kg bodyweight/day) which was followed 5 days later by PDT. The dose of prednisolone was then tapered by 10 mg weekly. During follow-up, patients would receive another PDT treatment if there was any sign of CNV activity on fluorescein angiography.

Only 5 eyes of 5 female patients were treated over the 12-month study period. Mean BCVA improved from 28.4 ETDRS letters at baseline to 38.8 ETDRS letters at the final visit. Mean number of PDT treatments was only two (range 1–3). All cases showed signs of decreased CNV activity both clinically and angiographically at the final visit. The study concluded that PDT combined with systemic oral prednisolone appears to be safe and effective as a primary treatment for subfoveal CNV secondary to PIC [46].

Bevacizumab Versus Photodynamic Therapy for Choroidal Neovascularization in Multifocal Choroiditis [47]
This study was a prospective, pilot, randomized trial comparing the effect of PDT vs intravitreal bevacizumab therapy in patients with multifocal choroiditis (MC) complicated by subfoveal CNV.

Twenty-seven eyes of 27 patients were randomized to PDT treatment (13 eyes) or bevacizumab treatment (14 eyes). At 12 months examination, 5 eyes (36%) treated with bevacizumab gained more than 3 lines compared to none in the PDT group. Final central retinal thickness dropped significantly in both groups compared to baseline values. A mean of 1.7 treatments (range, 1.0–3.0) were performed in the PDT subgroup compared to a mean number of 3.8 (range, 3–7) intravitreal bevacizumab injections at the final 12-month visit. The study concluded that better functional outcome can be achieved using intravitreal bevacizumab injection rather than PDT for the treatment of subfoveal CNV secondary to MC [47].

22.3.5 CNV's Associated with Central Serous Chorioretinopathy

22.3.5.1 Photodynamic Therapy

Photodynamic Therapy with Verteporfin in Subfoveal Choroidal Neovascularization Secondary to Central Serous Chorioretinopathy [48]
This was a prospective interventional, non-comparative case series of patients with subfoveal CNV secondary to central serous chorioretinopathy (CSC) treated with PDT. The diagnosis of CSC was based on the patient's history and fluorescein and indocyanine green angiographic findings.

Photodynamic therapy was administered to 26 eyes of 24 patients. The decision for additional PDT treatments was based on follow-up fluorescein angiography which was done on each visit. The patients were followed-up for a mean of 22.2 months (range, 6–36 months). No dropouts were encountered at the 6-month follow-up, 24 (92%) of 26 eyes were available for the 1-year follow-up, and only 19 (73%) eyes were available at the 2-year follow-up. There was an obvious treatment benefit in visual acuity gains at 6 months after PDT. After 24 months, 9 (47%) of 19 eyes had 3 lines or more visual improvement, 8 (42%) eyes had stable visual acuity, and 2 (11%) eyes had lost 3 lines or more. Change in visual acuity from baseline to 12 and 24 months was statistically significant. The mean number of PDT treatments needed per patient was 2.6 (range, 1–7). None of the patients had systemic or ocular adverse effects. This case series concluded that PDT with verteporfin is a safe and effective treatment for subfoveal CNV secondary to CSC and more than 75% of patients will have stable or improved visual acuity 2 years after treatment [48].

Treatment of Choroidal Neovascularization in Central Serous Chorioretinopathy by Photodynamic Therapy with Verteporfin [49]

This was a prospective, consecutive, nonrandomized, and interventional study on patients with subfoveal or juxtafoveal CNV secondary to CSC to evaluate the safety and efficacy of PDT with verteporfin as a treatment modality.

Ten eyes were included in the study with a mean follow-up of 12.6 months (range, 6–21 months). At the last follow-up, six (60%) eyes gained 2 or more lines in visual acuity testing, 4 (40%) eyes had the final BCVA within 1 line of their initial BCVA, but none of the patients suffered a loss of 2 or more lines in vision. The mean LogMAR BCVA improvement after PDT was 2.4 lines. The study concluded that PDT with verteporfin therapy for CNV's secondary to CSC is a safe, well-tolerated treatment option and achieves a stable or improved vision [49].

22.3.6 CNV's Associated with Pattern Dystrophy (PD)

22.3.6.1 Anti-Vascular Endothelial Growth Factor Agents

Intravitreal Bevacizumab for Subfoveal Choroidal Neovascularization Associated with Pattern Dystrophy [50]

This was a prospective, nonrandomized, open-label, interventional study on patients with subfoveal CNV secondary to pattern dystrophy (PD). The aim was to assess the effects of treatment with intravitreal bevacizumab. The treatment protocol was to administer a loading dose of three consecutive injections monthly, then patients were followed up monthly and injections were administered "as needed" during a 24-month follow-up period.

Twelve patients were included in the study. At the 12-month follow-up, 7 (58%) patients gained at least 3 lines, 11 (92%) patients gained at least 1 line, and 1 patient showed stabilization of BCVA. At the 24-month follow-up, data regarding BCA remained unchanged except for a single patient (8%) who lost one line compared to baseline value. The CMT decreased from 276 ± 95 μm at baseline to 199 ± 34 μm at the 24-month follow-up ($P = 0.016$). No ocular or systemic side effects were noted. The study concluded that intravitreal bevacizumab injection for subfoveal CNV associated with PD is a valuable treatment [50].

Key Learning Points

- Laser photocoagulation treatment for juxtafoveal, extrafoveal, and peripapillary CNV's secondary to POHS is superior to no treatment.
- Krypton laser photocoagulation is not superior to Argon laser photocoagulation in the setting of extrafoveal CNV's secondary to POHS.
- Argon laser photocoagulation for idiopathic CNV's was beneficial but benefit was less pronounced than that in the POHS trial.
- Systemic steroids prior to PDT was better than PDT alone in patients with idiopathic and inflammatory CNV's.
- Intravitreal bevacizumab is safe and effective in patients with idiopathic CNV's.
- Intravitreal ranibizumab was safe and effective in treating CNV's and improving visual acuity regardless of the etiology.
- PDT appears safe and effective in treating inflammatory CNV's and CNV's secondary to CSCR.
- Intravitreal anti-VEGF agents appear safe and effective in treating inflammatory CNV's and CNV's secondary to CSCR.
- Intravitreal anti-VEGF agents had greater beneficial effects than PDT therapy in patients with inflammatory CNV's.

References

1. Neri P, Lettieri M, Fortuna C, Manoni M, Giovannini A. Inflammatory choroidal neovascularization. Middle East Afr J Ophthalmol. 2009;16(4):245–51.
2. Dhingra N, Kelly S, Majid MA, Bailey CB, Dick AD. Inflammatory choroidal neovascular membrane in posterior uveitis-pathogenesis and treatment. Indian J Ophthalmol. 2010;58(1):3–10.
3. Bansal R, Bansal P, Gupta A, Gupta V, Dogra MR, Singh R, et al. Diagnostic challenges in inflammatory

choroidal neovascular membranes. Ocul Immunol Inflamm. 2017;25(4):554–62.
4. Cohen SY, Laroche A, Leguen Y, Soubrane G, Coscas GJ. Etiology of choroidal neovascularization in young patients. Ophthalmology. 1996;103(8):1241–4.
5. Cheung CMG, Lai TYY, Ruamviboonsuk P, Chen SJ, Chen Y, Freund KB, et al. Polypoidal choroidal vasculopathy: definition, pathogenesis, diagnosis, and management. Ophthalmology. 2018;125(5):708–24.
6. Schlaegel TF. Ocular histoplasmosis. New York: Grune & Stratton; 1977.
7. Makley TA Jr, Long JW, Suie T. Therapy of chorioretinitis presumed to be caused by histoplasmosis. Int Ophthalmol Clin. 1975;15(3):181–96.
8. Schlaegel TF Jr. Corticosteroids in the treatment of ocular histoplasmosis. Int Ophthalmol Clin. 1983;23(2):111–23.
9. Gass J. Stereoscopic atlas of macular diseases. St. Louis, MO: Mosby; 1987.
10. Watzke RC, Leaverton PE. Light coagulation in presumed histoplasmic choroiditis. Controlled clinical study. Arch Ophthalmol. 1971;86(2):127–32.
11. Argon laser photocoagulation for ocular histoplasmosis. Results of a randomized clinical trial. Arch Ophthalmol. 1983;101(9):1347–57.
12. Argon laser photocoagulation for neovascular maculopathy. Three-year results from randomized clinical trials. Macular Photocoagulation Study Group. Arch Ophthalmol. 1986;104(5):694–701.
13. Argon laser photocoagulation for neovascular maculopathy. Five-year results from randomized clinical trials. Macular Photocoagulation Study Group. Arch Ophthalmol. 1991;109(8):1109–14.
14. Krypton laser photocoagulation for neovascular lesions of ocular histoplasmosis. Results of a randomized clinical trial. Macular Photocoagulation Study Group. Arch Ophthalmol. 1987;105(11):1499–507.
15. Laser photocoagulation for juxtafoveal choroidal neovascularization. Five-year results from randomized clinical trials. Macular Photocoagulation Study Group. Arch Ophthalmol. 1994;112(4):500–9.
16. Persistent and recurrent neovascularization after krypton laser photocoagulation for neovascular lesions of ocular histoplasmosis. Macular Photocoagulation Study Group. Arch Ophthalmol. 1989;107(3):344–52.
17. Laser photocoagulation for neovascular lesions nasal to the fovea. Results from clinical trials for lesions secondary to ocular histoplasmosis or idiopathic causes. Macular Photocoagulation Study Group. Arch Ophthalmol. 1995;113(1):56–61.
18. Gutman FA. The natural course of active choroidal lesions in the presumed ocular histoplasmosis syndrome. Trans Am Ophthalmol Soc. 1979;77:515–41.
19. Marshall J, Bird AC. A comparative histopathological study of argon and krypton laser irradiations of the human retina. Br J Ophthalmol. 1979;63(10):657–68.
20. Argon green vs krypton red laser photocoagulation for extrafoveal choroidal neovascularization. One-year results in ocular histoplasmosis. The Canadian Ophthalmology Study Group. Arch Ophthalmol. 1994;112(9):1166–73.
21. Fine SL, Wood WJ, Isernhagen RD, Singerman LJ, Bressler NM, Folk JC, et al. Laser treatment for subfoveal neovascular membranes in ocular histoplasmosis syndrome: results of a pilot randomized clinical trial. Arch Ophthalmol. 1993, 111(1):19–20.
22. Saperstein DA, Rosenfeld PJ, Bressler NM, Rosa RH Jr, Sickenberg M, Sternberg P Jr, et al. Photodynamic therapy of subfoveal choroidal neovascularization with verteporfin in the ocular histoplasmosis syndrome: one-year results of an uncontrolled, prospective case series. Ophthalmology. 2002;109(8):1499–505.
23. Rosenfeld PJ, Saperstein DA, Bressler NM, Reaves TA, Sickenberg M, Rosa RH Jr, et al. Photodynamic therapy with verteporfin in ocular histoplasmosis: uncontrolled, open-label 2-year study. Ophthalmology. 2004;111(9):1725–33.
24. Saperstein DA, Rosenfeld PJ, Bressler NM, Rosa RH Jr, Sternberg P Jr, Aaberg TM Sr, et al. Verteporfin therapy for CNV secondary to OHS. Ophthalmology. 2006;113(12):2371.e1–3.
25. Thomas MA, Grand MG, Williams DF, Lee CM, Pesin SR, Lowe MA. Surgical management of subfoveal choroidal neovascularization. Ophthalmology 1992;99(6):952–68; discussion 75-6.
26. Hawkins BS, Bressler NM, Bressler SB, Davidorf FH, Hoskins JC, Marsh MJ, et al. Surgical removal vs observation for subfoveal choroidal neovascularization, either associated with the ocular histoplasmosis syndrome or idiopathic: I. Ophthalmic findings from a randomized clinical trial: Submacular Surgery Trials (SST) Group H Trial: SST Report No. 9. Arch Ophthalmol. 2004;122(11):1597–611.
27. Hawkins BS, Miskala PH, Bass EB, Bressler NM, Childs AL, Mangione CM, et al. Surgical removal vs observation for subfoveal choroidal neovascularization, either associated with the ocular histoplasmosis syndrome or idiopathic: II. Quality-of-life findings from a randomized clinical trial: SST Group H Trial: SST Report No. 10. Arch Ophthalmol. 2004;122(11):1616–28.
28. Walia HS, Shah GK, Blinder KJ. Treatment of CNV secondary to presumed ocular histoplasmosis with intravitreal aflibercept 2.0 mg injection. Can J Ophthalmol. 2016;51(2):91–6.
29. Argon laser photocoagulation for idiopathic neovascularization. Results of a randomized clinical trial. Arch Ophthalmol. 1983;101(9):1358–61.
30. Krypton laser photocoagulation for idiopathic neovascular lesions. Results of a randomized clinical trial. Macular Photocoagulation Study Group. Arch Ophthalmol. 1990;108(6):832–7.
31. Chan WM, Lam DS, Wong TH, Lai TY, Kwok AK, Tam BS, et al. Photodynamic therapy with verteporfin for subfoveal idiopathic choroidal neovascularization: one-year results from a prospective case series. Ophthalmology. 2003;110(12):2395–402.
32. Giovannini A, Neri P, Mercanti L, Brue C. Photodynamic treatment versus photodynamic treatment associated with systemic steroids for idiopathic choroidal neovascularisation. Br J Ophthalmol. 2007;91(5):620–3.

33. Li XX, Tao Y. Small laser spot versus standard laser spot photodynamic therapy for idiopathic choroidal neovascularization: a randomized controlled study. Chin Med J. 2012;125(24):4424–8.
34. Kumar A, Prakash G, Singh RP. Transpupillary thermotherapy for idiopathic subfoveal choroidal neovascularization. Acta Ophthalmol Scand. 2004;82(2):205–8.
35. Mandal S, Garg S, Venkatesh P, Mithal C, Vohra R, Mehrotra A. Intravitreal bevacizumab for subfoveal idiopathic choroidal neovascularization. Arch Ophthalmol. 2007;125(11):1487–92.
36. Zhang H, Liu ZL, Sun P, Gu F. Intravitreal bevacizumab for treatment of subfoveal idiopathic choroidal neovascularization: results of a 1-year prospective trial. Am J Ophthalmol. 2012;153(2):300–6.e1.
37. Lai TYY, Staurenghi G, Lanzetta P, Holz FG, Melissa Liew SH, Desset-Brethes S, et al. Efficacy and safety of ranibizumab for the treatment of choroidal neovascularization due to uncommon cause: twelve-month results of the Minerva study. Retina. 2018;38(8):1464–77.
38. Browning AC, Chung AK, Ghanchi F, Harding SP, Musadiq M, Talks SJ, et al. Verteporfin photodynamic therapy of choroidal neovascularization in angioid streaks: one-year results of a prospective case series. Ophthalmology. 2005;112(7):1227–31.
39. Neri P, Salvolini S, Mariotti C, Mercanti L, Celani S, Giovannini A. Long-term control of choroidal neovascularisation secondary to angioid streaks treated with intravitreal bevacizumab (Avastin). Br J Ophthalmol. 2009;93(2):155–8.
40. Iacono P, Battaglia Parodi M, La Spina C, Bandello F. Intravitreal Bevacizumab for nonsubfoveal choroidal neovascularization associated with angioid streaks: 3-year follow-up study. Am J Ophthalmol. 2016;165:174–8.
41. Ladas ID, Kotsolis AI, Ladas DS, Niskopoulou M, Georgalas I, Papakonstantinou D, et al. Intravitreal ranibizumab treatment of macular choroidal neovascularization secondary to angioid streaks: one-year results of a prospective study. Retina. 2010;30(8):1185–9.
42. Flaxel CJ, Owens SL, Mulholland B, Schwartz SD, Gregor ZJ. The use of corticosteroids for choroidal neovascularisation in young patients. Eye (Lond). 1998;12(Pt 2):266–72.
43. Parodi MB, Iacono P, Spasse S, Ravalico G. Photodynamic therapy for juxtafoveal choroidal neovascularization associated with multifocal choroiditis. Am J Ophthalmol. 2006;141(1):123–8.
44. Parodi MB, Iacono P, Mansour A, Benedetto U, Knutsson KA, Bandello F, et al. Intravitreal bevacizumab for juxtafoveal choroidal neovascularization secondary to multifocal choroiditis. Retina. 2013;33(5):953–6.
45. Battaglia Parodi M, Iacono P, Zucchiatti I, Bandello F. Choroidal neovascularization associated with multiple evanescent white dot syndrome treated with intravitreal ranibizumab. Ocul Immunol Inflamm. 2018;26(4):608–11.
46. Fong KC, Thomas D, Amin K, Inzerillo D, Horgan SE. Photodynamic therapy combined with systemic corticosteroids for choroidal neovascularisation secondary to punctate inner choroidopathy. Eye (Lond). 2008;22(4):528–33.
47. Parodi MB, Iacono P, Kontadakis DS, Zucchiatti I, Cascavilla ML, Bandello F. Bevacizumab vs photodynamic therapy for choroidal neovascularization in multifocal choroiditis. Arch Ophthalmol. 2010;128(9):1100–3.
48. Ergun E, Tittl M, Stur M. Photodynamic therapy with verteporfin in subfoveal choroidal neovascularization secondary to central serous chorioretinopathy. Arch Ophthalmol. 2004;122(1):37–41.
49. Chan WM, Lam DS, Lai TY, Yuen KS, Liu DT, Chan CK, et al. Treatment of choroidal neovascularization in central serous chorioretinopathy by photodynamic therapy with verteporfin. Am J Ophthalmol. 2003;136(5):836–45.
50. Parodi MB, Iacono P, Cascavilla M, Zucchiatti I, Kontadakis DS, Bandello F. Intravitreal bevacizumab for subfoveal choroidal neovascularization associated with pattern dystrophy. Invest Ophthalmol Vis Sci. 2010;51(9):4358–61.

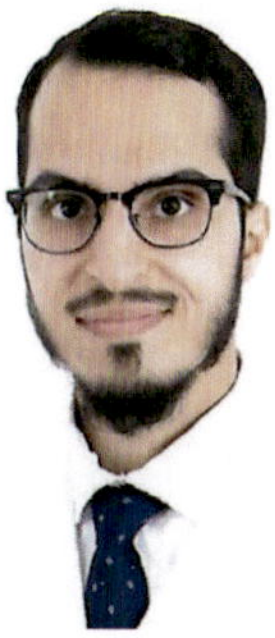

Tariq Alzahem is currently the Chief Resident in his last year in King Saud University Ophthalmology Training Program. He was awarded as The Resident of The Year in 2017 and 2018. He was also awarded the Ideal Student Prize at the level of King Saud University in 2014. Tariq is planning to be a clinical scientist in the field of Surgical Retina where his professional experience and education will allow him to make an immediate contribution as an integral part of a progressive institution.

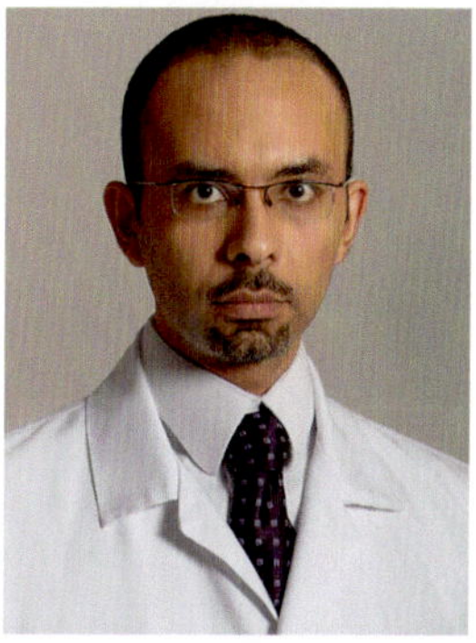

Marwan A. Abouammoh is a full Professor of Ophthalmology at King Saud University, Riyadh, Saudi Arabia. He is a graduate of Riyadh's Joint Ophthalmology residency program and has completed a 2-year vitreoretinal fellowship at King Khaled Eye Specialist Hospital. He did a further year of fellowship training at Queen's University, Kingston, Ontario where he also studied and practiced medical/scientific reasoning, health outcomes, and safety of novel treatments for macular degeneration and diabetic retinopathy. He is currently involved in clinical-based research related to Retina and Ophthalmology and actively contributes to original clinical trials, systematic reviews, and meta-analyses.

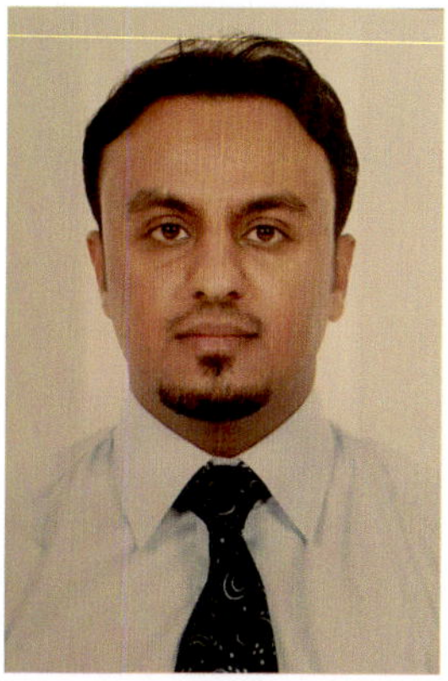

Nayef Alswaina is an Ophthalmology consultant with a sub-specialization and interest in surgical retina. He finished his residency and subspecialty program from Riyadh ophthalmology program (King Khaled Eye Specialist Hospital and King Abdulaziz University Hospital). Currently, he is working as an Assistant Professor at the Department of Ophthalmology, College of Medicine, Qassim University, Saudi Arabia.

Reading Centers for Clinical Trials of Choroidal Neovascularization (CNV): Present Role and Future Opportunities

23

René Rückert, Lala Ceklic, and Marion R. Munk

23.1 Introduction

Photographic reading centers play an important role in the objective, independent, and scientific justified development of novel diagnostic and therapeutic modalities for various eye pathologies, and in particular for new therapies of retinal diseases including choroidal neovascularization (CNV). In the recent decade, we all were witnesses of the development and launch of various improved and enhanced diagnostic tools. TD-OCT was a breakthrough in retina imaging, introduction of SD-OCT exponentially increased the spatial resolution of retinal images. OCT-A as a new imaging tool nowadays allows the noninvasive assessment of vascular structures in the retina that needed invasive procedures during FA including risk-associated injection of fluorescein until recently. With (experimental) Enhanced Deep Imaging (EDI)—OCT and Swept-Source (SS)—OCTs we are now able to even detect and quantify structures that were out of reach for non-invasive in vivo diagnosis and follow-up just a few years ago.

Pharmaceutical companies—big pharma and a growing number of small biotechs—develop (-ed) various drugs and devices which can prevent blindness and improve vision of patients affected by CNV such as the approved anti-VEGF drugs ranibizumab and aflibercept. Besides the current domination of CNV therapy by those two approved (and one off-label) VEGF blockers, new treatment modalities are under research in clinical trials. As global clinical trials for the approval or the label-extension of approved drugs require prospective and double-masked trials, and independent, expert processing and analyzing of retina images, retina imaging reading centers are a mainstay of current ophthalmic drug development. Experienced reading centers use masked analysis which prevents research outcomes from being influenced by various biases such as patient expectations (placebo effect), investigators expectancy (observer bias), and sponsor expectations. Professional reading centers can support protocol writing and definition of clinical endpoints for clinical trials.

A significant number of reading centers exist around the world, many are smaller with a focus on academic studies, plus several larger and more

R. Rückert
Eyegnos Consulting for Ophthalmic Drug Development, Bern, Switzerland

L. Ceklic
Bern Photographic Reading Center, Inselspital, University Hospital Bern, Bern, Switzerland

M. R. Munk (✉)
Bern Photographic Reading Center, Inselspital, University Hospital Bern, Bern, Switzerland

Department of Ophthalmology, Inselspital, University Hospital Bern, Bern, Switzerland

Department of Ophthalmology, Feinberg School of Medicine, Northwestern University, Chicago, IL, USA

J. Chhablani (ed.), *Choroidal Neovascularization*, https://doi.org/10.1007/978-981-15-2213-0_23

professionalized reading centers that have sufficient capacity for large, global, multicenter trials with 4-digit patient numbers. Such large studies are needed for late-stage trials to assess the efficacy of new drugs to treat retinal diseases such as exudative age-related macular degeneration (AMD).

Photographic Reading Centers apply professional administrative measures and standard operational procedures (SOP's) to assure GCP/ICH guidelines are followed and highest ethical standards are applied, to generate data which are the basis for regulatory submission. They apply measures to assure that images are properly labeled, that personal information are removed in order to de-identify patients, that image acquisition is complete, and that the images are of adequate quality for analysis. IT experts and engineers are the basis for development and support of the digital image transfer and long-term storage. Furthermore, reading centers usually offer certification and real-time teaching for investigators and photographers in clinical studies, thereby contributing to the education and general improvement in the quality of day-by-day diagnostic and of clinical research in ophthalmology. During the clinical studies, the digital images are assessed and analyzed by trained graders.

Ophthalmic reading centers collect data in a harmonized fashion and thereby produce data sets of high quality that were the basis for regulatory filings and countless post hoc analyses of global clinical studies. Such high-quality image data sets are furthermore the basis for new big data-driven research and support the development of automated, artificial intelligence (AI)-based analysis tools.

23.2 Roles and Responsibilities of Imaging Reading Centers

The purpose of reading centers is to assure that all steps in collecting, processing, and analyzing data and images are independent and non-biased by the sponsor of clinical studies following strict standard operating procedures. Such image analysis data are the basis for the evaluation of morphological changes and the statistical analysis of imaging endpoints and/ or can be used to identify biomarker at baseline or during the course of a therapeutic study—to assess and quantify biomarker of high/low-responders and many more aspects of a patient's data.

Photographic Reading Centers must base their work on principles of Good Clinical Practice.

Development of numerous retinal imaging techniques and need for more precise and more detailed imaging of CNV and possible morphologic risk factors require imaging experts that receive permanent training and managing of a reading center requires cooperation of retina experts, biomedicine engineers, and IT. Excellent training of image readers in the pathogenesis and detection of CNV leads to optimal results of the evaluation of retinal images.

The role of reading centers has expanded vastly in the past years—beyond simple analysis of images as service provider to pharma companies—to a real partnership model in drug development including the following service and expert support:

23.2.1 Pre-trial Support

- Clinical trial design and imaging endpoint consulting and development
- Development of clinical site manual for imaging procedures
- Training and certification of clinical sites

23.2.2 Trial Support

- Internal validation of key grading criteria across modalities/different imaging devices.
- Clinical site support for quality assurance.
- Real-time sponsor and CRO access to clinical trial reads and reports.
- Detection of safety signals in ongoing studies including support for independent data safety monitoring committees (IDMCs).

23.2.3 Post-trial Support

- Sponsor-tailored data outputs.
- Support of statistical analysis.
- Support for writing study report and regulatory filing documents.
- Research and post hoc analyses for additional data generation.

For evaluating CNV related to AMD, essential retinal imaging methods are 3 field fundus color photography (CF), fluorescein angiography (FA), indocyanine green angiography (ICGA; optional, in order to identify Type 3 neovascularization, polypoidal choroidal vasculopathy, and subclinical neovascularization, respectively), optical coherence tomography (OCT) and optical coherence tomography-angiography (OCT-A).

23.3 CNV Image Reading Modalities

Retinal Imaging reading centers were in the past initially established to read color fundus and FA images. Recent technical development of OCT devices has expanded the spectrum of analyses as OCT has become a mainstay of retinal disease diagnostic in particular also for CNV. Retina image reading centers accept and assess most of the current standard image modalities and devices for the analysis of morphologic outcome measures. Below, we describe in more detail some of the standard assessment and parameters analyzed by reading centers.

23.4 Color Fundus Photography for CNV in AMD

Most prospective clinical trials require detailed and objective analyses of fundus photographs. Thus, standard requirements for data processing for color fundus (CF) are stereoscopic three (3-) fields images with focus on posterior pole and optic disk (M1), macula (M2), and temporal to the macula field (M3) with angle of 30° and 55° or based on latest developments in imaging devices: ultra widefield imaging (105° and 180°).

The Age-Related Eye Disease Study (AREDS) was a multicenter prospective cohort study of the clinical course, prognosis, and risk factors for AMD. An important goal of AREDS has been the development of a severity scale for AMD, to provide baseline risk categories, to allow tracking of progression along the scale, and to define surrogate outcomes for progression to advanced AMD [1, 2]. AREDS started in 1992 and ran until 2005 and enrolled 4613 study participants. The AREDS Report No.17 from 2005 established an AREDS severity scale and risk factors were evaluated by human graders and reading of stereoscopic 3-field fundus photography's and recent publication by Burlina and co-authors are based on deep machine learning. This study used 67,401 color fundus images from the 4613 study participants. The weighted kappa scores were 0.77 for the 4-step and 0.74 for the 9-step AMD severity scales, which confirms that the concordance and reproducibility of artificial intelligence image grading are relatively high and reliable [2].

23.5 Fluorescein Angiography in CNV

Fluorescein angiography (FA) has been used to define lesion size and type of CNV. It allows the distinction between well-demarcated classic CNV, and ill-defined occult CNV. The location and exact boundaries of occult CNV often are difficult to determine precisely on FA, i.e., due to obscuration of the neovascular membrane by overlying turbid exudates, blood and/or pigment, and rapid fluorescein pooling beneath a serous PED.

According to angiographic patterns, as analyzed by photographic reading centers, CNVs are classified and described as below [3, 4]:

1. Classic CNV: Hyperfluorescence in the early phases of the angiogram, maintains well-demarcated borders, and leaks late thus obscuring its borders.
2. Occult CNV: A lesion whose borders cannot be determined and relatively late hyperfluorescence or lesion that increases by time.
3. Fibrovascular pigment epithelial detachment (PED); a form of occult CNV: A lesion, well-

demarcated or poorly demarcated, that is elevated solidly and hyperfluoresces irregularly to different degrees.
4. Late leakage of undetermined source (LLUS); a form of occult CNV: A lesion that demonstrates irregular, indistinct, late, and sub-RPE leakage [4].

CNV could be located relative to the center of fovea [4]:

1. Extrafoveal (the border of the CNV is 200–1500 μm from the center of the fovea)
2. Juxtafoveal (the border of the CNV is 1–199 μm from the center of the fovea)
3. Subfoveal

Prior to the anti-VEGF era, the location and the type of CNV lesion were of uppermost importance, as lesion type and location determined appropriate treatment such as laser treatment, assessed in the macular photocoagulation study (MPS), or photodynamic therapy, assessed in the TAP, VIP, and VIM trials [5, 6]. Nowadays, with the anti-VEGF treatments established as the standard of care, lesion type, and location may impact treatment response and long-term outcomes. The location of CNV lesion (subfoveal and juxtafoveal vs. extrafoveal) may determine inclusion and exclusion in AMD clinical trials. The importance of reading centers is supported by research performed early in the new decade of retina drug development, demonstrating only moderate interobserver agreement for CNV categorization between clinicians and poor agreement among diverse retina specialists for categorization and localization of CNV on fluorescein angiograms. There was only a moderate intra-observer agreement for both treatment decision and lesion categorization in past studies. And, there was only moderate agreement between observers and the reading center for angiographic CNV categorization [7–10]. Those data supported and build the basis for funding retina reading centers in order to reduce intra-observer variability and to harmonize image analysis in large, multicenter, and multicounty clinical studies.

Determining the CNV size and type in fluorescein angiograms are required for proper treatment and prognosis of the disease. Computer-assisted methods for CNV segmentation can be supportive not only to reduce the burden of manual segmentation but also to reduce inter- and intra-observer variability. The set of model parameters at each pixel are used to segment the image into regions of homogeneous parameters. Thus, development of computer-assisted systems for determining CNV lesion is important to avoid inter- and intra-observer variability among human graders [11]. For nAMD trials, FAs are usually performed at baseline, 1 year and 2 years, which is in most of the nAMD trials at the end of study visit.

23.6 Optical Coherence Tomography in CNV Due to AMD

Traditionally, FA has been considered the reference standard to detect CNV activity, but FA is costly and invasive with associated risks due to the fluorescein injection. Invention and widespread introduction of OCT as noninvasive method have revolutionized retinal diagnostic, treatment assessment and follow-up and improved analysis of CNV and definition of possible biomarkers as prognostic factors. Unfortunately, there is substantial disagreement between OCT and FA findings in detecting active disease in patients with CNV due to AMD during disease monitoring [12]. Recently published data show that OCT was useful in quantitatively evaluating subretinal and intraretinal fluid, assessing the possible subfoveal location of neovascularization, and in monitoring CNV before and after treatment. OCT was unable to detect CNV beneath serous pigment epithelial detachments. OCT may have the potential to accurately defining the boundaries in a subset of angiographically occult CNV [3, 13]. Unlike FA, which is two-dimensional but is a dynamic assessment (i.e., includes the time after injection as additional information/parameter) and detects leakage, lesion size, and localization, OCT provides a three-dimensional but non-dynamic snapshot of structural information on chorioretinal layers and the presence of fluid in the retina, and in subretinal pigment epithelial spaces, which are considered a surrogate for leakage. OCT is used to determine both the presence and activity of CNV and the need for anti-VEGF treatment/retreatment in clinical trials and routinely in clinical practice [14–16].

New choroidal blood vessels may extend into the sub-RPE space (type 1) or into the subretinal space (type 2) [4, 17]. Bleeding and exudation which may occur with further expansion of the lesion, lead to visual impairment and other functional symptoms. Alternatively, abnormal blood vessels may originate from an intraretinal location and grow into the subretinal space [4]. This pattern of growth has been named retinal angiomatous proliferation (RAP), or type 3 neovascularization [17]. Reading center usually assesses and defines the extent of CNV in the clinical images. CNV, when analyzed with OCT, could be described as thickening and fragmentation of the highly reflective RPE-choriocapillaris band [4]. Serous, hemorrhagic, or fibrovascular detachments of RPE represent RPE band elevations with shadowing of the structures beneath the elevated area [4, 18]. Neurosensory retinal detachment appears as elevation of moderately reflective band above the RPE band [4].

OCT imaging is standard procedure for managing CNV and inter-grader and intra-grader reproducibility are very high [19]. SD OCT showed high sensitivity (85.7–98.3%) and specificity (84.2–100%) compared to FA in the diagnosis of the CNV subtype [18]. Usually, in clinical nAMD trials, OCTs are performed at each study visit throughout the study, to assess disease activity and treatment needs. In some trials it is up to the investigator's discretion to decide whether CNV is active, in other trials disease activity will be assessed by the reading center and the (re-) treatment plan will be adapted accordingly. Although many predictive biomarkers can be assessed by OCT, the main surrogate markers on OCT are still central retinal thickness (CRT), presence of subretinal fluid, and presence of intraretinal fluid. Further parameters such as the presence of epiretinal membranes, vitreomacular adhesion, or—traction, subretinal hyperreflective material, macular atrophy, reticular pseudodrusen et al. will be in fact assessed by the reading centers and maybe important biomarkers for treatment response and (long-) term outcome, but are usually in the best case exploratory outcome parameters or often just used for post hoc analyses. The evaluation of CRT as one of the key secondary outcome parameters in nAMD trials was challenging in the earlier days, when TD-OCTs, as well as SD-OCTs, were used. The segmentation software of TD-OCTs devices used the internal limiting membrane (ILM) and the external limiting membrane (ELM) to obtain CRT values, while SD-OCT devices automatically segmented the ILM and the RPE or Bruch's membrane for CRT and retinal volume values, which resulted in an about 50–70 μm lower CRT measurements of TD-OCT's compared to SD-OCTs [20–22]. Nowadays only SD-OCTs or SS-OCTs are used for nAMD trials; however, also the current state-of-the-art OCT devices from different manufacturers still employ different segmentation borders, segmenting, i.e., the RPE or the Bruch's membrane, which also results in slightly different measurements [23, 24]. These mean differences range of 14–37 μm, while CRT is measured with SS-OCTs is, in general, lower than with SD-OCT. The two dominating OCT devices in clinical studies use their own software for CRT measurements, and so the Heidelberg Spectralis® software provides thicker CRT values than Zeiss Cirrus® software. One way how to overcome these differences is custom-made software applying the same segmentation for all imported OCTs scans, which are regularly used in a reading center setting.

In the era of emerging "Big data" machine deep learning, machine learning, and AI attracts many investigators to develop efficient and accurate system for screening, monitoring, management, and prediction systems for various treatment options. Most of those developments are based on the large image databases of retinal reading centers. It is very important to detect risk factors and early signs of CNV disease. Given that OCT imaging is the single most common diagnostic test performed on a daily basis in retinal clinics, its advantages are the features as noninvasive, quick, and highly sensitive method. Those features potentially lend itself to automation with deep-learning techniques. Based on many investigations, it is possible to detect small constraints like hard drusen automatically with relatively high accuracy [25, 26]. Several groups have successfully utilized deep learning in segmentation of OCT scans for the detection of morphological features such as intraretinal fluid (IRF) or subretinal fluid (SRF) from various retinovascular diseases [27, 28]. Having a system that can reliably produce diagnostic evaluations that match the physician's standards may help to increase direct face-time with patients, alleviate administrative burden, reduce administrative practice costs and, ultimately, improve day-to-day clinic efficiency. For developing such systems, reading centers play a crucial role in acquiring and analyzing large pools of imaging data, in order to precisely build a foundation of AI software's ability to become a more effective, accurate and reliable tool for screening, monitoring, and analyzing CNV [29, 30]. Automated classifiers may be also used in reading centers as additional graders or ultimately to replace human graders in the near future.

23.7 Optical Coherence Tomography Angiography for CNV

Optical coherence tomography angiography (OCT-A) is a recently introduced, noninvasive imaging technique that generates volumetric angiography images in a matter of seconds. Using OCT-A allows the clinician to visualize CNV noninvasively and may provide a method for identifying and guiding the treatment of CNV. The specificity of CNV detection on OCT-A compared with FA seems to be high [31]. OCT-A is a noninvasive imaging technique that can be used to visualize blood flow comprising CNV. Although OCT-A can reliably detect CNV, the morphologic appearance of CNV on OCT-A does not reliably correlate with clinical activity of CNV [32]. OCT-A allows identification of distinct CNV-specific vascular patterns at the level of the outer retinal layer and choriocapillaris. Correlation with clinical and functional parameters may be useful to better understand the pathology and guide efficient therapeutic strategies [33]. OCT-A provides noninvasive measurement of the area of neovascular lesions in AMD. Sustained growth of type 1 CNV can be identified in the majority of lesions (80%) that display characteristic patterns of progression despite ongoing anti-VEGF therapy [34]. According to FA, CNV was classified as classic predominantly classic, minimally classic, and occult. In a recently published study, corresponding to FA in OCT-A scans, 46.4% (26/56 eyes) had well-circumscribed vessels, and 53.6% (30/56 eyes) showed poorly circumscribed vessels. There were 11 false positives and 7 false negatives using OCT-A. The specificity of OCT-A for the detection of CNV was 67.6%, with sensitivity of 86.5%. OCT-A may help in the noninvasive diagnosis of CNV and may provide a method for monitoring the evolution of CNV [35]. OCT-A has its rationale as a fast, noninvasive screening tool for CNV in asymptomatic patients [36]. There is a notable prevalence of subclinical CNV in fellow eyes with unilateral exudative CNV, and significantly greater choriocapillaris nonperfusion adjacent to all CNV lesions. There is a trend for increased choriocapillaris nonperfusion in exudative AMD eyes as compared with their fellow subclinical CNV eyes [37]. OCT-A was generally less successful in detecting CNV than ICGA in patients who were included in this study based on FA and OCT. Types 1 and 2 CNV area were significantly smaller in OCT-A than in ICGA. However, OCT-A detected all type 1 lesions except for one, indicating that the SD-OCT-A signal is limited by detection limits of blood flow velocity rather than lesion type [38]. Treatment-naive eyes and treated eyes with CNV secondary to neovascular AMD respond differently to anti-VEGF therapy. This should be taken into account when performing OCT-A image analysis in clinical studies and when using OCT-A for CNV follow-up or planning therapeutic strategies [39]. There are a number of promising OCT-A parameters that can be used to diagnose the presence of CNV and to monitor the activity and progression of the lesion, pre- and post-treatment morphological characteristics, CNV dimensions, and other quantitative, computed parameters such as vessel density. However, as this methodology has been introduced only recently to the market and clinic, all OCT-A data and analysis require further validation before they can be widely used [40]. Manufacturers provide OCT-A software with their devices. Unfortunately, recent studies have shown that the inter-device agreement and comparability is rather low. This is contributed to, i.e., divergent segmentations, different algorithms to generate flow motion, and due to different post-acquisition processing software [41, 42]. Therefore, comparability and pooling of acquired data, in particular quantitative metrics for clinical trials, is a difficult task and currently a key challenge for reading centers in clinical trials. OCT-A is still in the focus of many investigators worldwide and knowledge from OCT-A imaging is still developing. Again though, image reading center will play a key role in collecting and analyzing large pools of OCT-A data in order to improve knowledge and familiarity with this new addition to the retina (CNV) imaging tools. Current ongoing nAMD trials have included OCT-A parameters as exploratory outcome parameters in their protocols.

23.8 Increased Complexity and Challenges in CNV Studies

The complexity of retina image analysis has increased significantly over the last years. New morphologic features are usually initially identified in small academic studies using new technology or advanced detection methods. Subsequently, such new possible imaging endpoints and pathologic morphologic features of retinal diseases need to be verified—and that is where reading centers can (and do) play a very significant role with post hoc analyses of existing studies using data from their large imaging database. Once verified as significant or interesting to evaluate disease progress or treatment outcome, such marker can be incorporated in a prospective way in new clinical trials for CNV treatments as exploratory endpoints.

One impressive example of the increased complexity of image analysis by reading centers is given in Table 23.1, with the listed outcome parameter in two selected Phase 3/3b/4 studies as

Table 23.1 Secondary imaging/morphologic endpoints in pivotal AMD/CNV trials—2008 versus 2018 (from: www.clinicaltrials.gov)

VIEW2 Study Aflibercept in AMD, Study start: April 2008	MERLIN Study Brolucizumab in AMD, Study start: October 2018
• Mean change from baseline in Choroidal Neovascularization (CNV) area at week 52—LOCF; CNV area values measured in square millimeters; lower values represent better outcomes.	• Change in Central Subfield Thickness (CST) from baseline to each post-baseline visit; CST will be assessed using Spectral Domain Optical Coherence Tomography (SD-OCT) images. • Intraretinal fluid (IRF) at each post-baseline visit; IRF will be assessed using SD-OCT images. The number of subjects with IRF (present, absent) will be reported for each post-baseline visit. • Subretinal fluid (SRF) at each post-baseline visit; SRF will be assessed using SD-OCT images. The number of subjects with SRF (present, absent) will be reported for each post-baseline visit. • Sub-retinal pigment epithelium (sub-RPE) fluid in patients with sub-RPE fluid at baseline; sub-RPE fluid will be assessed using SD-OCT images. The number of subjects with sub-RPE fluid in subjects with sub-RPE fluid at baseline (present, absent) will be reported for each post-baseline visit. • Fluid-free status (no IRF, SRF, or sub-RPE fluid) at each post-baseline treatment visit; IRF, SRF, and sub-RPE fluid will assessed using SD-OCT images. The number of subjects with fluid-free status (no IRF, SRF, or sub-RPE) will be reported for each post-baseline visit. • Time to first dry retina (no IRF or SRF) finding; IRF and SRF will be assessed using SD-OCT images. A dry retina is defined as no IRF or SRF at the visit. • Time to first sustained dry retina (no IRF or SRF at ≥2 consecutive visits) finding; IRF and SRF will be assessed using SD-OCT images. A sustained dry retina is defined as no IRF or SRF at 2 or more consecutive visits.

revealed on the www.clinicaltrials.gov website. In 2008, the VIEW studies for approval of aflibercept in AMD contained exactly one imaging endpoint as a secondary outcome, the MERLIN study, which just started—10 years later—to evaluate the efficacy of brolucizumab, a new generation anti-VEGF for the treatment of nAMD, lists seven (!) imaging/OCT endpoints as secondary outcome measures, all of which have to be evaluated and assessed by a central reading center (Table 23.1).

Both studies assess the therapeutic efficacy in CNV/neovascular AMD:

- Vascular Endothelial Growth Factor (VEGF) Trap-Eye: Investigation of Efficacy and Safety in Wet Age-Related Macular Degeneration (AMD) (VIEW 2); https://clinicaltrials.gov/ct2/show/NCT00637377
- Study of Safety and Efficacy of Brolucizumab 6 mg Dosed Every 4 Weeks Compared to Aflibercept 2 mg Dosed Every 4 Weeks in Patients With Retinal Fluid Despite Frequent Anti-VEGF Injections (MERLIN) in AMD; https://clinicaltrials.gov/ct2/show/NCT03710564

Such examples demonstrate the successful development and introduction of high-resolution imaging devices and the acceptance and contribution of research, often led by reading centers; in improving the knowledge and recognition of relevant parameters for diagnosis and treatment of CNV. Nevertheless, it also shows that the number of the morphological secondary surrogate outcome parameters may have increased but are still solely based on the presence of sub-RPE, intra- or subretinal fluid.

One key issue remains for drug developers and the retina community: the very conservative view of regulatory agencies on imaging outcomes in clinical studies. FDA and EMA usually accept functional parameter (BCVA) as primary outcome in AMD/CNV studies, all imaging and morphologic data are seen by regulators as just secondary surrogate or rather supportive exploratory outcome parameter.

Reading centers can play an essential role in educating regulators about the importance of imaging also on documenting the efficacy of new treatments. New developments, as a recent (April 08, 2019) conducted workshop at the FDA to discuss (beyond other modalities)—the importance of OCT-based imaging as valid and essential endpoints in ophthalmic clinical studies, can be seen as a move in the right direction.

23.9 Artificial Intelligence in Image Analysis

Artificial intelligence (AI) is a general term that implies the use of a computer to model intelligent behavior with minimal human intervention. Recent developments in the ophthalmology community and in reading centers are automated algorithms, which use AI to analyze and quantify morphologic characteristics of the (retina-) images. Those AI-based software assessments might be the future for analyzing many diagnostic imaging methods. Whether and when such automated segmentation and assessment of images will be accepted by regulatory agencies such as EMA or FDA for pivotal trials remain to be seen, though. However, automation could ease the work of reading center experts and the growing demand for analyses (see above). AI could support the analysis—and maybe 1 day replace the human trained experts as the final decision maker of diagnosis, pathology, or treatment need or treatment success. Especially, the fact that well-trained algorithms already outperform single human graders, raise hope that soon very accurate automated grading software will be available, at least for CF imaging and OCT.

Implementation of automated algorithms would save time and support fast screening of images. AI might also be helpful for improving vthe reproducibility of human graders and prevent inconsistencies between image analysis for different patients and/or patients' follow-up through the course of a clinical trial.

Nowadays, AI-assisted medical screening and diagnosis based on retinal images are emerging, especially in retinal diseases, including morphologic feature identification and auxiliary diagnosis support. AI has broad application across many medical fields, it holds significant promises for use in use in ophthalmology and will dramatically change the diagnostic and treatment pathways for many eye conditions such as AMD and diabetic retinopathy. For example, detection of CNV on stereo color fundus (CF) photography's could be easily missed. CF alone could identify reliably pigmentary changes, drusen, and hemorrhage which are highly correlated to CNV [43]. Based on those highly correlated morphologic characteristics, AI systems could be very efficiently implemented. There are a variety of approaches to program AI systems to automatically detect and measure pathologic features in images of the eye. All of them analyze pixels or group of pixels in CF photographs, FA images, and in OCT / OCT-A images. The simplest form of AI is simple automated detectors, but recent advancements in the field led to basic machine learning, advanced machine learning, and deep machine learning algorithms [44]. High-quality images, based on homogenous and reliable image acquisition, and the high expertise of photographic reading centers (with their unique asset of large image database and world-leading human image analysis know-how) are an essential basis for developing AI systems for high reliability and reproducibility of such automated output. Such systems and algorithms can be included in the respective imaging devices to support decision making and to guide treatment—also for not so experienced ophthalmologists. Recommendations for treatment needs can be based on AI big data analysis built-in directly in the imaging device to support ophthalmologists in the future in their proper and efficient decision-making process for further treatment and monitoring needs in patients with, i.e., CNV and high-risk AMD.

23.10 Conclusion

Photographic reading centers established pools of retinal images in CNV and the purpose of those institutions is the proper analysis of morphologic data and development of modern, efficient, accurate, and reproducible analysis tools. Deep learning, machine learning, artificial intelligence are projects that are based on large pools of digital retina images and serve to develop a more efficient and precise system of early detection, early treatment, and objective final outcome evaluation. Reading Centers have a crucial role in the development of such systems and tools. A growing trend and demand in clinical medicine are to develop standards which could be practically applicable worldwide. Today globally there is intensive investment and development of various devices for the screening (including home-based OCTs) and clinical use in ophthalmology. For evaluating and assessing real applicability, there is a need for objective, reproducible, and highly accurate data. For high-quality clinical trials, reading centers are important players for initiating trials, obtaining precious results and directions, and helping in submissions and regulatory filling. The future of large, professional reading centers is to be a driver of AI-based analysis and development of more precise and more predictive diagnostic and analysis systems for various diseases, including but not limited to CNV. The final goal of all developments and investigations led by reading center experts is to improve health care facilities, support effective education of various professional individuals involved in the process of screening, diagnosis, and treatment of blinding diseases and finally the prevention of blindness worldwide.

Key Learning Points

1. Reading centers are an essential part of successful drug development and regulatory approval in retinal diseases.
2. Large Phase 3 studies require professional reading center structure and management.

3. Complexity in image acquisition and image analysis in retinal diseases has significantly increased over the last decade.
4. Comparability of images from different devices/manufacturers is poor and need to be improved with the help of large data sets from reading centers.
5. Reading centers can drive and support harmonization of nomenclature and analysis of newly developed imaging devices such as OCT-A.
6. Reading centers can play an essential role in the development of automated, AI-based image analysis algorithms.
7. Overall, imaging experts at reading centers support widespread use and progress in regulatory acceptance and scientific advancement of retinal imaging.

References

1. Davis MD, Gangnon RE, Lee LY, Hubbard LD, Klein BE, Klein R, Ferris FL, Bressler SB, Milton RC, Age-Related Eye Disease Study Group. The age-related eye disease study severity scale for age-related macular degeneration: AREDS report no. 17. Arch Ophthalmol. 2005;123(11):1484–94.
2. Burlina PM, Joshi N, et al. Use of deep learning for detailed severity characterization and estimation of 5-year risk among patients with age-related macular degeneration. JAMA Ophthalmol. 2018;136(12):1359–66.
3. Malamos P, Sacu S, et al. Correlation of high-definition optical coherence tomography and fluorescein angiography imaging in neovascular macular degeneration. Invest Ophthalmol Vis Sci. 2009;50(10):4926–33.
4. Wu L, Dahl AA. Choroidal Neovascularization (CNV) Workup. https://emedicine.medscape.com/article/1190818-workup#c6
5. Moisseiev J, Alhalel A, Masuri R, Treister G. The impact of the macular photocoagulation study results on the treatment of exudative age-related macular degeneration. Arch Ophthalmol. 1995;113(2):185–9.
6. Argon laser photocoagulation for neovascular maculopathy. Three-year results from randomized clinical trials. Macular Photocoagulation Study Group. Arch Ophthalmol. 1986;104:694–701.
7. Holz FG, Jorzik J, et al. Agreement among ophthalmologists in evaluating fluorescein angiograms in patients with neovascular age-related macular degeneration for photodynamic therapy eligibility (FLAP-study). Ophthalmology. 2003;110(2):400–5.
8. Zayit-Soudry S, Alfasi M, et al. Variability among retina specialists in evaluating fluorescein angiograms of patients with neovascular age-related macular degeneration. Retina. 2007;27(6):798–803.
9. Jefferys JL, Alexander J, et al. Reproducibility of gradings of retinal photographs in eyes with subfoveal choroidal neovascularization and age-related macular degeneration in the macular photocoagulation study. Ophthalmic Epidemiol. 2008;15(3):191–201.
10. Muni RH, Altaweel M, et al. Agreement among Canadian retina specialists in the determination of treatment eligibility for photodynamic therapy in age-related macular degeneration. Retina. 2008;28(10):1421–6.
11. Abdelmoula WM, Shah SM, et al. Segmentation of choroidal neovascularization in fundus fluorescein angiograms. IEEE Trans Biomed Eng. 2013;60(5):1439–45.
12. Castillo MM, Mowatt G, et al. Optical coherence tomography for the monitoring of neovascular age-related macular degeneration: a systematic review. Ophthalmology. 2015;122(2):399–406.
13. Hee MR, Baumal CR, et al. Optical coherence tomography of age-related macular degeneration and choroidal neovascularization. Ophthalmology. 1996;103(8):1260–70.
14. Fung AE, Lalwani GA, et al. An optical coherence tomography-guided, variable dosing regimen with intravitreal ranibizumab (Lucentis) for neovascular age-related macular degeneration. Am J Ophthalmol. 2007;143(4):566–83.
15. Kaiser PK, Blodi BA, et al. Angiographic and optical coherence tomographic results of the MARINA study of ranibizumab in neovascular age-related macular degeneration. Ophthalmology. 2007;114(10):1868–75.
16. Wilde C, Patel M, et al. The diagnostic accuracy of spectral-domain optical coherence tomography for neovascular age-related macular degeneration: a comparison with fundus fluorescein angiography. Eye (Lond). 2015;29(5):602–9. quiz 610
17. Freund KB, Ho IV, et al. Type 3 neovascularization: the expanded spectrum of retinal angiomatous proliferation. Retina. 2008;28(2):201–11.
18. Mathew R, Pefkianaki M, et al. Correlation of fundus fluorescein angiography and spectral-domain optical coherence tomography in identification of membrane subtypes in neovascular age-related macular degeneration. Ophthalmologica. 2014;231(3):153–9.
19. Joeres S, Tsong JW, et al. Reproducibility of quantitative optical coherence tomography subanalysis in neovascular age-related macular degeneration. Invest Ophthalmol Vis Sci. 2007;48(9):4300–7.
20. Mylonas G, Ahlers C, Malamos P, Golbaz I, Deak G, Schuetze C, Sacu S, Schmidt-Erfurth U. Comparison of retinal thickness measurements and segmentation performance of four different spectral and time

domain OCT devices in neovascular age-related macular degeneration. Br J Ophthalmol. 2009 Nov;93(11):1453–60.
21. Grover S, Murthy RK, Brar VS, Chalam KV. Comparison of retinal thickness in normal eyes using stratus and Spectralis optical coherence tomography. Invest Ophthalmol Vis Sci. 2010 May;51(5):2644–7.
22. Kakinoki M, Sawada O, Sawada T, Kawamura H, Ohji M. Comparison of macular thickness between cirrus HD-OCT and stratus OCT. Ophthalmic Surg Lasers Imaging. 2009;40(2):135–40.
23. Sander B, Al-Abiji HA, Kofod M, Jørgensen TM. Do different spectral domain OCT hardwares measure the same? Comparison of retinal thickness using third-party software. Graefes Arch Clin Exp Ophthalmol. 2015 Nov;253(11):1915–21.
24. Tan CS, Chan JC, Cheong KX, Ngo WK, Sadda SR. Comparison of retinal thicknesses measured using swept-source and spectral-domain optical coherence tomography devices. Br J Ophthalmol. 2015 Mar;99(3):354–8.
25. Dufour PA, Abdillahi H, et al. Pathology hinting as the combination of automatic segmentation with a statistical shape model. Med Image Comput Comput Assist Interv. 2012;15(Pt 3):599–606.
26. Dufour PA, Ceklic L, et al. Graph-based multi-surface segmentation of OCT data using trained hard and soft constraints. IEEE Trans Med Imaging. 2013;32(3):531–43.
27. Prahs P, Radeck V, et al. OCT-based deep learning algorithm for the evaluation of treatment indication with anti-vascular endothelial growth factor medications. Graefes Arch Clin Exp Ophthalmol. 2018;256(1):91–8.
28. Schlegl T, Waldstein SM, et al. Fully automated detection and quantification of macular fluid in OCT using deep learning. Ophthalmology. 2018;125(4):549–58.
29. Bogunovic H, Waldstein SM, et al. Prediction of anti-VEGF treatment requirements in neovascular AMD using a machine learning approach. Invest Ophthalmol Vis Sci. 2017;58(7):3240–8.
30. Schmidt-Erfurth U, Waldstein SM, et al. Prediction of individual disease conversion in early AMD using artificial intelligence. Invest Ophthalmol Vis Sci. 2018;59(8):3199–208.
31. de Carlo TE, Bonini Filho MA, et al. Spectral-domain optical coherence tomography angiography of choroidal neovascularization. Ophthalmology. 2015;122(6):1228–38.
32. Liang MC, de Carlo TE, et al. Correlation of spectral domain optical coherence tomography angiography and clinical activity in neovascular age-related macular degeneration. Retina. 2016;36(12):2265–73.
33. Sulzbacher F, Pollreisz A, et al. Identification and clinical role of choroidal neovascularization characteristics based on optical coherence tomography angiography. Acta Ophthalmol. 2017;95(4):414–20.
34. Xu D, Davila JP, et al. Long-term progression of type 1 neovascularization in age-related macular degeneration using optical coherence tomography angiography. Am J Ophthalmol. 2018;187:10–20.
35. Gong J, Yu S, et al. The diagnostic accuracy of optical coherence tomography angiography for neovascular age-related macular degeneration: a comparison with fundus fluorescein angiography. J Ophthalmol. 2016; https://doi.org/10.1155/2016/7521478.
36. Park MM, Rebhun CB, et al. Diagnosing choroidal neovascularization in asymptomatic individuals using optical coherence tomography angiography. Ophthalmic Surg Lasers Imaging Retina. 2017;48(7):596–8.
37. Treister AD, Nesper PL, et al. Prevalence of subclinical CNV and choriocapillaris nonperfusion in fellow eyes of unilateral exudative AMD on OCT angiography. Transl Vis Sci Technol. 2018;7(5):19.
38. Told R, Sacu S, et al. Comparison of SD-optical coherence tomography angiography and Indocyanine green angiography in type 1 and 2 neovascular age-related macular degeneration. Invest Ophthalmol Vis Sci. 2018;59(6):2393–400.
39. Miere A, Oubraham H, et al. Optical coherence tomography angiography to distinguish changes of choroidal neovascularization after anti-VEGF therapy: monthly loading dose versus Pro Re Nata Regimen. J Ophthalmol. 2018;2018:3751702.
40. Cole ED, Ferrara D, et al. Clinical trial endpoints for optical coherence tomography angiography in neovascular age-related macular degeneration. Retina. 2016;36(Suppl 1):S83–92.
41. Munk MR, Giannakaki-Zimmermann H, et al. OCT-angiography: a qualitative and quantitative comparison of 4 OCT-A devices. PLoS One. 2017;12(5):e0177059.
42. Corvi F, Pellegrini M, Erba S, Cozzi M, Staurenghi G, Giani A. Reproducibility of vessel density, fractal dimension, and foveal avascular zone using 7 different optical coherence tomography angiography devices. Am J Ophthalmol. 2018;186:25–31.
43. Mokwa NF, Ristau T, et al. Grading of age-related macular degeneration: comparison between color fundus photography, fluorescein angiography, and spectral domain optical coherence tomography. J Ophthalmol. 2013; https://doi.org/10.1155/2013/385915.
44. Roach L. Artificial intelligence. EyeNet Mag 2017; 77–83.

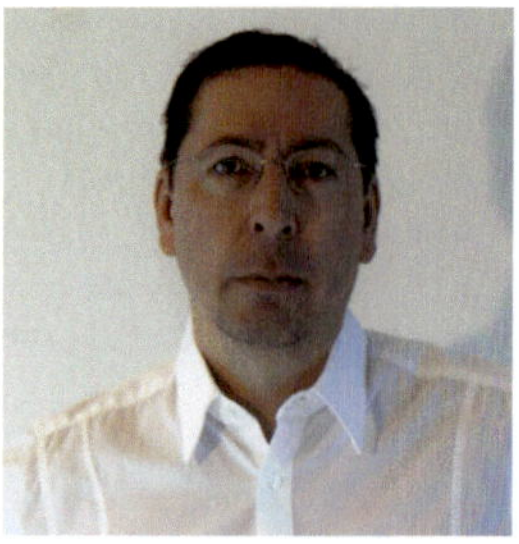

René Rückert earned his MD degree with distinction from Charité Medical School, Berlin, Germany and MBA from Warwick Business school, United Kingdom. He is a trained immunologist, and board-certified in biochemistry. After many years in academic basic research he joined Bayer Healthcare in Berlin to establish the Ophthalmology franchise and to lead global development programs for Eylea, later he led the global development clinical programs for Lucentis at Novartis in Switzerland. Dr. Rückert is now an independent consultant for ophthalmic drug development with his own company—eyegnos consulting, based in Switzerland.

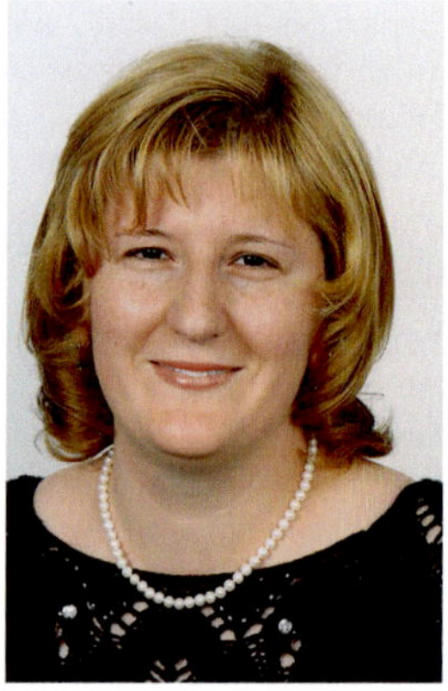

Lala Ceklic MD is grader at Bern Photographer Reading Center university of Bern, Bern Switzerland. She also serves as consultant ophthalmologist at own private practice at Pale-E. Sarajevo, Bosnia, and Herzegovina. Her primary research interest is primarily in retina. She has published 18 peer-reviewed papers (https://www.ncbi.nlm.nih.gov/pubmed/?term=lala+ceklic). She has been awarded by Helmerich Foundation, American Academy of Ophthalmology—Rotary foundation, International Council of Ophthalmology and Society of Ophthalmology Europeana. International member of American Academy of Ophthalmology, Euretina and Association of medical doctors of Serbia and Republic of Srpska.

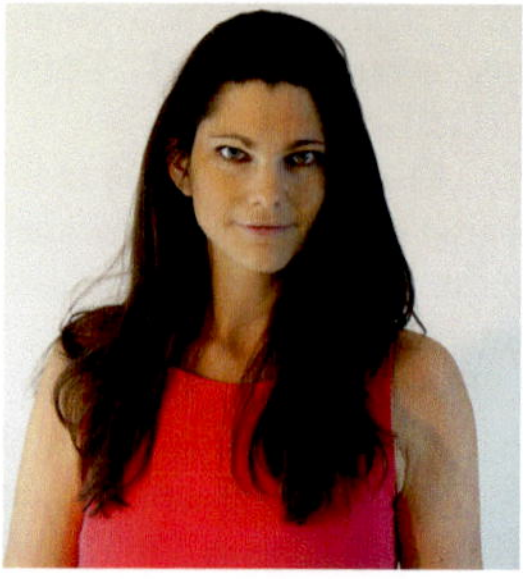

Marion R. Munk is a trained MD, PhD, Assoc. Prof. and Uveitis and Medical Retina specialist at the University Clinic Bern in Switzerland and Managing Director at the Bern Photographic Reading Center. She is adjunct Lecturer at the Northwestern University, Chicago, USA. She did her residency and fellowships at Department of Ophthalmology, Univ. Clinic Vienna, Northwestern University, Chicago and Univ. Clinic Bern and at Department of Rheumatology, Charite, Univ. Clinic of Berlin. Marion is author of >90 scientific articles and book chapters. Her major research interests cover image processing, image analyses, macular diseases, and posterior uveitis. She is a member of the Editorial Board of IOVS, Acta Ophthalmologica, Ocular Inflammation and Infection, and BMC Ophthalmology and is providing peer-review for a long list of scientific journals within Ophthalmology.

Part IV

Therapy and Rehabilitation

24 Anti-Vascular Endothelial Growth Molecules

Eduardo Tomazoni
and Eduardo Buchelle Rodrigues

24.1 Introduction

Pathological angiogenesis and increased vascular permeability are involved with important eye diseases like diabetic retinopathy (DR) and age-related macular degeneration (AMD) [1]. The vascular endothelial growth factor (VEGF) family coordinates these tissue modifications [2]. This chapter will cover angiogenesis mechanism, evolution of therapy with monoclonal antibody, monoclonal antibodies (mAbs), antibody fragments, recombinant fusion protein, novel drugs, and future perspectives.

24.2 Angiogenesis Mechanism

In 1971, Judah Folkman wrote that angiogenesis mechanism is a highly integrated ecosystem started by pro-angiogenic factors with the aim to maintain a healthy organism or recover an injured tissue trough a preexisting vessel [3]. After some years, abnormal vessels growth-up was recognized as the common denominator to several systemic and eye diseases like: AMD, DR, central retina vein occlusion (CRVO), infections and inflammatory ocular diseases, trauma, angioid streaks (AS), prematurity retinopathy (PR), neovascular glaucoma, high myopia, idiopathic macular telangiectasia (IMT), and hereditary retinal diseases [4].

Choroidal neovascularization begins with regulations of VEGF gene expression that is activated mostly by tissue hypoxia, cytokines, and cell differentiation and transformation [5]. These proangiogenic environments occur in association with fibroblasts, myofibroblasts, lymphocytes, and macrophages [6]. The breaks through Bruch's membrane lead to ingrowth of new vessels from the choriocapillaris layer into the subretinal pigment epithelial space [7].

Angiogenesis regard to a bridging new vessel from existing vessels. This growth depends on VEGF that acts signaling vessel formation and creating a mature and interconnected support network in vascular periphery [8]. A sequential activation of receptors Tie1, Tie2, and platelet-derived growth factor (PDGF) receptor-β (PDGRF-β) by numerous binders in endothelial and mural cells are required in the process of angiogenesis, with VEGF representing the critical rate-limiting step in physiological cases [9]. VEGF-A (usually called only by VEGF) is a 45-kDa homodimeric glycoprotein belonging to a family of cytokines that also includes: VEGF-B, VEGF-C, VEGF-D, VEGF-E, VEGF-F, and placental growth factor (PGF) [10]. VEGF-A exists as six mRNA splice

E. Tomazoni
Department of Ophthalmology, Visum Retina Clinic, Florianópolis, SC, Brazil

E. B. Rodrigues (✉)
Department of Ophthalmology, Saint Louis University School of Medicine, Saint Louis, MO, USA

J. Chhablani (ed.), *Choroidal Neovascularization*, https://doi.org/10.1007/978-981-15-2213-0_24

variants coded in gene 6q21.3—isoforms 121, 145, 165, 183, 189, and 206 (Fig. 24.1), depending upon the number of amino acids present on exons 6 and 7 [11, 12].

Besides VEGF, other molecules involved in angiogenesis bioassays (either directly promoting endothelial cell proliferation or indirectly via recruitment of inflammatory cells) include (Fig. 24.2): fibroblast growth factor (FGF), angiopoietins, epidermal growth factor, transforming growth factor (TNF)-α and β, angiogenin, and several others that can be founded in Angiogenesis Foundation website: angio.org/about-angiogenesis).

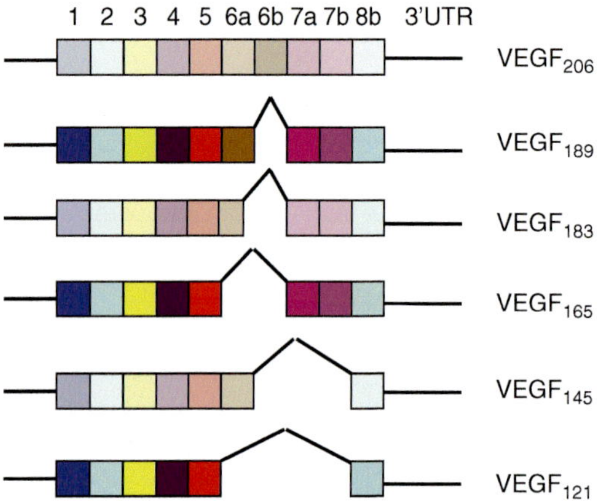

Fig. 24.1 The main difference between VEGF forms resides on exons 6a, 6b, 7a, and 7b, which consists of heparan sulfate subunit (HSPGs) (Adapted from Ferrara N [4])

The FGF family involves 20 factors categorized into six subfamilies, and display affinity to surface heparan sulfate proteoglycans (HSPGs) acting via receptors tyrosine kinases (FGFR 1, 2, 3, and 4) through alternative splicing [13]. Angiopoietins are a group of three structurally linked proteins (Ang-1, 2, and 3) that acts on vascular differentiation through angiogenesis and maintenance of blood and lymphatic vessels [13]. In vivo injection of Ang-2 neutralizing antibody (named αvβ5-integrin) inhibited astrocyte loss in early diabetic retinopathy patients [14]. The major signalling pathways in angiogenesis are presented schematically in Fig. 24.3.

24.3 Evolution of Therapy with Monoclonal Antibody

Paul Ehrilich in the early XX wrote, "By injecting one animal with the cells of another, we can produce substances in the serum of the first, which have a specific damaging or destructive influence on these cells. This possibility has within a short time extended the theoretical doc-

Fig. 24.2 Schematic view of neovascularization steps

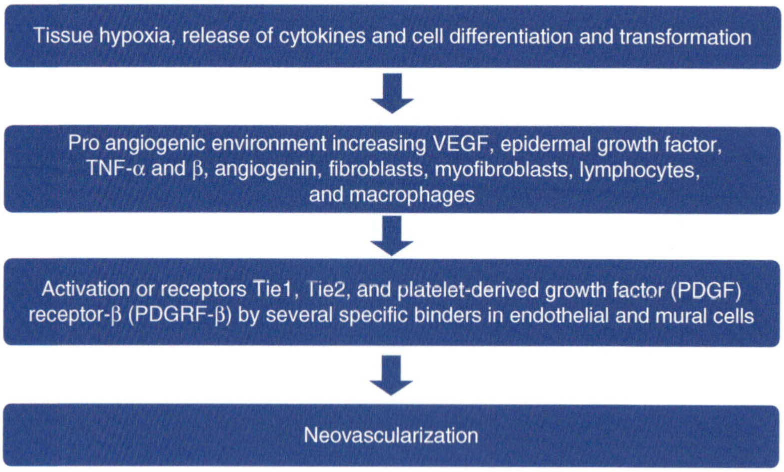

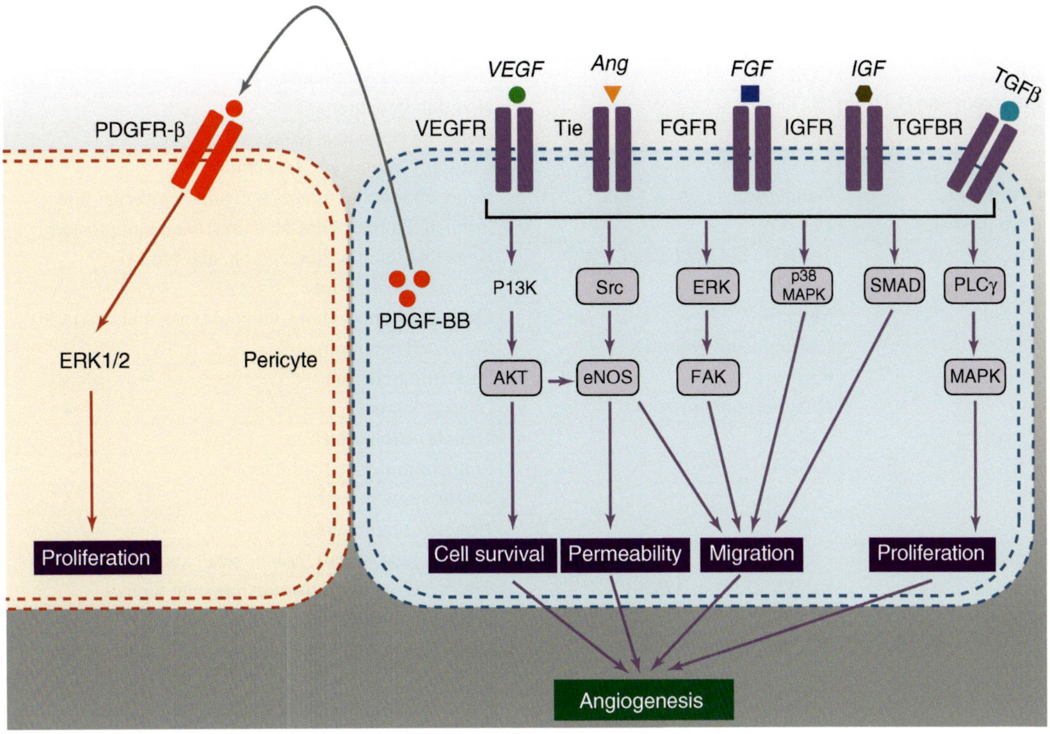

Fig. 24.3 Schematic diagram of major signalling pathways in angiogenesis. Special thanks to Patriek NM

trines of immunity in various directions." [15]. These models of therapy were recognized later by "passive serotherapy" that initially produced a good response, however, after a relatively short period of time, the patient experienced severe side effects [16].

During the 1960s and 1970s, Lloyd Old and Ted Boyse revolutionized the understanding of the immune system introducing the concept of surface cell differentiation antigens (cluster of differentiation: CD) using cytotoxic tests and distinguish lineage and functional subsets of leukocytes in mice [17]. Assorted discoveries were possible after this contribution, including the major histocompatibility complex (MHC), leukemia, and Ly series (markers to distinguish between helper and cytotoxic T cells) [18]. Finally, Köhler and Milstein in 1975 described a method for the hybridoma project: cloned cell lines producing monoclonal antibodies [18]. Table 24.1 presents some examples of antigens and their respective expressed tumors. Only after identifying the expressed antigen, the antibodies can be produced to reach the control of the disease.

The first therapy using antibody produced by hybridoma project was Murine antibody, with target CEA and CD3 in patients with solid tumors and hematologic tumors [17]. To avoid the immune response Winter and cols changed the regions Gc and Fv of Murine antibodies to human germline amino acids [19]. Currently, new strategies are used to decrease the immune response, like smaller antibodies, fusion proteins, and

Table 24.1 Antigens and their respective expressed tumors

Antigen class	Antigens	Tumor types expressing antigen
Cluster of differentiation (CD) antigens	CD20	Non-Hodkin lymphoma
	CD30	Hodgkin lymphoma
	CD33	Acute myelogenous leukemia
	CD52	Chronic lymphocytic leukemia
Glycolipids	Gangliosides (GM2, GD2, GD3)	Neuroectodermal tumors and other epithelial tumors
Carbohydrates	Lewis-Y^2	Epithelial tumors (breast, colon, lung, and prostate)
Glycoproteins	TAG-72, EpCAM, and CEA	Epithelial tumors (lung, colon, and breast)
	gpA33	Colorectal carcinoma
	Mucins	Epithelial tumors (lung, colon, breast, and ovarian)
	Carbonic anhydrase IX	Renal cell carcinoma
	PSMA	Prostate carcinoma
	Folate-binding protein	Ovarian tumors
Vascular targets	VEGF	Tumour vascularization
	VEGFR	Epithelium-derived solid tumors
	αVβ3	Tumor vascularization
	A5β1	Tumor vascularization
Growth factors	ErbB1/EGFR	Glioma, lung, breast, colon, head, and neck tumors
	RrbB2/HER2 and ErbB3	Breast, colon, lung, ovarian, prostate tumors
	c-MET	Epithelial tumors (breast, ovary, and lung)
	IGF1R	Lung, breast, head and neck, prostate, thyroid, and glioma
	EphA3	Lung, kidney, colon, melanoma, glioma, and hematological malignancies
	TRAIL-R1, TRAIL-R2	Solid tumors (colon, lung, pancreas) and hematological malignancies
	RANKL	Prostate cancer and bone metastases
Stromal and extracellular matrix antigens	FAP	Epithelial tumors (colon, breast, lung, head and neck, and pancreas)
	Tenascin	Glioma and epithelial tumors (breast and prostate)

Adapted from: Scott AM, James PA, and Wolchok JD. Monoclonal antibodies in cancer therapy [17]

bispecific antibody [17]. Figure 24.4 presents the pathways used by antibodies against overexpressed cell antigens.

The first drug (or antigen) that acts against overexpressed VEGF approved by Food and Drug Administration (FDA) was pegaptanib Sodium (MACUGEN®), and due to its low effectiveness (acts only by blocking the forms $VEGF_{165}$ and $VEGF_{188}$), this drug was supplanted [20, 21]. Ranibizumab and bevacizumab blocks six forms of VEGF-A ($VEGF_{121}$, $VEGF_{145}$, $VEGF_{165}$, $VEGF_{183}$, $VEGF_{189}$, and $VEGF_{206}$) [21]. Aflibercept blocks six types of VEGF-A, VEGF-B, and PGF, inhibited the activation of VEGFRs 1 and 2 [21, 22]. Until the publication of this chapter, the current pharmacological drugs approved by FDA to ophthalmologic use are pegaptanib sodium (MACUGEN®), ranibizumab (Lucentis®), and aflibercept (Eylea®), with bevacizumab (Avastin®) having his ophthalmological uses off label for choroidal neovascularization and macular edema [22] (Fig. 24.5). As of mid-2019, the company's Biologics Licences Application (BLA) for brolucizumab (RTH258) was accepted for treatment of wet AMD by the US Food and Drug Administration (FDA). Systemic anti-VEGF agents are presented in Table 24.2.

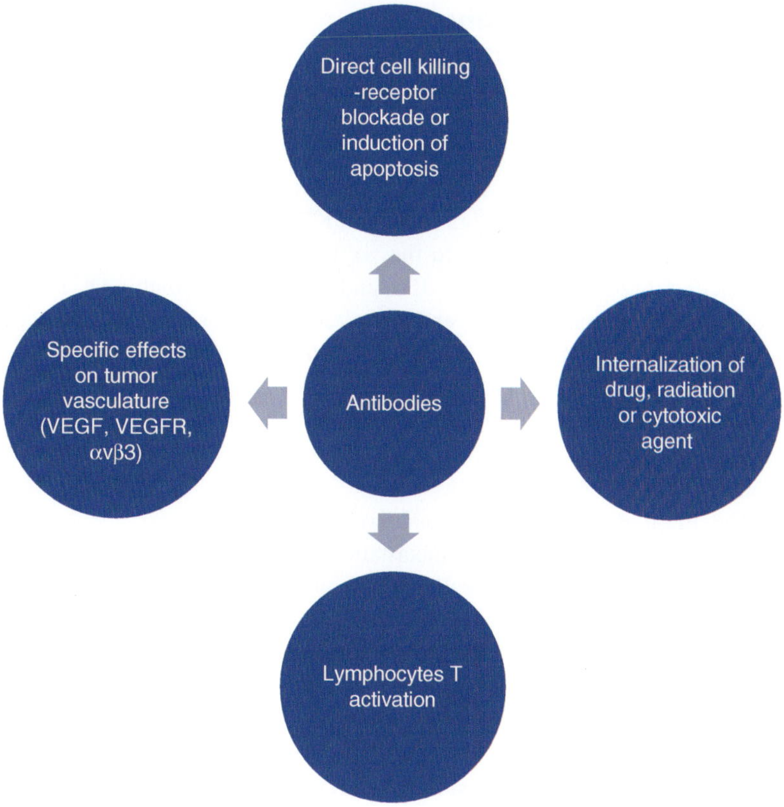

Fig. 24.4 Pathways used by antibodies against overexpressed cells' antigens. Adapted from Scott et al. [17]

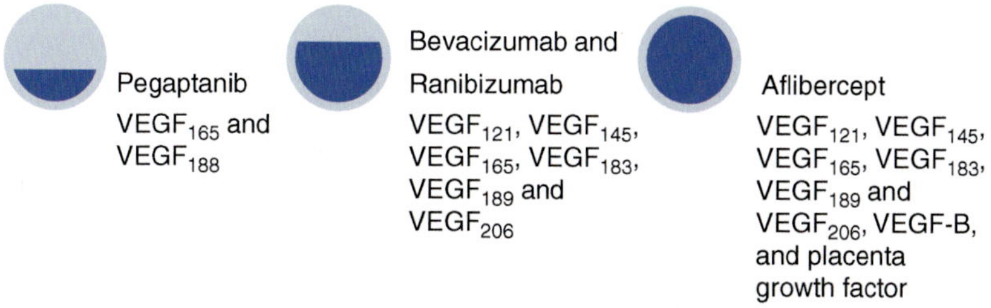

Fig. 24.5 Drugs and their respective site of action. Pegaptamib acts against two forms of VEGF (165 and 188); Bevacizumab and Ranibizumab block six forms of VEGF-A (121, 145, 165, 183, 189, and 206); Aflibercept acts blocking six forms of VEGF-A (121, 145, 165, 183, 189, and 206), VEGF-B, and placental growth factor. Adapted from Nicholas Papadopoulos et al. [21] and Anu Joseph [22]

Table 24.2 Available anti-VEGF treatment for systemic conditions

Systemic anti-VEGF			
• Bevacizumab	• Cabozantinib	• Pazopanib	• Regorafenib
• Ziv-Aflibercept	• Sorafenib	• Sutinib	• Vandetanib

Adapted from Angiogenesis Foundation website

24.4 Monoclonal Antibodies (mAb's): Bevacizumab Humanized IgG1 (Avastin®)

The bevacizumab (Avastin®) humanized IgG1 is a recombinant monoclonal antibody of 149 kDa that binds to receptors Flt-1 and KDR of VEGF. Bevacizumab binds to the six forms of VEGF-A (121, 145, 165, 183, 189, and 206). Composed by human structure and complementary structures of Murine antibody, the molecule of bevacizumab is produced on ovarian mammary cells of Chinese Hamsters in an expression system containing the antibiotic Gentamicin [23, 24].

The FDA approves bevacizumab to several types of cancers, like colorectal metastatic carcinoma, cervical cancer, peritoneal primary cancer, fallopian tubes cancer, and epithelial ovarian cancer [23]. Although several studies have shown satisfactory results in the treatment of ocular diseases, intravitreal injection of bevacizumab remains off label [24].

The CATT study (comparison of age-related macular degeneration treatment trials) suggests the efficiency and safety of bevacizumab when compared to ranibizumab, with the similar gain of letters (15 letters) on both groups, and the regimens "as needed" or "extended" have the same results in one year of follow-up [25].

24.5 Antibodies Fragments: Ranibizumab (Lucentis®)

The ranibizumab (Lucentis®) is a fragment of bevacizumab with 48 kDa of weight produced by *Escherichia coli* bacteria into a recipient contending the antibiotic Tetracycline by the portion Fc of bevacizumab catted out. The Fab part binds to VEGF through the VEGFR1 and VEGFR2 on the endothelial cells' surface. Ranibizumab also inhibiting the degradation products of VEGF-A [26]. Currently, FDA approves Ranibizumab for DMRI, CRVO, CME, DR, and macular choroidal neovascularization [27].

The studies MARINA and ANCHOR prove the superiority of ranibizumab under photodynamic therapy (PDT) and placebo in patients with DMRI [28, 29]. The EXCITE study confirms the safety and efficiency of ranibizumab [30]. The study SUSTAIN evaluates the sustained improvement by ranibizumab on gains in visual acuity [31]. Finally, the study PrONTO suggests that monthly OCT reduces the necessity of injections in "treat as needed" scheme with ranibizumab [32].

24.6 Recombinant Fusion Protein: Aflibercept (Eylea®)

The aflibercept (Eylea®) is a recombinant fusion protein constituted by portions of human VEGFR1 (Ig domain 2), VEGFR2 (Ig domain 3), and extracellular domains fused to the Fc portion of human IgG1. The aflibercept is formed by dimeric glycoprotein associated with glycosides that result in a total molecular weight of 115 kDa that binds to VEGF-A, VEGF-B, and placental growth factor (PGF). The molecule is produced in recombinant Chinese hamster ovary cells. The drug is administered 2 mg per eye and achieves the high plasma concentration at day 2 (0.081 mcg/mL), with total plasma washout after 2 weeks of administration. There are no signs of the drug in the plasma after 4 weeks of intravitreal injection. Currently, FDA approved aflibercept for the treatment of wet AMD, DME, dosing schedule (doses are given at least every 12 weeks, and additional doses as needed in patients with wet AMD and DME), and diabetic retinopathy without macular edema [33].

24.7 Novel Agents

24.7.1 Ziv-aflibercept

Ziv-aflibercept (Zaltrap, Sanofi-Aventis US, LLC, Bridgewater, NewJersey, USA and Regeneron Pharmaceuticals, Inc., Tarrytown,

New York, USA) was approved by FDA in 2012 for treatment of metastatic colorectal carcinoma in specific conditions. Ziv-aflibercept is a VEGF-trap (like the aflibercept) that acts selectively on VEGF-A, VEGF-B, and PGF. The clinical trials using rabbits showed no complications after the intravitreal injection of 0.05 ml (25 mg/ml) of ziv-aflibercept [34]. Using twice of clinical doses, ziv-aflibercept reduces Müller cells function on electroretinogram exam. This abnormality was not present for bevacizumab, ranibizumab, or aflibercept [35].

The first human use of ziv-aflibercept was in a patient with refractory neovascular AMD. The patients received 1.25 mg (0.05 ml) of the drug, and after 30 days of the injection was not any damage to the retina and visual acuity improvements were observed [36]. In 2019, a review of prospective, retrospective, case study, and case series trials, suggest that ziv-aflibercept have the same safety profile, and effectiveness in patients with diabetic macular edema and neovascular AMD, regarding to (1) reduction retinal fluid or central foveal thickness and (2) maintenance or improvement of visual acuity [37].

24.7.2 Brolucizumab

Brolucizumab (RTH258, Alcon Research Ltd., a Novartis Company, Fort Worth, TX) is an anti-VEGF single-chain antibody fragment (scFv) with 26.3 kDa of weight and consisting of 252 amino acids with activeness against all VEGF-A isoforms. In nonhuman primates, after intravitreal infection of brolucizumab the drug readily reaches the RPE and choroid layer with minimal subsequent systemic exposure [38].

The study HAWK and HARRIER [39] compared brolucizumab with aflibercept to treat neovascular AMD in patients without previous treatment. The patients were randomized and received intravitreal brolucizumab 3 mg (HAWK) or 6 mg or aflibercept 2 mg. After 3 monthly doses, patients with brolucizumab-treated eyes received an injection every 12 weeks if disease was not present and 8 weeks if present. Aflibercept-treated eyes received a dose every 8 weeks. Patients that received brolucizumab 6 mg maintained on 12-week dosing interval through week 48, and anatomic outcomes favored brolucizumab also. Overall safety was similar on both drugs [39]. In 2019 was announced by the US Food and Drug Administration (FDA) that the company's Biologics License Application (BLA) for brolucizumab (RTH258) was accepted for the treatment of wet age-related macular degeneration (AMD).

24.7.3 Faricimab

Faricimab (developed by Roche, Basel, Switzerland and Genentech, South San Francisco, CA, USA) is a bispecific antibody that acts simultaneously binding both VEGF-A and Ang-2. Patients with diabetic macular edema (DME) have a multifactorial angiogenic factors and inflammatory pathways, that can respond to other agents besides anti-VEGF drugs. The Ang-2 receptor stimulation increases permeability and migration of the endothelial cells that contribute to angiogenesis in patients with DME. Blocking those two receptors (VEGF-A and Ang-2) possibly improves the efficacy and durability during treatment of diabetic macular edema. The BOULEVARD study compared faricimab with ranibizumab and demonstrated a statistically significant gain of 3.6 letters ($P = 0.03$) and central subfield thickness reduction in treatment-naïve patients with faricimab [40]. The clinical trials YOSEMITE and RHINE, until the publication of this chapter, are investigating the efficacy, durability and safety of the faricimab [40].

24.7.4 Conbercept

The conbercept (Lumitin; Chengdu Kanghong Biotech CO, Ltd., Chengdu, China) is an anti-VEGF molecule produced in China with 141-kDa of weight. Conbercept is a fusion protein that binds to the same receptors that aflibercept binds (VEGF-A, VEGF-B, and Placental Growth factor), plus the fourth binding domain of VEGFR2. The capacity of binding in the fourth domain of VEGFR2 theoreticaly extends the half-life of the conbercept, decreasing VEGF levels over 60 days on animals' experiments [41]. Conbercept proves to have the same efficacy of ranibizumab for the treatment of diabetic macular edema [42], retinopathy of prematurity [43], and macular edema secondary to branch retinal vein occlusion [41].

24.8 Future Perspectives

In conclusion, new drugs have aloud much progress in choroidal neovascularization. Nowadays, there are several monoclonal antibodies and fusion proteins available for the management of naïve and complex cases. Future drugs should further elucidate and improve clinical outcomes.

In the next years, generic biosimilars could be the mostly used anti-VEGF drugs due to a high potential cost-efficient choice [44]. Biosimilars are medicines manufactured by or extracted from a biological source. The first patent to be expired is for ranibizumab in 2020 for the United States (US) and 2023 for Europe. There are many companies developing biosimilars for ranibizumab (Table 24.3). Aflibercept has its patent expiration date set for the year 2020 in the United States, however, there are indications that the patent may be extended until the year of 2023 in the United States and 2025 in Europe.

Table 24.3 Ranibizumab biosimilars under development

Ranibizumab biosimilars			
Formycon	Samsung Bioepis	Pfenex	BioCND
German company		Pfizer company	The Republic of Korea-based company
Phase 3 clinical trial for FYB201 in 2019. Probable release date: 2020.	Phase 3 clinical trial for SB11. Probable release date: 2020.	Phases 1 and 2 conducted in 2016 for PF582.	Phase 3 clinical trial of BCD 300 in 2019. Probable release date: 2020.

Source: https://www.formycon.com/en/press-release/formycon-and-bioeq-achieve-important-milestone-biosimilar-ranibizumab-candidate-fyb201-shows-efficacy-comparable-to-the-reference-product-in-phase-iii-study/, https://clinicaltrials.gov/ct2/show/NCT03150589?term=sb11&rank=1, https://www.pfenex.com/products/, and https://adisinsight.springer.com/drugs/800048500

Key Learning Points

A pro-angiogenic environment increases not only VEGF, but also angiopoietins and other molecules involved in angiogenesis. The anti-VEGF drugs are one way to reduce the choroidal neovascularization, but more drugs with different targets are in development with the same purpose.

Nowadays, overexpressed VEGF is the main target of the drugs. The FDA approved drugs anti-VEGF are ranibizumab and aflibercept, and brolucizumab will probably also be approved in the coming years.

The Faricimab is the first available drug that binds to VEGF and Angiopoietin-2, theoretically reducing the effects of choroidal neovascularization with more intensity.

The biosimilars are coming in the next few years with the end of the patents of ranibizumab and aflibercept, probably resulting on a lower price with generics.

References

1. Witmer AN, et al. Vascular endothelial growth factors and angiogenesis in eye disease. Prog Retin Eye Res. 2003;22:1–29.
2. Adamis AP, David TS, Kiang-Tech Y, Tet-Kin Y, Lawrence FB, Brygida B, Patricia ADA, Folkman J. Synthesis and secretion of vascular permeability factor/vascular endothelial growth factor by human retinal pigment epithelial cells. Biochem Biophys Res Commun. 1993;193(2):631–8.
3. Folkman J. Tumor angiogenesis: therapeutic implications. N Engl J Med. 1971;285(21):1182–6.
4. Garner A. Vascular diseases. In: Garner A, Klintworth GK, editors. Pathobiology of ocular diseases. New York: Dekker; 1994. p. 1625–710.
5. Ferrara N, Davis-Smyth T. The biology of vascular endothelial growth factor. Endocr Rev. 1997;18(1):4–25.
6. Killingsworth MC, Sarks JP, Sarks SH. Macrophages related to Bruch's membrane in age-related macular degeneration. Eye (Lond). 1990;4:613–21.
7. Heriot WJ, Henkind P, Bellhorn RW, Burns MS. Choroidal neovascularization can digest Bruch's membrane. Opthalmology. 1984;91(12):1603–8.
8. Jain Rakesh K. Molecular regulation of vessel maturation. Nat Med. 2003;9(6):685–93.
9. Ferrara N. Vascular endothelial growth factor: basic science and clinical progress. Endocr Soc. 2004;25(4):581–611.
10. Adamis AP. Retinal Pharmacotheraphy, vol. 4. Basel: Karger AG; 2010. p. 23–36.
11. Harper SJ, Bates DO. VEGF-A splicing: the key to anti-angiogenic therapeutics? Nat Rev Cancer. 2008;8:880–7.
12. Robinson CJ, Stringer SE. The splice variants of vascular endothelial growth factor (VEGF) and their receptors. J Cell Sci. 2001;114:853–65.
13. Patriek NM, Ramya A, Howard LP, Krishna KS. Friends turned foes: angiogenic growth factors beyond angiogenesis. Biomol Ther. 2017;7:74.
14. Yun JH, Park SW, Kim JH, Park YJ, Cho CH, Kim JH. Angiopoietin 2 induces astrocyte apoptosis via αvβ5-integrin signaling in diabetic retinopathy. Cell Death Dis. 2016;7:e2101.
15. Ehrlich P. Studies in immunity. New York: Wiley; 1910. p. p23.
16. Ritz J, Schlossman SF. Utilization of monoclonal antibodies in the treatment of leukemia and lymphoma. Blood. 1982;59(1):1–11.
17. Scott AM, James PA, Wolchok JD. Monoclonal antibodies in cancer therapy. Cancer Immun. 2012;12:p14.
18. Moticka EJ. Learn about Ly antigen – T lymphocyte subpopulations. In: Moticka EJ, editor. A historical perspective on evidence-based immunology. Amsterdam: Elsevier; 2016. p. p197–205.
19. Riechmann L, Clark M, Waldmann H, Winter G. Reshaping human antibodies for therapy. Nature. 1988;332:323–7.
20. Goldbaum M, Cunningham ET Jr. Aptamers and intramers: pegaptanib. In: Nguyen QD, editor. Retinal pharmacotherapy, vol. 38. Maryland Heights, MO: Elsevier; 2010. p. 265–72.
21. Ppadopoulos N, Martin J, Ruan Q, Rafique A, Rosconi MP, Shi E, Pyles EA, Yancopoulos GD, Stahl N, Wiegand SJ. Binding and neutralization of vascular endothelial growth factor (VEGF) and related ligands by VEGF trap, ranibizumab and bevacizumab. Angiogenesis. 2012;15:171–85.
22. Joseph A. Intravitreal injections: a brief note. Kerala J Opthalmol. 2018;30(1):63–6.
23. Avastin (bevacizumab) Information. Update 29 June 2011. https://www.fda.gov/drugs/postmarket-drug-safety-information-patients-and-providers/avastin-bevacizumab-information
24. Avastin (bevacizumab) injection, for intravenous use. Initial US approval. 2004. Revised June 2019. https://www.gene.com/download/pdf/avastin_prescribing.pdf
25. The CATT Research Group. Ranibizumab and bevacizumab for neovascular age-related maucular degeneration. N Engl J Med. 2011;364:1897–908.
26. Ursula S-E. Therapeutic monoclonal antibodies and fragments: ranibizumab. In: Nguyen QD, editor. Retinal Pharmacotherapy, vol. 33. Maryland Heights, MO: Elsevier; 2010. p. 226–9.
27. LUCENTIS® (ranibizumab), for intravitreous injection. Initial U.S. approval. 2006. Revised Jan 2017 https://www.accessdata.fda.gov/drugsatfda_docs/label/2017/125156s111lbl.pdf
28. Rosenfeld PJ, Brown DM, Heier JS, Boyer DS, Kaiser PK, Chung CY, Kim RY. Ranibizumab for neovascular age-related macular degeneration. N Engl J Med. 2006;355:1419–31.

29. Brown DM, Michaels M, Kaiser PK, Heirer JS, Sy JP, Ianchulev T, ANCHOR Study Group. Ranibizumab versus verteporfin photodynamic therapy for neovascular age-related macular degeneration: two-year results of the ANCHOR study. Ophthalmology. 2009 Jan;116(1):57–65.e5.
30. Schmidt-Erfurth U, Eldem B, Guymer R, Korobelnik JF, Schlingemann RO, Axer-Siegel R, Wiedmann P, Simader C, Gekkieva M, Weichselberger A, EXCITE Study Group. Efficacy and safety of monthly versus quarterly ranibizumab treatment in neovascular age-related macular degeneration: the EXCITE study. Ophthalmology. 2011 May;118(5):831–9.
31. Holz FG, Amoaku W, Donate J, Guymer RH, Kellner U, Schlingemann RO, Weichselber A, Staurenghi G, SUSTAIN Study Group. Safety and efficacy of a flexible dosing regimen of ranibizumab in neovascular age-related macular degeneration: the SUSTAIN study. Ophthalmology. 2011 Apr;118(4):663–71.
32. Lalwani GA, Rosenfeld PJ, Fung AE, Dubovy SR, Michels S, Feuer W, Davis JL, Flynn HW Jr, Esquiabro M. A variable-dosing regimen with intravitreal ranibizumab for neovascular age-related macular degeneration: year 2 of the PrONTO Study. Am J Ophthalmol. 2009 Jul;148(1):43–58.e1.
33. EYLEA® (aflibercept) approval history. Initial U.S. approval. 2011. https://www.drugs.com/history/eylea.html
34. de Oliveira Dias JR, Badaró E, Novais EA, Colicchio D, Chiarantin GM, Matioli M. Preclinical investigations of intravitreal ziv-aflibercept. Ophthalmic Surg Lasers Imaging Retina. 2014;45:577–84.
35. del Carpio JC, Moustafa MTM, Ramirez CA, et al. Effects of ra-nibizumab, bevacizumab, Aflibercept and ziv-aflibercept on cultured human retinal Müller cells. Report presented at: The Annual Meeting of the Association for Research in Vision and Ophthalmology (ARVO) 2014–Orlando, Fla, May 4–8, 2014.
36. de Oliveira Dias JR, Xavier CO, Maia A, de Moraes NS, Meyer C, Farah ME, et al. Intravitreal injection of ziv-aflibercept in patient with refractory age-related macular degeneration. Ophthalmic Surg Lasers Imaging Retina. 2015;46:91–4.
37. Barmas-Alamdari D, D'Souza HS, Kapoor KG, Wagner AL. Intravitreal Ziv-Aflibercept: a comprehensive review. Semin Ophthalmol. 2019;34(6):420–45.
38. Nimz EL, Vanà Land CW, Yàñez JA, Chastain JE. Intraocular and systemic pharmacokinetics of brolucizumab (RTH258) in nonhuman primates. Program number: 4996. Poster Board Number: B0202. ARVO 2016 Annual Meetings Abstracts.
39. Dugel PU, Koh A, Ogura Y, Jaffe GJ, Schmidt-Erfurth U, Brown DM, Gomes AV, Warburton J, Weichselberger A, Holz FG. HAWK and HARRIER: Phase 3, multicenter, randomized, double-masked trials of brolucizumab for neovascular age-related macular degeneration. Presented at: American Academy of Ophthalmology Annual Meeting, November 11–14, 2017, New Orleans, Louisiana.
40. Sahn J, Patel SS, Dugel PU, Khanani AM, Jhaveri CD, Wykoff CC, Hershberger VS, Pauly-Evers M, Sadikhov S, Szczesny P, Schwab D, Nogoceke E, Osborne A, Weikert R, Fauser S. Simultaneous inhibition of angiopoietin-2 and vascular endothelial growth factor-A with faricimab in diabetic macular edema: BOULEVARD phase 2 randomized trial. Ophthalmology. 2019 Aug;126(8):1155–70.
41. Li F, Sun M, Guo J. Comparison of conbercept with ranibizumab for the treatment of macular edema secondary to branch retinal vein occlusion. Curr Eye Res. 2017;42(8):1174–8.
42. Xu Y, Rong A, Xu W, Niu Y, Wang Z. Comparison of 12-month therapeutic effect of conbercept and ranibizumab for diabetic macular edema: a real-life clinical practice study. BMC Ophthalmol. 2017;17:158.
43. Jin E, Yin H, Li X, Zhao M. Short-term outcomes after intravitreal injections of conberceptversus ranibizumab for the treatment of retinopathy of prematurity. Retina. 2018;38(8):1595–604.
44. Sharma A, Reddy P, Kuppermann BD, Bandello F, Lowenstein A. Biosimilars in ophthalmology: "is there a big change on the horizon?". Clin Ophthalmol. 2018;12(12):2137–43.

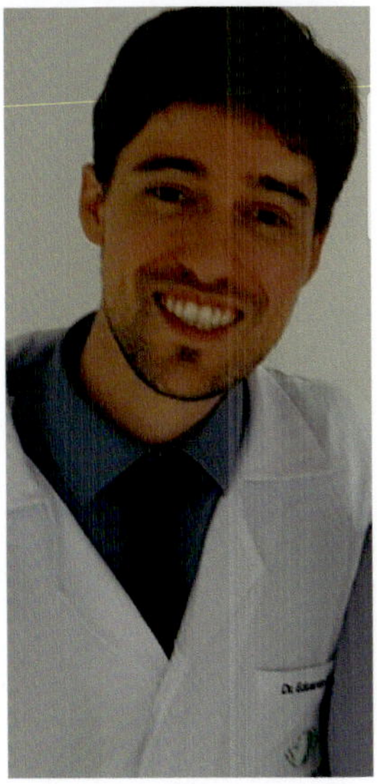

Eduardo Tomazoni is a medical doctor who graduated from the University of Joinville Region in 2013. He concluded his ophthalmology residency in 2019 at Governador Celso Ramos Hospital, in Florianópolis-SC, Brazil. He became a member of the Brazilian Ophthalmology Society in 2019. Currently, he is doing Retina and Vitreous and Ocular Oncology fellowship at Lumine Institute, Florianópolis-SC, Brazil. He is also a reviewer in the International Journal of Retina and Vitreous.

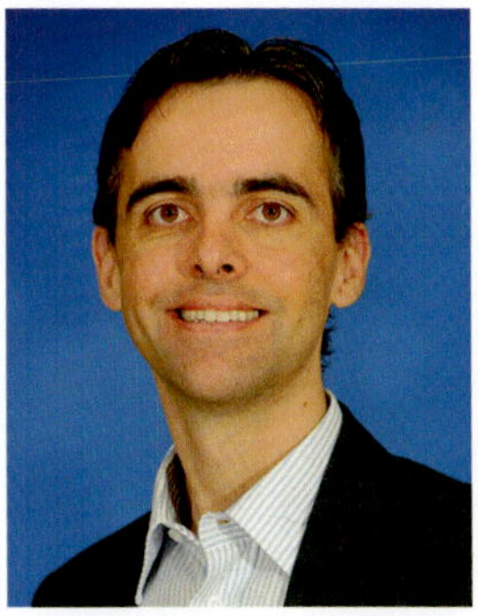

Eduardo Buchelle Rodrigues is an Assistant Professor of Ophthalmology, Saint Louis University, Saint Louis, USA. He graduated in medicine at the Federal University of Santa Catarina in 1998. Prof. Buchele Rodrigues finished his doctoral and postdoctoral degrees at the Federal University of São Paulo. He has published around 160 scientific articles in international journals of impact such as *Archives of Ophthalmology*, *American Journal of Ophthalmology*, and *Retina*. He is one of the editors of the major international book on the use of medications in the treatment of retinal diseases, Retinal Pharmacotherapy, published in 2010. He is Co-Editor In-Chief of the *International Journal of Retina and Vitreous*. He has conducted more than 250 paper presentations in national and international conferences, received 19 awards in congress by presenting work including the prestigious Paul Kayser Award of the Retina Research Foundation through the Pan-American Association of Ophthalmology. He is a member of the medical societies of the area as BRAVS, PAAO, ASRS, Club Jules Gonin, CBO, and AAO.

Surgical Interventions 25

Elizabeth D. Marlow and Tamer H. Mahmoud

25.1 Introduction

Age-related macular degeneration (AMD) was the leading cause of irreversible severe vision loss among adults aged more than 50 years in the United States prior to the emergence of anti-vascular endothelial growth factor (VEGF) therapy, and it remains one of the most important causes of vision loss among Caucasians in developed countries [1, 2]. Nonexudative or dry macular degeneration causes localized RPE dysfunction, sub-RPE drusenoid deposits, and geographic atrophy [1]. The majority of severe vision loss occurs due to the exudative or wet form of the disease, which accounts for two-thirds of AMD cases and is typified by submacular choroidal neovascular (CNV) networks leading to subretinal fluid, bleeding, and fibrotic scar formation [3]. No treatment for nonexudative AMD exists, though vitamin supplementation has shown to be effective at decreasing rates of progression and conversion to exudation.

Prior to anti-VEGF, the primary treatment options for exudative AMD were retinal photocoagulation for non-fovea involving CNV and photodynamic therapy with verteporfin for subfoveal CNV in eyes with good vision. Laser photocoagulation carried an immediate loss of vision in exchange for the reduced long-term decline in visual function. Neither treatment option restored vision nor prevented recurrent CNV with its attendant complications.

Amidst a paucity of therapeutic options, efforts were devoted to developing surgical approaches for AMD. This chapter reviews the evolution of vitreoretinal surgical techniques and principles in the management of exudative AMD with a focus on subretinal hemorrhage, excision of submacular CNV, macular translocation, and transplantation of retinal pigment epithelium (RPE), choroid, and retina to restore or improve vision. The role of adjuvants such as tPA, anti-VEGF, and gas will also be discussed.

Although some techniques have been abandoned with time due to limited benefit and invasiveness, surgical management remains an option for select AMD patients with advanced disease or subretinal hemorrhage. An understanding of the historic progression toward our current surgical practice lends valuable perspective to the contemporary vitreoretinal surgeon with an eye to future advances such as stem cell and gene therapy, which will once again emphasize subretinal procedures.

25.2 Submacular Hemorrhage

Submacular hemorrhage (SMH) is a rare complication of CNV that can markedly diminish vision and has limited potential for spontaneous

E. D. Marlow · T. H. Mahmoud (✉)
Associated Retinal Consultants, Royal Oak, MI, USA

J. Chhablani (ed.), *Choroidal Neovascularization*, https://doi.org/10.1007/978-981-15-2213-0_25

recovery [4]. The degree of visual impairment caused by SMH is proportionate to the initial size and thickness of the bleed, and typically deteriorates over time [5]. Bennet et al. [6] showed that patients with SMH due to AMD had an average VA of 20/1700 at final follow-up. Moreover, hemorrhage impairs absorption of laser energy and thus precluded treatment of the causative CNV in the era of laser photocoagulation [7–9]. All studies support that the clot volume and time to evacuation have prognostic significance and, in general, clots should be evacuated within 1 week.

Animal models of subretinal hemorrhage (SRH) have elucidated multiple mechanisms inflicting permanent damage to retinal photoreceptors, which is the principle cause of vision loss: hemoglobin-derived iron toxicity that worsens with the amount of hemorrhage and duration of exposure, separation of the photoreceptors from underlying RPE, impaired diffusion of oxygen from the choroid, shearing effects from clot contraction [10]. Anatomic changes following subretinal hemorrhage include fibrous tissue proliferation, atrophic scar formation, and RPE tear [5].

Toth et al. [11] demonstrated in a cat model that retinal damage from SRH is partially mediated by fibrin formation leading to tearing of photoreceptor inner and outer segments. Fibrin formation and photoreceptor trauma were diminished with the delivery of subretinal tissue plasminogen activator (tPA), even without hemorrhage evacuation. In feline eyes, the use of tPA in conjunction with a small retinotomy for clot evaluation showed better preservation of outer retinal architecture compared to eyes that were untreated or had clots evacuated without adjuvant tPA [12, 13]. Tissue plasminogen activator is well-tolerated in the subretinal space, and was shown in rabbits to provide rapid clearance of SRH via a mechanism beyond simple dilutional effects, principally by minimizing clot contraction [14].

The origin of submacular surgery in humans began in 1988 with Eugene de Juan and Machemer accessing the subretinal space to remove fibrous complications of CNV, which produced improvement in visual acuity [15]. Despite the value of prompt evacuation of SRH suggested by histologic studies, an initial case series of surgical removal of massive SMH and associated fibrosis without tPA resulted in poor visual function and high rates of complication, including retinal detachment. The greatest visual acuity gains were observed in those patients undergoing clearance within 1 week of hemorrhage [16]. Given the visual recovery noted by de Juan and Machemer with CNV removal, these results highlighted that functional outcome were dependent on minimizing surgical trauma yet limited by the underlying macular degenerative changes. As methods for the management of SMH evolved, tandem efforts were underway to advance surgical techniques for CNV excision, which is discussed later in this chapter.

25.2.1 TPA-Assisted Evacuation

Initial techniques utilizing fluid–air exchange and active suction through a retinotomy to evacuate clots frequently caused inadvertent enlargement of the retinotomy. The introduction of subretinal tPA in the clearance of SRH facilitated aspiration through retinotomies; although smaller, less invasive retinotomies were attempted, they required prolonged waiting time for tPA-induced clot liquefaction and were generally less successful than the larger retinotomies that were ultimately utilized [17, 18]. Still, a comparison of outcomes among patients with large SMH due to multiple etiologies undergoing prompt pars plana vitrectomy (PPV) with mechanical clot extraction versus tPA-assisted (10–40 mcg dose) drainage showed that AMD-related hemorrhages portend a worse visual prognosis compared to other causes, and that the use of tPA did not improve visual outcomes over mechanical extraction [19]. Limitations in visual outcomes for all patients were proposed to be from photoreceptor shearing during clot evacuation, as elucidated in animal models, with underlying macular degenerative changes leading to worse visual outcomes in AMD-associated hemorrhages compared to other causes.

Intravitreal perfluorocarbon liquid (PFCL) was applied in combination with tPA to provide passive, mechanical extrusion of hemorrhage through a smaller retinotomy into the vitreous cavity thereby reducing iatrogenic retinal damage [20]. The majority of eyes achieved improved vision (88%) with adjuvant PFCL, although the procedure was complicated by retinal detachment (14%), epiretinal membrane formation (14%), and recurrent submacular hemorrhage (18%).

Less invasive techniques for large SMH include intravitreal tPA to induce clot liquefaction in the absence of a direct communication into the subretinal space followed by pneumatic displacement, thereby minimizing outer retinal damage caused by clot extraction. Heriot et al. [21] first introduced this technique for use in an outpatient clinic setting in 1996. Although animal data did not support the capacity for tPA to diffuse into the subretinal space [22], multiple studies in humans have shown visual acuity gains in a majority of patients [23–25].

Subsequent studies by Haupert et al. [26] showed that subretinal tPA followed by intravitreal gas provided good, and in some cases superior, displacement compared to intravitreal tPA. This was a retrospective study of 11 eyes with thick SMH in the setting of exudative AMD who underwent vitrectomy and subretinal injection of 25 μg/0.1 mL or 50 μg/0.1 mL of tPA followed by fluid gas exchange. The hemorrhage was successfully displaced in all 11 eyes. Baseline VA was 20/200 to HM, and best postoperative VA showed improvement in eyes eyes with four eyes being 20/80 or better. However, final postoperative VA was not significantly different from preoperative VA, likely due to recurrent hemorrhage (27%) and disease progression. Olivier et al. [27] applied the same technique with lower concentrations of tPA (125 μg/mL) and larger subretinal volumes to achieve greater hemorrhage displacement. With this technique, subfoveal blood displacement was achieved in 25 of 29 eyes with significant improvement in postoperative visual acuity at 3 months. Further studies showed long-term visual acuity gains were achieved in a majority of patients, but remained predictably limited by the progression of underlying disease and recurrent hemorrhages [28].

A retrospective comparison of PPV combined with either intravitreal or subretinal administration of tPA showed greater displacement rates when tPA was delivered directly into the subretinal space with equivalent VA outcomes [29]. A similar retrospective, nonrandomized study of 18 patients by Bell et al. [30] comparing PPV with subretinal tPA versus intravitreal tPA with pneumatic showed no significant difference in visual acuity outcomes at 1 year.

A comparison of outcomes between intravitreal tPA versus vitrectomy combined with subretinal tPA is limited by patient selection as many physicians deliver clinic-based therapy for less severe hemorrhages. Still, the literature to date supports intravitreal tPA combined with pneumatic as an effective and less invasive treatment option for non-massive SRH.

It should be noted that clot liquefaction induced by intravitreal tPA is more variable and dose-dependent than with subretinal administration. Intravitreal tPA has also been shown to cause vitreous opacification, and at high doses (100 μg) may provoke large, self-resolving exudative retinal detachments, which were not observed with 25 μg or 50 μg dose [31]. Recently tenecteplase has been explored as an alternative to tPA for its superior fibrin specificity, and has shown promising early results in SMH due to exudative AMD [32]. Future studies will be required to compare this agent to the well-established efficacy of tPA.

25.2.2 Anti-VEGF as Monotherapy and Adjuvant

In the era preceding anti-VEGF, the capacity for surgical techniques to improve visual acuity was stunted by a high incidence of recurrent hemorrhage and progression of underlying exudative AMD. When anti-VEGF became available for intraocular applications, its role as monotherapy or in combination with pneumatic displacement were established as effective treatment options for submacular hemorrhage [33]. Some studies have reported that anti-VEGF in combination with pneumatic displacement delivers superior visual outcomes compared to monotherapy for thicker hemorrhages [34].

Anti-VEGF has also been applied as an adjuvant to subretinal tPA and pneumatic tamponades with the aim of preventing repeat bleeding and maintaining visual acuity gains from hemorrhage displacement. A study by Chang et al. [35] showed that among 101 eyes with exudative AMD undergoing vitrectomy with subretinal tPA and gas tamponade, those eyes that received postoperative intravitreal anti-VEGF injections showed greater visual acuity improvement at 6 months postoperatively compared to those eyes that did not. The rate of displacement away from the fovea was 82%, and both groups achieved significant improvement in postoperative visual acuity with a minimum follow-up of 3 months.

The compatibility of tPA with anti-VEGF agents varies. Bevacizumab has proven efficacy and stability when co-administered with tPA into the subretinal space [36–38]. Klettner et al. [39] studied the impact of recombinant tPA and plasmin on aflibercept and ranibizumab when the agents were incubated together by evaluating resultant antibody fragments with electrophoresis, and quantifying antiangiogenic activity with VEGF-ELISA. Ranibizumab was not cleaved or functionally compromised by either tPA or plasmin, supporting its stability when co-applied with tPA in the presence of plasmin for submacular hemorrhage. While aflibercept was not cleaved or inhibited by tPA, additional fragments appeared after incubation with plasmin and its VEGF-binding ability was inhibited by plasmin at clinical doses. A retrospective case series of 45 eyes by González-López et al. [40] showed that small gauge vitrectomy with subretinal tPA and ranibizumab for SMH secondary to AMD followed by pro re nata monthly intravitreal ranibizumab injections resulted in visual acuity improvement in 73% of patients, though follow-up was limited in some cases (12.9 ± 10.8 months).

In addition, anti-VEGF can be combined with tPA and pneumatic displacement without performing vitrectomy. A retrospective analysis by Guthoff et al. [41] compared intravitreal tPA and gas versus intravitreal bevacizumab, tPA, and gas in 38 patients with recent (within 31 days) SRH and showed significantly better visual acuity at 4 weeks among eyes that received intravitreal anti-VEGF. This benefit persisted at 7 months with 50% of eyes receiving anti-VEGF being restored to reading vision compared to none in the tPA and gas-only group.

Comparison of outcomes in retrospective studies of intravitreal versus subretinal tPA injection with gas when either technique is combined with intravitreal anti-VEGF are hampered by the limitations previously discussed. It remains common clinical practice to triage eyes with more severe hemorrhages to undergo vitrectomy while less substantial bleeds are frequently managed in clinic. A prospective study by de Jong et al. [42] randomized 24 patients with recent (<14 days) SMH (250 μm to 1250 μm thickness at the fovea) to receive either intravitreal injection tPA, gas, and bevacizumab, versus vitrectomy with subretinal tPA, gas and intravitreal bevacizumab. The median reduction in subretinal blood volume at 6 weeks postoperatively was not significantly different between the two groups: 97% in the intravitreal tPA group versus 100% in the subretinal tPA group. Larger prospective, randomized clinical trials will be needed to further evaluate the difference between subretinal versus intravitreal tPA in the era of anti-VEGF.

25.2.3 PFCL

As previously mentioned, PFCL can mechanically displace SRH into the vitreous cavity through a small retinotomy [20], but it can also be left within the vitreous cavity postoperatively for a period of 7–17 days to provide prolonged displacement [43]. Concerns regarding the use of PFCL as an intraocular tamponade for a prolonged period include risk of inflammation and increased intraocular pressure, but a limited duration of intraocular exposure can provide the benefits of prolonged mechanical displacement without significant complications.

25.2.4 Positioning

With the application of expansile gas and heavy liquids for displacement of SMH, greater consideration was given to optimizing the forces acting on the hemorrhage through postoperative patient positioning. Initial studies utilizing pneumatics universally applied prone positioning with the thought that intravitreal gas would exert maximal upward force on the macula leading to hemorrhage displacement away from the fovea. However, an analysis of the biophysical forces of intravitreal gas provided by Stopa and Lincoff [44] led to the adoption of upright positioning with improved outcomes.

To summarize this analysis, one can start with a fundamental understanding of Archimedes' principle as it applies to both liquids and gases, which states that a body immersed in fluid experiences a buoyant (upward) force equal to the weight of the fluid it has displaced. The relative weight of the body and fluid determine if the body floats, remains in equilibrium, or sinks. Hemorrhage and vitreous have nearly equal weights, and thus no displacement occurs in the natural course of SMH. When the hemorrhage is fully immersed in gas (albeit separated by the neurosensory retina), then there is a strong driving force to displace the hemorrhage. In the upright position, gravity is acting maximally in the subretinal space to drive the hemorrhage downward. In contrast, there is no gravitational force acting to displace the hemorrhage in the prone position. The effects of intraocular pressure and gas surface tension are distributed equally across the surface of the hemorrhage and thus do not induce displacement.

Of key importance is the concept that the hemorrhage must be fully immersed in gas. As the volume of gas injection is limited in the absence of vitrectomy, the patient's head must be positioned to provide adequate coverage of the hemorrhage, while continuing to maximize gravitational force parallel to the desired direction of displacement (i.e., inferiorly).

25.2.5 Subretinal Air

A recent innovation has been the use of subretinal air to provide greater SMH displacement and earlier visual acuity improvement compared to intravitreal gas alone. In this technique developed by Martel and Mahmoud [45], pars plana vitrectomy is followed by simultaneous injection of subretinal rTPA (12.5 ug/0.1 mL, total 50 ug), 0.1 mL bevacizumab (2.5 mg), and filtered air. The injection is delivered via a 41-gauge extendable subretinal cannula that is inserted at the superior margin of the SMH, and is connected to a syringe attached to the fluid control unit of the vitrectomy machine. While the rTPA enzymatically lysis the clot to reduce friction of RBCs on the photoreceptors, the total injected subretinal volume also serves to reduce mechanical friction. The injected 0.5 mL of fluid creates space for the liquefied clot to be displaced inferiorly. The introduction of air (typically 0.2 mL) into the subretinal space dramatically reduces the buoyancy of the hemorrhage within the subretinal space and allows sequestration of air into the central macular region. As the ratio of gravitational force to buoyancy is increased, so is the degree and rapidity of hemorrhage displacement inferiorly. A partial fluid–air exchange is then followed by nonexpansile concentration of sulfur hexafluoride (SF_6 20%), which will serve to keep the subretinal air within the macula rather than tracking superiorly. The patient is then positioned upright. Risks of the procedure include iatrogenic hole creation and inadvertent displacement of SMH into the fovea. In one case, a 55-year-old with baseline VA of 20/80 who suffered at large SMH due to exudative AMD that reduced vision to count fingers (CF), the above protocol effectively displaced the SMH and vision recovered to 20/100 within 1 month postoperatively.

Subsequent elaboration of this technique was provided in a prospective study by Kadonosono [46] in which a 47-gauge microneedle (50 μm outer diameter) connected to a 10-mL syringe attached to the viscous fluid control unit of the vitrectomy machine was used to inject a 0.4-mL volume of TPA (62.5 μg/0.1 mL; total dose 250 μg) into the submacular space at a pressure of 15 mmHg. In contrast to Martel and Mahmoud's [45] technique that simultaneously injected a therapeutic cocktail of TPA, air, and anti-VEGF, Kadosono techniques allow the tPA to sit for one minute, after which 0.4 mL filtered air is injected with 4–6 mmHg pressure. No anti-VEGF was used, and a fluid air exchange was not performed. Patients maintained prone positioning overnight. This technique allowed subfoveal blood displacement in all eyes, and visual acuity improved by over two lines in 11 of 13 eyes with average gains being significantly improved compared to baseline at 1 and 3 months postoperatively.

A retrospective study examined ten eyes with SMH due to AMD that had undergone vitrectomy followed by submacular injection of TPA (12.5 ug/0.1 mL), bevacizumab (2.5 mg/0.1 mL and air (0.3 mL) followed by gas tamponade with 20% SF6 and postoperative upright positioning. At 6 month follow-up, visual acuity improved in 80% of patients, and bleed occurred in two eyes, which was treated with intravitreal tPA, anti-VEGF, and 20% SF6 [47].

In 2018, the initial findings of a multicenter retrospective study of 24 eyes undergoing displacement of SMH due to exudative AMD of polypoidal choroidal vasculopathy with vitrectomy, subretinal injections of air and tPA (125 mg/mL) followed by partial fluid–air exchange and gas tamponade coupled with either preoperative, intraoperative, or postoperative intravitreal injection of anti-VEGF were published [48]. Complete displacement of SMH from the foveal center was achieved in all eyes, with 75% having displacement outside the arcades and additional 20% beyond the equator. Visual functional significantly improved in 95.8% of eyes postoperatively. In addition, 74% of sub-RPE hemorrhages were also displaced, which was noted to be more efficient in cases of smaller sub-RPE and submacular hemorrhage. In massive SRH, subretinal air does not adequately localize to the height of the sub-RPE hemorrhage to provide mechanical displacement and flattening in prone positioning (Fig. 25.1).

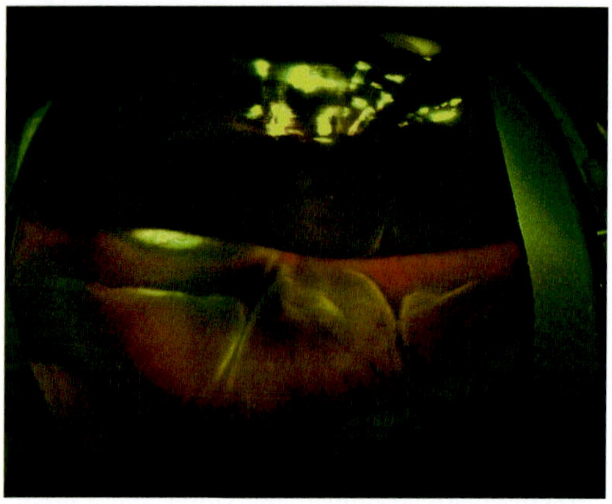

Fig. 25.1 Postoperative day 1 image from a patient with subretinal air, intravitreal gas, inferior subretinal fluid, and displaced subretinal hemorrhage. The intravitreal gas prevents superior migration of the subretinal air while the patient is in the upright position, allowing for maximum displacement of the subretinal hemorrhage. *Text quoted from original publication* [48]

In the same study by Sharma et al. [48], none of the surgeons had prior experience injecting subretinal air. Macular hole formation is a potential complication of any subretinal injection near the macula, and patients with SMH are predisposed due to the effect of SMH on foveal tissue. One of the 24 eyes included developed an intraoperative macular hole where the subretinal air was delivered superior to the macula. Complications on subsequent cases were avoided by administering the subretinal injection closer to the inferior arcade and directing the injection toward the inferior retina (Fig. 25.2). This allows the subretinal air and tPA to move into the inferior periphery and does not expose the fovea to the mechanical force of injection, when the risk of macular hole formation is greatest. The air then moves passively to displace the hemorrhage when the patient is upright.

25.2.6 Emerging Techniques

Recent advances in subretinal surgery include the creation of increasingly small retinotomies, automated injection techniques, and new small gauge intravitreal devices that can deliver subretinal therapy without the need for vitrectomy.

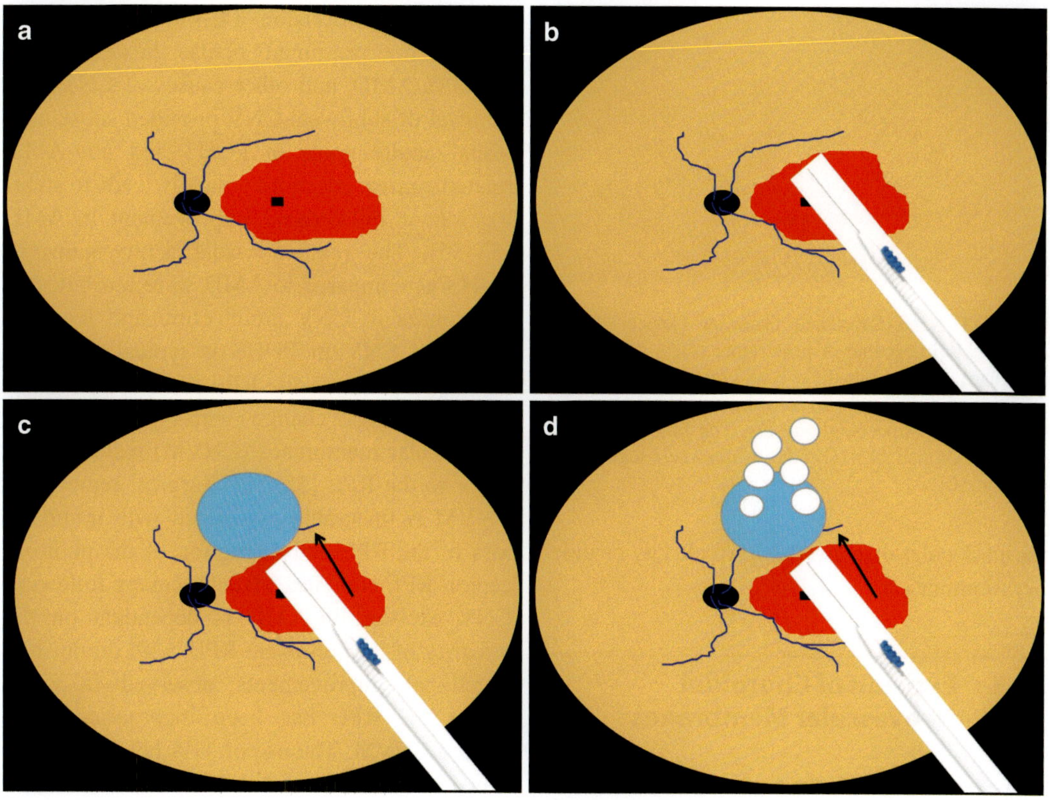

Fig. 25.2 Depiction of subretinal air injection from surgeon's view. (**a**) Submacular hemorrhage. (**b**) Subretinal delivery device is oriented toward the inferior periphery. (**c, d**) The subretinal air and pharmacologic agents are delivered near the inferotemporal arcade, avoiding mechanical trauma to the fovea during injection, which poses the greatest risk for iatrogenic macular hole formation. The air then moves passively to displace the hemorrhage when the patient is upright

Injection of pharmacologic agents or gas into the subretinal space may be performed manually with an assistant pushing an insulin syringe plunger while the surgeon holds the syringe body. Flexible tubing can be attached to the subretinal cannula to minimize the translation of surgeon tremor to instruments in the subretinal space, but great care must still be taken to avoid iatrogenic trauma or induction of a macular hole with rapid subretinal injection. Recent studies have shown better control of automated administration via 41-gauge cannula and insulin syringe coupled to the viscous fluid control of the standard vitrectomy systems, typically with 6–10 PSI [48, 49]. The controlled introduction of liquids and gas into the subretinal space may minimize photoreceptor trauma.

The most recent advancement to facilitate delivery of pharmacologic agents and air into the subretinal space is the Nano Subretinal Gateway Device developed by Mahmoud et al. [50]. It consists of an external very thin needle-like tip and an inner extendable, flexible cannula 25% smaller than the 41G (Fig. 25.3). The outer needle has a sharp tip capable of penetrating the sclera through pars plana to establish intraocular access without a traditional sclerotomy with a cannula. Once inside the vitreous cavity, the internal cannula is extended when the needle is close to the retinal surface, and its beveled tip creates a retinotomy for access to the subretinal space. Pharmacologic agents are delivered through automated injection as described above, and the retinotomy is self-sealing. Visualization

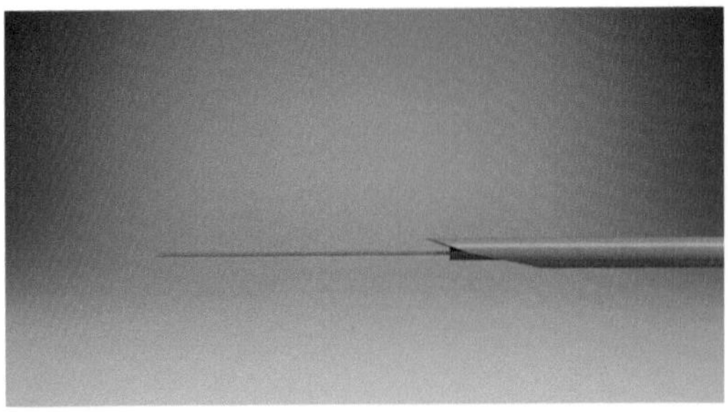

Fig. 25.3 Nano Subretinal Gateway Device. A thin needle-like tip capable of penetrating sclera through the pars plana. Once inside the eye, an inner, flexible cannula is extended and penetrates into the subretinal space for delivery of pharmacologic agents. The inner cannula is 25% smaller than the 41G and provides a self-sealing retinotomy [50]

for intraocular maneuvers is provided by chandelier illumination.

25.3 Excision of Choroidal Neovascular Membranes

As previously noted, the functional gains in the management of CNV-related complications are often limited by the progression of underlying macular degeneration. Photocoagulation of subfoveal CNV diminished visual acuity loss over time with the distinct drawback of immediately decreased vision at the time of treatment, as shown in the Macular Photocoagulation Study Group [7]. Excision of subfoveal CNV in an effort to restore vision and stop disease progression was first reported by Thomas et al. [51] in 1992. The surgical technique utilized in Thomas' and similar studies published in the same year involved a pars plana vitrectomy, induction of posterior vitreal detachment, and the creation of 200 μm retinotomy with diathermy, typically temporal to the fovea. A blunt 30G needle was used to inject subretinal balanced salt solution to create a localized neurosensory retinal detachment. Once in the subretinal space, an angled pick facilitated dissection of the CNV from the RPE and was then extracted through the retinotomy with forceps. Following fluid–air exchange, the retinotomy was sealed with diathermy or laser photocoagulation [51, 52].

The surgical excision of CNVM has been performed for presumed ocular histoplasmosis (POHS), AMD, and other causes of CNV. The removal of subfoveal CNV provided substantial visual acuity gains in POHS and non-AMD related causes, but more typically leads to stabilization or mild visual improvement in AMD [53–55]. The relative visual acuity gains in POHS as compared to AMD were attributed to differences in CNV architecture and localization. The CNV in POHS is typically type 2, existing anterior to the RPE. In contrast, AMD often has diffuse changes with type 1 choroidal neovascular membranes (CNVM) residing posterior to the RPE [55, 56]. Surgical removal of CNVM is invariably associated with traumatic loss of the RPE and disruption of the photoreceptor–RPE complex. Visual recovery following CNV excision in AMD is dependent on the integrity of the subfoveal RPE, with diminished functional improvements observed in cases where the RPE has been incorporated into mature CNVM. The use of TPA before surgical excision of subfoveal membranes has shown no benefit in mitigating this limitation [14].

Maintenance of long-term visual improvements in AMD remained limited by CNVM recurrence with a rate of 20% over a 2-year follow-up period, and rarely produced reading vision [57]. Consequently, criteria for patient selection for surgical excision versus laser photocoagulation were considered, and a surgical approach was primarily utilized in more advanced disease with low baseline visual acuity (generally under 20/200), large CNVM occupying the foveal avascular zone, and exudative lesions [56].

Following CNVM excision, decreased choroidal perfusion observed on fluorescein and indocyanine green angiography was indicative of choriocapillaris atrophy that may have contributed to limited visual acuity outcomes. In contrast, large and medium choroidal vessels remained perfused [58]. The cause of choriocapillaris atrophy was unknown, but may have been related to the underlying disease process or surgical trauma. Histologic analysis of surgically removed tissue showed the universal presence of RPE, but an infrequent appearance of choriocapillaris [58, 59]. It was proposed that the removal of overlying RPE may cause subsequent choroidal atrophy with proposed mechanisms including inadequate RPE repopulation, abnormalities of the repopulated RPE cells, or permanent changes to the denuded Bruch's membrane [58, 59]

The submacular surgery trials were the seminal study that compared complications and visual acuity changes in eyes undergoing surgical removal versus laser photocoagulation of recurrent extrafoveal or juxtafoveal CNV due to neovascular AMD. In this prospective, randomized, multicenter study by Bressler et al. [60], no significant advantage to submacular surgery in terms of visual acuity or size of the central macular lesions was found. A total of 70 patients were enrolled and among these, 65% (31 eyes) in the laser arm and 50% (14 eyes) of the surgical group had visual acuity at 2 years after enrollment that was better or no more than one line worse than at baseline. The similarity in ophthalmic outcomes in the two treatment arms was also reflected in health-related quality of life metrics [61]

25.4 Foveal Translocation

25.4.1 Exudative AMD

Given the limitations in visual acuity gains following CNVM removal in exudative AMD that was attributed in part to loss of foveal RPE function, an alternative therapeutic intervention was to relocate the foveal retina to overlie healthy RPE.

The initial strategy for macular translocation involved a PPV, the creation of a total retinal detachment with 360-degree retinectomy and excision of the CNVM, followed by rotation of the foveal neural retina onto adjacent, intact RPE, and subsequent silicone oil tamponade. The first demonstration of this technique by Machemer in 1993 [62] involved three patients in whom the fovea was rotated between 30 to 80 degrees to overlay healthy RPE. One patient demonstrated improvement in vision, albeit with excyclotorsion of images.

Future elaborations on this surgical technique varied the extent of the retinectomy and reduced the degree of macular rotation [63, 64]. This modification, which was termed "Limited Macular Translocation" involved only 15–25 degree rotation of the retina, and was associated with fewer postoperative complications such as retinal detachment and PVR [65]. In this procedure, a partial thickness scleral resection was created in the supratemporal or infratemporal equatorial region, followed by a retinotomy to induce a subtotal retinal detachment, before finally suturing the edges of the resected sclera. Others performed scleral imbrication or infolding rather than resection [65–67]. Either approach served to shorten the length of the globe in one meridian so that the fovea no longer rested on the CNVM when the retina was reattached [68]. Visual acuity gains were seen in 40% of eyes, but persistence and recurrence of CNVM remained common causes of vision loss. A review of a visual acuity gains following limited macular translocation showed that the foveal sensory retina does recover when overlaid onto healthy RPE up to 5 years after surgery when combined with CNVM excision or photocoagulation [69]. As with full macular translocation, metamorphopsia, and image tilt remained common complaints and complications included PVR, complex RD, epiretinal membrane, macular hole, corneal astigmatism, and constricted visual field [70, 71].

The macular translocation with 360-degree retinectomy (MTS360) carried the advantage of avoiding scleral dissection while providing access to the subretinal space for CNVM excision and evacuation of submacular hemorrhage. In other studies, the CNV was treated with macular photocoagulation rather than excision [67].

Considering the profound changes in RPE–retina anatomy and frequent torsional diplopia following macular translocation, the functional outcomes were surprisingly good. Long-term follow-up of MTS360 retinectomy and silicone oil tamponade showed stabilization or improvement in visual acuity and reading speed for most patients. At 12 months after MTS360, a majority of patients maintained their preoperative vision, and in a study by Abdel et al. [72], 33% of patients showed improvement (three or more lines logMar) [73]). Another study by Aisenbrey et al. [71] included patients with submacular hemorrhage and showed similar outcomes at 1 year. Among eyes undergoing MTS360 with compensatory muscle surgery followed for an average of 21 months, two-thirds of patients experienced visual acuity gains consistent with reading vision and nearly one-third showed stable vision (within 1 Snellen line); deterioration of vision was observed infrequently (6%) [74]. Overall, a majority of patients with 20/80 vision or better at baseline were likely to retain this level of vision 12 months after surgery [75]. Central visual fields also improved following macular translocation [76].

Cyclotropia and diplopia affected approximately 50% of patients and was effectively mitigated by extraocular muscle surgery, either at the time of surgery or early in the postoperative period [72, 77]. Infrared eye tracking showed that the majority of eyes had improvement in central scotoma following macular translocation and adequate foveal function to produce a single, stable focus for fixation. Saccadic function was impaired, but oculomotor limitations did not significantly impede reading behavior [78].

In all of these techniques, recurrence of CNVM remained a common complication that curtailed long-term gains in visual function. Recurrences were noted to have a predisposition to involve the newly repositioned fovea, which led to the hypothesis that the development of CNV may occur via foveal signaling [79], though this was not supported by later studies. As expected, choroidal perfusion in individuals who underwent macular translocation without CNV excision showed no change in choroidal perfusion following surgery [80]. Nonetheless, long-term follow-up showed that half of the patients who underwent MTS360 had a stable or improved vision at 3 years [81].

The Macular Relocation in Age-related Neovascular disease (MARAN) trial sought to assess the efficacy of macular relocation in neovascular AMD as compared to observation or photodynamic therapy (PDT). Limited recruitment was attributed to inherent risks of the surgical arm as well as the emergence of new pharmacologic treatment options, namely anti-VEGF. Among the small number of patients recruited, no significant difference was seen in the surgical versus observation or PDT arm [82]. Another small study comparing full macular translocation vs PDT in the treatment of neovascular AMD also showed lack of difference between the two methods [83]. With the introduction of anti-VEGF, macular translocation was used with decreasing frequency and only for select patients.

25.4.2 Nonexudative AMD

In the evolution of surgical techniques to manage AMD, few therapeutic options had emerged for the nonexudative form of AMD. Geographic atrophy (GA) accounts for severe vision loss in 40% of patients with AMD [84]. Vitamin supplementation in the form of AREDS was introduced in 1991, and no other therapeutic intervention has shown the ability to slow or stabilize disease progression [85]. The concept of foveal translocation away from the area of RPE atrophy held the attractive possibility of improving visual function for patients with nonexudative AMD.

Macular translocation was applied to nonexudative AMD and GA and showed visual acuity gains [76, 86]. As GA has been reported to have an average growth rate of 139 microns per year in one direction [86, 87], the macula had to be translocated a sufficient distance to avoid the spread of atrophy to involve the fovea at its new site. The posterior retina was typically rotated about 40 degrees upward until the fovea was positioned approximately two-thirds of a disk diameter away from the border of the RPE lesion. Geographic atrophy was shown to recur subfoveally in a variable portion of patients with nonexudative AMD who underwent macular translocation [88]. A comparison of outcomes for MTS360 for the management of exudative versus nonexudative AMD showed that the prevalence of postoperative subfoveal RPE atrophy was higher in the nonexudative group compared to the exudative group due to recurrence of GA lesions [89]. There was not a significant difference in mean preoperative or postoperative VA between nonexudative versus exudative AMD groups.

25.5 Transplantation

25.5.1 RPE Transplantation

As techniques to excise choroidal neovascular complexes elaborated in the early 1990s, the importance of RPE integrity to visual recovery became increasingly apparent, thus directing efforts toward the simultaneous transplantation of RPE. The fundamental rationale is to transport healthy RPE and choroid from the periphery to the fovea. As the technique has evolved, multiple studies have shown its capacity to stabilize vision loss, improve visual acuity, and increase reading speed for several years following surgery.

The initial techniques created a retinal flap to access the subfoveal RPE then used an autologous pedicle RPE flap that was rotated into place or homologous RPE cells and Bruch's membrane, which was ultimately covered with the same retinal flap [90]. Alternatively, RPE grafts harvested from the edge of the RPE defect where CNV was excised were transplanted onto the denuded Bruch's membrane with the neurosensory retina relaid on top; these RPE grafts exhibited autofluorescence and patients demonstrated improved central visual function with the ability to fixate [91]. Larger series showed that best-corrected visual acuity remained improved in over half of eyes, and was stable in 35% over an average of 17 months follow-up [92].

However, the encouraging results of studies with a follow-up of 2 years or less were not perpetuated at longer intervals. Although macular translocation of the RPE demonstrated anatomical longevity up to 5–6 years, there was ultimate loss of foveal fixation and graft autofluorescence [93].

Transplantation of suspended peripheral RPE cells using poly-L-lysine to promote adhesion in the bed of the choroid after CNV extraction was technically feasible but associated with high rates of PVR and no functional improvement [94]. A comparison of grafts consisting of RPE-choroid sheets versus RPE cell suspension overlaying healthy choroid showed comparable anatomic and functional outcomes [95].

25.5.2 Transplantation of Alternative Tissue

Alternative sources of tissue to replace RPE were also considered. Transplantation of iris pigment epithelium (IPE) after removal of CNV demonstrated that autologous IPE cells are tolerated in the subretinal space and could be considered in cases with diffuse RPE degeneration [96, 97]. Human fetal RPE (15–17 week gestational) was also cultured and transplanted as a monolayer into the subretinal space with viability for up to 3 months [98]. Still, the majority of RPE transplantations for the management of neovascular AMD utilize an autologous graft harvested from the periphery.

25.5.3 RPE–Choroid Transplantation in Wet AMD

The observation of choriocapillaris atrophy in eyes that underwent CNV excision, and the demonstrated visual improvements with RPE transplantation, paved the way for the creation of RPE–choroid transplants. The first subfoveal RPE-choroid transplantation of a graft harvested from the nasal midperiphery was performed in 2003. An average of two Snellen line visual acuity increase and graft survival was noted 1 year postoperatively [99]. Although harvest sites for RPE–choroid grafts were generally from the nasal periphery, RPE–choroidal translocation with pedicle flap to maintain a connection with adjacent choroidal blood supply was also successfully demonstrated [100]. There is no correlation between superior or inferior periphery donor sites and the incidence of PVR after transplantation [101].

One large series of 84 eyes undergoing autologous free RPE–choroid grafts showed modest visual acuity gains that continued to slightly improve up to 4 years after surgery, with fixation located on the graft [102]. Long-term follow-up showed that RPE–choroid grafts in eyes with exudative AMD were sustained at 7 years with minimal complication rates and CNVM recurrence under 10% [103]. Full-thickness RPE–choroid grafts were also successfully transplanted [104]. However, functional outcomes in eyes that underwent successful autologous RPE–choroid transplantation appeared limited by overlying neuroretinal damage [105].

A smaller series in exudative AMD showed more heterogeneous results with frequent postoperative complications [106]. The variable results between studies highlight the lack of standardization for patient selection to undergo RPE–choroid transplants, and the uncertainty of what preoperative features of exudative AMD (e.g., submacular hemorrhage) may predispose to favorable postoperative outcomes. Preoperative factors shown to carry better postsurgical prognosis were predominantly classic and occult lesions; in contrast, minimally classic or large (>50%) hemorrhagic lesions showed less visual acuity improvement [102].

Histologic evidence of angiogenesis leading to revascularization of autologous RPE–choroid grafts has been demonstrated in porcine models with bridging vessels between the recipient layer and graft identified from 1 week to 3 months after surgery [107]. This integration occurred regardless of the integrity of Bruch's membrane. Angiographic studies assessing revascularization of the RPE–choroid graft in patients showed that the vast majority of grafts revascularized as early as 1 week after surgery and persisted up to 3 years [108].

25.5.4 RPE–Choroid Transplantation in Dry AMD

Similar work in nonexudative AMD showed that RPE–choroid grafts vascularized in the majority of eyes, including those with GA, and that visual outcomes were not clearly related to the type AMD [109]. A separate study of ten patients demonstrated no recurrence of RPE atrophy with graft survival at 3 years, but limited visual benefit due to postoperative complications and patient selection. Notably, individuals with extrafoveal fixation preoperatively were not able to convert to foveal fixation following transplantation despite graft viability [110].

25.5.5 Retina–RPE–Choroid Transplants

Subretinal surgery for exudative AMD leads to damage to RPE and Bruch's membrane and variable retinal trauma, which may compound preexisting outer retinal atrophy from AMD. Visual acuity following successful RPE-choroid transplantation is limited by this neurosensory damage [104]. Autologous transplantation of neurosensory retina has demonstrated efficacy in the management of large, refractory macular holes with the capacity to integrate with the adjacent neurosensory retina and improve vision [111–113].

The combination of this technique with the RPE–choroid graft in advanced exudative AMD was first presented by Parolini et al. [114] who reported on outcomes in nine eyes where the RPE–choroid and retinal grafts were placed subretinal (n = 5), intraretinal to cover an area of an iatrogenically induced macular hole (n = 1), and preretinal (n = 1). In this study, the average follow-up was 7 ± 5.5 months and the visual acuity changed from being an average of CF preoperatively to approximately 20/800 postoperatively (Fig. 25.4). Vision was stable in five eyes and improved in four eyes. Complications included graft atrophy (n = 1) and dislocation (n = 1). Future studies to establish the long-term survival of these grafts the visual function improvements they offer remain to be established [114].

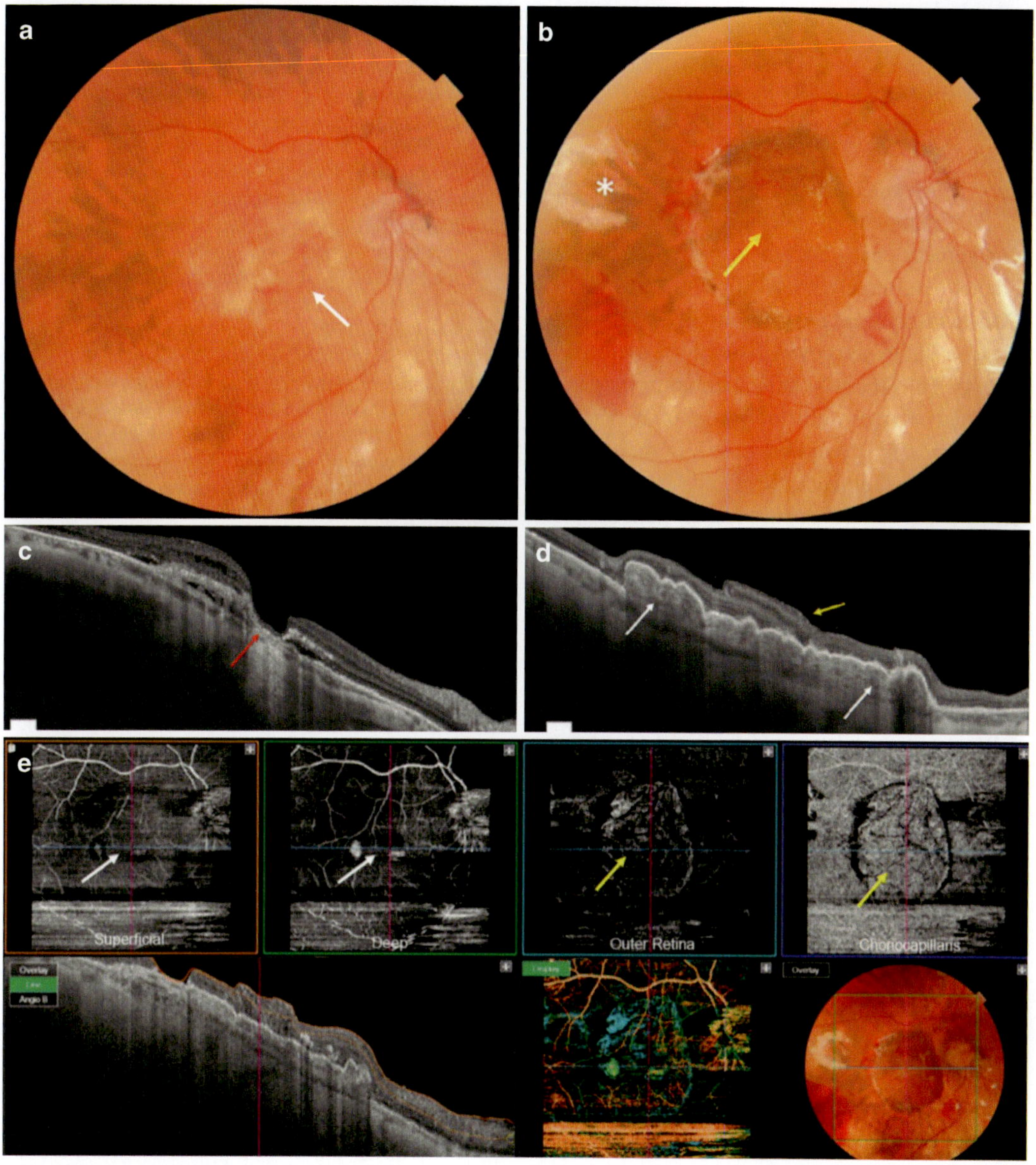

Fig. 25.4 Patient with advanced exudative AMD (**a**) with RPE atrophy in the macular region (white arrow). OCT (**c**) showing lamellar MH configuration with a very thin residual foveal floor, significant loss of outer retinal layers and RPE atrophy (red arrow), overlying intraretinal fluid, and subretinal hyporeflective spaces. Postoperative photograph 1 month after surgery (**b**) showing the choroidal–RPE graft in the center of the macular region and the neurosensory retinal graft covering the MH (yellow arrow). The temporal harvest site of the neurosensory retinal graft is shown with the white asterisk. Postoperative OCT 3 months after surgery (**d**) showing RPE–choroidal patch in the macula area, with rounded hyporeflective round spaces because of the dilatation of choroidal vessels inside the graft (white arrows). The neurosensory retinal graft (yellow arrow) seems well integrated into the MH and is partly lying over the original retina, separated by a hyperreflective line. Postoperative OCT angiography (**e**, scan area 66 mm) 3 months after surgery. The choroidal graft (yellow arrows) is visualized on the en face images at the level of the outer retina and choriocapillaris. The superficial and deep retinal vasculature seems grossly preserved in the area of the original overlying neurosensory retina (white arrows); however, the scan is limited by artifact and segmentation errors. *Text quoted from original publication* [114]

25.6 Conclusion

Efforts directed at the surgical management of exudative AMD have spurred profound advances in vitreoretinal surgery technology and technique. With the emergence of anti-VEGF therapy for the treatment of exudative AMD, surgical management has become limited to select patients. Fortunately, the medical management of AMD in our current era is minimally invasive and provides stable, improved vision for a majority of patients. Thick large submacular hemorrhage displacement remains the most common surgical indication for complications of neovascular AMD, with better anatomical and functional outcomes using newer techniques. In patients with advanced disease, retina–RPE–choroid transplantation remains a treatment option that will continue to be refined through surgical device innovation and less invasive techniques.

Key Learning Points

- Displacement rather than removal of submacular hemorrhage improves visual recovery and is facilitated by delivery of subretinal TPA and gas.
- Newer techniques of displacement using subretinal TPA, subretinal air, with and without antiVEGF results in 100% displacement far away from the fovea, preserving the central visual field.
- Minimally invasive, nanovitreoretinal gateway devices allow subretinal access for delivery of pharmacologic agents with less iatrogenic trauma and may circumvent the need for vitrectomy.
- Transplantation of retina, RPE, and choroidal grafts for improved central visual acuity is an area of active development in the surgical management of exudative AMD.

References

1. Bressler NM, Bressler SB, Fine SL. Age-related macular degeneration. Surv Ophthalmol. 1988;32: 375–413.
2. Klein R, Klein BE, Jensen SC, Meuer SM. The five-year incidence and progression of age-related maculopathy: the Beaver Dam Eye Study. Ophthalmology. 1997;104:7–21.
3. la Cour M, Kiilgaard JF, Nissen MH. Age-related macular degeneration: epidemiology and optimal treatment. Drugs Aging. 2002;19:101–33.
4. Avery RL, Fekrat S, Hawkins BS, Bressler NM. Natural history of subfoveal subretinal hemorrhage in age-related macular degeneration. Retina. 1996;16:183–9.
5. Scupola A, Coscas G, Soubrane G, Balestrazzi E. Natural history of macular subretinal hemorrhage in age-related macular degeneration. Ophthalmologica. 1999;213:97–102.
6. Bennett SR, Folk JC, Blodi CF, Klugman M. Factors prognostic of visual outcome in patients with subretinal hemorrhage. Am J Ophthalmol. 1990;109:33–7.
7. Macular Photocoagulation Study Group. Laser photocoagulation of subfoveal neovascular lesions of age-related macular degeneration. Updated findings from two clinical trials. Arch Ophthalmol. 1993;111:1200–9.
8. Virgili G, Bini A Laser photocoagulation for neovascular age-related macular degeneration. Cochrane Database Syst Rev CD004763. 2007.
9. Macular Photocoagulation Study Group. Subfoveal neovascular lesions in age-related macular degeneration. Guidelines for evaluation and treatment in the macular photocoagulation study. Arch Ophthalmol. 1991;109:1242–57.
10. Glatt H, Machemer R. Experimental subretinal hemorrhage in rabbits. Am J Ophthalmol. 1982;94:762–73.
11. Toth CA, Morse LS, Hjelmeland LM, Landers MB 3rd. Fibrin directs early retinal damage after experimental subretinal hemorrhage. Arch Ophthalmol. 1991;109:723–9.
12. Benner JD, Hay A, Landers MB 3rd, Hjelmeland LM, Morse LS. Fibrinolytic-assisted removal of experimental subretinal hemorrhage within seven days reduces outer retinal degeneration. Ophthalmology. 1994;101:672–81.
13. Toth CA, Benner JD, Hjelmeland LM, Landers MB 3rd, Morse LS. Ultramicrosurgical removal of subretinal hemorrhage in cats. Am J Ophthalmol. 1992;113:175–82.
14. Lewis H, Resnick SC, Flannery JG, Straatsma BR. Tissue plasminogen activator treatment of experimental subretinal hemorrhage. Am J Ophthalmol. 1991;111:197–204.
15. de Juan E Jr, Machemer R. Vitreous surgery for hemorrhagic and fibrous complications of age-related macular degeneration. Am J Ophthalmol. 1988;105:25–9.
16. Vander JF, Federman JL, Greven C, Slusher MM, Gabel VP. Surgical removal of massive subretinal hemorrhage associated with age-related macular degeneration. Ophthalmology. 1991;98:23–7.
17. Claes C, Zivojnovic R. Efficacy of tissue plasminogen activator (t-PA) in subretinal hemorrhage removal. Bull Soc Belge Ophtalmol. 1996;261:115–8.
18. Peyman GA, Nelson NC Jr, Alturki W, Blinder KJ, Paris CL, Desai UR, Harper CA 3rd. Tissue plasmino-

gen activating factor assisted removal of subretinal hemorrhage. Ophthalmic Surg. 1991;22:575–82.
19. Ibanez HE, Williams DF, Thomas MA, Ruby AJ, Meredith TA, Boniuk I, Grand MG. Surgical management of submacular hemorrhage. A series of 47 consecutive cases. Arch Ophthalmol. 1995;113:62–9.
20. Kamei M, Tano Y, Maeno T, Ikuno Y, Mitsuda H, Yuasa T. Surgical removal of submacular hemorrhage using tissue plasminogen activator and perfluorocarbon liquid. Am J Ophthalmol. 1996;121:267–75.
21. Heriot WJ. Intravitreal gas and TPA: an outpatient procedure for submacular hemorrhage. Case Rep Ophthalmol Med. 1996:4. https://doi.org/10.1155/2016/9809583.
22. Kamei M, Misono K, Lewis H. A study of the ability of tissue plasminogen activator to diffuse into the subretinal space after intravitreal injection in rabbits. Am J Ophthalmol. 1999;128:739–46.
23. Hassan AS, Johnson MW, Schneiderman TE, Regillo CD, Tornambe PE, Poliner LS, Blodi BA, Elner SG. Management of submacular hemorrhage with intravitreous tissue plasminogen activator injection and pneumatic displacement. Ophthalmology. 1999;106:1900–6. discussion 1906–7
24. Chen CY, Hooper C, Chiu D, Chamberlain M, Karia N, Heriot WJ. Management of submacular hemorrhage with intravitreal injection of tissue plasminogen activator and expansile gas. Retina. 2007;27:321–8.
25. Hattenbach LO, Klais C, Koch FH, Gümbel HO. Intravitreous injection of tissue plasminogen activator and gas in the treatment of submacular hemorrhage under various conditions. Ophthalmology. 2001;108:1485–92.
26. Haupert CL, McCuen BW 2nd, Jaffe GJ, Steuer ER, Cox TA, Toth CA, Fekrat S, Postel EA. Pars plana vitrectomy, subretinal injection of tissue plasminogen activator, and fluid-gas exchange for displacement of thick submacular hemorrhage in age-related macular degeneration. Am J Ophthalmol. 2001;131:208–15.
27. Olivier S, Chow DR, Packo KH, MacCumber MW, Awh CC. Subretinal recombinant tissue plasminogen activator injection and pneumatic displacement of thick submacular hemorrhage in age-related macular degeneration. Ophthalmology. 2004;111:1201–8.
28. Kamei M, Tano Y. Tissue plasminogen activator-assisted vitrectomy: surgical drainage of submacular hemorrhage. Dev Ophthalmol. 2009;44:82–8.
29. Hillenkamp J, Surguch V, Framme C, Gabel V-P, Sachs HG. Management of submacular hemorrhage with intravitreal versus subretinal injection of recombinant tissue plasminogen activator. Graefes Arch Clin Exp Ophthalmol. 2010;248:5–11.
30. Bell JE, Shulman JP, Swan RJ, Teske MP, Bernstein PS. Intravitreal versus subretinal tissue plasminogen activator injection for submacular hemorrhage. Ophthalmic Surg Lasers Imaging Retina. 2017;48:26–32.
31. Hesse L, Schmidt J, Kroll P. Management of acute submacular hemorrhage using recombinant tissue plasminogen activator and gas. Graefes Arch Clin Exp Ophthalmol. 1999;237:273–7.
32. Lee JP, Park JS, Kwon OW, You YS, Kim SH. Management of Acute Submacular Hemorrhage with intravitreal injection of Tenecteplase, anti-vascular endothelial growth factor and gas. Korean J Ophthalmol. 2016;30:192–7.
33. Cho HJ, Koh KM, Kim JH, Kim HS, Han JI, Lew YJ, Lee TG, Kim JW. Intravitreal ranibizumab injections with and without pneumatic displacement for treating submacular hemorrhage secondary to neovascular age-related macular degeneration. Retina. 2015;35:205–12.
34. Shin JY, Lee J-M, Byeon SH. Anti-vascular endothelial growth factor with or without pneumatic displacement for submacular hemorrhage. Am J Ophthalmol. 2015;159:904–14.e1.
35. Chang W, Garg SJ, Maturi R, Hsu J, Sivalingam A, Gupta SA, Regillo CD, Ho AC. Management of thick submacular hemorrhage with subretinal tissue plasminogen activator and pneumatic displacement for age-related macular degeneration. Am J Ophthalmol. 2014;157:1250–7.
36. Shah SP, Hubschman JP, Gonzales CR, Schwartz SD. Submacular combination treatment for management of acute, massive submacular hemorrhage in age-related macular degeneration. Ophthalmic Surg Lasers Imaging. 2009;40:308–15.
37. Klettner A, Puls S, Treumer F, Roider J, Hillenkamp J. Compatibility of recombinant tissue plasminogen activator and bevacizumab co-applied for neovascular age-related macular degeneration with submacular hemorrhage. Arch Ophthalmol. 2012;130:875–81.
38. Hillenkamp J, Klettner A, Puls S, Treumer F, Roider J. Subretinal co-application of rtPA and bevacizumab for exudative AMD with submacular hemorrhage. Compatibility and clinical long-term results. Ophthalmologe. 2012;109:648–56.
39. Klettner A, Grotelüschen S, Treumer F, Roider J, Hillenkamp J. Compatibility of recombinant tissue plasminogen activator (rtPA) and aflibercept or ranibizumab coapplied for neovascular age-related macular degeneration with submacular haemorrhage. Br J Ophthalmol. 2015;99:864–9.
40. González-López JJ, McGowan G, Chapman E, Yorston D. Vitrectomy with subretinal tissue plasminogen activator and ranibizumab for submacular haemorrhages secondary to age-related macular degeneration: retrospective case series of 45 consecutive cases. Eye. 2016;30:929–35.
41. Guthoff R, Guthoff T, Meigen T, Goebel W. Intravitreous injection of bevacizumab, tissue plasminogen activator, and gas in the treatment of submacular hemorrhage in age-related macular degeneration. Retina. 2011;31:36–40.
42. de Jong JH, van Zeeburg EJT, Cereda MG, van Velthoven MEJ, Faridpooya K, Vermeer KA, van Meurs JC. Intravitreal versus subretinal administration of recombinant tissue plasminogen activator combined with gas for acute submacular hemorrhages due

to age-related macular degeneration: an exploratory prospective study. Retina. 2016;36:914–25.
43. Fleissig E, Barak A, Goldstein M, Loewenstein A, Schwartz S. Massive subretinal and subretinal pigment epithelial hemorrhage displacement with perfluorocarbon liquid using a two-step vitrectomy technique. Graefes Arch Clin Exp Ophthalmol. 2017;255:1341–7.
44. Stopa M, Lincoff A, Lincoff H. Analysis of forces acting upon submacular hemorrhage in pneumatic displacement. Retina. 2007;27:370–4.
45. Martel JN, Mahmoud TH. Subretinal pneumatic displacement of subretinal hemorrhage. JAMA Ophthalmol. 2013;131:1632–5.
46. Kadonosono K, Arakawa A, Yamane S, Inoue M, Yamakawa T, Uchio E, Yanagi Y. Displacement of submacular hemorrhages in age-related macular degeneration with subretinal tissue plasminogen activator and air. Ophthalmology. 2015;122:123–8.
47. Kumar A, Roy S, Bansal M, Tinwala S, Aron N, Temkar S, Pujari A. Modified approach in management of submacular hemorrhage secondary to wet age-related macular degeneration. Asia Pac J Ophthalmol. 2016;5:143–6.
48. Sharma S, Kumar JB, Kim JE, Thordsen J, Dayani P, Ober M, Mahmoud TH. Pneumatic displacement of submacular hemorrhage with subretinal air and tissue plasminogen activator: initial United States experience. Oph Retina. 2018;2:180–6.
49. Novelli FJD, Preti RC, Monteiro MLR, Nóbrega MJ, Takahashi WY. A new method of subretinal injection of tissue plasminogen activator and air in patients with submacular hemorrhage. Retina. 2017;37:1607–11.
50. Mahmoud T. Nanovitreoretinal subretinal gateway device to displace submacular hemorrhage: access to the subretinal space without vitrectomy. Retina. 02/2019; https://doi.org/10.1097/IAE.0000000000002669.
51. Thomas MA, Grand MG, Williams DF, Lee CM, Pesin SR, Lowe MA. Surgical management of subfoveal choroidal neovascularization. Ophthalmology. 1992;99:952–68. discussion 975–6
52. Skaf AR, Mahmoud T. Surgical treatment of age-related macular degeneration. Semin Ophthalmol. 2011;26:181–91.
53. Berger AS, Kaplan HJ. Clinical experience with the surgical removal of subfoveal neovascular membranes. Short-term postoperative results. Ophthalmology. 1992;99:969–75. discussion 975–6
54. Benson MT, Callear A, Tsaloumas M, Chhina J, Beatty S. Surgical excision of subfoveal neovascular membranes. Eye. 1998;12(Pt 5):768–74.
55. Thomas MA, Dickinson JD, Melberg NS, Ibanez HE, Dhaliwal RS. Visual results after surgical removal of subfoveal choroidal neovascular membranes. Ophthalmology. 1994;101:1384–96.
56. Sabates FN, Fletcher DC. Surgical excision of subfoveal neovascular membranes in age-related macular degeneration. Am J Ophthalmol. 1992;114:241–2.
57. Ormerod LD, Puklin JE, Frank RN. Long-term outcomes after the surgical removal of advanced subfoveal neovascular membranes in age-related macular degeneration. Ophthalmology. 1994;101:1201–10.
58. Thach AB, Marx JL, Frambach DA, LaBree LD, Lopez PF. Choroidal hypoperfusion after surgical excision of subfoveal neovascular membranes in age-related macular degeneration. Int Ophthalmol. 1996;20:205–13.
59. Nasir MA, Sugino I, Zarbin MA. Decreased choriocapillaris perfusion following surgical excision of choroidal neovascular membranes in age-related macular degeneration. Br J Ophthalmol. 1997;81:481–9.
60. Bressler NM, Bressler SB, Hawkins BS, Marsh MJ, Sternberg P Jr, Thomas MA, Submacular Surgery Trials Pilot Study Investigators. Submacular surgery trials randomized pilot trial of laser photocoagulation versus surgery for recurrent choroidal neovascularization secondary to age-related macular degeneration: I. Ophthalmic outcomes submacular surgery trials pilot study report number 1. Am J Ophthalmol. 2000;130:387–407.
61. Bressler NM, Bressler SB, Hawkins BS, Marsh MJ, Sternberg P Jr, Thomas MA, Submacular Surgery Trials Pilot Study Investigators. Submacular surgery trials randomized pilot trial of laser photocoagulation versus surgery for recurrent choroidal neovascularization secondary to age-related macular degeneration: II. Quality of Life Outcomes Submacular Surgery Trials Pilot Study report number 2. Am J Ophthalmol. 2000;130:408–18.
62. Machemer R, Steinhorst UH. Retinal separation, retinotomy, and macular relocation: II. A surgical approach for age-related macular degeneration? Graefes Arch Clin Exp Ophthalmol. 1993;231:635–41.
63. Fujikado T, Ohji M, Kusaka S, Hayashi A, Kamei M, Okada AA, Oda K, Tano Y. Visual function after foveal translocation with 360-degree retinotomy and simultaneous torsional muscle surgery in patients with myopic neovascular maculopathy. Am J Ophthalmol. 2001;131:101–10.
64. Ninomiya Y, Lewis JM, Hasegawa T, Tano Y. Retinotomy and foveal translocation for surgical management of subfoveal choroidal neovascular membranes. Am J Ophthalmol. 1996;122:613–21.
65. Fujii GY, de Juan E Jr, Pieramici DJ, Humayun MS, Phillips S, Reynolds SM, Melia M, Schachat AP. Inferior limited macular translocation for subfoveal choroidal neovascularization secondary to age-related macular degeneration: 1-year visual outcome and recurrence report. Am J Ophthalmol. 2002;134:69–74.
66. Mateo C, Moreno J, Rosales G, Lechuga M, Castillo R, Vaz F, Corcóstegui B. Two-year results of macular translocation with scleral infolding in myopic choroidal neovascularisation. Semin Ophthalmol. 2004;19:29–42.
67. Pieramici DJ, De Juan E Jr, Fujii GY, Reynolds SM, Melia M, Humayun MS, Schachat AP, Hartranft CD. Limited inferior macular translocation for the treatment of subfoveal choroidal neovascularization secondary to age-related macular degeneration. Am J Ophthalmol. 2000;130:419–28.

68. de Juan E Jr, Loewenstein A, Bressler NM, Alexander J. Translocation of the retina for management of subfoveal choroidal neovascularization II: a preliminary report in humans. Am J Ophthalmol. 1998;125:635–46.
69. Oshima H, Iwase T, Ishikawa K, Yamamoto K, Terasaki H. Long-term results after limited macular translocation surgery for wet age-related macular degeneration. PLoS One. 2017;12:e0177241.
70. Ohji M, Fujikado T, Saito Y, Hosohata J, Hayashi A, Tano Y. Foveal translocation: a comparison of two techniques. Semin Ophthalmol. 1998;13:52–62.
71. Aisenbrey S, Lafaut BA, Szurman P, et al. Macular translocation with 360 degrees retinotomy for exudative age-related macular degeneration. Arch Ophthalmol. 2002;120:451–9.
72. Abdel-Meguid A, Lappas A, Hartmann K, Auer F, Schrage N, Thumann G, Kirchhof B. One year follow up of macular translocation with 360 degree retinotomy in patients with age related macular degeneration. Br J Ophthalmol. 2003;87:615–21.
73. Toth CA, Freedman SF. Macular translocation with 360-degree peripheral retinectomy impact of technique and surgical experience on visual outcomes. Retina. 2001;21:293–303.
74. Pertile G, Claes C. Macular translocation with 360 degree retinotomy for management of age-related macular degeneration with subfoveal choroidal neovascularization. Am J Ophthalmol. 2002;134:560–5.
75. Mruthyunjaya P, Stinnett SS, Toth CA. Change in visual function after macular translocation with 360 degrees retinectomy for neovascular age-related macular degeneration. Ophthalmology. 2004;111:1715–24.
76. Eckardt C, Eckardt U. Macular translocation in nonexudative age-related macular degeneration. Retina. 2002;22:786–94.
77. Eckardt C, Eckardt U, Conrad HG. Macular rotation with and without counter-rotation of the globe in patients with age-related macular degeneration. Graefes Arch Clin Exp Ophthalmol. 1999;237:313–25.
78. Uppal G, Feely MP, Crossland MD, Membrey L, Lee J, da Cruz L, Rubin GS. Assessment of reading behavior with an infrared eye tracker after 360° macular translocation for age-related macular degeneration. Invest Ophthalmol Vis Sci. 2011;52:6486–96.
79. Baer CA, Rickman CB, Srivastava S, Malek G, Stinnett S, Toth CA. Recurrent choroidal neovascularization after macular translocation surgery with 360-degree peripheral retinectomy. Retina. 2008;28:1221–7.
80. Cekiç O, Ohji M, KesercI B, Sawa M, Zheng Y, Hayashi A, Ikuno Y, Nakata K, Gomi F, Tano Y. Evaluation of choroidal perfusion of the new central macular area by dilution analysis of indocyanine green angiography after macular translocation. Retina. 2004;24: 210–4.
81. Aisenbrey S, Bartz-Schmidt KU, Walter P, Hilgers RD, Ayertey H, Szurman P, Thumann G. Long-term follow-up of macular translocation with 360 degrees retinotomy for exudative age-related macular degeneration. Arch Ophthalmol. 2007;125:1367–72.
82. Joussen AM, Wong D, Walter P, et al. Surgical management of subfoveal choroidal neovascular membranes in age-related macular degeneration by macular relocation: experiences of an early-stopped randomised clinical trial (MARAN Study). Eye. 2010;24:284–9.
83. Gelisken F, Voelker M, Schwabe R, Besch D, Aisenbrey S, Szurman P, Grisanti S, Herzau V, Bartz-Schmidt KU. Full macular translocation versus photodynamic therapy with verteporfin in the treatment of neovascular age-related macular degeneration: 1-year results of a prospective, controlled, randomised pilot trial (FMT-PDT). Graefes Arch Clin Exp Ophthalmol. 2007;245:1085–95.
84. Owen CG, Fletcher AE, Donoghue M, Rudnicka AR. How big is the burden of visual loss caused by age related macular degeneration in the United Kingdom? Br J Ophthalmol. 2003;87:312–7.
85. Age-Related Eye Disease Study Research Group. The age-related eye disease study (AREDS): design implications. AREDS report no. 1. Control Clin Trials. 1999;20:573–600.
86. Sunness JS, Gonzalez-Baron J, Applegate CA, Bressler NM, Tian Y, Hawkins B, Barron Y, Bergman A. Enlargement of atrophy and visual acuity loss in the geographic atrophy form of age-related macular degeneration. Ophthalmology. 1999;106:1768–79.
87. Schatz H, McDonald HR. Atrophic macular degeneration: rate of spread of geographic atrophy and visual loss. Ophthalmology. 1989;96:1541–51.
88. Khurana RN, Fujii GY, Walsh AC, Humayun MS, de Juan E Jr, Sadda SR. Rapid recurrence of geographic atrophy after full macular translocation for nonexudative age-related macular degeneration. Ophthalmology. 2005;112:1586–91.
89. Cahill MT, Mruthyunjaya P, Bowes Rickman C, Toth CA. Recurrence of retinal pigment epithelial changes after macular translocation with 360 degrees peripheral retinectomy for geographic atrophy. Arch Ophthalmol. 2005;123:935–8.
90. Peyman GA, Blinder KJ, Paris CL, Alturki W, Nelson NC Jr, Desai U. A technique for retinal pigment epithelium transplantation for age-related macular degeneration secondary to extensive subfoveal scarring. Ophthalmic Surg. 1991;22:102–8.
91. Stanga PE, Kychenthal A, Fitzke FW, Halfyard AS, Chan R, Bird AC, Aylward GW. Retinal pigment epithelium translocation after choroidal neovascular membrane removal in age-related macular degeneration. Ophthalmology. 2002;109:1492–8.
92. Binder S, Stolba U, Krebs I, et al. Transplantation of autologous retinal pigment epithelium in eyes with foveal neovascularization resulting from age-related macular degeneration: a pilot study. Am J Ophthalmol. 2002;133:215–25.
93. MacLaren RE, Bird AC, Sathia PJ, Aylward GW. Long-term results of submacular surgery combined with macular translocation of the retinal pigment epithelium in neovascular age-related macular degeneration. Ophthalmology. 2005;112:2081–7.

94. van Meurs JC, ter Averst E, Hofland LJ, van Hagen PM, Mooy CM, Baarsma GS, Kuijpers RW, Boks T, Stalmans P. Autologous peripheral retinal pigment epithelium translocation in patients with subfoveal neovascular membranes. Br J Ophthalmol. 2004;88:110–3.
95. Falkner-Radler CI, Krebs I, Glittenberg C, Povazay B, Drexler W, Graf A, Binder S. Human retinal pigment epithelium (RPE) transplantation: outcome after autologous RPE-choroid sheet and RPE cell-suspension in a randomised clinical study. Br J Ophthalmol. 2011;95:370–5.
96. Thumann G, Aisenbrey S, Schraermeyer U, Lafaut B, Esser P, Walter P, Bartz-Schmidt KU. Transplantation of autologous iris pigment epithelium after removal of choroidal neovascular membranes. Arch Ophthalmol. 2000;118:1350–5.
97. Lappas A, Foerster AMH, Weinberger AWA, Coburger S, Schrage NF, Kirchhof B. Translocation of iris pigment epithelium in patients with exudative age-related macular degeneration: long-term results. Graefes Arch Clin Exp Ophthalmol. 2004;242:638–47.
98. Algvere PV, Berglin L, Gouras P, Sheng Y. Transplantation of fetal retinal pigment epithelium in age-related macular degeneration with subfoveal neovascularization. Graefes Arch Clin Exp Ophthalmol. 1994;232:707–16.
99. van Meurs JC, Van Den Biesen PR. Autologous retinal pigment epithelium and choroid translocation in patients with exudative age-related macular degeneration: short-term follow-up. Am J Ophthalmol. 2003;136:688–95.
100. Angunawela RI, Williamson TH, Khan MAJ, Chong V. Choroidal translocation with a pedicle following excision of a type 1 choroidal neovascular membrane. Br J Ophthalmol. 2005;89:386.
101. van Zeeburg EJT, Maaijwee K, van Meurs JC. There is no relation between the occurrence of proliferative vitreoretinopathy and the location of the donor site after transplantation of a free autologous retinal pigment epithelium-choroid graft. Acta Ophthalmol. 2014;92:228–31.
102. Maaijwee K, Heimann H, Missotten T, Mulder P, Joussen A, van Meurs J. Retinal pigment epithelium and choroid translocation in patients with exudative age-related macular degeneration: long-term results. Graefes Arch Clin Exp Ophthalmol. 2007;245:1681–9.
103. van EJT Z, KJM M, TOAR M, Heimann H, van Meurs JC. A free retinal pigment epithclium-choroid graft in patients with exudative age-related macular degeneration: results up to 7 years. Am J Ophthalmol. 2012;153:120–7.e2.
104. Cereda MG, Parolini B, Bellesini E, Pertile G. Surgery for CNV and autologous choroidal RPE patch transplantation: exposing the submacular space. Graefes Arch Clin Exp Ophthalmol. 2010;248:37–47.
105. Parolini B, Alkabes M, Baldi A, Pinackatt S. Visual recovery after autologous retinal pigment epithelium and choroidal patch in a patient with choroidal neovascularization secondary to ANGIOID streaks: long-term results. Retin Cases Brief Rep. 2016;10:368–72.
106. Degenring RF, Cordes A, Schrage NF. Autologous translocation of the retinal pigment epithelium and choroid in the treatment of neovascular age-related macular degeneration. Acta Ophthalmol. 2011;89:654–9.
107. Maaijwee KJM, van Meurs JC, Kirchhof B, Mooij CM, Fischer JH, Mackiewicz J, Kobuch K, Joussen AM. Histological evidence for revascularisation of an autologous retinal pigment epithelium--choroid graft in the pig. Br J Ophthalmol. 2007;91:546–50.
108. Maaijwee K, Van Den Biesen PR, Missotten T, Van Meurs JC. Angiographic evidence for revascularization of an rpe-choroid graft in patients with age-related macular degeneration. Retina. 2008;28:498–503.
109. Joussen AM, Heussen FMA, Joeres S, Llacer H, Prinz B, Rohrschneider K, Maaijwee KJM, van Meurs J, Kirchhof B. Autologous translocation of the choroid and retinal pigment epithelium in age-related macular degeneration. Am J Ophthalmol. 2006;142:17–30.
110. Caramoy A, Liakopoulos S, Menrath E, Kirchhof B. Autologous translocation of choroid and retinal pigment epithelium in geographic atrophy: long-term functional and anatomical outcome. Br J Ophthalmol. 2010;94:1040–4.
111. Grewal DS, Mahmoud TH. Autologous neurosensory retinal free flap for closure of refractory myopic macular holes. JAMA Ophthalmol. 2016;134:229–30.
112. Thomas AS, Mahmoud TH. Subretinal transplantation of an autologous retinal free flap for chronic retinal detachment with proliferative vitreoretinopathy with and without macular hole. Retina. 2018;38(Suppl 1):S121–4.
113. Grewal DS, Charles S, Parolini B, Kadonosono K, Mahmoud TH. Autologous retinal transplant for refractory macular holes: multicenter international collaborative study group. Ophthalmology. 2019;126:1399. https://doi.org/10.1016/j.ophtha.2019.01.027.
114. Parolini B, Grewal DS, Pinackatt SJ, Baldi A, Di Salvatore A, Besozzi G, Finzi A, Cardillo D, Mahmoud TH. Combined autologous transplantation of neurosensory retina, retinal pigment epithelium and choroid free grafts. Retina. 2018;38(Suppl 1):S12–22.

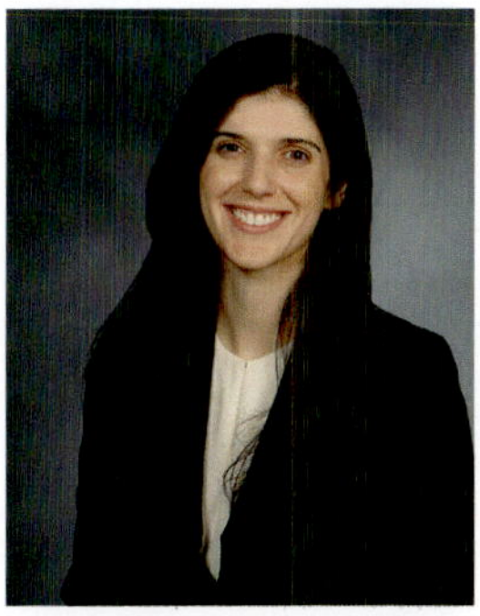

Elizabeth D. Marlow M.D. is completing her fellowship in vitreoretinal surgery at Associated Retinal Consultants/William Beaumont Hospital with plans to practice in the San Francisco Bay Area. She is originally from Washington State and completed her ophthalmology residency at Weill Cornell Medical Center/New York–Presbyterian Hospital. Interests include diabetic eye disease and complex retinal detachment repair.

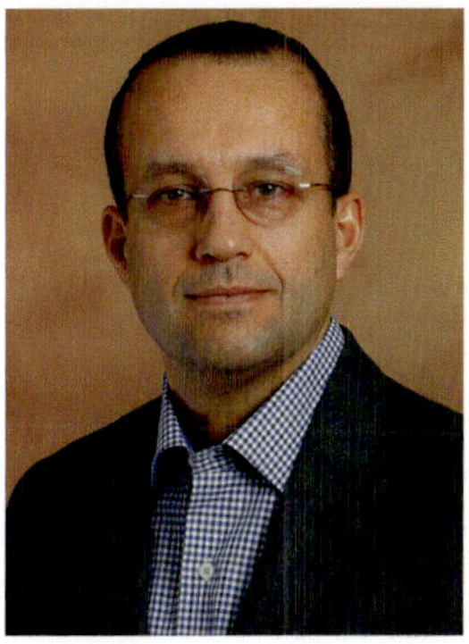

Tamer H. Mahmoud is a professor of Ophthalmology at Oakland University William Beaumont School of Medicine. He was the program director of the vitreoretinal surgery fellowship at the Duke University Eye Center and a tenured associate professor at Duke. He has developed many surgical techniques including the use of subretinal air to displace submacular hemorrhage and performed the first human autologous retinal transplantation. He also introduced chandelier buckles to the United States and developed the ILM retracting door technique for macular holes. In 2019, he developed the Nanovitreoretinal Surgery Platform.

Mahmoud finished his internship, residency, and vitreoretinal fellowship at Duke. He is a member of the AAO, ARVO, ASRS, the Club Jules Gonin, the Macula Society, and the Retina Society. He received the Edward K. Isbey, Jr., M.D. award for "Excellence in Clinical Care, Ethics, and Research" from Duke, the Retina Research Foundation Award from ARVO, the "Senior Honor Award" from ASRS, The "Achievement Award" from the AAO, the prestigious Robert A. Machemer Research Award from Duke, the "Distinguished Teacher of the Year Award" from the Kresge Eye Institute and the "Golden Globe Award" for residents' education from Duke.

26 Home Monitoring for Age-Related Macular Degeneration

Voraporn Chaikitmongkol

26.1 Introduction

Age-related macular degeneration remains the leading cause of central visual loss and blindness in individuals aged 50 or older in North America and other regions worldwide [1]. The primary etiology of visual deterioration in neovascular AMD eyes associated with the development of choroidal neovascularization (CNV). Patients with neovascular AMD could experience various visual symptoms in their central visual field, i.e. blurry vision, metamorphopsia, and scotoma. Intravitreous anti-VEGF injection has been dramatically improved visual functions of eyes with neovascular AMD [2–5]. Ninety percent of neovascular AMD patients receiving anti-VEGF therapy could avoid moderate or more severe visual loss over a 2-year treatment with anti-VEGF. However, not more than one-third of treated patients achieved moderate visual gain [2–5]. The main predictors for favorable treatment outcomes include the presenting level of visual acuity and size of the CNV lesion at the time of treatment initiation [6–8]. According to the CATT subgroup analysis, eyes presenting with good baseline visual acuity (20/25 to 20/40) were eyes that achieved the best mean visual acuity at one year [6]. Therefore, early recognition of CNV development when visual acuity is least affected is crucial for AMD treatment. Delay in treatment may lead to irreversible damage and poor visual outcome [9].

Patients at risk to develop neovascular AMD are those with intermediate stage of AMD, either bilateral large drusen (125 μm or larger in diameter) or large drusen in one eye and advanced AMD (neovascular AMD or central geographic atrophy) in the fellow eye, whom typically are scheduled for fundus evaluations every 6–12 months or only 1–2 times per year. Due to the longer durations between clinic visits in these patients, recognition of visual function changes by the patients themselves is very important as such recognition would urge them to be evaluated by an ophthalmologist sooner than regular schedules. Then, they will be able to receive prompt treatment if there is a presence of CNV and result in excellent visual acuity. The home-monitoring device for AMD, therefore, plays an essential role in assisting patients in detecting subtle changes in their visual functions at an early stage of CNV development.

The idea to detect an early stage of macular abnormalities has been established since 1940s when the Amsler grid was developed by Mark Amsler. Subsequently, the Amsler grid has become the only self-monitoring tool used worldwide for more than 70 years despite an absence of effective treatment for AMD. Until the past

V. Chaikitmongkol (✉)
Retina Division, Department of Ophthalmology, Chiang Mai University, Chiang Mai, Thailand

J. Chhablani (ed.), *Choroidal Neovascularization*, https://doi.org/10.1007/978-981-15-2213-0_26

decade when there are advancements in therapeutic options for neovascular AMD, the importance of an early detection of CNV has been re-emphasized and many home-monitoring devices for AMD have been invented.

This chapter will describe the testing principles and scientific evidence on the validity of each home-monitoring device for AMD including the Amsler grid, preferential hyperacuity perimeter (ForeseeHome device), shape discrimination hyperacuity test (myVisionTrack), and other self-measured visual function tests designed for personal electronic devices, e.g., smartphone or tablet device, which are recently available.

26.2 The Amsler Grid

The Amsler grid was first introduced by Marc Amsler, a Swiss ophthalmologist, in 1947 and subsequently publicized around 1950 as a method for macular function testing [10]. Amsler had been interested in developing methods for patients to detect early symptoms of maculopathy, i.e., metamorphopsia and relative scotoma, which typically fails to be revealed by the perimeter and the Bjerrum screen [11]. Amsler designed a square-shaped grid as his testing tool "since it is a matter of making apparent some kind of deformation, we must present to the patient a precise and regular contour which forms as simple a figure as possible, the alterations of which he can access without difficulty" [11].

The original Amsler grid was drawn as a 10-cm. square white grids on a black background (Fig. 26.1). The square was subdivided every 5 mm. by vertical and horizontal parallel lines. Each small 5-mm. square subtends an angle of one degree at 28–30 cm. distance. The entire grid is thus 20 degrees high and 20 degrees wide [11]. The field spans ten degrees from the fixation center. To start testing, simply place the Amsler grid 28–30 cm. from an eye under good illumination. Refractive errors, if presents, should be corrected with reading glasses or contact lens. The patient is instructed to close one eye, look at the center of the grid, and asked if they notice any distorted line, blurry or missing square, or greyish or blackish spot.

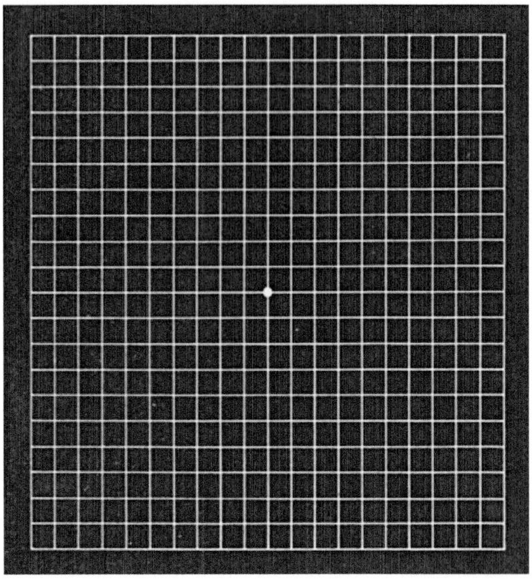

Fig. 26.1 The original Amsler grid (white lines on a black background)

The Amsler grid testing is a simple, inexpensive, and practical testing method that patients can be used easily at home. However, there were studies suggesting poor validity of the Amsler grid testing for detection macular pathologies [12, 13]. Regarding scotoma detection, Schuchart et al. evaluated the Amsler grid testing in 55 patients with vision loss in the macular region and ten normally sighted subjects. Results revealed nearly half of the standard and threshold scotomas were not detected by the Amsler grid testing. In addition, for scotomas of six degrees or less in diameter, 77% of standard and 87% of threshold scotomas were not detected by the Amsler grid [13]. The poor validity of the Amsler Grid may be a result of difficulty with fixation and the perceptual completion phenomenon. The perceptual completion phenomenon is an ability of the brain to "fill in" a scotoma with the same color and texture as the surrounding background, as similar to visual perceptions when part of an image falls on a blind spot of the visual field. Therefore, it appears that the Amsler grid is less efficient in assessing the extent of scotomas, while may still be useful for early detection of metamorphopsia [14].

Modified versions of the original Amsler grid have been developed, including a version with white lines on a black background. However, Augustin et al. evaluated a role of this modified Amsler grid in 182 patients with dry and exudative age-related macular degeneration and a history of metamorphopsia, compared with the original Amsler grid, and found that for overall study population, the original Amsler grid provided significantly better results than the modified version ($p < 0.05$). For patients with visual acuity ranging from 0.1 to 0.3 (20/63 to 20/200 Snellen equivalent), there was no significant difference across groups. However, for patients with visual acuity of 0.5 (20/40 Snellen equivalent) or better, the original Amsler grid was significantly more informative and reliable than the modified version [15]. Therefore, in case that the Amsler grid is still considered as part of home-monitoring tools in clinical practice, the original Amsler grid (white lines on a black background) might be preferred.

Recently, a systematic review and meta-analysis by Faes et al. had focused on the diagnostic accuracy of the Amsler grid and the preferential hyperacuity perimeter (PHP) in the screening of patients with AMD. Results revealed the pooled sensitivity of studies assessing the Amsler grid was 0.78 (95% confidence intervals (CI); 0.64–0.87), and the pooled specificity was 0.97 (95%CI; 0.91–0.99). The pooled sensitivity of studies assessing the PHP was 0.85 (95%CI; 0.80-0.89), and specificity was 0.87 (95%CI; 0.82-0.91). These results suggest promising test performance characteristics of both the Amsler grid and the PHP in terms of specificity. However, the Amsler grid has a relatively lower sensitivity in detecting neovascular AMD when compared with the PHP [16]. Also, the Amsler grid does not provide quantifiable measures of scotomas or visual field defects. Therefore, the Amsler grid cannot be used to monitor disease progression over time.

26.3 Home-Based Preferential Hyperacuity Perimeter (PHP)

The controversial role of the Amsler grid in detecting CNV in AMD leads to development of the PHP. Hyperacuity (or vernier acuity) is an ability to perceive a difference in the spatial localization of two or more stimuli [17]. This property would permit the detection of a metamorphopsia caused by the displacement of photoreceptors by the CNV or by the separation of the neurosensory retina or the retinal pigment epithelium related to neovascular AMD [18]. The PHP device presents artificial images with different degrees of distortion. Due to brain preferential awareness, the device user can detect more noticeable distortions and overlook the smaller ones. Regarding this brain mechanism, a quantified visual field map of the metamorphopsia for each eye was created along with longitudinal detections of visual field changes as well as deviation from the normative data. The first generation of devices using PHP technology was designed for supervised use in a clinical setting and previously shown to have high sensitivity and specificity in detecting CNV [19].

Following several modifications of the original PHP device, including decreasing in its physical size; enclosure of the screen viewer in a closed hood in order to control distance from the display, ambient light conditions, and occlusion of the non-tested eye; and addition of infrared sensors to ensure correct positioning of the head, a home device or ForeseeHome was developed [19] for use in the detection and characterization of central and paracentral metamorphopsia in patients with AMD, as an aid in monitoring progression of disease factors causing metamorphopsia including but not limited to CNV. The ForeseeHome device has been approved by the US FDA in 2009 and becomes the first FDA approved home-monitoring device for AMD.

The ForeseeHome device tests the central area of the visual field of 14 degrees, with approximately 500 data points sampled rapidly 3–5 times (Fig. 26.2). The stimulus is a dot deviation signal

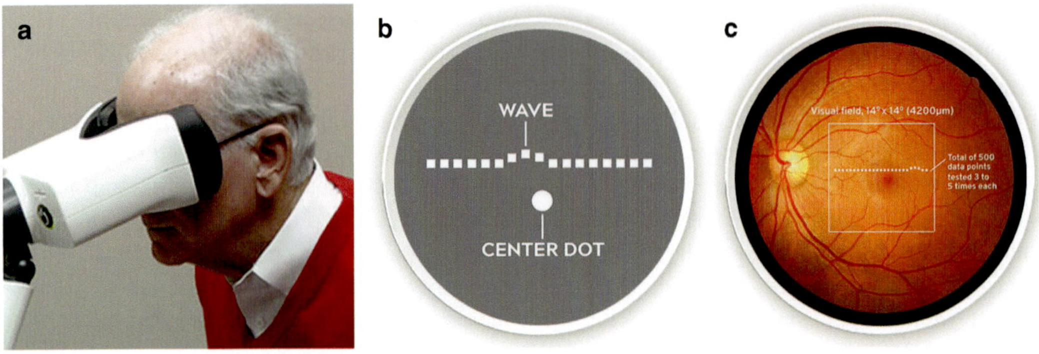

Fig. 26.2 The ForeseeHome device. The patient tests one eye at a time with the device. (**a**) The testing screen shows a dotted line with a wave or a bump in it, which appears briefly then disappears. The patient is instructed to use the device's mouse to click where the bump appeared on the screen and return the cursor to the center dot. A new dotted line will appear, and the test continues for approximately 3 min. Daily testing results are sent to the central monitoring center. (**b**) The device tests the central area of the visual field of 14 degrees with approximately 500 data points sampled rapidly 3–5 times. (**c**) (Reference: www.foreseehome.com; accessed June 24, 2019)

flashed in a pseudo-random predetermined order. During the course of the testing, the patient is presented with artificial distortions similar to those seen by individuals with neovascular AMD. The patient indicates where he/she perceives distortion along the dotted line using a computer mouse. When a signal is presented to the retina over a CNV lesion, the pathological distortion and the artificial distortion compete for the participant's attention. Preferential looking will subconsciously direct the user to select the more extreme distortion. Varying degree of the artificial distortions serves as control stimuli to quantify the extent of possible pathologic distortions originating from retinal pathology. A gray-scale map of the visual field is generated, and the intensity of the visual field defect is determined. Based on a comparison of this intensity with a normative database and the participant's baseline performance with the ForeseeHome device, the system determines whether there are visual responses that may be associated with the progression of AMD to CNV [20]. Participants are instructed to use the ForeseeHome device ideally every day to monitor each eye separately, which takes approximately 3 min per eye. Results of each home-testing session are transmitted via a cellular modem to a data monitoring center, when the monitoring center detects a significant change compared with baseline, the physician is alerted to recall the patient for an exam [20]. The sensitivity and specificity of the ForeseeHome monitoring device were shown to be similar to that of a clinical device using PHP technology that was used to determine visual field defects associated with AMD progression in an office setting in a cross-sectional study [12]. The ForeseeHome monitoring device plus standard care was evaluated in the HOME study (the randomized trial of a home monitoring system for early detection of CNV-Home Monitoring of the Eye (HOME) study) [21].

The HOME study was the unmasked, controlled, randomized clinical trial aimed to determine whether home monitoring with ForeseeHome device, using macular visual field testing with hyperacuity techniques and telemonitoring, results in earlier detection of CNV associated with neovascular AMD, reflected in better vision when compared with standard care. The study was conducted in 44 clinical sites of the Age-Related Eye Disease Study2 (AREDS2), a clinical trial of nutritional supplements for the treatment of AMD [22]. The enrolled participants were individuals at risk for developing CNV, with large drusen in both eyes (two study eyes) or large drusen in one eye (study eye) and advanced AMD in the fellow (non-study) eye, and best-corrected visual acuity of 20/60 or better in the study eye(s). Each participant was screened using a brief tutorial on the home monitoring device in the clinic to make sure that they could use the device and did not have any abnormalities preventing device monitoring in the future. Of 1970 participants who were screened, 1520 (77%) were enrolled and randomized to one of the two arms: 763 were randomized to device arm and 757 to standard care. Participants in the standard care arm received investigator-specific instructions to monitor any changes in their vision at home (Amsler grid may be recommended). Participants randomized to the device arm received the same standard care instruction, and also received a home monitoring device, with instructions for installation and use. Participants were encouraged to use the device on a daily basis, and results were transmitted automatically via cellular modem to a central data monitoring center. When the device testing suggested a change compared with the baseline measurement, an alert was sent from the monitoring center to the participant's clinical center prompting the staff to schedule a visit with the study ophthalmologist within 72 h. The development of CNV was evaluated and confirmed by an investigator, based on standardized ocular imaging with fundus photography, OCT, and FA [21].

Results showed the mean (SD) study follow-up period of 1.4 (0.6) years. Fifty-one patients in the device arm and 31 in the standard care arm developed CNV. Participants in the device arm demonstrating less impaired visual acuity or fewer letters lost from baseline at the time of CNV detection (median (interquartile range [IQR]):−4 [−11.0, −1.0] letters) compared with standard care arm (median [IQR]:−9 [−14.0, −4.0] letters) (p = 0.021). Also, as a secondary visual acuity outcome, a higher percentage of eyes maintained 20/40 or better visual acuity at the time of CNV diagnosis and initiation of treatment in the device arm (87%) compared with the standard care arm (62%) (p = 0.014). Among participants who used the device at the recommended frequency, the proportion of eyes that maintained BCVA of 20/40 or better was 94%. In the device arm, among 609 subjects who continue using the home device, the weekly usage throughout the study period was 4.4 times/week on average (SD, 1.7), and less than two times/week in 57 participants. Results from the HOME study suggest that individuals with higher risk to develop CNV would receive advantage from this home monitoring strategy to detect CNV development at an early stage and be able to achieve favorable visual outcomes after intravitreous anti-VEGF injections [21].

For clinical characteristics of eyes that newly developed CNV detected and alerted by the ForeseeHome device, a report of two cases demonstrated that the device alerts occurred when the patients had minimal or no visual symptoms and visual acuities were 20/32 or better; subtle cystoid abnormalities appeared on optical coherence tomography of both cases with minimal or no fluorescein angiogram leakage [23].

Although the ForeseeHome device has been proven in its efficacy in detecting early development of neovascular AMD, not every AMD patient can successfully use the device. According to the HOME study, eyes with preexisting visual field defects resulted in an approximate 20% screen failure rate. An additional 8% of the eyes could not establish baseline measurements after randomization, and 20% stopped monitoring at different time points during the study [21]. Individuals with difficulty using a computer mouse would not be able to use the ForeseeHome device as well.

The ForeseeHome device is currently available only in the United States by physician's prescription on a rental basis for individuals who are at risk to develop a neovascular form of AMD.

26.4 Handheld Shape Discrimination Hyperacuity Test on Smart Phone

The shape discrimination hyperacuity (SDH) test was developed by Wang et al. using perfect and distorted circular contour called radial frequency patterns [24] as visual stimuli, based on a hypothesis that patients with maculopathy have more difficulty performing visual tasks that require global integration of visual stimuli over a large retinal area than performing a localized task like visual acuity [25]. The optimal performance of SDH requires global visual integration [24]. By measuring SDH, a patient's ability to detect visual distortion at his/her own ability to integrate visual information can be quantified. SDH is significantly reduced in AMD [25], while less affected by normal aging [26].

Recently, a handheld SDH test (myVisionTrack; Vital Art and Science, Inc., Richardson, TX) has been implemented on a mobile platform (iOS; Apple Inc., Cupertino, CA). It received clearance by the US FDA in 2013 to be marketed as an at-home method for monitoring the progression of degenerative eye diseases, such as macular degeneration and diabetic retinopathy.

The myVisionTrack app displays side-by-side circles on the screen (Fig. 26.3); firstly, one circle is significantly different from the others (for example, with a wavy or jagged edge). To perform a self-check, the patient covers one eye and then touches/selects what he or she determines to be the "differently-shaped" circle. Each time the patient makes a selection, subsequent screens display additional circles with increasingly subtle differences among all circles. The test is then repeated with the other eye. The device stores the self-check test results, tracks eye disease progression, and automatically alerts a health care provider if a significant deterioration of visual function is suspected.

Wang et al. compared the handheld SDH (hSDH) (MyVisionTrack app) on a mobile device with a previously established desktop SDH (dSDH) in 100 subjects, results suggested that the hSDH test on a mobile device was highly correlated with PC-based testing methods ($r = 0.88$, $p < 0.0001$). The mobile app is also sensitive to the severity of maculopathy. The mean hSDH measurement of eyes with advanced AMD or with severe to very severe nonproliferative diabetic retinopathy (NPDR) was significantly worse than that of the eyes with intermediate AMD or with mild-to-moderate NPDR ($p < 0.0001$). Ninety-eight percent of 46 patients with maculopathy who completed the usability survey reported that the hSDH test was easy to use [27].

A prospective study had evaluated the feasibility of the handheld SDH (myVisionTrack) in 160 patients with neovascular AMD in at least one eye from 24 centers in the United States. Approximately two-thirds of participants aged 75 years or older. Results demonstrated that 84.7% on average complied with daily myVisionTrack

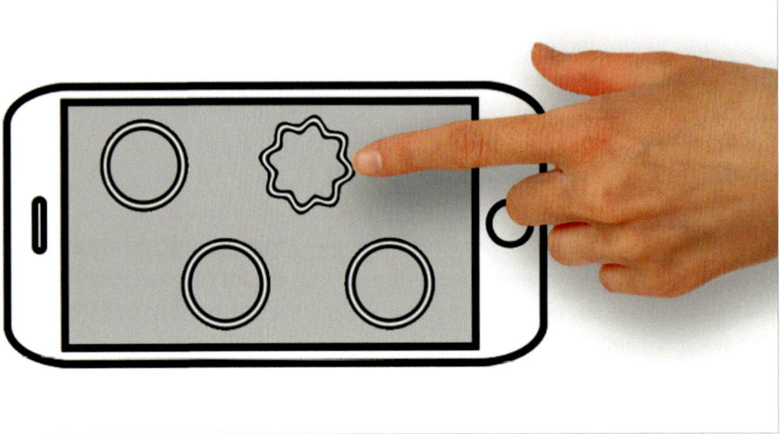

Fig. 26.3 The myVisionTrack (handheld shape discrimination hyperacuity test) on an iOS mobile platform. To start testing, the patient covers one eye and then selects what he/she determines to be the "differently-shaped" circle. Each time the patient makes a selection, subsequent screens display additional circles with increasingly subtle differences among all circles. The test is then repeated with the other eye. The device stores the self-check test results, tracks eye disease progression, and automatically alerts a health care provider if a significant deterioration of visual function is suspected (Reference: www.myvisiontrack.com; accessed June 24, 2019)

testing, and 98.9% complied with at least weekly myVisionTrack testing [28]. However, reports on the validity of myVisionTrack in detecting changes associated with AMD from this study have not yet been published.

26.5 Self-Measured Hyperacuity Test on A Tablet Device

The Hyperacuity App (HAC) is a test developed for use on an iPad (Apple, Cupertino, California). The aim of the app is to be intuitive and easy to use for individuals without cognitive impairment up to the age of 90 years while quantitatively assessing the individual's vision.

The app introduces challenges as a presence of distortion in the line. The distortion is shown for 200 milliseconds before the distortion becomes straight. The subject then selects on the line where he/she believes the distortion was. The selections are required to be within a certain perpendicular distance of the line to be considered. Audio feedback is given for each selection to confirm that a valid selection was accomplished. After a valid selection, the screen clears to black. Subjects are then required to select the center of the empty screen for the next challenge in order to refocus the fovea on the center. Challenges are randomized during each test and can be either horizontal or vertical. Some challenges are randomized to have no distortions. Subjects are asked to select the center of the screen if no distortion is seen. A score is then calculated from the data collected based on a grading system created prior to the study that was optimized to detect errors in distortion perception.

In 2016, a cross-sectional study performed to explore the HAC as a screen for the progression of disease in 33 AMD subjects. Results showed that the HAC had high sensitivity (92.3%) and moderate specificity (61.5%) in distinguishing between patients who required treatment and those who did not require treatment. The researcher determined whether each subject would receive an anti-VEGF treatment based on the OCT findings [29].

Future studies with a larger sample size or a longitudinal study may be warranted to determine whether changes in HAC score compared to baseline correlates with the changes in OCT.

26.6 Self-Measured Retinal Sensitivity on A Tablet Device

The PsyPad platform is a central retinal sensitivity testing developed for use on a tablet device (iPad; Apple, Cupertino, California).

Adams et al. determined its feasibility in 38 participants with intermediate AMD to monitor retinal sensitivity, the benefits of weekly reminders, and the comparison with clinic-based results. The sensitivity results obtained in the home mirrored those obtained in formal clinic-based perimetry. However, there was a high level of inactivity (45%) mainly due to noncompatible devices and other technology access issues [30].

Another study by Wu et al. compared the central retinal sensitivity measured by the Psypad platform on a tablet device with standardized microperimetry in 30 participants with AMD. The average test duration on PsyPad was 53.9 ± 7.5 s. The mean central retinal sensitivity was not significantly different between PsyPad (25.7 ± 0.4 dB) and microperimetry (26.1 ± 0.4 dB, $P = 0.094$), and the 95% limits of agreement between the two measures were between −4.12 and 4.92 dB [31].

Ho et al. evaluated the feasibility of the Psypad platform to identify alterations in retinal sensitivity and correlations with underlying pathology in 53 neovascular AMD eyes receiving treatment and in 21 at-risk fellow eyes. Results demonstrated that the decreased retinal sensitivity associated with the presence of atrophy ($p < 0.01$), retinal pigment epithelium disruption ($p < 0.01$), and absent ellipsoid zone ($p < 0.01$), but not with the presence of subretinal fluid ($p = 0.94$) nor intraretinal fluid ($p = 0.52$). There were differences in retinal sensitivity between locations of the intact retina to that of retinal pathology associated with AMD [32].

Future studies with a more significant number of sample sizes might be warranted to evaluate the validity of the Psypad platform in detecting changes in central retinal sensitivity associated with an early development of CNV or reactivation of CNV during treatments.

26.7 Home-Based Self-Measuring OCT

In an office-setting, optical coherence tomography (OCT) imaging has become the mainstay in AMD management, as OCT assists physicians in being able to identify even subtle disease activity, i.e., subretinal or intraretinal fluid both in quantitative and in qualitative methods, and far better than fundus examination alone. The use of OCT device as part of home monitoring for AMD would increase the sensitivity and specificity of early CNV diagnosis.

Although the home-based OCT device is currently not available in the market, some investigators have explored the possibility of using a home-based self OCT scan. Mansour et al. evaluated the image quality of self-OCT by the ophthalmologist and optometrists. Results demonstrated that self-OCT scans of the macula could be performed with excellent image quality, but image decentration is a common finding [33]. Recently, Maloca et al. have reported the safety and feasibility of a novel sparse OCT device for patient-delivered retina home monitoring in AMD patients and to compare the device to an OCT device that is commercially available. Results demonstrated the feasibility and safety of this home-based OCT monitoring under real-life settings and suggesting the potential clinical benefit of the device. However, the device tested in this study was just the prototype, which required further modification and evaluation as a portable self-measuring OCT device in the future [34].

26.8 Summary

Main predictors for favorable final vision in eyes with neovascular AMD receiving intravitreous anti-VEGF therapy include a good visual acuity (20/40 or better) and smaller size of CNV lesions at the time of treatment initiation [6, 8]. Therefore, the earliest detection of CNV developments when the visual acuity remains unaffected is considered the ultimate goal for home-monitoring devices for AMD patients.

In the past decade, a number of home-monitoring devices for AMD have been researched and developed. However, only two (the ForeseeHome and the MyVisionTrack) have been approved by the US FDA, and only one (the ForeseeHome monitoring program) was proven in a large randomized clinical trial to be beneficial for individuals at high risk to develop neovascular AMD (large drusen in both eyes, or large drusen in one eye and advanced AMD in the fellow eye) to detect CNV at an earlier stage and would increase the patients' opportunities to achieve better outcomes following intravitreous anti-VEGF treatment, compared with standard care alone (with aids include the Amsler grid) [21].

Given the increasing popularity of personal electronic devices, e.g., smartphone, tablet usage among individuals of any age group including those aged 50 years or older who may be at risk for neovascular AMD, many applications for iPhone or tablet device have been developed for people to monitor visual functions at home. Nevertheless, substantial evidence to support their reliability or efficacy in detecting newly developed CNV or changes in the macula is very limited at this time. Home-based self-measuring OCT may be a potential home-monitoring device in the future but required further developments and validations.

In the meantime, while the efficacy-proven ForeseeHome AMD monitoring program is available only in the United States and other devices are still under investigation, the Amsler grid may still play a role in addition to regular eye care as a simple and inexpensive home-monitoring tool for AMD. Though its efficacy in detecting early CNV is relatively lower when compared with recent technologies, the Amsler grid may still be beneficial for AMD patients living in countries or regions where the efficacy-proven home-monitoring program is not available or those with limited access to smartphones or tablet devices. As a physician, in addition to prescribing home-monitoring devices to patients at risk for neovascular AMD, it is also crucial to raise the patients' awareness on the changes of their visual functions, emphasize importance of early detection of CNV with timely anti-VEGF treatments, and the importance of regular usage of any available home-monitoring devices (daily or at least once weekly), to be able to detect the CNV as early as possible and be able to stabilize or maximize their visual functions after receiving anti-VEGF treatments.

Key Learning Points

- Early detection of CNV when vision remains unaffected is crucial for neovascular AMD eye to achieve favorable visual outcomes after anti-VEGF treatments.
- Scotoma sometimes not detected when using the Amsler grid due to the perceptual completion phenomenon of the brain.
- According to the HOME study, participants in the device arm (ForeseeHome device plus standard care) had a significantly better vision when CNV was detected compared with the standard care arm.
- A number of self-measured visual function tests designed for personal electronic devices, i.e., smartphone and tablet devices are available, but strong evidence to support their validity in detecting changes in AMD eyes is very limited.
- Patients' awareness and regular usage of any home-monitoring device (daily or at least once weekly) would increase an opportunity for early detection of CNV.

References

1. Wong WL, Su X, Li X, Cheung CMG, Klein R, Cheng C-Y, et al. Global prevalence of age-related macular degeneration and disease burden projection for 2020 and 2040: a systematic review and meta-analysis. Lancet Glob Health. 2014 Feb;2(2):e106–16.
2. Rosenfeld PJ, Brown DM, Heier JS, Boyer DS, Kaiser PK, Chung CY, et al. Ranibizumab for neovascular age-related macular degeneration. N Engl J Med. 2006 Oct 5;355(14):1419–31.
3. Brown DM, Michels M, Kaiser PK, Heier JS, Sy JP, Ianchulev T, et al. Ranibizumab versus verteporfin photodynamic therapy for neovascular age-related macular degeneration: two-year results of the ANCHOR study. Ophthalmology. 2009 Jan;116(1):57–65.e5.
4. Schmidt-Erfurth U, Kaiser PK, Korobelnik J-F, Brown DM, Chong V, Nguyen QD, et al. Intravitreal aflibercept injection for neovascular age-related macular degeneration: ninety-six-week results of the VIEW studies. Ophthalmology. 2014 Jan;121(1):193–201.
5. Comparison of Age-related Macular Degeneration Treatments Trials (CATT) Research Group, Martin DF, Maguire MG, Fine SL, Ying G, Jaffe GJ, et al. Ranibizumab and bevacizumab for treatment of neovascular age-related macular degeneration: two-year results. Ophthalmology. 2012 Jul;119(7):1388–98.
6. Ying G, Huang J, Maguire MG, Jaffe GJ, Grunwald JE, Toth C, et al. Baseline predictors for one-year visual outcomes with ranibizumab or bevacizumab for neovascular age-related macular degeneration. Ophthalmology. 2013 Jan;120(1):122–9.
7. Ying G, Maguire MG, Daniel E, Ferris FL, Jaffe GJ, Grunwald JE, et al. Association of baseline Characteristics and early vision response with 2-year vision outcomes in the comparison of AMD treatments trials (CATT). Ophthalmology. 2015 Dec;122(12):2523–2531.e1.
8. Blinder KJ, Bradley S, Bressler NM, Bressler SB, Donati G, Hao Y, et al. Effect of lesion size, visual acuity, and lesion composition on visual acuity change with and without verteporfin therapy for choroidal neovascularization secondary to age-related macular degeneration: TAP and VIP report no. 1. Am J Ophthalmol. 2003 Sep;136(3):407–18.
9. Lim JH, Wickremasinghe SS, Xie J, Chauhan DS, Baird PN, Robman LD, et al. Delay to treatment and visual outcomes in patients treated with anti-vascular endothelial growth factor for age-related macular degeneration. Am J Ophthalmol. 2012 Apr;153(4):678–686.e2.
10. Marmor MF. A brief history of macular grids: from Thomas Reid to Edvard Munch and Marc Amsler. Surv Ophthalmol. 2000 Feb;44(4):343–53.
11. Amsler M. Earliest symptoms of diseases of the macula. Br J Ophthalmol. 1953 Sep;37(9):521–37.
12. Fine AM, Elman MJ, Ebert JE, Prestia PA, Starr JS, Fine SL. Earliest symptoms caused by neovascular membranes in the macula. Arch Ophthalmol. 1986 Apr;104(4):513–4.
13. Schuchard RA. Validity and interpretation of Amsler grid reports. Arch Ophthalmol. 1993 Jun;111(6):776–80.
14. Achard OA, Safran AB, Duret FC, Ragama E. Role of the completion phenomenon in the evaluation of Amsler grid results. Am J Ophthalmol. 1995 Sep;120(3):322–9.
15. Augustin AJ, Offermann I, Lutz J, Schmidt-Erfurth U, Tornambe P. Comparison of the original Amsler grid with the modified Amsler grid: result for patients with age-related macular degeneration. Retina Phila Pa. 2005 Jun;25(4):443–5.

16. Faes L, Bodmer NS, Bachmann LM, Thiel MA, Schmid MK. Diagnostic accuracy of the Amsler grid and the preferential hyperacuity perimetry in the screening of patients with age-related macular degeneration: systematic review and meta-analysis. Eye. 2014 Jul;28(7):788–96.
17. Goldstein M, Loewenstein A, Barak A, Pollack A, Bukelman A, Katz H, et al. Results of a multicenter clinical trial to evaluate the preferential hyperacuity perimeter for detection of age-related macular degeneration. Retina Phila Pa. 2005 May;25(3):296–303.
18. Preferential Hyperacuity Perimetry Research Group. Preferential hyperacuity perimeter (PreView PHP) for detecting choroidal neovascularization study. Ophthalmology. 2005 Oct;112(10):1758–65.
19. Loewenstein A, Ferencz JR, Lang Y, Yeshurun I, Pollack A, Siegal R, et al. Toward earlier detection of choroidal neovascularization secondary to age-related macular degeneration: multicenter evaluation of a preferential hyperacuity perimeter designed as a home device. Retina Phila Pa. 2010 Aug;30(7):1058–64.
20. Chew EY, Clemons TE, Bressler SB, Elman MJ, Danis RP, Domalpally A, et al. Randomized trial of the ForeseeHome monitoring device for early detection of neovascular age-related macular degeneration. The home monitoring of the eye (HOME) study design – HOME study report number 1. Contemp Clin Trials. 2014 Mar;37(2):294–300.
21. Chew EY, Clemons TE, Bressler SB, Elman MJ, Danis RP, Domalpally A, et al. Randomized trial of a home monitoring system for early detection of choroidal neovascularization home monitoring of the eye (HOME) study. Ophthalmology. 2014 Feb;121(2):535–44.
22. Age-Related Eye Disease Study 2 Research Group. Lutein + zeaxanthin and omega-3 fatty acids for age-related macular degeneration: the age-related eye disease study 2 (AREDS2) randomized clinical trial. JAMA. 2013 May 15;309(19):2005–15.
23. Chaikitmongkol V, Bressler NM, Bressler SB. Early detection of choroidal neovascularization facilitated with a home monitoring program in age-related macular degeneration. Retin Cases Brief Rep. 2015;9(1): 33–7.
24. Wilkinson F, Wilson HR, Habak C. Detection and recognition of radial frequency patterns. Vis Res. 1998 Nov;38(22):3555–68.
25. Wang Y-Z, Wilson E, Locke KG, Edwards AO. Shape discrimination in age-related macular degeneration. Invest Ophthalmol Vis Sci. 2002 Jun;43(6):2055–62.
26. Wang YZ. Effects of aging on shape discrimination. Optom Vis Sci Off Publ Am Acad Optom. 2001 Jun;78(6):447–54.
27. Wang Y-Z, He Y-G, Mitzel G, Zhang S, Bartlett M. Handheld shape discrimination hyperacuity test on a mobile device for remote monitoring of visual function in maculopathy. Invest Ophthalmol Vis Sci. 2013 Aug 13;54(8):5497–505.
28. Kaiser PK, Wang Y-Z, He Y-G, Weisberger A, Wolf S, Smith CH. Feasibility of a novel remote daily monitoring system for age-related macular degeneration using mobile handheld devices: results of a pilot study. Retina Phila. 2013 Oct;33(9):1863–70.
29. Chen JS, Adelman RA. Hyperacuity exam screens for choroidal neovascularization in age-related macular degeneration on a mobile device. Ophthalmic Surg Lasers Imaging Retina. 2016;47(8):708–15.
30. Adams M, Ho CYD, Baglin E, Sharangan P, Wu Z, Lawson DJ, et al. Home monitoring of retinal sensitivity on a tablet device in intermediate age-related macular degeneration. Transl Vis Sci Technol. 2018 Sep;7(5):32.
31. Wu Z, Guymer RH, Jung CJ, Goh JK, Ayton LN, Luu CD, et al. Measurement of retinal sensitivity on tablet devices in age-related macular degeneration. Transl Vis Sci Technol. 2015 Jun;4(3):13.
32. Ho CYD, Wu Z, Turpin A, Lawson DJ, Luu CD, McKendrick AM, et al. A tablet-based retinal function test in Neovascular age-related macular degeneration eyes and at-risk fellow eye. Transl Vis Sci Technol. 2018 Mar;7(2):2.
33. Mansour AM. Self-optical coherence tomography and angiography. Case Rep Ophthalmol. 2017 Apr;8(1):108–15.
34. Maloca P, Hasler PW, Barthelmes D, Arnold P, Matthias M, Scholl HPN, et al. Safety and feasibility of a novel sparse optical coherence tomography device for patient-delivered retina home monitoring. Transl Vis Sci Technol. 2018 Jul;7(4):8.

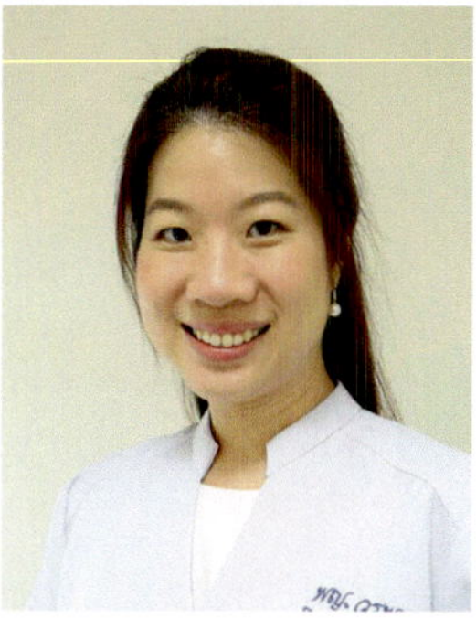

Voraporn Chaikitmongkol received her medical degree in 2005 and an ophthalmology degree in 2010 from Chiang Mai University, Thailand. Following her vitreoretinal fellowship training in 2011, she subsequently joined the faculty at the Department of Ophthalmology, Chiang Mai University. In 2012, Dr. Chaikitmongkol did her post-doctoral clinical research fellowship at the Retina Division, Wilmer Eye Institute, Johns Hopkins University School of Medicine (USA); medical retina training with Professor Neil M. Bressler and Professor Susan B. Bressler (2012–2014), and visual neurophysiology training with Professor Hendrik P.N. Scholl (2013–2014). Her research interest involves the diagnosis and treatments of polypoidal choroidal vasculopathy, age-related macular degeneration, diabetic macular edema, diabetic retinopathy, and novel retinal imaging modalities. Dr. Chaikitmongkol is currently an Assistant Professor in Ophthalmology at the Faculty of Medicine, Chiang Mai University, Chiang Mai, Thailand. Dr. Chaikitmongkol has recently received the Japanese Ophthalmological Society International Young Investigator Award 2019.

Rehabilitation

27

Yogeshwari Bansal

Age-related macular degeneration (AMD) is the leading cause of visual impairment in the Western world [1, 2] and presents a substantial healthcare burden currently after Diabetic Retinopathy in the adult age group. AMD causes visual impairments of reduced visual acuity, central scotoma, and reduced contrast sensitivity which cause multiple disabilities [3] of walking difficulty, difficulty in recognizing faces, and near tasking problems of difficulty in reading and writing, mobile operations and other activities of daily living (ADL) which do affect the quality of life [4, 5]. Despite medical advancements of anti-VEGF therapy, there are limitations. Patients need low vision rehabilitation (LVR) during orter the therapy. LVR aims at minimizing visual disabilities by helping them to make use of their dual vision that can be used with the help of certain magnifiers and techniques to make the best use of remaining eyesight.

A person with low vision exists with visual impairment even after treatment and /or standard refractive correction, and has a best-corrected visual acuity of less than 6/18 to light perception in the better eye, or a total visual field less than 10 degrees from the point of fixation, but who wants to and is potentially able to use, vision for the planning and/or execution of a task. In AMD, it is the central visual acuity that is reduced while peripheral visual fields are intact until and unless it is combined with some other disease such as glaucoma, etc.

The treating ophthalmologist needs to identify and refer patients with AMD to LVR department for LVR counseling, rather than referring only patients with less than 6/18 vision. As patients with AMD have functional difficulties even when the vision is 6/18 or better. At this stage, the patients need counseling about understanding the disease process and prognosis, visual requirements need to be discussed to set the goals, contrast acuity needs to be checked to work on contrast enhancement by improving the lighting conditions, environment modifications if need so and simple higher plus near addition in near glasses to help them in reading. This is called LVR counseling or conventional LVR that could be done by all the clinical practicing Optometrists.

Patients by Low vision definition need "Enhanced LVR" that includes prescription of Low vision devices or aids (LVD/LVA). LVA includes various optical magnifiers and nonoptical aids, projection magnifiers, different computer Software program, and mobile applications. It will include environment modi-

Y. Bansal (✉)
Heading Department of Optometry, ICARE Eye Hospital & Postgraduate Institute, Noida, Uttar Pradesh, India
e-mail: yogeshwari@icarehospital.org

J. Chhablani (ed.), *Choroidal Neovascularization*, https://doi.org/10.1007/978-981-15-2213-0_27

fications and rehabilitators' counseling to help them in social issues such as depression, loss of independence, reduced confidence level, and dependency issues. Mild-to-Moderate cases of low vision, that is Snellen acuity of 3/60 to 6/24, can be helped a lot with the help of LVA and patients can function independently but severe cases of vision impairment, with visual acuity less than 3/60, need some help from their family members as well to perform their daily routine activities.

27.1 LVA in AMD

Functional vision problems for distance and near need to be identified and tabulated at the time of LVR. Most commonly for distance, the patient is going to have problems in recognizing faces at home and outside. Common challenges include watching television at home, navigation within the house, and inability to see the clock. So, for distance functional vision improvement, magnification needs to be explained which means closer the object is to the patient, it becomes bigger. In this magnification, the closer object subtends a larger visual angle and larger image at the retina. Keeping a larger TV screen, clock with larger numbers or talking watches, nail trimmers with a magnifier attached to it are a few examples of nonoptical magnifiers that are useful in AMD.

Optical magnifiers for distance will include telescope and watch television.

Spectacle mounted telescope, head-mounted telescope, and head-mounted magnifier are better carried in old age group [1]. Head-mounted telescope like Ocutech is US FDA approved for driving as well.

Optical magnifiers work on linear and angular magnification and create a virtual and enlarged image that is defined in X. 2X means the image is twice the object size. All the magnifiers are marked with X according to the power of the system and X amount required by the patient is decided by the trial of the optical magnifier. Though different magnification formulas calculate X required that depend upon best-corrected visual acuity(BCVA).One easy Kestenbaum formula will calculate magnification (X), which is reciprocal of BCVA like 6/24 visual acuity means 4x. Optical magnifiers can provide up to 12–20X but higher magnification will reduce the field of vision. So, projection magnifiers are to be used which can provide higher magnification with better field of vision.

Nonoptical magnifiers work on contrast enhancement. Maximum contrast is like jet black on white gives maximum contrast and is more visible and watching the white screen in a dark room is more sharper. The reading acuity can be increased by keep reading text as bigger, bolder, and brighter. I always prefer Big B (Photos 27.1, 27.2, 27.3, 27.4, and 27.5).

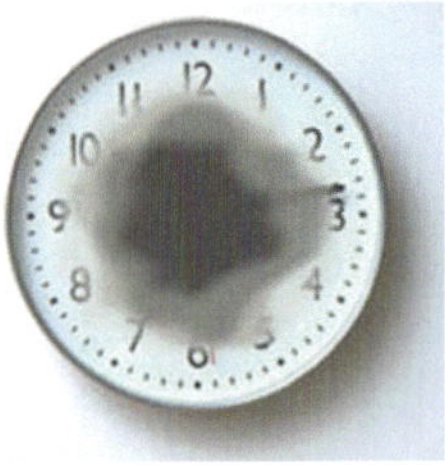

Photo 27.1 Central scotoma

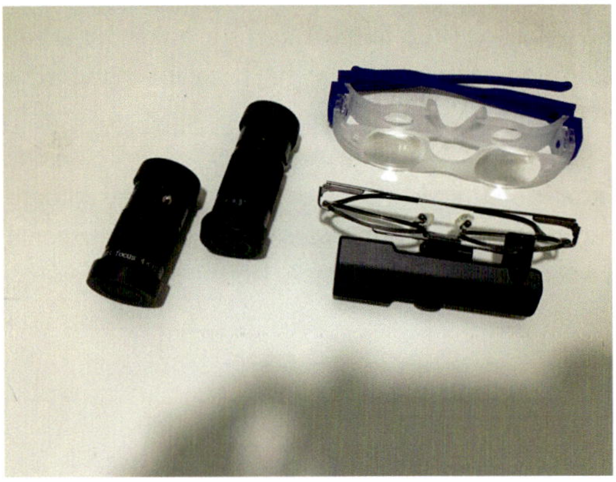

Photo 27.2 Distance optical magnifier- telescope-4x, 6x, see tv and Ocutech

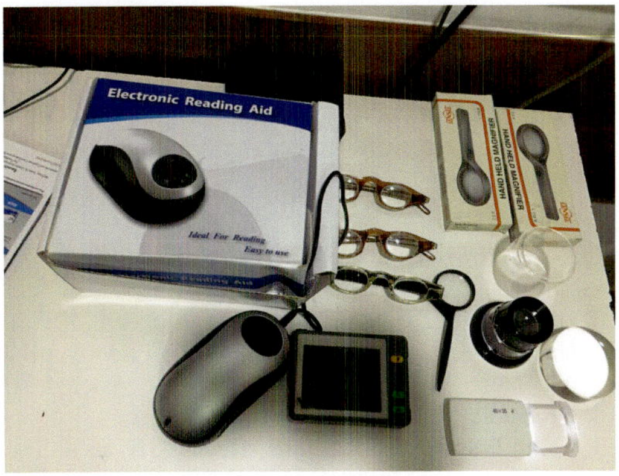

Photo 27.3 Near magnifiers—optical and projection magnifiers

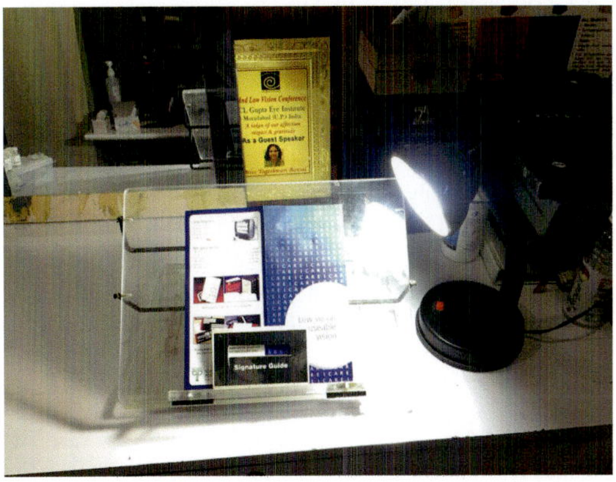

Photo 27.4 Reading stand with table lamp

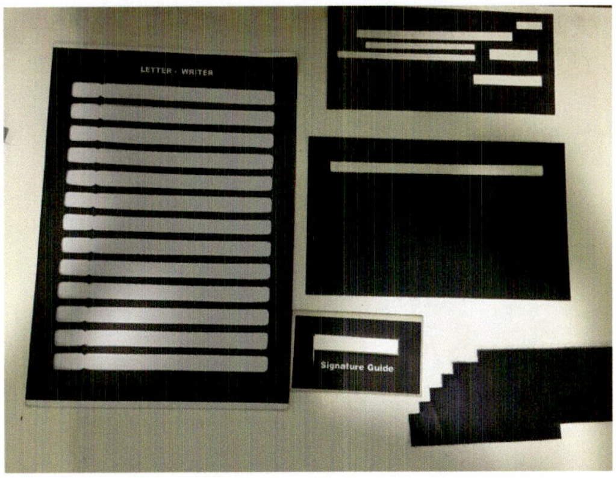

Photo 27.5 Non optical aids- typoscope, notex, cheque guide

27.2 Central Scotoma

AMD patients are the most unhappy in doing even simple near tasks like reading [6] newspaper, signing a cheque, writing a letter, mobile operation, threading a needle, etc. As there is macular involvement causing central scotoma, near tasking is the most affected. But rest of the visual field is spared so magnifiers work well as they enlarge the image and image falls on the seeing area now, away from the scotomatous area.

Near optical magnifiers like spectacle magnifiers(SM), handheld illuminated magnifiers (HHM), stand and dome magnifiers, pocket magnifiers, bar magnifiers along with chest magnifier work well. Nonoptical aids include reading stand or riser, typoscope, letter writer, cheque guide, and signature guide. Near projection magnifiers and desktop magnifiers like Merlyn also are very useful in severe visual impairment. Close circuit televisions (CCTV) are of immense help in moderate to severe VI*^. When optical magnifiers do not work then projection magnifiers definitely help in reading. There is SARA reader also which is talkative assistance technology based, which converts text into audio and the patient can listen to it. Kindle books and e-books are also available, which are more useful than textbooks as size and contrast can be increased on the screen.

Socioeconomic and behavioral issues are taken care of through counseling by the Optometrist or Rehabilitator that plays a very important role in LVR. The patient needs to continue his or her hobbies and profession not to feel left out. This assurance has to be provided to the patient along with the family member through successful case examples and testimonials.

Eccentric viewing is a good technique to see better in AMD. This makes use of extrafoveal peripheral area called preferred retinal locus (PRL) [7] to see by turning your head as and when the central area is affected. So all patients of AMD should have Amsler grid charting done if possible to localize the extent of damage and the technique followed.

Walking cane with sensors and light and audible clues is an excellent support for walking in old age group. Besides, peer group discussions among AMD, Facebook groups can be a booster for them as some people come out with great ideas and innovations and can be the resource providers for the other patients. Larger screen size mobiles with magnifier option in smart phones along with flashlight features and various apps in Android and Apple give a lot of assistance to AMD patients.

To reduce the complaints of glare and photophobia, filters and photochromatic glasses are advised. Usually, yellow filter reduce glare indoors in AMD.

My personal experience has seen a lot of satisfactory clinical improvement in AMD as most of the patients can read newspaper N10–N8 print with the help of optical LVA or Projection magnifier [5] but the depression is high and confidence level is so low sometimes that they are unable to make use of that device. So the identification and referral of AMD patient have to be earlier to avoid that burnout stage. The ARMD patients need to accept their disabilities and we need to make them accept the remedies so as to spread the basic message of early referral to low vision specialists.

References

1. Evans J, Wormald R. Is the incidence of registrable age-related macular degeneration increasing? Br J Ophthalmol. 1996;80:9–14.
2. Harvey PT. Common eye diseases of elderly people: identifying and treating causes of vision loss. Gerontology. 2003;49:1–11.
3. Rubin GS, Bandee-Roche K, Huang GH, et al. The association of multiple visual impairments with self-reported visual disability: SEE project. Invest Ophthalmol Vis Sci. 2001;42:64–72.
4. Williams RA, Brody BL, Thomas RG, et al. The psychosocial impact of macular degeneration. Arch Ophthalmol. 1998;116:514–20.
5. Mangione CM, Gutierrez PR, Lowe C, et al. Influence of age-related maculopathy on visual functioning and health-related quality of life. Am J Ophthalmol. 1999;128:45–53.
6. Crossland MD, Culham LE, Rubin GS. Predicting reading fluency in macular disease. Optom Vis Sci. 2005;82(1):11–7.
7. Crossland MD, Culham LE, et al. Fixation stability and reading speed in patients with newly developed macular disease. Ophthalmic Physiol Opt. 2004;24(4):327–33.

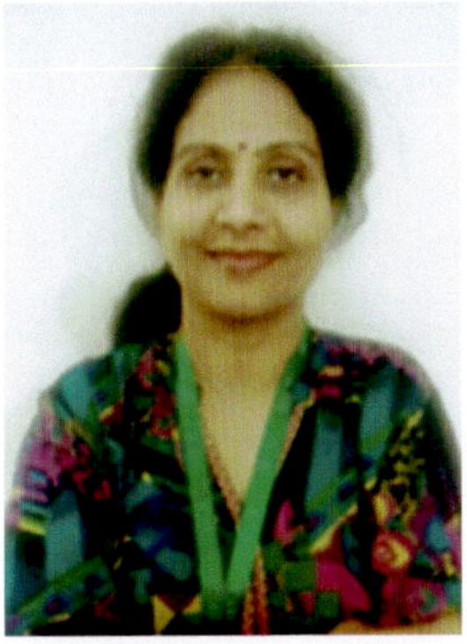

Yogeshwari Bansal has a Master's degree in Optometry from Vinayaka University, India and Bachelor's degree in Optometry from AIIMS, New Delhi, India. She completed her Fellowship in optometry from L. V. Prasad Eye Institute, Hyderabad, India in 1993–1994. She is also a Fellow of IACLE, Australia. Her areas of interest and excellence are contact lenses and low visual aids besides comprehensive optometry. Currently she is heading the Optometry Department at ICARE Eye Hospital and Post Graduate Institute, Noida, India with 35 full-time optometrists in the team. She has co-authored many thesis works at ICARE besides a few publications. She is an academician and active key speaker and chairperson in many national-level optometry CMEs. She has organized LVA workshops in-house and other tertiary hospitals.

28 Gene Therapy for Choroidal Neovascularization

Joo Yong Lee and Joon Hyung Yeo

28.1 Introduction

The United States Food and Drug Administration (FDA) has recently approved gene therapy for treating *RPE65* mutation-associated retinal dystrophy (a.k.a. Leber's congenital amaurosis). This has garnered considerable attention for its possibilities for treating inherited retinal disease (IRD) such as choroideremia, Usher's disease, retinitis pigmentosa (RP), Stargardt disease, and X-linked retinoschisis [1, 2].

In gene therapy, mutated disease-causing genes are replaced with healthy genes, mutated genes that do not function properly are deactivated, and/or new genes are introduced into the system for the treatment of a particular condition. Of the various methods of gene therapy, gene augmentation therapy may be employed for treating IRD through inserting a new gene which can produce missing functioning products; it can also treat choroidal neovascularization (CNV) through producing a number of proteins including anti-angiogenic proteins, amongst others that have a therapeutic effect, in sufficient quantity following genes being transferred to targeted cells. Successful gene therapies for LCA have boosted interest in employing it to treat age-related macular degeneration (AMD), which is extremely common and has a considerable social and economic impact. Neovascular AMD (nAMD) has a complex pathogenesis and CNV develops due to imbalances between pro-angiogenesis and anti-angiogenesis factors. Many factors may be employed as therapeutic targets to treat CNV, including VEGF receptor 1, soluble fms-like tyrosine kinase-1 (sFLT-1), pigment epithelium-derived factor (PEDF), and vascular endothelial growth factor (VEGF). This section will encompass a discussion of the latest advances in AMD gene therapy and ongoing clinical testing.

J. Y. Lee (✉) · J. H. Yeo
Department of Ophthalmology, Asan Medical Center, University of Ulsan College of Medicine, Seoul, South Korea
e-mail: ophthalmo@amc.seoul.kr

28.2 Viral Vectors

Several means of delivering genes, both viral and nonviral, have been created in the last 20 years. Because target cells have close associations with nearby nontarget cells, and in some instances can be problematic to access, viral vectors have a number of advantages in comparison to nonviral treatments. These include electroporation and transfection, which can allow cellular tropism to be altered via pseudotyping and which incorporates enhanced safety. Additionally, when tissue-specific promoters are incorporated, transgene expression may be kept solely within the targeted cells.

Some of the most widely used viral vectors are lentivirus, gamma-retrovirus, adeno-associated

J. Chhablani (ed.), *Choroidal Neovascularization*, https://doi.org/10.1007/978-981-15-2213-0_28

virus (AAV), and adenovirus. Viral vectors are chosen specifically for individual applications; the type chosen is dependent on several elements, including the vector's cloning capacity, tissue tropism, and safety profiles, including insertional oncogenesis and genotoxicity. Adenovirus vectors, especially third-generation/helper-dependent vectors, possess high cloning capacities (around 35 kb) and are capable of transducing a broad variety of cell types, which includes quiescent tissues. The adenoviral vector genome generally stays within the nucleus as an episome, rarely integrating. Nevertheless, the employment of first-generation vectors has been hampered because they can activate the inflammatory response [3, 4]. Second-generation vectors are not as immunogenic, and helper-dependent adenoviral vectors are the safest by a considerable margin [5, 6].

At present, the most commonly employed gene delivery vehicles in ocular gene therapy are AAV vectors. AAV vectors usually exhibit low immunogenicity, which makes the vector system highly suitable in the gene therapy treatment of numerous human conditions. As with adenoviral vectors, the genome of AAV vectors is generally maintained as an episome, and they transduce quiescent tissues [7]. In addition, multiple serotypes are available, with each one offering enhanced tropism related to a specific tissue, e.g., AAV2 transduces the central nervous system (CNS), the liver, the retina, and skeletal muscle; AAV8 transduces the retina, the liver, the heart, the pancreas, and the CNS [8]. There are numerous other features displayed by AAV vectors that make it particularly suitable for ocular gene therapies. Among such features are abilities to transduce nondividing cells, low levels of retinal toxicity, the fact that it is generally nonintegrating, and that in human trials it has shown to have good levels of safety and tolerability [9, 10]. The possible value of using AAV vectors in AMD gene therapy is clear from the success of past clinical trials with IRDs. It is notable that the FDA granted recent approval for Luxturna™, a novel gene therapy for subjects with genetic eye diseases. Nevertheless, there are limitations to AAV vectors, including restricted transgene capacities (4.5–5.0 kb) and problems with eliminating risks of humoral immune responses with subjects with a viral exposure history [11]. A pair of clinical trials employing AAV2 vectors for human rational gene therapy offered contradictory results with regard to serum neutralizing antibody (NAb) levels and viral vector efficacy [12, 13]. In one of these trials AAV2-sFLT01 was tested to see how tolerable and safe it was for subjects with advanced nAMD; the second trial tested the same treatment for subjects with Leber's hereditary optic neuropathy (LHON). The AMD patient study found that there was a negative correlation between the presence of NAbs to AAV2 and AAV2-sFLT01's capacity for the production of sFLT01 protein. However, the research on subjects suffering LHON found that high NAbs serum levels do not necessarily limit the capacity of AAV2 vectors to effectively deliver genes. Looking at the findings of Lee et al., such contradictory outcomes may be explainable through the variations in the maintenance status of the blood–retinal barrier (BRB) depending upon the disease targeted [14]. These researchers demonstrated that NAbs levels in the vitreous humor may be elevated in instances of BLB disruption; they proposed that a number of retinal diseases that have associations with BRB breakdown could be disruptive to the retina's immune-privileged characteristics and could affect absolute values of NAbs within the vitreous humor.

Either equine infectious anemia virus (EIAV) or human immunodeficiency virus 1 (HIV1) can be used to derive lentiviral factors [15], having cloning capacities reaching 10 kb [16]. Lentiviral factors can be employed when an application requires the vector genome to be integrated within the host genome; it has seen extensive use in transduction for hematopoietic stem cells [17]. Lentiviruses have increased in popularity in recent times due to the fact that they are capable of transducing quiescent tissues, dividing cells, and have a superior safety profile to gamma retroviruses because vector genomes do not exhibit preferences between promoter or enhancer regions and therefore have a lower likelihood of being genotoxic [18, 19].

28.3 Route of Administration

There are numerous features of the eye that make it an extremely useful model for AMD gene therapy, including:

(a) There is a tight blood–ocular barrier that imposes limitations on the new genetic material being disseminated throughout the system.
(b) The eye is immune-privileged, meaning inflammatory responses to new genetic material will be limited.
(c) The targeted retinal cells are easily accessible for direct delivery of genetic materials and for noninvasive monitoring of the progression of disease and response to therapy.
(d) When the other eye remains untreated it can act as a control against which the therapeutic response can be measured [20].

At present, there are two ways in which genetic material can be introduced to targeted rational tissue, both by injection, either subretinal or intravitreal. The most highly researched method is pars plana vitrectomy (PPV), then retinotomy and subretinal injections of viral vectors. There is no standardization regarding the exact retinal location in the eye (generally the injection is made in the subretinal gap between the retinal pigment epithelium and the photoreceptors) for injection, nor the dosage or volume of viral vector, nor the quantity of retinotomies used to deliver the vector or the location of the injection. This method is more invasive and causes temporary detachment of the retina, but it does provide a means of direct delivery of viral vectors in the targeted tissue. Following this, the target cell (e.g., RPE or photoreceptor cells) becomes infected with the virus, which makes the host cells undertake transcription and translation of the genetic material carried with the virus into therapeutic proteins. The alternative means of intravitreal injection of viral vectors has been tried by some researchers. Although this technique is not as invasive and has the potential to cause fewer undesirable complications, it is generally seen as less effective in delivering viral vectors straight to target tissue [21, 22]. Viral vector diffusion can be limited by a number of physical blocks between the vitreous and the targeted retinal cells, including the inner retina (especially the dense interphotoreceptor matrix) and the inner limiting membrane (ILM). A number of attempts have been made to mitigate this problem: Petrs-Silva et al. found that intravitreal injections of capsid-mutated AAV2 in mouse retinas promoted the efficiency of transduction [23]; Dalkara et al. demonstrated that transduction could be enhanced in a number of different retinal cell types by mildly digesting ILM and a nonspecific protease in combination with AAV intravitreal injections [24]. Lee et al. found that AAV vectors' transduction efficiency could be enhanced using prior laser photocoagulation after intravitreal injection [25]. This positive result of laser pretreatment could be caused by the fact that basic thermal disruption in the ILM opens up access to every retinal layer surrounding the burned area, or it may be due to Müller cell endfeet movement increasing due to Müller cell stress responses.

Because variations in inflammatory responses have been demonstrated, depending on which ocular compartment the injection targets, subretinal injection has been considered safe 1 year after readministration [26]. Contrastingly, intravitreal injection with animal models is responsible for stimulating NAbs formation [27].

28.4 nAMD Gene Therapy

nAMD has a complicated pathogenesis involving a number of pathways making contributions to pathologic endothelial proliferation, especially in causing imbalances between pro-angiogenesis and anti-angiogenesis elements. A number of widely recognized elements include relative PEDF deficiencies, VEGF overexpression, and the secreted extracellular domain of sFLT-1, the VEGF receptor 1, being downregulated [28]. Many other elements also have involvement with AMD pathogenesis, e.g., angiostatin and anti-angiogenic endostatin (Table 28.1).

Table 28.1 List of ongoing or recently completed human gene therapy trials for age-related macular degeneration

Therapy and delivery method	Mechanism of gene therapy	Targeted disease	Clinicaltrials.gov Number	Sponsor	Study phase
Intravitreal AdGVPEDF.11D	PEDF expression with anti-angiogenesis	nAMD	NCT00109499	GenVec	Phase I
Subretinal rAAV. sFLT-1	Cellular expression of VEGF-binding receptor FLT1	nAMD	NCT01494805	Lions Eye Institute Avalanche Biotechnologies, Inc.	Phase I Phase II
Intravitreal AAV2-sFLT01	Cellular expression of VEGF-binding receptor FLT1	nAMD	NCT01024998	Sanofi Genzyme	Phase I
Subretinal AAV-8-based anti-VEGF (RGX-314)	Monoclonal antibody binds VEGF	nAMD	NCT03066258	Regenxbio Inc.	Phase I
Subretinal lentiviral vector expressing endostatin and angiostatin (RetinoStat)	Angiogenesis inhibition	nAMD	NCT01301443 NCT01678872	Oxford BioMedica	Phase I
Intravitreal Bevasiranib	Downregulation of VEGF production	nAMD	NCT00722384 NCT00259753	OPKO Health	Phase I Phase II
Intravitreal Sirna-027	Knockdown of the Flt-1	nAMD	NCT00363714	Allergan	Phase I
Intravitreal PF-04523655	Hypoxia-inducible RTP801 gene inhibition	nAMD	NCT00713518	Quark Pharmaceuticals	Phase II

28.4.1 PEDF

An early use of intraocular gene therapy for AMD took place in a phase I trial in 2006 (NCT00109499) with advanced AMD 1 being treated with the PEDF gene delivered by AAV [29]. PEDF is an anti-angiogenic peptide that occurs naturally which has been shown to have a positive effect in the prevention and regression of neovascularization with AMD models in mice [30, 31]. For a phase I clinical trial, 28 subjects suffering severe nAMD were given single intravitreal injections of adenoviral vector expressing human PEDF (AdPEDF.11). No serious side effects were reported, although 25% of subjects suffered transient intraocular inflammation. Because there was no control group and the sample size was limited it was not possible to draw conclusions about visual outcomes, although subjects receiving 10^8 particle units or more generally displayed stability, while those receiving less than this demonstrated decreases in visual acuity and CNV lesions increased in size. This research suggests that the size of dose may be influential [29].

28.4.2 Anti-VEGFs

Following on from this, attention switched in terms of gene therapy for AMD two investigating sFLT-1, which is regarded as having anti-angiogenic effects through two means: the first is the way in which inactive heterodimers are formed with membrane-bound VEGF receptor 1 (Flt-1) and VEGF receptor 2 (Flk-1); the second is the direct binding and sequestration of VEGF [32–34]. Additionally, because the expression of sFLT-1 is endogenous, the system should not be identified as being a harmful antigen in the target tissue and so when expressed from an AAV vector no inflammatory response should occur. CNV formation was successfully prevented in preclinical primate and rodent testing using a subretinal recombinant AAV (rAAV) with sFLT-1 injection [35–38]. Avalanche Biotechnologies, collaborating with the Australian Lions Eye Institute (NCT01494805) undertook investigations of both the safety and efficacy of subretinal rAAV sFLT-1 using clinical trials involving humans. In 2015 they published the outcomes of the phase I trial, following up with a report on 3-year outcomes in 2017 [39, 40]. This experimentation incorporated administering PPV and following up with subretinal injections of low-dose (1×10^{10} vector genomes (vg)) or high-dose (1×10^{11} vg) vector. Every subject was given ranibizumab injections at the start of the program and four weeks post-surgery, with further injections being provided when necessary in accordance with preset active nAMD criteria. The report on 3-year follow-up stated that the site of the subretinal injection showed no scarring, chorioretinal atrophy, or RPE cell proliferation [41]. It was not possible to undertake visual/anatomical outcome statistical analysis because of the small size of the sample. Nevertheless, subjects receiving the low dose, and the control group, needed more intravitreal ranibizumab injections than those receiving the high dose. As the safety elements of the phase I trial were within acceptable parameters, further investigations were pursued. In line with previous research, subjects in the phase IIa clinical trial were randomly assigned subretinal rAAV.sFLT-1 gene therapy (1×10^{11} vg) or no treatment, with both groups being given injections of ranibizumab as identical points in time. Avalanche Biotechnologies released preliminary data in a press release in June 2015 reporting that the group receiving a high dosage of rAAV.sFLT-1 gained just 2.2 letters in their mean change for best-corrected visual acuity (BCVA); control group results, in comparison with phase I results, were significantly lower, with 9.3 letters being lost in comparison with the baseline. Publication of further results occurred in December 2016, and in March 2019 the 3-year outcomes of the combined phases I and IIa were published [42, 43]. As with phase I, no systemic side effects were demonstrated and no significant ocular damage was found from the treatment.

For controls, there was a 61.5–41.0 change in median BCVA for ETDRS letters; for the group receiving treatment the change was from 58.5 to 47.0. At no point were any statistically significant variations between data points revealed. The number of ranibizumab treatments ranged from 5.0 to 15.2, with the median number being 10.5, for those receiving gene therapy; for the control group the number ranged from 1.0 to 22.0, with a median number of 7.0 [43]. The group receiving treatment and the control group both showed significant underperformance in this trial in comparison to the benchmark MARINA (7.2 ETDRS letter improvement) and ANCHOR (11.3 ETDRS letter improvement) [41, 43].

The intravitreal delivery of AAV2-sFLT01 was investigated by Sanofi Genzyme (NCT01024998). The sFLT1 employed was similar to the one used by the Avalanche research, apart from it only encoding the VEGF-binding domain of sFlt1 with links to a human IgG1 heavy chain Fc domain and the expression employed the chicken β-actin (CBA) promoter [44]. This research employed a CBA promoter that fused the cytomegalovirus (CMV) immediate-early enhancer and the chicken-actin promoter; when macaques were given intravitreal injections, they demonstrated increases in gene expression in ganglion and Muller cells [45]. For a phase I trial, 19 subjects having serious nAMD were given one intravitreal AAV2-SFLT01 injection of one of four doses (2×10^8 vg, 2×10^9 vg, 6×10^9 vg, and 2×10^{10} vg); one group was given the maximum tolerated dose (2×10^{10} vg) [13]. In total, there were 10 adverse events involving five patients, including a retinal tear, retinal hemorrhage, and one subject aged 91 years dying 12 months following the end of the research. However, it is important to note that none of these events are believed to have any relationship to vector administration. Adverse events were experienced by two of the maximum tolerated dosage groups that were classified as being caused by the research drug: one subject developed pyrexia that resolved itself within 180 min; a second subject developed an intraocular inflammation within a month of administration which underwent successful treatment with topical steroids.

Reginexbio also has a new AAV8 vector in development, RGX-314, which can express a soluble anti-VEGF monoclonal antibody within transduced retinal cells. Publicly available information states that in primate eyes that underwent treatment with RGX-314 the anterior chamber showed a maximal expression of therapeutic protein of 4992 ng/mL (Avalanche therapy showed maximum expression of 0.217 ng/mL, and Genzyme 528 ng/mL) [35, 46]. In March 2017 a phase I open-label dose-escalation trial began (NCT03066258). This clinical trial, which currently continues, is undertaking the assessment of three doses of RGX-314 with 18 patients who had received previous treatment for nAMD. The primary endpoint incorporates a safety assessment at 26 weeks. The secondary endpoints, to be assessed at 106 weeks, include central retinal thickness, changes to BCVA, areas of CNV and leakage, and mean numbers of anti-VEGF injections.

RNA interference (RNAi) offers an alternative to inhibiting VEGF on a protein basis. A trio of research studies are investigating intravitreal injection of chemically modified short-interfering RNA (siRNA) molecules. Bevasiranib (a.k.a. Cand5) the earliest nAMD treatment using siRNA agents, is an RNA duplex, 21 nucleotides in length, intended for targeting VEGF messenger RNA (mRNA). With intravitreal injection, this agent induces catalytic destruction of mRNA, which silences gene expression. It has no effect on extant VEGF protein, which suggests that it may provide a synergistic effect in administration combined with anti-VEGF therapies. The early results of the phase I and II bevasiranib clinical trials (NCT00722384/NCT00259753) have shown considerable potential in treating nAMD [47]. However, as yet there are no data in the literature presenting the results in detail. A phase III clinical trial was not completed due to the unlikelihood of it meeting its primary endpoint. For that trial, a comparison was made between how safe and efficacious bevasiranib, administered at 8- or 12-week intervals following a triple injection for initial pretreatment, was in comparison to ranibizumab-only treatment (NCT00499590). The preliminary outcomes of this clinical trial offer indications that bevasiranib shows no effect until 6 weeks after treatment has commenced, suggesting that it could be useful to employ combination therapies with bevasiranib as an adjunct [47]. It may be that bevasiranib's effects appear so late due to the way in which it works. Because it is not involved in the elimination of extant VEGF but is responsible for the inhibition of fresh VEGF molecules synthesizing, it may be necessary to neutralize extant VEGF in the eye with a direct action anti-VEGF agent prior to initiating the treatment with bevasiranib.

Sirna-027 (a.k.a. AGN 211745) is an RNA duplex, 21 nucleotides in length, capable of targeting a conserved region of Flt-1 mRNA molecules in humans, mice, rats, and cynomolgus monkeys [48]. As Flt-1 is a receptor for P1GF and VEGF, receptor knockdown may be more influential than inhibiting single ligands. Pathological neovascularization was reduced in a laser-induced CNV model with mice by Sirna-027 [49]. Successful completion of a phase I clinical trial has already occurred (NCT00363714). Nevertheless, when Ambati et al. demonstrated that CNV in mice models could be suppressed by a number of siRNAs, which included Sirna-027 and bevasiranib, through specific RNAi effects and the activation of the cell surface Toll-like receptor-3, the phase II study was abandoned (NCT00395057) [50].

The hypoxia-inducible RTP801 gene is targeted by a different RNAi (PF-04523655, an RNA duplex 19 nucleotides long); there is clear target validation for the RNAi molecules mentioned above. Inhibiting RTP801 causes suppression of the rapamycin (m-TOR) pathway in mammalian targets, which may reduce synthesis VEGF-A. Inhibiting m-TOR can additionally cause the downstream response of endothelial cells regarding VEGF activation to be decreased due to intracellular signaling being downregulated [51–53]. There were promising outcomes from a phase II clinical trial (NCT00713518), demonstrating that monotherapy with combination therapy with ranibizumab was superior to both ranibizumab and PF-04523655 monotherapy. There were no identifiable safety issues [54].

28.4.3 Angiostatin/Endostatin

Preclinical safety research employing RetinoStat (Oxford Biomedica) has supported initial clinical trials of LV gene therapy vectors for subjects suffering nAMD (NCT01301443) [55, 56]. RetinoStat employs the nonhuman, nonreplicating recombinant equine infectious anemia lentivirus (EIAV-LV). This treatment is given to humans subretinally, chiefly transducing target RPE cells and leading to strong angiostatic proteins, human endostatin, and angiostatin, being expressed [57, 58]. RetinoStat has been created for expressing both of these proteins because each has a synergistic effect on the formation of new blood vessels [59, 60]. Phase 1 trials took 21 subjects with severe refractory nAMD. The subject was given a subretinal viral dose after PPV of either 2.4×10^4, 2.4×10^5, or 8.0×10^5 transduction units. During the study, the eyes that had been treated exhibited continuously high levels of expression of endostatin and angiostatin. 71% of patients experienced leakage reductions on FA. Nevertheless, significant reductions against baseline levels for intra-/subretinal fluid only occurred with one patient [61]. These results were not particularly promising, but because patients with advanced nAMD were enrolled in this trial, the improvements might have been limited. The surgery caused patients to develop retinal tears and one to develop a macular hole; these were managed without further complications. No adverse effects related to the lentiviral vector were noted.

28.5 Conclusions

Gene therapy demonstrates considerable promise as a therapy for several diseases, including genetic disorders and also chronic and refractory retinal disease. Nevertheless, a number of issues still exist in relation to using gene therapy as an approved treatment. The first important issue relates to the ability to deliver a gene to the correct cell. Once the gene is delivered in the target cell, it must be activated to function properly. The second issue is that when a gene has been delivered it may have off-target influences, with the new gene being inserted into other genes and disrupting their activities, harming the patient. The final issue is how to avoid immune responses: the host may regard newly introduced genes as being harmful antigens and so initiate harmful immune responses.

Should gene therapy prove itself to be significantly more effective and safer than the treatments currently available, it has the potential to provide therapy for nAMD and IRD through the induction of the expression of therapeutic proteins over a long period spurred by just one round of therapy.

Key Learning Points

- The usage of gene therapy in a clinical context has recently started to be applied to neovascular age-related macular degeneration (nAMD). Such therapies could mitigate the heavy treatment loads experienced with chronic intravitreal therapies and may offer improvements to the unsatisfactory visual results of "real-world" undertreatment with anti-vascular endothelial growth factor (anti-VEGF).
- Adeno-associated virus (AAV) vectors are frequently employed in gene therapy to deliver genes due to the fact that they are nonpathogenic, offer low risk of inflammation, can transduce nondividing cells, have low levels of retinal toxicity (when dosed appropriately), and trials on human subjects have an extremely good safety record.
- At present, there are two ways in which a viral vector can be administered for targeting of retinal cells, either intravitreal injections or subretinal injections.
- In relation to nAMD, assessments are being made of gene therapy as a means of chronically expressing anti-angiogenic proteins, e.g., fms-like tyrosine kinase-1 and pigment epithelium-derived factor, and also endostatin, aflibercept, angiostatin, and ranibizumab.
- If gene therapy is to be approved for the treatment of nAMD than a number of concerns must be resolved, including the triggering of adverse immune responses, target cell delivery, and off-target incidents.

References

1. Bennett J. Taking stock of retinal gene therapy: looking back and moving forward. Mol Ther. 2017;25(5):1076–94.
2. Hafler BP. Clinical progress in inherited retinal degenerations: gene therapy clinical trials and advances in genetic sequencing. Retina. 2017;37(3):417–23.
3. Morral N, O'Neal W, Zhou H, Langston C, Beaudet A. Immune responses to reporter proteins and high viral dose limit duration of expression with adenoviral vectors: comparison of E2a wild

type and E2a deleted vectors. Hum Gene Ther. 1997;8(10):1275–86.
4. Gao GP, Yang Y, Wilson JM. Biology of adenovirus vectors with E1 and E4 deletions for liver-directed gene therapy. J Virol. 1996;70(12):8934–43.
5. Morral N, O'Neal W, Rice K, Leland M, Kaplan J, Piedra PA, et al. Administration of helper-dependent adenoviral vectors and sequential delivery of different vector serotype for long-term liver-directed gene transfer in baboons. Proc Natl Acad Sci USA. 1999;96(22):12816–21.
6. Morral N, Parks RJ, Zhou H, Langston C, Schiedner G, Quinones J, et al. High doses of a helper-dependent adenoviral vector yield supraphysiological levels of alpha1-antitrypsin with negligible toxicity. Hum Gene Ther. 1998;9(18):2709–16.
7. Kay MA, Nakai H. Looking into the safety of AAV vectors. Nature. 2003;424(6946):251.
8. Lisowski L, Tay SS, Alexander IE. Adeno-associated virus serotypes for gene therapeutics. Curr Opin Pharmacol. 2015;24:59–67.
9. Daya S, Berns KI. Gene therapy using adeno-associated virus vectors. Clin Microbiol Rev. 2008;21(4):583–93.
10. Stieger K, Cronin T, Bennett J, Rolling F. Adeno-associated virus mediated gene therapy for retinal degenerative diseases. Methods Mol Biol. 2011;807:179–218.
11. Surace EM, Auricchio A. Versatility of AAV vectors for retinal gene transfer. Vis Res. 2008;48(3):353–9.
12. Guy J, Feuer WJ, Davis JL, Porciatti V, Gonzalez PJ, Koilkonda RD, et al. Gene therapy for leber hereditary optic neuropathy: low- and medium-dose visual results. Ophthalmology. 2017;124(11):1621–34.
13. Heier JS, Kherani S, Desai S, Dugel P, Kaushal S, Cheng SH, et al. Intravitreous injection of AAV2-sFLT01 in patients with advanced neovascular age-related macular degeneration: a phase 1, open-label trial. Lancet. 2017;390(10089):50–61.
14. Lee S, Kang IK, Kim JH, Jung BK, Park K, Chang H, et al. Relationship between neutralizing antibodies against adeno-associated virus in the vitreous and serum: effects on retinal gene therapy. Transl Vis Sci Technol. 2019;8(2):14.
15. Everson EM, Trobridge GD. Retroviral vector interactions with hematopoietic cells. Curr Opin Virol. 2016;21:41–6.
16. Kumar M, Keller B, Makalou N, Sutton RE. Systematic determination of the packaging limit of lentiviral vectors. Hum Gene Ther. 2001;12(15):1893–905.
17. Booth C, Gaspar HB, Thrasher AJ. Treating immunodeficiency through HSC gene therapy. Trends Mol Med. 2016;22(4):317–27.
18. Zufferey R, Dull T, Mandel RJ, Bukovsky A, Quiroz D, Naldini L, et al. Self-inactivating lentivirus vector for safe and efficient in vivo gene delivery. J Virol. 1998;72(12):9873–80.
19. Shaw A, Cornetta K. Design and potential of non-integrating lentiviral vectors. Biomedicine. 2014;2(1):14–35.
20. Streilein JW. Ocular immune privilege: therapeutic opportunities from an experiment of nature. Nat Rev Immunol. 2003;3(11):879–89.
21. Yu-Wai-Man P. Genetic manipulation for inherited neurodegenerative diseases: myth or reality? Br J Ophthalmol. 2016;100(10):1322–31.
22. Cheng L, Toyoguchi M, Looney DJ, Lee J, Davidson MC, Freeman WR. Efficient gene transfer to retinal pigment epithelium cells with long-term expression. Retina. 2005;25(2):193–201.
23. Petrs-Silva H, Dinculescu A, Li Q, Min SH, Chiodo V, Pang JJ, et al. High-efficiency transduction of the mouse retina by tyrosine-mutant AAV serotype vectors. Mol Ther. 2009;17(3):463–71.
24. Dalkara D, Kolstad KD, Caporale N, Visel M, Klimczak RR, Schaffer DV, et al. Inner limiting membrane barriers to AAV-mediated retinal transduction from the vitreous. Mol Ther. 2009;17(12):2096–102.
25. Lee SH, Colosi P, Lee H, Ohn YH, Kim SW, Kwak HW, et al. Laser photocoagulation enhances adeno-associated viral vector transduction of mouse retina. Hum Gene Ther Methods. 2014;25(1):83–91.
26. Bennett J, Ashtari M, Wellman J, Marshall KA, Cyckowski LL, Chung DC, et al. AAV2 gene therapy readministration in three adults with congenital blindness. Sci Transl Med. 2012;4(120):120ra15.
27. Li Q, Miller R, Han PY, Pang J, Dinculescu A, Chiodo V, et al. Intraocular route of AAV2 vector administration defines humoral immune response and therapeutic potential. Mol Vis. 2008;14:1760–9.
28. Campochiaro PA. Gene transfer for ocular neovascularization and macular edema. Gene Ther. 2012;19(2):121–6.
29. Campochiaro PA, Nguyen QD, Shah SM, Klein ML, Holz E, Frank RN, et al. Adenoviral vector-delivered pigment epithelium-derived factor for neovascular age-related macular degeneration: results of a phase I clinical trial. Hum Gene Ther. 2006;17(2):167–76.
30. Mori K, Duh E, Gehlbach P, Ando A, Takahashi K, Pearlman J, et al. Pigment epithelium-derived factor inhibits retinal and choroidal neovascularization. J Cell Physiol. 2001;188(2):253–63.
31. Mori K, Gehlbach P, Ando A, McVey D, Wei L, Campochiaro PA. Regression of ocular neovascularization in response to increased expression of pigment epithelium-derived factor. Invest Ophthalmol Vis Sci. 2002;43(7):2428–34.
32. Bouck N. PEDF: anti-angiogenic guardian of ocular function. Trends Mol Med. 2002;8(7):330–4.
33. Ohno-Matsui K, Morita I, Tombran-Tink J, Mrazek D, Onodera M, Uetama T, et al. Novel mechanism for age-related macular degeneration: an equilibrium shift between the angiogenesis factors VEGF and PEDF. J Cell Physiol. 2001;189(3):323–33.
34. Luo L, Uehara H, Zhang X, Das SK, Olsen T, Holt D, et al. Photoreceptor avascular privilege is shielded by soluble VEGF receptor-1. elife. 2013;2:e00324.
35. Lai CM, Estcourt MJ, Himbeck RP, Lee SY, Yew-San Yeo I, Luu C, et al. Preclinical safety evaluation of subretinal AAV2.sFlt-1 in non-human primates. Gene Ther. 2012;19(10):999–1009.

36. Lai CM, Brankov M, Zaknich T, Lai YK, Shen WY, Constable IJ, et al. Inhibition of angiogenesis by adenovirus-mediated sFlt-1 expression in a rat model of corneal neovascularization. Hum Gene Ther. 2001;12(10):1299–310.
37. Lai CM, Estcourt MJ, Wikstrom M, Himbeck RP, Barnett NL, Brankov M, et al. rAAV.sFlt-1 gene therapy achieves lasting reversal of retinal neovascularization in the absence of a strong immune response to the viral vector. Invest Ophthalmol Vis Sci. 2009;50(9):4279–87.
38. Drga V, Plack CJ, Yasin I. Frequency tuning of the efferent effect on cochlear gain in humans. Adv Exp Med Biol. 2016;894:477–84.
39. Rakoczy EP, Lai CM, Magno AL, Wikstrom ME, French MA, Pierce CM, et al. Gene therapy with recombinant adeno-associated vectors for neovascular age-related macular degeneration: 1 year follow-up of a phase 1 randomised clinical trial. Lancet. 2015;386(10011):2395–403.
40. Constable IJ, Lai CM, Magno AL, French MA, Barone SB, Schwartz SD, et al. Gene therapy in neovascular age-related macular degeneration: three-year follow-up of a phase 1 randomized dose escalation trial. Am J Ophthalmol. 2017;177:150–8.
41. Brown DM, Kaiser PK, Michels M, Soubrane G, Heier JS, Kim RY, et al. Ranibizumab versus verteporfin for neovascular age-related macular degeneration. N Engl J Med. 2006;355(14):1432–44.
42. Constable IJ, Pierce CM, Lai CM, Magno AL, Degli-Esposti MA, French MA, et al. Phase 2a randomized clinical trial: safety and post hoc analysis of subretinal rAAV.sFLT-1 for wet age-related macular degeneration. EBioMedicine. 2016;14:168–75.
43. Rakoczy EP, Magno AL, Lai CM, Pierce CM, Degli-Esposti MA, Blumenkranz MS, et al. Three-year follow-up of phase 1 and 2a rAAV.sFLT-1 subretinal gene therapy trials for exudative age related macular degeneration. Am J Ophthalmol. 2019;204:113–23.
44. Pechan P, Rubin H, Lukason M, Ardinger J, DuFresne E, Hauswirth WW, et al. Novel anti-VEGF chimeric molecules delivered by AAV vectors for inhibition of retinal neovascularization. Gene Ther. 2009;16(1):10–6.
45. Yin L, Greenberg K, Hunter JJ, Dalkara D, Kolstad KD, Masella BD, et al. Intravitreal injection of AAV2 transduces macaque inner retina. Invest Ophthalmol Vis Sci. 2011;52(5):2775–83.
46. Maclachlan TK, Lukason M, Collins M, Munger R, Isenberger E, Rogers C, et al. Preclinical safety evaluation of AAV2-sFLT01—a gene therapy for age-related macular degeneration. Mol Ther. 2011;19(2):326–34.
47. Singerman L. Combination therapy using the small interfering RNA bevasiranib. Retina. 2009;29(6 Suppl):S49–50.
48. Shen J, Samul R, Silva RL, Akiyama H, Liu H, Saishin Y, et al. Suppression of ocular neovascularization with siRNA targeting VEGF receptor 1. Gene Ther. 2006;13(3):225–34.
49. Krzystolik MG, Afshari MA, Adamis AP, Gaudreault J, Gragoudas ES, Michaud NA, et al. Prevention of experimental choroidal neovascularization with intravitreal anti-vascular endothelial growth factor antibody fragment. Arch Ophthalmol. 2002;120(3):338–46.
50. Kleinman ME, Yamada K, Takeda A, Chandrasekaran V, Nozaki M, Baffi JZ, et al. Sequence- and target-independent angiogenesis suppression by siRNA via TLR3. Nature. 2008;452(7187):591–7.
51. Sabers CJ, Martin MM, Brunn GJ, Williams JM, Dumont FJ, Wiederrecht G, et al. Isolation of a protein target of the FKBP12-rapamycin complex in mammalian cells. J Biol Chem. 1995;270(2):815–22.
52. Corradetti MN, Inoki K, Guan KL. The stress-inducted proteins RTP801 and RTP801L are negative regulators of the mammalian target of rapamycin pathway. J Biol Chem. 2005;280(11):9769–72.
53. Dumont FJ, Su Q. Mechanism of action of the immunosuppressant rapamycin. Life Sci. 1996;58(5):373–95.
54. Nguyen QD, Schachar RA, Nduaka CI, Sperling M, Klamerus KJ, Chi-Burris K, et al. Evaluation of the siRNA PF-04523655 versus ranibizumab for the treatment of neovascular age-related macular degeneration (MONET Study). Ophthalmology. 2012;119(9):1867–73.
55. Igarashi T, Miyake K, Kato K, Watanabe A, Ishizaki M, Ohara K, et al. Lentivirus-mediated expression of angiostatin efficiently inhibits neovascularization in a murine proliferative retinopathy model. Gene Ther. 2003;10(3):219–26.
56. Lai LJ, Xiao X, Wu JH. Inhibition of corneal neovascularization with endostatin delivered by adeno-associated viral (AAV) vector in a mouse corneal injury model. J Biomed Sci. 2007;14(3):313–22.
57. Binley K, Widdowson PS, Kelleher M, de Belin J, Loader J, Ferrige G, et al. Safety and biodistribution of an equine infectious anemia virus-based gene therapy, RetinoStat((R)), for age-related macular degeneration. Hum Gene Ther. 2012;23(9):980–91.
58. Balaggan KS, Binley K, Esapa M, Iqball S, Askham Z, Kan O, et al. Stable and efficient intraocular gene transfer using pseudotyped EIAV lentiviral vectors. J Gene Med. 2006;8(3):275–85.
59. Scappaticci FA, Smith R, Pathak A, Schloss D, Lum B, Cao Y, et al. Combination angiostatin and endostatin gene transfer induces synergistic anti-angiogenic activity in vitro and antitumor efficacy in leukemia and solid tumors in mice. Mol Ther. 2001;3(2):186–96.
60. Yokoyama Y, Dhanabal M, Griffioen AW, Sukhatme VP, Ramakrishnan S. Synergy between angiostatin and endostatin: inhibition of ovarian cancer growth. Cancer Res. 2000;60(8):2190–6.
61. Campochiaro PA, Lauer AK, Sohn EH, Mir TA, Naylor S, Anderton MC, et al. Lentiviral vector gene transfer of endostatin/angiostatin for macular degeneration (GEM) study. Hum Gene Ther. 2017;28(1):99–111.

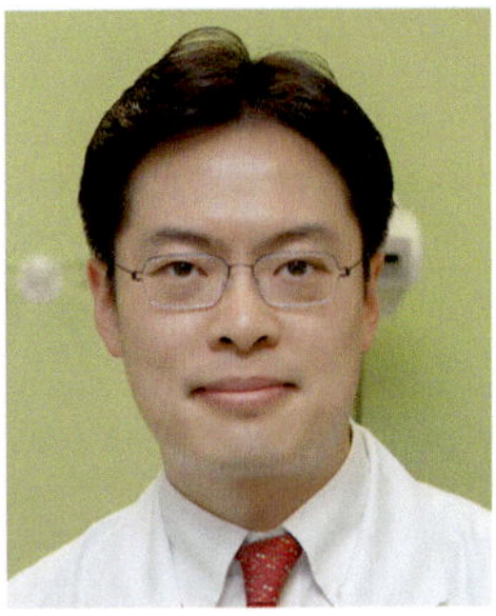

Dr. Joo Yong Lee is the Associate Professor of Ophthalmology and a member of the vitreoretinal faculty at Asan Medical Center and University of Ulsan College of medicine. Dr. Lee received his medical degree at Seoul National University and his ophthalmology residency training at Asan Medical Center in Seoul, Korea. He completed a 2-year clinical vitreoretinal fellowship at Asan Medical Center. He joined the faculty at Asan Medical Center in 2009.

He has published over 50 articles in peer-reviewed journals and has an active clinical and basic science research program. Dr. Lee treats patients with a variety of medical and surgical vitreoretinal diseases. His clinical research interests include novel medical and surgical therapies of age-related macular degeneration, retinitis pigmentosa, and other posterior segment disorders. He has been a pioneer in the development of stem cell-based cell therapy and gene delivery to the retina to treat ocular disease. He has participated in numerous clinical trials of new therapies for vitreoretinal diseases. He directs a basic research program to develop a new treatment option for age-related macular degeneration and retinitis pigmentosa and investigate the mechanisms responsible for uveitis.

Dr. Lee serves on the Editorial Board of the journal of *Retina* and reviews manuscripts for a variety of ophthalmology journals.

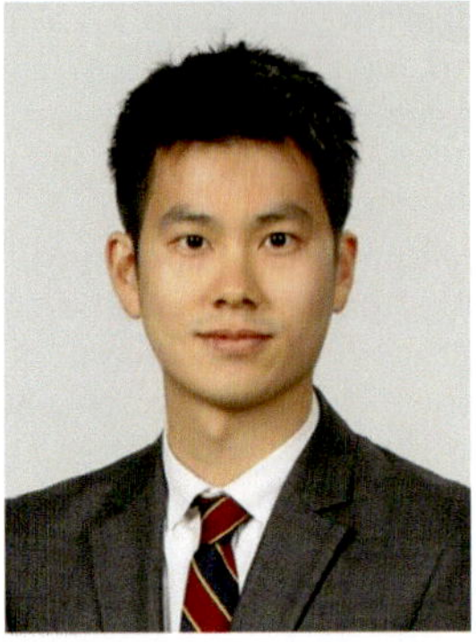

Joon Hyung Yeo graduated from Chung-Ang University, South Korea. He subsequently completed his ophthalmology residency at the Chung-Ang University Hospital in Seoul. He then concluded a vitreoretinal fellowship at the Asan Medical Center under the mentorship of Drs. Young Hee Yoon and Joo Yong Lee.

His research and clinical interests involve diabetic retinopathy, novel medical and surgical therapies of age-related macular degeneration, hereditary retinal dystrophy including retinitis pigmentosa, and gene therapy. He has participated in numerous clinical trials of new therapies for vitreoretinal diseases.

29 Radiotherapy for Choroidal Neovascularization

David Pérez González, Matias Iglicki, and Dinah Zur

29.1 Introduction

Age-related macular degeneration (AMD) is the leading cause of blindness in people over 65-years old [1]. Currently, the main objective to treat choroidal neovascularization (CNV) in neovascular AMD is focused on reducing the amount of vasoproliferative factors, mainly vascular endothelial growth factor (VEGF) [2].

The prognosis of patients with neovascular AMD was radically favored with the onset of anti-VEGF intravitreal therapy. Ranibizumab and aflibercept are approved for intravitreal use in the treatment of CNV secondary to AMD. Bevacizumab has been widely used off-label in clinical practice, showing comparable visual outcomes [3, 4]. However, treatment with anti-VEGF agents does not cure the disease; nonetheless, it reduces the rate of progression and establishes good visual outcomes in most patients. With an aging population, projections indicate that there will be 200 million AMD patients globally by 2020. This situation is causing a tremendous burden on patients needing multiple medical visits and injections over years, as well as an increasing heavy economic burden on healthcare systems and providers. In this sense, reducing the number of injections without compromising outcomes would be desirable. These are part of the objectives aimed to reach with the use of radiotherapy [5].

29.2 Basic Principles in Radiotherapy for Neovascular AMD

When energy of sufficient level is emitted to a cell surface or tissue, electrons separate from their respective atoms; this process is known as ionization. The ionization of oxygen atoms produces reactive oxygen species with consequent damage to DNA molecules and eventually cell death [6, 7]. Albeit all the cells in the area to be radiated are at risk to be damaged, the effect of radiation is specific and relatively localized as only cells with active replication retain the capacity for DNA repair. Endothelial cells in particular are much more radiosensitive than any other mesenchymal cell in the body [8, 9].

Ionizing radiation is especially promising as a synergic treatment in neovascular AMD due to its anti-angiogenic properties by decreasing capillary permeability, increasing vascular flow rate, decreasing cellular stasis, influencing capillary closure, and also due to

D. Pérez González · D. Zur (✉)
Ophthalmology Division, Tel Aviv Medical Center, Affiliated to the Sackler Faculty of Medicine, Tel Aviv University, Tel Aviv, Israel

M. Iglicki
Private Retina Practice, University of Buenos Aires, Buenos Aires, Argentina

J. Chhablani (ed.), *Choroidal Neovascularization*, https://doi.org/10.1007/978-981-15-2213-0_29

its important anti-inflammatory as well as anti-fibrotic effects [7, 10].

29.3 Current Approaches for Radiotherapy in AMD

In medical practice, two types of radiotherapy can be differentiated: Brachytherapy, where the radiation source is placed directly or as close as possible to the treatment site, and teletherapy in which the radiation is emitted from a distant source and is projected toward the tissue or area of interest [5, 10, 11].

The use of radiation in other ocular pathologies has been noted since many years ago. It was until 1993 when its implementation directly associated with the treatment of choroidal neovascularization in AMD began. Early clinical studies showed contradictory results [12–15].

The use of anti-VEGF has a rapid mechanism of action, however poor durability. On the other hand, radiotherapy has a slow-acting effect but provides a long time of action. This builds the scientific rationale to consider a synergistic response when combining radiotherapy and anti-VEGF treatment [6].

There are currently two systems to approach radiation therapy in AMD: the epimacular brachytherapy (Vidion Anti-Neovascular Epimacular Brachytherapy (EMBT), System NeoVista Inc. Fremont, CA), and stereotactic radiation (IRay Radiotherapy System Oraya Therapeutics Inc. Newark, CA) [10].

29.3.1 Epimacular Brachytherapy for Neovascular AMD

This approach aims to provide treatment in a localized manner, i.e., adjacent to the vascular proliferation site. This technique uses beta radiation, whose dose declines with increasing distance from the source of emission, limiting exposure, and allaying damage to adjacent ocular structures [7, 10]. Epimacular brachytherapy is an invasive procedure since it is delivered through pars plana vitrectomy. Once the vitreous has been removed, the surgeon places the source of emission above the area to be treated, using a dedicated device. The probe with the emission source is held in place during 4–5 min, transmitting 24 Gray (Gy) to the macular lesion [6, 10]. The success of the procedure mainly depends on the hand skills of the surgeon, i.e., accurate and stable localization of the emission probe, which is not easy at all, and minimal distance changes or time variance can rely on poor or less effective outcomes (Fig. 29.1).

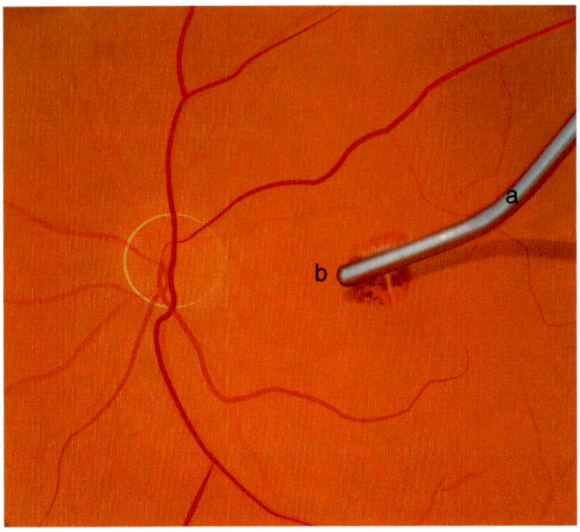

Fig. 29.1 Once the vitrectomy is performed, the probe (**a**) is held by the surgeon above the lesion (**b**) for approximately 4–5 min. The distance and the location of the probe are hands skills dependent and crucial for the success of the treatment. Image courtesy of Estephania Tirado Torrero

While this approach bares the known complications of vitrectomy, it should be noted that there is good evidence that the removal of the vitreous ameliorates oxygenation of the inner retinal layers [16]. In addition, the simultaneous application of brachytherapy provides a synergistic action in the production of reactive oxygen species with double-stranded DNA and hereby prevention of further formation of neovascular membranes [6, 17].

29.3.1.1 Major Trials in Brachytherapy for Neovascular AMD

One of the pivotal studies demonstrating the safety and efficacy of brachytherapy for AMD arose in 2009 [18]. This was a non-randomized, multicenter feasibility study. Thirty-four treatment-naïve patients with subfoveal predominantly classic, minimally classic, or occult CNV lesions due to AMD were included. They received a single intraocular treatment of either 15-Gy or 24-Gy beta radiation, using strontium-90 with an intraocular delivery device. Patients were evaluated for 12 months; at the end of the study, there were no adverse effects associated with radiation exposure. A higher percentage of patients who received 24-Gy of radiation (76%) improved or maintained their visual acuity. The authors concluded proper short-term safety and efficacy of intraocular epiretinal delivery of beta radiation [18].

A 3-year follow-up study evaluated the long-term safety and visual acuity outcomes of brachytherapy combined with intravitreal bevacizumab [19]. A total of 34 subjects were included and followed for 24 months. Based on the beneficial effects of higher radiation doses shown in the earlier trial, each subject received 24-Gy beta radiation treatment with a simultaneous intravitreal bevacizumab injection, and a second dose 1 month after brachytherapy. Further treatment with bevacizumab was bestowed as a pro-re-nata (PRN) regimen.

No radiation retinopathy events were identified over the follow-up period. However, compared to the prior study, there was a higher percentage of cataract formation. At 24 months, 50% of the patients exhibited two grades of progression according to LOCS II classification system and a total of five eyes underwent cataract extraction.

Mean best-corrected visual acuity (BCVA) demonstrated an average gain of +15.0 letters at 12 months and drop to −4.9 letters from baseline at 24 months. The drop in mean gain at month 24 was mainly attributable to cataract formation. At month 36, mean VA improved to +3.9 letters, which can be explained by cataract extraction performed in part of the phakic eyes during the third year of follow-up. Moreover, at 36 months, 90% of the patients showed stability, 53% gained more than one letter, and 21% gained more than 15 letters. Although EMBT is an invasive procedure, patients in this study needed only a small number of subsequent bevacizumab injections over 3 years. The authors hypothesize that if not treated by EMBT, these patients would have needed a high number of reinjections in order to reach those visual outcomes [19].

The MERITAGE Study

Shortly after these two pivotal studies, the role of brachytherapy for patients who have been previously treated with multiple anti-VEGF injections for neovascular AMD was investigated. The MERITAGE study was a prospective, multicenter, interventional, noncontrolled clinical trial which was initiated in the United Kingdom and then subsequently expanded to the United States and Israel [20].

Fifty-three patients with AMD requiring frequent anti-VEGF injections were enrolled. Participants received a 24-Gy dose of beta radiation delivered via pars plana vitrectomy, followed by ranibizumab injections administered monthly if needed (PRN). Optical coherence tomography (OCT) monitoring was performed monthly to evaluate anatomical response. After a single treatment with radiation therapy, 81% maintained stable vision with an average of 3.49 ranibizumab injections over 12 months. This finding was of particular interest since vitrectomy is believed to reduce the clearance of some intravitreal drugs [21]. The MERITAGE study proved a reduction in CNV activity by the need for less frequent anti-VEGF injections. However, it was not possible to determine if this could be translated to fewer hospital visits, as all patients in this prospective trial were monitored monthly by OCT. [20] Twenty-four months' results showed that 68.1% of participants maintained stable visual acuity and received a mean of 8.7 ranibizumab retreatment injections over 24 months [22].

The CABERNET Study

This was a multicenter, randomized, active-controlled, phase III clinical trial that evaluated the safety and efficacy of epimacular brachytherapy (EMBT) in conjunction with anti-VEGF therapy in naïve neovascular AMD patients [23].

Four hundred ninety-four patients with classic, minimally classic, and occult lesions were enrolled and then randomized (2:1) to EMBT or a ranibizumab monotherapy control arm. The EMBT group received two monthly loading injections of 0.5 mg ranibizumab. The control arm received three mandated, monthly loading injections of ranibizumab, and then fixed quarterly injections.

The results of this study were controversial: after 24 months of follow-up, 77% of the EMBT group and 90% of the control group lost fewer than 15 letters. The EMBT group did not meet the superiority margin, predefined as a gain of ≥15 letters in vision (16% for the EMBT group vs. 26% for the control group). While there was a statistically significant difference for patients with occult lesions, none was found predominantly classic and minimally classic lesions. Mean visual acuity change was −2.5 letters in the EMBT group and +4.4 letters in the control arm. Although the EMBT group received less injections (6.2 ranibizumab injections vs. 10.4 in the control arm), the data in this trial did not support the routine use of EMBT in patients with naïve neovascular AMD despite the good safety profile [23].

The MERLOT Study

This study evaluated the safety and efficacy of EMBT in patients with chronic neovascular AMD previously treated with ranibizumab with the main hypothesis that the use of EMBT will reduce the number of intravitreal injections and will maintain a non-inferior visual acuity [24]. A total of 363 patients were enrolled in order to receive either pars plana vitrectomy with 24-Gy EMBT and continued ranibizumab injections as needed or monotherapy with PRN ranibizumab injections.

After 12 months, the mean number of PRN injections was 4.8 in the EMBT arm and 4.1 in the ranibizumab monotherapy arm. The proportion of participants losing fewer than 15 letters was 84% in the EMBT arm compared to 92% in the ranibizumab arm. In the EMBT arm, the mean total lesion and CNV size increased significantly more than in the ranibizumab group. Hence, the results of the MERLOT study did not support the hypothesis established previously. On the contrary, patients who underwent EMBT received more intravitreal injections, and had a remarkably worse visual acuity than those on ranibizumab monotherapy.

These results differ in some proportion from what was shown in the MERITAGE study, where a reduction in the frequency of injections was found for patients undergoing adjuvant treatment with EMBT. The reasons for these differences may be associated with the surgical technique, probe accuracy, surgeon's hand skills, or for some other unidentified factors.

The MERLOT study group concluded a lack of support for EMBT in chronic, active CNV patients with AMD [24].

29.3.1.2 Other Trials Involving Brachytherapy for Neovascular AMD

A retrospective study evaluated the clinical feasibility, safety, and efficacy of EMBT for CNV in AMD for unresponsive eyes after repeated anti-VEGF injections in real-life conditions [1]. A total of 22 patients were treated with EMBT and retreated with anti-VEGF injections on an as-needed basis if subretinal or intraretinal fluid was detected on OCT.

At 12 months, half of the patients maintained stable visual acuity, 40% showed improvement, and only 10% presented decrease in vision with loss of more than 3 Snellen lines. The average number of injections before treatment with EMBT was 13.8, compared to 5.5 ± 4.4 during 12 months after. It is important to mention that there was lacking data about the exact number of anti-VEGF injections patients received during the 1-year period prior EMBT treatment, and therefore, there was no standard analysis in relation to the reduction of injection frequency 12 months before and after EBMT. The authors concluded that EMBT was safe and feasible for use in clinical practice, and could help in cases of resistant disease with a poor response even after multiple anti-VEGF injections [1].

In 2013, a novel brachytherapy device called SMD-1 was proposed using a less invasive sub-Tenon retrobulbar approach. A small study included 6 patients who received 24-Gy radiation delivered over 5.5 min using the SMD-1 brachytherapy probe [25]. After removal of the probe, patients received concomitant anti-VEGF injections with further PRN regimen. After 12 months of follow-up, three out of the six patients showed stabilization and improvement of visual acuity. Although this approach seems less invasive, the technique was used only in a very small number of patients, and results so far are inconclusive.

29.3.2 Stereotactic Radiotherapy for Neovascular AMD

Consideration for teletherapy in neovascular AMD began around the 1990s. Initial studies generally used a large amount of radiation with little precision range over the area to be treated, so the results were not favorable, especially compared to those achieved since the introduction of anti-VEGF injections. A Cochrane Database Systematic review that analyzed around 30 studies using teletherapy concluded that at that time, the use of this approach did not provide enough evidence to be recommended as a treatment in patients with neovascular AMD [26, 27].

Recently, the way in which teletherapy is used has evolved. Nowadays specifically with the IRay system (formerly Oraya Therapeutics Inc., Newark, CA), the radiation source is precisely direct to the site of interest from different angles, minimizing damage to healthy surrounding tissues [5]. This device uses a low-voltage X-ray source which does not require the same degree of radiation shielding as the first linear accelerators that were investigated in the past.

The IRay technique uses a robotically controlled delivery system which is connected to the patient through a contact lens with a suction force of approximately 25 mmHg. Once placed on the patient, 2–3 separate beams of radiation are emitted entering the globe through the lower portion of the pars plana, overlapping the predicted foveal center. When the beam of radiation enters the eye, it disperses, reducing exposure and damage to adjacent ocular structures, mainly the lens and the optic nerve. During the procedure, the patient can be monitored through a small window, and the eye is continuously tracked. If an unexpected movement occurs an inbuilt safety feature interrupts the process allowing the physician to avoid misdirected beams into the eye [10, 28] (Fig. 29.2).

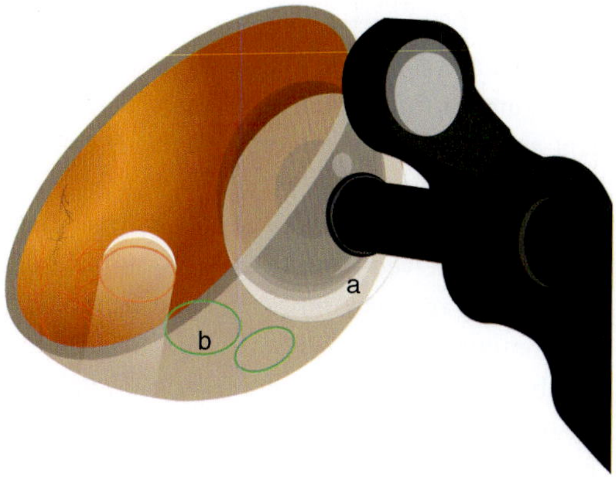

Fig. 29.2 The IRay technique uses a robotically controlled delivery system which is connected to the patient through a contact lens (**a**) with a suction force of approximately 25 mmHg. Once placed on the patient, 2–3 separate beams of radiation are emitted entering the globe through the lower portion of the pars plana (**b**), overlapping the predicted foveal center. Image courtesy of Estephania Tirado Torrero

29.3.2.1 Main Trials in Stereotactic Radiotherapy for Neovascular AMD

The INTREPID Study

This was a large randomized, double-masked, sham-controlled, multicenter, clinical trial with the main objective to determine the safety and efficacy of stereotactic radiotherapy (SRT) for patients with neovascular AMD [9].

A total of 230 participants who received more than three anti-VEGF injections (ranibizumab or bevacizumab) during the year prior to recruitment and still requiring injections at the time of the study were considered.

Patients received 16-Gy, 24-Gy, or sham SRT. All received injections of ranibizumab using a PRN regimen during the first 12 months, then continued with either bevacizumab or ranibizumab also with PRN regimen with a total follow-up of 24 months. Interestingly, the number of injections was significantly reduced with the use of SRT during the first 12 months. Results during the second year were markedly favorable showing that 15% of patients who received SRT did not require any injection, and 43% received three or fewer injections.

During the second year, 3% of the participants showed microvascular abnormalities; however, the vision was not affected because most of these lesions did not involve the fovea.

Albeit 2-year results showed promising results, potential long-term complications of radiation exposure remain a major concern with SRT and need to be further investigated [29–31].

Although both, the CABERNET and INTREPID studies showed improvement in vision, it is important to point out that the technique of radiation transmission is different and might impact the outcomes. EBMT used in the CABERNET study bares the limitations of surgeon-dependent procedures as detailed above [32]. On the contrary, stereotactic radiation eliminates the human error factor during the treatment.

The STAR Study

This is a multicenter, double-masked, randomized, sham-controlled 24-months clinical trial and one of the most recent studies, with an ongoing recruitment phase at the time of writing this chapter. Patients with chronic and active neovascular AMD are enrolled with the aim to evaluate the efficacy of SRT in this population. Participants are randomized to receive a single session of SRT with 16-Gy or sham, with a concomitant baseline ranibizumab injection, and then continue under the PRN regimen.

The primary outcome will be the number of injections needed over the 2-year follow-up period. Accordingly, additional visits will be considered at 36 and 48 months to evaluate the development of radiation retinopathy. The estimated primary completion date will be estimated in October 2021, with the final results for March 2024 [33].

29.3.3 Main Complications Associated with Radiotherapy in Neovascular AMD

Complications due to radiotherapy vary depending on the method and the amount of energy emitted to each ocular structure. The use of radiotherapy in patients with neovascular AMD differs from other modalities, and then, the rate and severity of complications are offbeat. Also, with the advance of new techniques that sharpened the precision and diminished extension to unwanted structures, these complications are becoming less frequent. By far, the most affected structures are the lens, the optic nerve, and the retina.

The reported thresholds for clinically observable radiation damage in the lens and progression of cataracts are around 2-Gy. Usually, brachytherapy and stereotactic radiotherapy will not exceed the amount of 0.13-Gy emitted to the lens. Radiation retinopathy is usually observed with levels around 33 to 55-Gy. Generally, with the new treatment modalities the amount of emission to the retinal surface outside the fovea will not exceed 24-Gy. Recent studies report mostly microvascular abnormalities without showing decreased visual acuity and even remission of these changes during the follow-up is possible [31].

Optic neuropathy is usually observed after exposure to a much greater amount of radiation considering thresholds above 55-Gy. The amount of radiation with new modalities will not exceed 2.4-Gy [7, 19, 34].

Although there is evidence that the use of radiotherapy seems safe, caution is advised as clinically visible structural damage caused by radiation can appear several years after exposure. Further studies evaluating the rate of long-term complications are needed in order to establish a better understanding of the potential and risks for radiotherapy as an adjuvant treatment in neovascular AMD.

Key Learning Points and Conclusions

1. The adjuvant use of radiation (i.e., brachytherapy and stereotactic radiotherapy) in the treatment of choroidal neovascularization due to neovascular AMD is to minimize the number of anti-VEGF injections, without reducing their effectiveness.
2. Epimacular brachytherapy requires the use of vitrectomy. The emission source is placed just above the macular lesion for 4–5 min.
3. Stereotactic radiotherapy is a less invasive procedure, although more microvascular changes have been seen after its use.
4. The main studies investigating brachytherapy are MERITAGE, CABERNET, and MERLOT. While injection frequency was reduced after epimacular brachytherapy in the MERITAGE and CABERNET trials, the MERLOT study revealed contradictory results with less improvement using this modality.
5. The main studies for stereotactic radiotherapy are INTREPID, which showed favorable results, and STAR, the most recent one that still ongoing.
6. More studies are needed, not only to prove effectiveness but also to investigate long-term safety.

Acknowledgment To Estephania Tirado Torrero for graphical illustrations.

References

1. Zur D, Loewenstein A, Barak A. One-year results from clinical practice of epimacular strontium-90 brachytherapy for the treatment of subfoveal choroidal neovascularization secondary to AMD. Ophthalmic Surg Lasers Imaging Retina. 2015 Mar;46(3):338–43.
2. Kaiser PK. Emerging therapies for neovascular age-related macular degeneration. Ophthalmology. 2013 May;120(5):S11–5.
3. Villegas VM, Aranguren LA, Kovach JL, Schwartz SG, Flynn HW. Current advances in the treatment of neovascular age-related macular degeneration. Expert Opin Drug Deliv. 2017 Feb;14(2):273–82.
4. Michels S, Rosenfeld P, Puliafito C, Marcus E, Venkatraman A. Systemic bevacizumab (avastin) therapy for neovascular age-related macular degeneration twelve-week results of an uncontrolled open-label clinical study. Ophthalmology. 2005 Jun;112(6):1035–1047.e9.
5. Ranjbar M, Kurz M, Holzhey A, Melchert C, Rades D, Grisanti S. Stereotactic radiotherapy in neovascular age-related macular degeneration. Medicine (Baltimore). 2016 Dec;95(52):e5729.
6. Casaroli-Marano R, Alforja S, Giralt J, Farah ME. Epimacular brachytherapy for wet AMD: current perspectives. Clin Ophthalmol. 2014 Aug;8:1661.
7. Kishan AU, Modjtahedi BS, Morse LS, Lee P. Radiation therapy for neovascular age-related macular degeneration. Int J Radiat Oncol. 2013 Mar;85(3):583–97.
8. Johnson LK, Longenecker JP, Fajardo LF. Differential radiation response of cultured endothelial cells and smooth myocytes. Anal Quant Cytol. 1982 Sep;4(3):188–98.
9. Kirwan JF, Constable PH, Murdoch IE, Khaw PT. Beta irradiation: new uses for an old treatment: a review. Eye. 2003 Mar;17(2):207–15.
10. Petrarca R, Jackson TL. Radiation therapy for neovascular age-related macular degeneration. Clin Ophthalmol. 2011 Jan;5:57.
11. Taddei PJ, Chell E, Hansen S, Gertner M, Newhauser WD. Assessment of targeting accuracy of a low-energy stereotactic radiosurgery treatment for age-related macular degeneration. Phys Med Biol. 2010 Dec;55(23):7037–54.
12. Journal B. Editorials Treatment of age-related subfoveal neovascular membranes by teletherapy. 1993;261–2.
13. Bergink GJ, Hoyng CB, van der Maazen RW, Vingerling JR, van Daal WA, Deutman AF. A randomized controlled clinical trial on the efficacy of radiation therapy in the control of subfoveal choroidal neovascularization in age-related macular degeneration: radiation versus observation. Graefes Arch Clin Exp Ophthalmol. 1998 May;236(5):321–5.

14. A prospective, randomized, double-masked trial on radiation therapy for neovascular age-related macular degeneration (RAD study). Ophthalmology. 1999 Dec;106(12):2239–47.
15. Sivagnanavel V, Evans JR, Ockrim Z, Chong V. Radiotherapy for neovascular age-related macular degeneration. In: Sivagnanavel V, editor. Cochrane database of systematic reviews. Chichester: Wiley; 2004.
16. Stefansson E, Landers MB 3rd, Wolbarsht ML. Increased retinal oxygen supply following panretinal photocoagulation and vitrectomy and lensectomy. Trans Am Ophthalmol Soc. 1981;79:307–34.
17. Nordsmark M, Overgaard M, Overgaard J. Pretreatment oxygenation predicts radiation response in advanced squamous cell carcinoma of the head and neck. Radiother Oncol. 1996 Oct;41(1):31–9.
18. Avila MP, Farah ME, Santos A, Kapran Z, Duprat JP, Woodward BW, et al. Twelve-month safety and visual acuity results from a feasibility study of intraocular, epiretinal radiation therapy for the treatment of subfoveal CNV secondary to AMD. Retina [Internet]. 2009 Feb;29(2):157–69. Available from http://www.ncbi.nlm.nih.gov/pubmed/19202425
19. Ávila MP, Farah ME, Santos A, Carla L, Fuji G, Rossi J, et al. Three-year safety and visual acuity results of epimacular 90strontium/90yttrium brachytherapy with bevacizumab for the treatment of subfoveal choroidal neovascularization secondary to age-related macular degeneration. Retina. 2012 Jan;32(1):10–8.
20. Dugel PUU, Petrarca R, Bennett M, Barak A, Weinberger D, Nau J, et al. Macular epiretinal brachytherapy in treated age-related macular degeneration: MERITAGE study: twelve-month safety and efficacy results. Ophthalmology [Internet]. 2012 Jul [cited 2014 Nov 13];119(7):1425–31. Available from http://www.ncbi.nlm.nih.gov/pubmed/22465819
21. Chin H-S, Park T-S, Moon Y-S, Oh J-H. Difference in clearance of intravitreal triamcinolone acetonide between vitrectomized and nonvitrectomized eyes. Retina. 2005;25(5):556–60.
22. Petrarca R, Dugel PU, Bennett M, Barak A, Weinberger D, Nau J, et al. Macular epiretinal brachytherapy in treated age-related macular degeneration (meritage). Retina. 2014 May;34(5):874–9.
23. Dugel PU, Bebchuk JD, Nau J, Reichel E, Singer M, Barak A, et al. Epimacular brachytherapy for neovascular age-related macular degeneration: a randomized, controlled trial (CABERNET). Ophthalmology [Internet]. 2013 Feb [cited 2014 Nov 13];120(2):317–27. Available from http://www.ncbi.nlm.nih.gov/pubmed/23174399
24. Jackson TL, Desai R, Simpson A, Neffendorf JE, Petrarca R, Smith K, et al. Epimacular brachytherapy for previously treated neovascular age-related macular degeneration (MERLOT). Ophthalmology. 2016 Jun;123(6):1287–96.
25. Balaggan K, Schindler R, Joffe L, Patel P, Stea B, Adnan Tufail LM. Novel minimally-invasive episcleral brachytherapy for the treatment of neovascular age-related macular degeneration (nAMD): results of a twelve month prospective phase i safety and tolerability evaluation. Invest Ophthalmol Vis Sci. 2013;54(15):3787.
26. Holz FG, Engenhart R, Bellmann C, Debus J, Völcker HE. Stereotactic radiation therapy for subfoveal choroidal neovascularization secondary to age-related macular degeneration. Front Radiat Ther Oncol. 1997;30:238–46.
27. Evans JR, Sivagnanavel V. Chong V. Cochrane Database Syst Rev: Radiotherapy for neovascular age-related macular degeneration; 2010 May.
28. Lee C, Chell E, Gertner M, Hansen S, Howell RW, Hanlon J, et al. Dosimetry characterization of a multibeam radiotherapy treatment for age-related macular degeneration. Med Phys. 2008 Oct;35(11):5151–60.
29. Jackson TL, Chakravarthy U, Slakter JS, Muldrew A, Shusterman EM, O'Shaughnessy D, et al. Stereotactic radiotherapy for neovascular age-related macular degeneration. Ophthalmology. 2015 Jan;122(1):138–45.
30. Jackson TL, Chakravarthy U, Kaiser PK, Slakter JS, Jan E, Bandello F, et al. Stereotactic radiotherapy for neovascular age-related macular degeneration. Ophthalmology. 2013 Sep;120(9):1893–900.
31. Jackson TL, Shusterman EM, Arnoldussen M, Chell E, Wang K, Moshfeghi DM. Stereotactic radiotherapy for wet age-related macular degeneration (INTREPID). Retina. 2015 Feb;35(2):194–204.
32. Dugel PU, Petrarca R, Bennett M, Barak A, Weinberger D, Nau J, et al. Macular epiretinal brachytherapy in treated age-related macular degeneration. Ophthalmology. 2012 Jul;119(7):1425–31.
33. Neffendorf JE, Desai R, Wang Y, Kelly J, Murphy C, Reeves BC, et al. StereoTactic radiotherapy for wet age-related macular degeneration (STAR): study protocol for a randomised controlled clinical trial. Trials. 2016;17(1):560.
34. Parsons JT, Bova FJ, Fitzgerald CR, Mendenhall WM, Million RR. Radiation retinopathy after external-beam irradiation: analysis of time-dose factors. Int J Radiat Oncol. 1994 Nov;30(4):765–73.

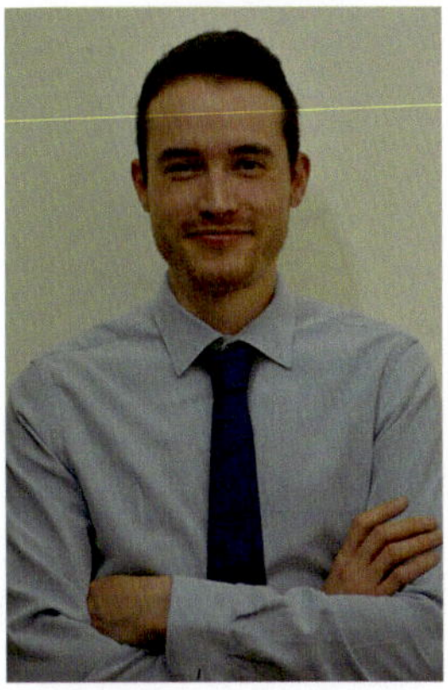

David Pérez González is a doctor from Mexico where he was raised and where he studied medicine at the Autonomous Popular University of the State of Puebla (UPAEP). At the end of the medical school, he continued his pre-graduate medical internship at the National Institute of Medical Sciences and Nutrition "Salvador Zubiran" (INCMNSZ) in Mexico City and then continued another year as an active member in the research area at his university. He completed his ophthalmology residency program at the Twenty-First Century National Medical Center in Mexico City, endorsed and certified by the National Autonomous University of Mexico (UNAM) for later being recognized as a certified active member of the Mexican Council of Ophthalmology and International Member in Training Candidate by the American Academy of Ophthalmology. He is currently conducting the Fellowship in Medical and Surgical Retina at Tel Aviv Medical Center affiliated with the Sackler Faculty of Medicine, Tel Aviv University.

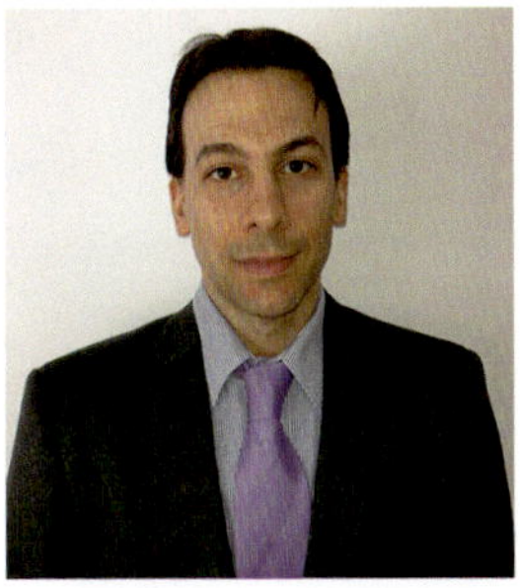

Matias Iglicki is a certified Teacher of Ophthalmology at the University of Buenos Aires. He was born in Buenos Aires, he went to Medical School at the university of Buenos Aires and he did his residency at the Hospital de Clinicas which depends on the university of Buenos Aires He has obtained a Degree Ophthalmology Specialist Physician Higher Course at the university of Buenos Aires His current activities involve, research, clinical as well as surgical practices, He went to the to conservartory of music where he lerned how to play the violin, he loves playing the violin and listening to classical music. He teaches graduate and postgraduate courses, and he is currently doing research about Diabetic Retinopathy at the university of Buenos Aires. He won an award from the university of Buenos Aires because his Project of Diagnosis of Diabetic Retinopathy by 'Telemedicine'" He has attended and delivered lectures in Buenos Aires and abroad. He have won the "best Resident award" when he was in his 1st year of his residency programme. This award was given by his colleagues. He has sat for every International Council of Ophthalmology standardized test, that is why he has got an Scholarship to did part of his Fellowship in Bern, Switzerland Nowadays he teaches at the University of Buenos Aires, performs surgeries and does research. He has won several awards about his diabetic macular edema projects, the latest in May 2017 for the ***IRG project*** *"Dexamethasone implant for diabetic macular edema in naïve compared to refractory cases: a retrospective 24 months study",* this award was given by the **Pan-American Association of Ophthalmology** at the Pan American Research Day in Baltimore, USA where ARVO 2017 took place.

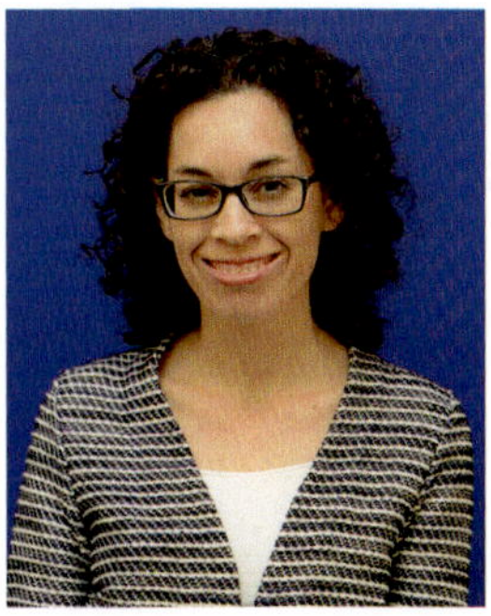

Dinah Zur is a Retina specialist at the Tel Aviv Medical Center and a Senior Lecturer at the Sackler Faculty of Medicine, Tel Aviv University, Tel Aviv, Israel. She was born and raised in Berlin, Germany, where she studied medicine at the Charite University Hospital. After her medical studies, she moved to Israel and completed residency in the Ophthalmology Division at the Tel Aviv Medical Center in Tel Aviv, and fellowship in Medical Retina at the Sankt Gertrauden Hospital, Charite, Berlin, Germany. Following this, she returned to Israel and since 2005 she is part of the Faculty at the Department of Ophthalmology at the Tel Aviv Medical Center.

She published more than 40 original papers; she is the author of reviews and book chapters and a reviewer in high impact journals. Her main field of interest is in retinal and choroidal imaging, retinal vascular diseases, and hereditary retinal diseases with focus on the identification of biomarkers in these conditions.

She is one of the initiators of the International Retina Group, which is an independent research group.

Moreover, she is coordinating the Continuing Medical Education in Ophthalmology at the Tel Aviv University.

Laser for Prevention of Choroidal Neovascularization

30

Jeffrey K. Luttrull and David Kent

30.1 Introduction

For most of the modern history of ophthalmology, laser treatment has been the primary treatment for macular disease [1]. Until the relatively recent advent of vascular endothelial growth factor (VEGF) inhibitors, ablative photocoagulation was the only treatment option for most eyes with choroidal neovascularization (CNV) [1–4]. Due to the risks of treatment-associated visual loss, location, and often poor definition of macular neovascular lesions, few patients with macular CNV were candidates for treatment. Of those, fewer still enjoyed any long-term treatment benefits [5].

While anti-VEGF medications have revolutionized the treatment of CNV, both due to their effectiveness and minimal risks of treatment-associated visual loss, other than Age-Related Eye Disease Study (AREDS) vitamin supplements, there remains no effective treatment, pharmacologic or otherwise, to prevent macular CNV [6, 7]. The history of macular laser treatment to prevent CNV is as long and as disappointing as the treatment of CNV itself. Recent studies indicate a change in this regard [8–11]. Spurred by a new understanding of retinal laser treatment, new information from both the laboratory and clinic suggests that laser for prevention of CNV should be effective, and is [11]. To understand the past failure, and future promise, of laser treatment to prevent CNV it is essential to understand exactly what is meant by "laser" treatment, and all that follows from it [8]. Our discussion of laser CNV prevention will focus on CNV complicating age-related macular degeneration (AMD). This is for two reasons: first, because AMD is the most important cause of visual loss due to CNV; and second, because only in AMD have notable efforts been made to prevent CNV by any means, and in particular, with laser [12, 13].

For over 50 years, photocoagulation was universally presumed to be the necessary and sufficient cause of all therapeutic benefits of retina laser treatment [14–16]. Low-intensity/high-density subthreshold diode micropulse laser (SDM) proved this presumption to be false by demonstrating therapeutically effective treatment in the total absence of laser-induced retinal damage (LIRD) [17–21]. As a watershed development in the history of retinal laser treatment, this discovery led to two key advances in our understanding of retinal laser treatment. These bear heavily on the following examination of the potential for the laser to prevent CNV. First, as

J. K. Luttrull (✉)
Ventura County Retina Vitreous Medical Group, Ventura, California, USA
e-mail: office@venturacountyretina.com

D. Kent
The Vision Clinic, Kilkenny, Ireland

J. Chhablani (ed.), *Choroidal Neovascularization*, https://doi.org/10.1007/978-981-15-2213-0_30

both unnecessary and the sole source of all risks, adverse treatment effects, and treatment limitations, we now understand photocoagulation (for other than cautery) to be a complication of retinal laser treatment. Second, abandonment of photocoagulation as the necessary precondition for therapy has led to, for the first time, a satisfying and useful understanding of the mechanism of action of retinal laser treatment as a physiologic "reset" phenomenon [22, 23]. Unlike prior unsuccessful attempts to explain the effects of retinal laser arising from photocoagulation, reset theory accounts for all clinically observed retinal laser effects. Further, in a fundamental test of any theory, reset theory has accurately predicted a new retinal laser application never conceived of in the photocoagulation era. These include reversal of anti-VEGF drug tolerance in neovascular AMD (NAMD); improved retinal and visual function following panmacular laser treatment in dry AMD, inherited retinopathies, and open-angle glaucoma; and neuroprotective effects in glaucomatous optic neuropathy [22–25].

Critical to a clear understanding of the retinal laser literature is a clear understanding of various retinal laser modes and their effects [8]. Complicating this task is historical imprecision and frequent misuse, unintentional and otherwise, of key clinical terminology that can obfuscate and mislead readers not keenly aware of these issues. The history of laser prevention of NAMD is particularly illustrative in this regard. Essential differences in the conception, design, expectations, claimed and actual effects of various laser modes account for both the past failures and future promise of retinal laser for the prevention of CNV. To draw out the key distinctions, the following discussion will divide the topic into two main headings: Laser for drusen; and laser *not* for drusen.

30.2 Laser for Drusen

As the hallmark of dry AMD, drusen are an important risk factor for progression and visual loss, particularly due to the development of CNV and NAMD [25–30]. As such, drusen are a clinically useful indicator of the degree of age-related macular dysfunction. The risk of age-related visual loss generally parallels the number, size, and proximity of drusen to the fovea [25–30]. Thus, drusen reduction has been a natural target for therapeutic intervention in dry AMD [31, 32].

Inflammatory disturbances of the macula in eyes with drusen, such as the development of CNV, other exudations, and focal chorioretinitis, including the iatrogenic chorioretinitis of macular photocoagulation, have long been noted to result in local disappearance of drusen in and around the inflammatory lesion [27, 30, 33, 34]. This suggested macular photocoagulation might be used therapeutically to reduce drusen and the risks of visual loss due to AMD [33, 35].

At the time of the first attempts to use photocoagulation to reduce drusen, the standard for photocoagulation intensity was established by the Early Treatment of Diabetic Retinopathy Study (ETDRS) and Macular Photocoagulation Study Group (MPSG) reports, which employed intense suprathreshold treatment resulting in clinically obvious white, full-thickness retinal burns [36, 37]. Recognition that drusen occurred at the level of the RPE suggested that less intense and thus less obviously clinically visible photocoagulation lesions (limited to the RPE and outer retina, or "threshold" intensity), barely visible, or even initially non-ophthalmoscopically "subthreshold" photocoagulation lesions, might be effective and reduce adverse treatment effects by reducing neurosensory retinal damage [32]. These less-severe lower intensity retinal burns were described, in comparison to the starkly white ETDRS and MPSG lesions, as "invisible" [38]. However, photocoagulation lesions acutely invisible or difficult to see ophthalmoscopically are virtually always immediately visible by fundus fluorescein angiography (FFA) and become clinically visible minutes to weeks after treatment. The contrast in lesion severity with conventional ETDRS and MPSG suprathreshold photocoagulation, however, led investigators to incorrectly assume a difference in substance, rather than style. This was (1) because LIRD was assumed to be essential to the therapeutic benefits of retinal laser treatment in general, and drusen reduction in particular could not be done without; and (2) over-estimation of the risk and adverse effect reduction associated with lower intensity retinal photocoagulation [31, 32, 35, 38].

The initial reports of macular laser treatment to reduce drusen were positive and encouraging [31, 32]. Treatment, directed at the drusen themselves, was effective in reducing drusen numbers and density, and improving visual acuity [31, 32, 35, 38]. With time, however, treated eyes began to demonstrate an increased propensity to develop new CNV thus converting to NAMD; worsening, rather than improving, the long-term visual prognosis [39–41]. Subsequent studies found that eyes demonstrating both the greatest drusen reduction and the greatest likelihood of CNV were those receiving the most intense macular photocoagulation [42, 43]. This realization brought about the effective end of interest in conventional (millisecond) continuous wave (CW) laser treatment for drusen [44].

It was recognized that LIRD to retinal architecture, particularly the Bruch's membrane/RPE complex, was a likely key predisposing factor to CNV, but possibly not necessary to achieve effective drusen reduction [9]. What to do? By shortening laser pulse duration the thermal effects of retinal laser treatment could be more selectively concentrated in the RPE [45, 46]. Microsecond CW exposures demonstrated the ability to selectively damage the outer retina and the homogeneously pigmented RPE of animals in laboratory studies [47–50]. Further shortening of the laser pulse to the nanosecond range can result in selective heating of the RPE melanosomes themselves [50]. However, shortening of pulse duration results in narrowing of the therapeutic range (TR), such that at nanosecond exposures, there is no TR. Instead, the threshold for RPE cell death is exceeded before the threshold for HSP activation (the cell dying before the HSPs can activate), the prime mediator of therapeutic retinal laser effects [8, 49]. In practice, this means that the effect of nanosecond laser (NSL) exposure is either no effect at all (below the TR threshold); or—at minimum—photodisruptive killing of the RPE by intracellular vaporization of RPE melanosomes. In this volatile, literally explosive setting, excess laser energy or RPE pigment density will necessarily result in collateral damage extending to the retina and Bruch's membrane [8]. Again, next to the severity of the suprathreshold full-thickness retinal burns from conventional standard photocoagulation in the ETDRS and MPSG reports, however, the LIRD resulting from short-pulse CW lasers, generally confined to the RPE and outer retina, still considered essential, seemed also negligible in comparison. By confining LIRD to the RPE and outer retina, it was hoped that drusen could be reduced without incurring either neurosensory retinal damage or increasing the risk of CNV, led to studies of both microsecond and nanosecond lasers, more selective for the RPE, as preventative treatments for AMD, and thus age-related CNV.

In 1999, Roider and coworkers reported two patients with soft drusen treated with 1.7-microsecond exposures of 527 nm laser with identical treatment parameters ("selective retinal laser therapy", or SRT, Lutronic, Billerica MA, USA), both clinically subthreshold, without visible laser spots at the time of treatment [51]. Both produced LIRD visible by FFA. However, in one eye the LIRD became visible clinically following treatment. In this eye, the drusen disappeared. In the other patient, no clinically visible LIRD developed later and there was no drusen reduction. The authors duly note that these eyes demonstrate the clinical variability of short pulse laser effects, a clinical manifestation of the narrow CW laser TR.

As noted above, NSL takes the quest for selective RPE destruction a step further. By shortening the pulse further, NSL maximizes the thermal energy uptake to the RPE melanosomes themselves, causing explosive vaporization of the melanosomes with internal cavitation of the RPE causing cell death (2RT®; Ellex Pty Ltd., Adelaide, Australia). In its idealized form, 2RT NSL seeks to limit LIRD to selective killing of the RPE, which they term "rejuvenation," without causing damage to adjacent structures such as photoreceptors and Bruch's membrane. Pilot studies of NSL demonstrated both drusen reduction and improvement in visual acuity without a notable increase in

CNV [9, 10]. At 24 months follow-up in a randomized clinical trial of comparing NSL to sham for dry AMD, the LEAD study found no overall effect of treatment [52]. Subgroup analyses showed drusen reduction in eyes with early, low-risk AMD, without an increase in CNV incidence, suggesting the success of the trial hypothesis. However, the 2RT NSL treatment response in eyes with high-risk AMD, those with the greatest risk of visual loss and with thus the most to gain from effective preventive treatment, was negative [52]. In these eyes, often identified by the presence of reticular pseudodrusen (RPD), NSL caused rapid progression of AMD and visual loss, particularly due to the development and/or progression of geographic atrophy. Of note is that LIRD was not considered an adverse treatment effect in the LEAD study. This is despite the fact that LEAD trial was performed to assess the effect of "non-damaging" 2RT NSL in AMD, a stated differentiator of the LEAD study from prior studies of laser for drusen (https://www.ellex.com/us/products/2rt/). Unfortunately, no fundus images accompanied the published report [52]. However, in a meeting presentation of LEAD study results by the investigators, all posttreatment fundus photographs presented demonstrated laser damage due to the NSL applications, clinically indistinguishable from conventional CW photocoagulation lesions (Guymer R, Marshall J, et al. The LEAD Study, presentation to the European Society of Retina specialists, Sept. 22, 2018, Vienna, Austria). The LEAD study authors did not explicitly correlate worsening of high-risk AMD with LIRD, but concluded that 2RT NSL was contraindicated in eyes with high-risk AMD [52].

Despite disappointing results, the LEAD study findings offer important insights. While it supports the concept that LIRD is necessary for drusen reduction (without establishing a benefit) it also suggests that avoidance or minimization of damage to Bruch's membrane may reduce the risk of CNV as an adverse treatment effect. However, it also demonstrates that that NSL is unreliable for this purpose, resulting in significant collateral damage in many, if not most, treated eyes leading to significant worsening of high-risk eyes. As with other studies of laser for drusen reduction, the LEAD study challenges the presumption that drusen reduction is a desirable end. Rather, the acceleration of visual loss due to age-related geographic atrophy (ARGA) in the LEAD study suggests 2RT appears to cause rapid decompensation of the most vulnerable eyes with high-risk AMD. This may be due to added physiologic stresses associated with the inflammation and healing response to the LIRD caused by NSL in these already tenuous eyes. Transmacular shock-waves produced by explosive photodisruption of the RPE, unique to NSL, may also contribute to RPE decompensation as far as 2 mm from an NLS application site (Chang DB, Luttrull JK; unpublished data, March 2019). The worsening of AMD, and particularly the progression of ARGA following laser for drusen in the LEAD study is not entirely unexpected. In the Cochrane meta-analysis of laser for drusen studies, Virgili and associates noted that, while little information could be gleaned from prior studies in this regard, available data suggested that ARGA worsened after laser for drusen [44]. In addition, a prospective clinical trial of microsecond SRT laser hoping to slow ARGA progression was abandoned early, due to the finding that treatment, designed to produce LIRD at the margins of the ARGA lesions, increased the rate of ARGA progression by 50% compared to untreated controls [53].

In sum, efforts to reduce the risks of visual loss in AMD with laser treatment have been driven by the recognized necessity of LIRD to achieve drusen reduction and the presumption of a resulting benefit. The failure of these efforts results from this very same LIRD, and casts doubt on the presumption of benefits from drusen reduction.

30.3 Laser *Not* for Drusen

The only treatment as yet proven to reduce the risk of developing age-related CNV in a multicenter prospective clinical trial is AREDS vitamin supplementation [6]. Interestingly, challenging the presumption of the need for drusen reduction, the success of AREDS treatment was not associated with any notable treatment effects on drusen or other morphologic features of AMD. The treatment benefits were consistent over time, reducing progression to advanced AMD by about 4% per year over the course of the study. Unlike short pulse lasers, the greatest benefit from AREDS supplements was seen in eyes at the greatest risk for visual loss [6]. As 90% of eyes with advanced AMD have CNV, it was a reduction in new CNV that accounted for most of the AREDS treatment benefits as the progression of ARGA was not affected. Thus, it was nutritionally derived improvement in retinal physiology alone that accounted for the benefits of AREDS study, and it did so, via CNV reduction, without reducing drusen or effecting any other alteration in macular anatomy [6].

All laser modes are capable of causing LIRD. Some, like NSL, cause it necessarily. For others, such as CW lasers, LIRD is prohibitively difficult to avoid and still accomplish effective treatment. Only a micropulsed laser (MPL) operated at a low duty-cycle (DC) can reliably and predictably preclude LIRD while maintaining therapeutic effectiveness [9]. The epitome of low-DC MPL reliably sublethal to the RPE is "low-intensity/high-density subthreshold diode micropulse laser" (SDM). SDM both established and defined the fundamental principles of modern retinal laser therapy. First; by employing a low-DC (5%) 810 nm near-infrared laser, SDM is reliably sublethal to the RPE ("low-intensity"), which it selectively targets. Despite this safety, it is an effective activator of RPE HSPs, the essential mediators of the therapeutic laser response. Second; the therapeutic response is amplified, maximized, and made clinically effective by confluent and complete treatment aimed at recruiting large areas of diseased retina ("high-density") to the normalizing process [9, 45, 46, 49, 50, 54, 55]. This is in contrast to the traditional focal or local application strategy used in conventional photocoagulation, which are abandoned in modern retinal laser therapy [37, 38]. Over time, the SDM treatment paradigm has evolved to the employment of just two treatment fields: "panmacular" treatment, consisting of confluent treatment of the entire retina between the major vascular arcades including the fovea; and "panretinal" treatment, consisting of confluent and complete treatment of all the retina outside the major vascular arcades [11, 20, 22–25, 46, 56, 57]. Panmacular treatment is used for all treatment indications. Panretinal treatment is added for generalized retinopathies, such as diabetic retinopathy or early retinitis pigmentosa, resulting in treatment of the entire retina, and thus all of the retinopathy, just as would be treated by medication (Figs. 30.1 and 30.4).

Initial studies of SDM demonstrated effective treatment for complications of diabetic retinopathy in the complete absence of LIRD [18–20, 46]. Like AREDS supplements, the absence of LIRD with SDM indicates, by exclusion, that SDM treatment benefits arise entirely from laser-induced improvements in retinal physiology elicited by sublethal thermal laser stimulation of the RPE [58]. Whereas the TR of CW laser is only 10× ANSI MPE, the same ANSI data show the TR of micropulse lasers, like SDM, to be much wider, 100×MPE or more [47]. SDM is thus safe and without any known adverse treatment effects [45, 47, 58]. Because of the broad SDM TR, treatment intensity need not be subjectively titrated on a per eye basis (effectively turning each treated eye into a dosimetry experiment), as decades of clinical experience have identified safe and effective SDM parameters that can be used effectively in all eyes of all patients without regard for pathology or pigment variation [8, 18–20, 45, 47, 57, 58]. Employment of "fixed" SDM laser parameters enhances treatment safety by eliminating the possibility for surgeon misjudgment, the most common cause of visual loss from modern retinal laser treatment [8].

As noted, SDM led to a new understanding of the therapeutic benefits of retinal laser treatment stemming from a physiologic "reset" effect on the RPE, normalizing retinal function largely independent of the underlying cause of dysfunction [23–25]. Making no unique contribution to treatment efficacy and solely responsible for all risks, limitations, and adverse effects of retinal laser treatment, photocoagulation, and all other forms of LIRD are now considered necessary complications of treatment [8, 21–24, 59].

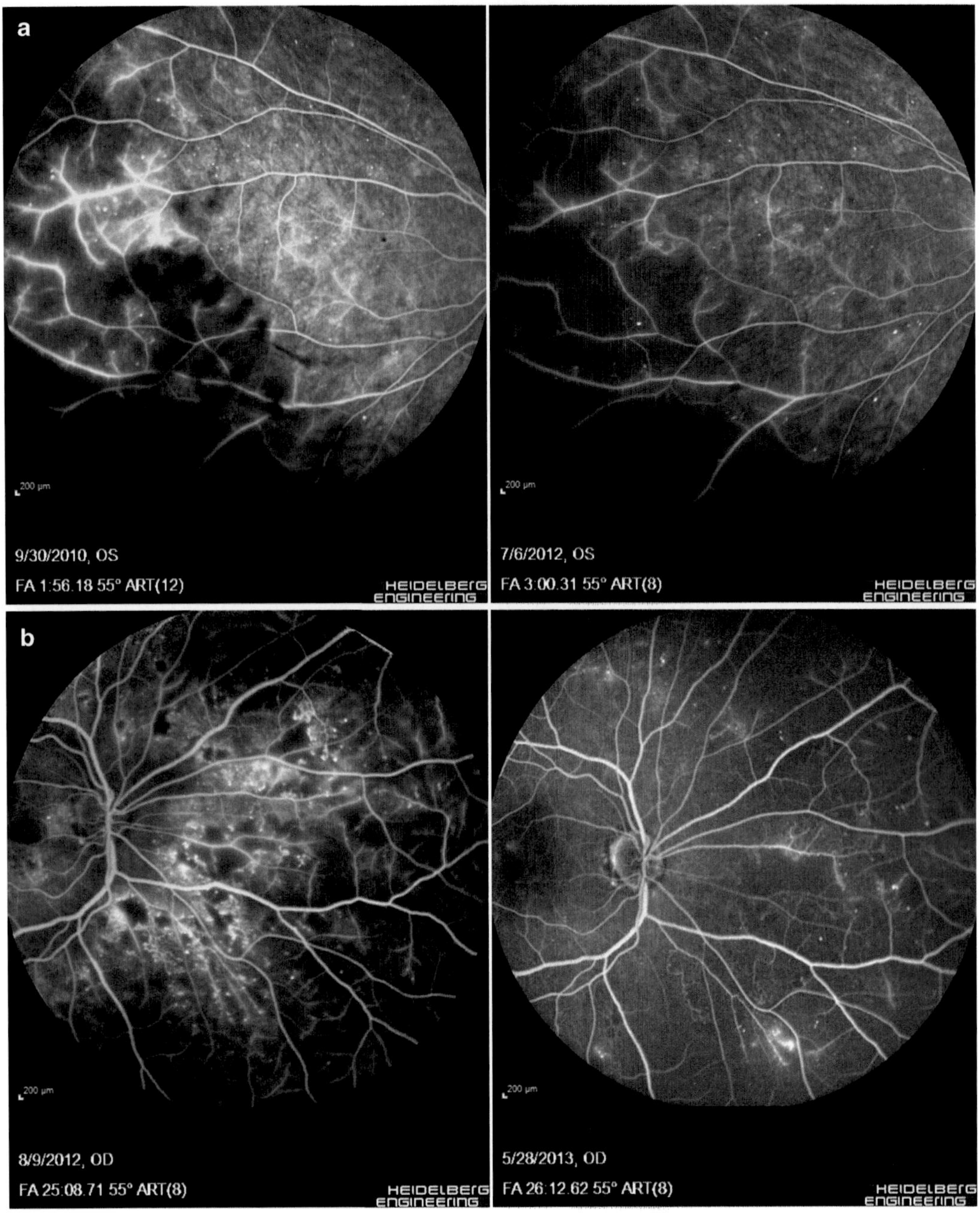

Fig. 30.1 Intravenous fundus fluorescein angiograms (FFA) of diabetic retinopathy (DR) following total retinal SDM laser (panmacular and panretinal) in three patients (**a**), (**b**) and (**c**). No VEGF inhibitors, steroids, or other medical treatment for DR was used. Left photo, before treatment; right photo after treatment. Note reduction in macro and microvascular leakage along with reversal/ diminution of retinopathy severity in each case

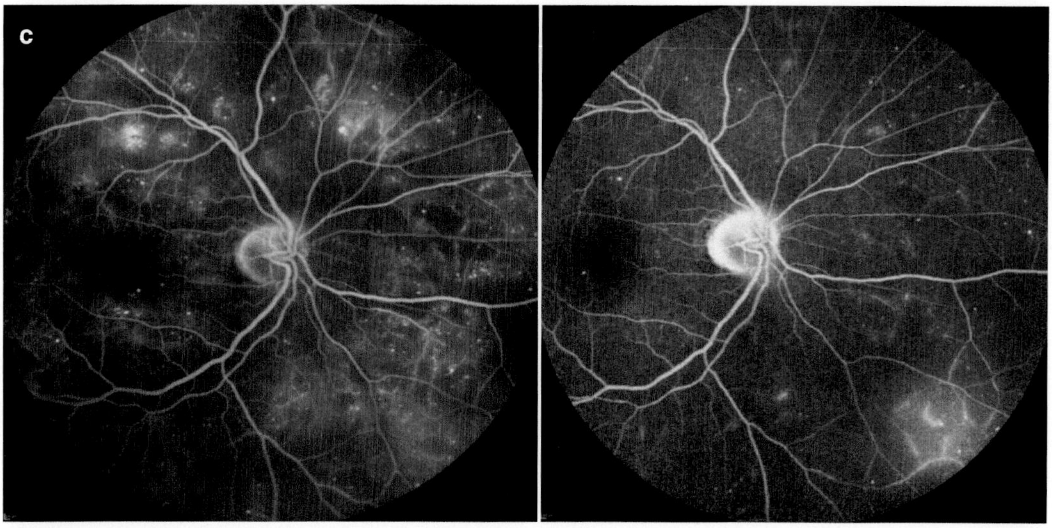

Fig. 30.1 (continued)

Reset theory indicated that SDM should improve retinal function not just in the conventional retinal laser indications such as diabetic macular edema, proliferative diabetic retinopathy, central serous chorioretinopathy, and retina vein occlusions; but in any chronic progressive retinopathy (CPR) of any cause [23–25]. In short, this is because all CRPs are neurodegenerations, and thus share many key features that are addressed by the reset effects of laser treatment [23, 24, 54, 55]. By addressing those fundamental commonalities, the reset phenomenon acts as a "non-specific trigger of disease-specific repair," improving both retinal and visual function in all CPRs, including AMD [23, 24].

In a pilot study of a large cohort of 547 eyes of 363 patients with dry AMD, panmacular SDM treatment was followed by a much lower than expected rate of new CNV [11]. In the absence of LIRD or any other adverse treatment effects, the annual incidence of new CNV following panmacular SDM in dry AMD was 0.87%, compared to 4% in the AREDS [6]. This 80% reduction in expected CNV was noted despite significantly higher risk factors for CNV in the panmacular SDM-treated group compared to the AREDS, particularly age (median 84 vs. 69 years) [6]. Adjusting only for the risk factor age, SDM treated eyes had an incidence of new CNV 93–98% lower than expected compared to the AREDS and other natural history studies of AMD [6, 11]. In a subsequent study of 111 eyes of 70 patients with ARGA from the same dry AMD cohort, SDM reduced the radial velocity of ARGA progression 55% per year compared to untreated controls ($p = 0.0002$) (pretreatment observation period avg. 2.7 years, posttreatment avg. 1.9 years) [56]. Echoing the AREDS, other than reducing the incidence of new CNV and slowing ARGA progression, panmacular SDM prophylaxis of dry AMD was not associated with any notable short-term effects on drusen or other macular morphology [11, 56]. The findings of these studies will inform the design of future confirmatory studies. However, the robust results of these pilot studies of panmacular SDM for dry AMD indicate that retinal laser treatment designed to preclude, rather than cause, LIRD may become an important tool in the prevention of visual loss due to AMD and age-related CNV in particular [11].

In sum, while retina-damaging laser increases the risk of CNV, non-damaging laser sublethal to RPE reduces that risk. While damaging laser appears to cause rapid progression of high-risk AMD; non-damaging laser, sublethal to the RPE, appears to slow progression significantly. Thus, contrary to traditional thinking (but as predicted

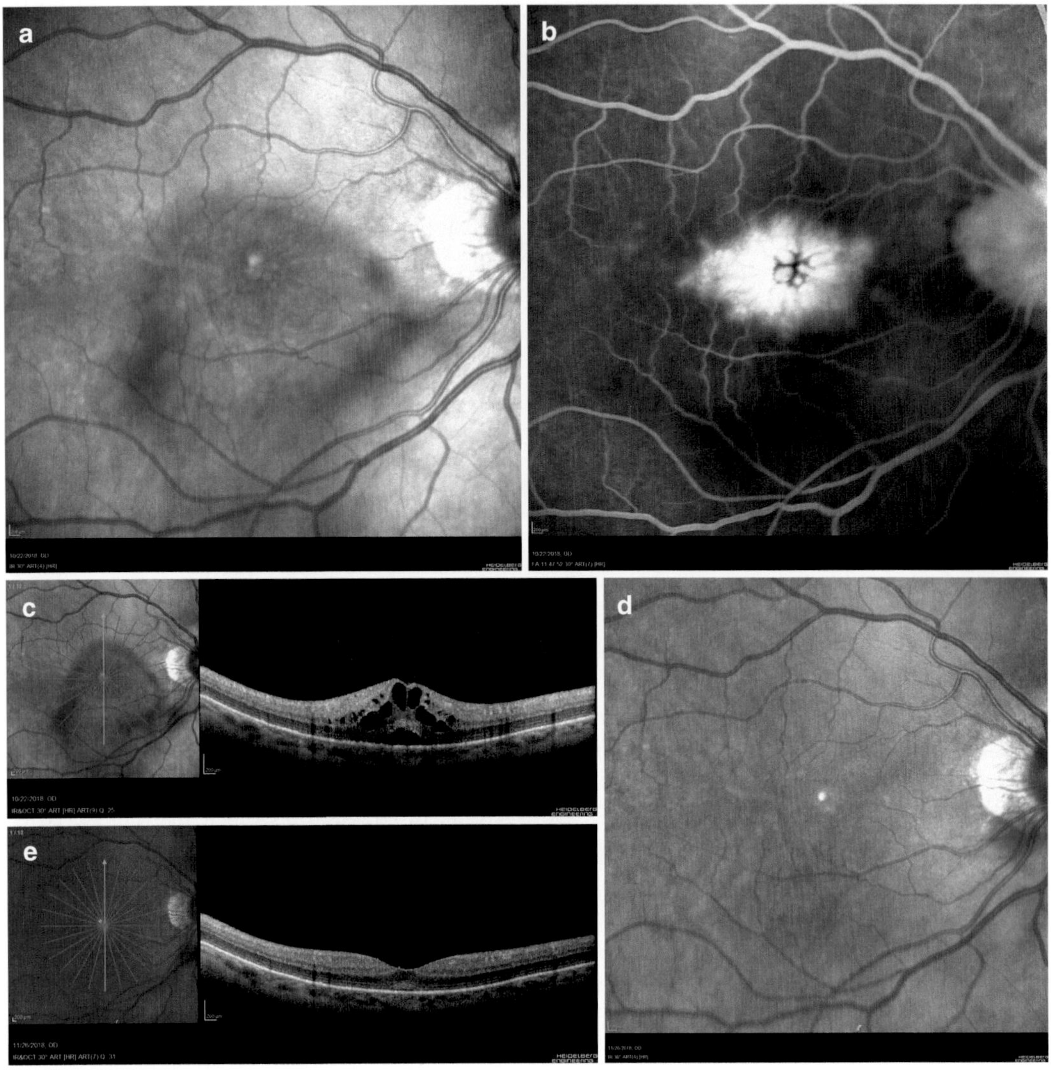

Fig. 30.2 Pseudophakic cystoid macular edema (CME). Unresponsive to combination of topical steroid and non-steroidal anti-inflammatory drops for 1 year. Drops discontinued and panmacular SDM performed. (**a**) Infrared (IR), (**b**) late phase FFA and (**c**) Spectral-domain optical coherence tomography (OCT) prior to treatment with severe CME. Visual acuity (VA) 20/200. (**d**) IR and (**e**) OCT 1 month following panmacular SDM. CME resolved. VA 20/30

by reset theory) it is successful avoidance of LIRD, and thus *avoidance* of drusen reduction, that appears key to the success or failure of laser for prevention of CNV in AMD. How do we account for this? First, by understanding AMD as a chronic progressive neurodegenerative disease; second, by taking into account the effects of retinal laser on retinal integrity and RPE function; third, by recognizing how the classical dynamics of wound repair are engaged by treatment; and fourth, by understanding the ability of laser to modulate both acute and chronic inflammation—one the healer, the other the driver, of the chronic disease process (Figs. 30.1, 30.2, 30.3, 30.4, 30.5).

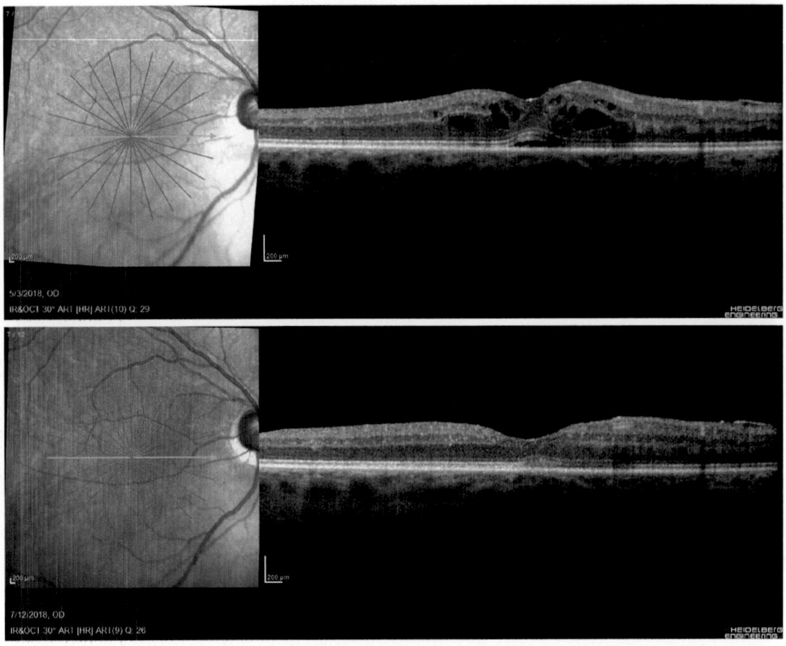

Fig. 30.3 Sarcoid uveitis with cystoid macular edema. History of severe steroid response in the fellow previously. Unresponsive to bevacizumab. Other VEGF inhibitors refused by insurance. Top: Prior to panmacular SDM treatment VA 20/30. Bottom, 1 month following panmacular SDM. VA 20/25

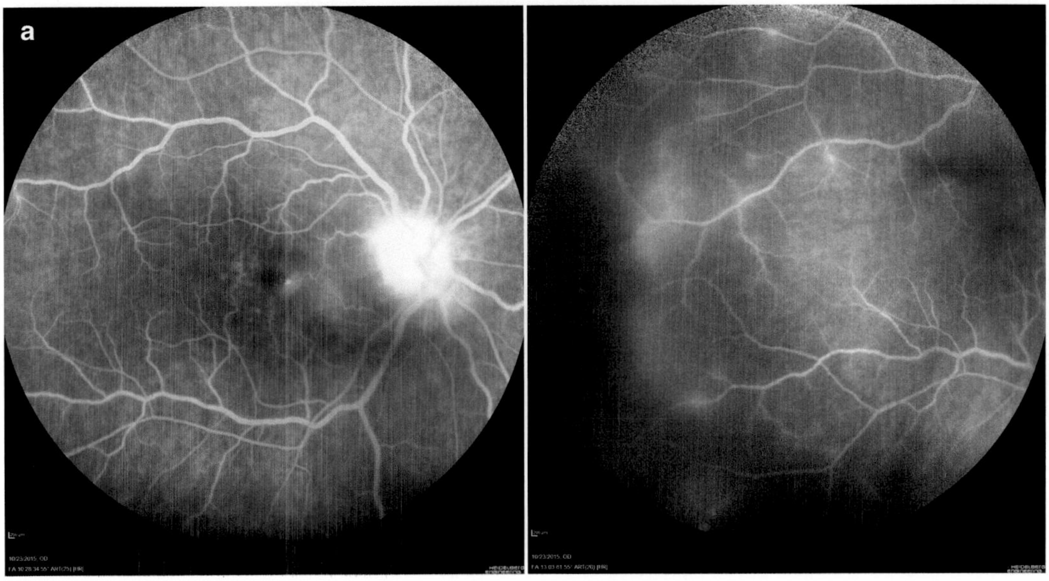

Fig. 30.4 Idiopathic retinal vasculitis, optic neuritis, and vitriitis. (**a**) FFA before treatment. (**b**) FFA 1 month following total retinal SDM laser. No other local or systemic medical treatment given. Note the decrease in inflammatory dye leakage from retinal vessels and optic nerve. VA prior to treatment 20/70; after, 20/50

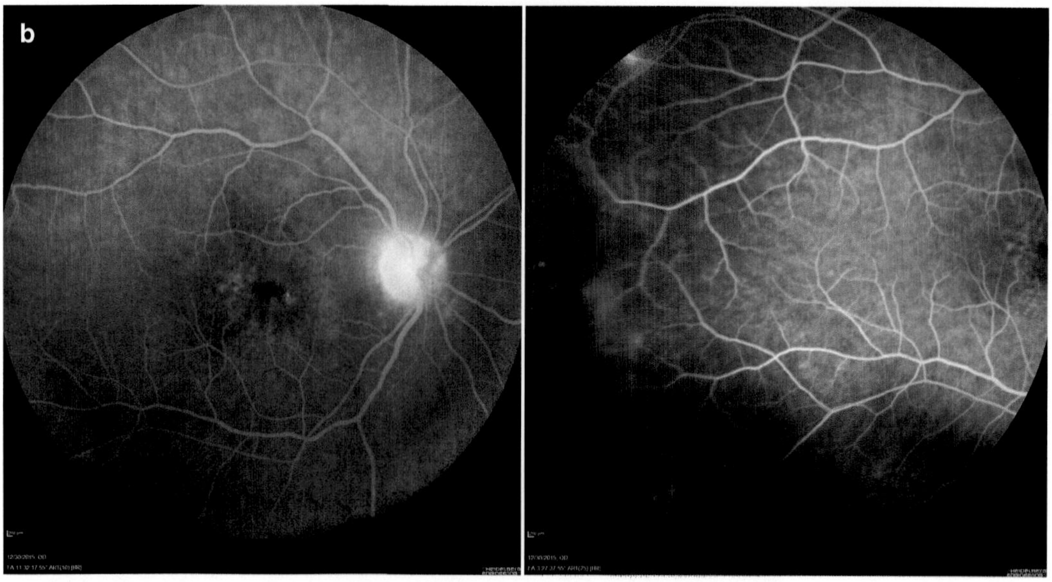

Fig. 30.4 (continued)

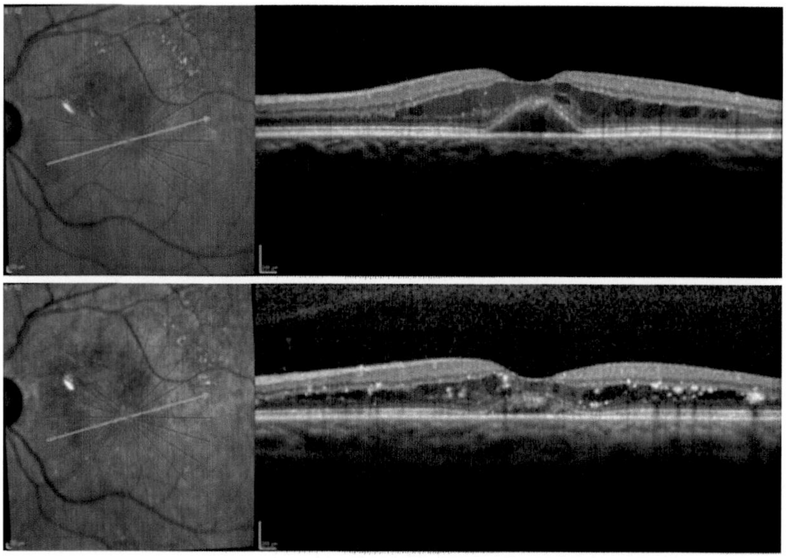

Fig. 30.5 Bevacizumab- and ranibizumab-resistant serous macular detachment associated with diabetic macular edema. No steroid therapy was given. Top: Before panmacular SDM. VA 20/200. Bottom: Three months after panmacular SDM. Note the decrease in macular edema and resolution of inflammatory serous macular detachment. VA 20/70

30.4 Dry AMD as a Model of Chronic Disease and Inflammaging

The association of aging with chronic inflammation, often referred to as "inflammaging," is now recognized as a significant component of virtually all chronic, age-related diseases, including AMD [60]. Unlike acute inflammation, inflammaging is low grade, chronic, persistent, and self-perpetuating, and leads to tissue degeneration [61]. To understand the mechanisms by which inflammaging is generated, we must first understand the essential role of the immune system in the maintenance of normal tissue function and homeostasis.

In healthy cells, there is constant surveillance and repair to maintain normal cell function and homeostasis [49, 62, 63]. However, in disease intracellular abnormalities often either escape repair and/or exceed the cell's ability to manage them successfully leading to a loss of normal function that is generally characteristic of the primary underlying disease process. Further, both normal and diseased tissues produce waste, or "self-debris," that includes damaged cells and macromolecules. In disease, the accumulation of this waste is excessive and thus progressive, ultimately compromising tissue structure and function [60]. At the tissue level, the mechanism employed to repair this damage and remove this waste is inflammatory-mediated (inflammation being a prerequisite of repair) and is dependent on resident macrophages and mast cells [64]. With aging this "housekeeping" function becomes less efficient, due mainly to the combination of increased generation of self-debris and inefficient removal, requiring additional inflammatory input to maintain the tissue in a physiologic (normal) or near physiologic working state, a process that is mediated but ultimately compromised by assembly of the "inflammasome." The inflammasome is a multiprotein stimulus-dependent oligomer that activates the inflammatory process by promoting secretion of pro-inflammatory cytokines and interleukins with dysregulation of inflammasomes being a feature of all chronic diseases [65]. This heightened inflammatory state, between basal physiologic inflammation and pathologic inflammation, is referred to as "para-inflammation" [64]. With further aging the inflammatory stakes continue to rise, eventually escalating to require mobilization of a systemic immune response that includes the recruitment of additional leukocytes and expression of systemic pro-inflammatory cytokines [66]. Thus, maintenance of tissue homeostasis in the aging human requires an increasing inflammatory response to address increased reparative demands that eventually moves beyond para-inflammation to a self-perpetuating and degenerative chronic inflammatory state referred to as "inflammaging" [60, 66].

A classic example of a disease with self-debris is AMD. In dry AMD, this debris is the phenotypic marker of disease and a clinically useful biomarker of the heightened inflammatory state within the retina, classically represented by drusen. Ultrastructurally, this is reflected by priming or activation of the NLRP3 inflammasome and the specific proteins known to be associated with inflammasome assembly [65]. Experimentally, identified proteins include C1q complement component in drusen extracts from AMD donor tissue, carboxyethylpyrrole-adducted proteins from the aging retina, and Alu RNA transcripts from the RPE of patients with ARGA [67–71]. This inflammasome-mediated damage to the retina in AMD may be further aggravated by inflammatory pyroptotic and apoptotic effects resulting from IL-1β and IL-18 expression [70]. In those individuals who have the genetic risk variant for complement factor H (CFH) or other complement risk variants, regulation of these factors is abnormal and excessive quantities of inflammatory complement components are generated and deposited in the retina. Thus, the chronic inflammatory state we recognize as AMD is driven by a number of factors, including complement dysfunction and inflammasome-mediated inflammation, with genetic and environmental (such as smoking) modifiers [72–85].

30.5 Acute Inflammation—Prelude to Repair

It is a basic tenet of biologic repair that an acute inflammatory response is necessary to activate the correct cascade of molecular events to generate successful and complete repair [81, 82]. In contrast, the molecular signature of all acquired age-related diseases, such as AMD, is the presence of chronic inflammation. Chronic inflammation, by definition, indicates that normal repair is not proceeding [61, 65, 81, 82, 86, 87]. Unimpeded, this can lead to tissue degeneration and vision loss via the end-stage AMD phenotypes we recognize clinically as ARGA and disciform scarring due to CNV. Thus, a desired goal of any therapy would be to intervene preventatively, prior to anatomic derangement and visual loss (end-stage disease markers), when the disease process is manifest only by the earliest detectable physiologic dysfunction and most amenable to repair [23]. If the chronic inflammatory disease bed that is AMD could be converted to an acute inflammatory lesion, would the resulting corrective molecular cascades allow for healing and repair sufficient to permit restoration and normalization of retinal function?

30.6 Laser—Prelude to Acute Inflammation

As discussed previously, clinical retinal laser effects can be generally divided into two types: damaging (lethal to at least the RPE) and non-damaging (sublethal to the RPE). These divisions reflect progression in our understanding of the mechanism of retinal laser treatment. As discussed, while photocoagulation was once the goal of retinal laser treatment, it is now clear that photocoagulation and indeed all forms and degrees of LIRD are unnecessary and detrimental; complications of treatment rather than the necessary and sufficient cause of therapeutic retinal laser effects. Within the context of LIRD there is a spectrum of damage that is also instructive. An extreme example of LIRD is the inadvertent rupture of Bruch's membrane. This can be seen with excessively intense photocoagulation, or even as the result of micro- or nanosecond laser damage limited to the outer retina, such as that reported in the LEAD study [52]. Clinically acute rupture of Bruch's membrane is heralded by the instantly recognizable audible "pop" and subretinal gas-bubble formation, with the simultaneous localized appearance of subretinal hemorrhage. Clinically undesirable as promoting the development of CNV, this observation has led to the use of laser rupture of Bruch's membrane to experimentally promote CNV animal models [88].

By any definition, whether clinically inadvertent or experimentally deliberate, laser-induced rupture of Bruch's membrane is a good example of an acute, brief, and once-off traumatic event that will result in activation of a classical tissue repair response [89]. As an extreme example of sorts, it also offers an important insight into the prior failures of laser treatment associated with LIRD to prevent CNV.

Classical tissue repair involves a sequence of key interactions that can be divided into the three overlapping phases of (1) inflammation, (2) tissue formation, and (3) tissue remodeling; involving cells, cytokines, and the extracellular matrix (ECM) [82, 90–92].

Ultimately, the degree of tissue remodeling and resultant scar tissue deposition is directly proportional to the severity of the initial injury: the greater the injury, the greater the degree of acute inflammation induced and the greater the degree of irreversible tissue damage and scar tissue formation. Scar tissue formation represents the restoration of tissue integrity, but without restoration of normal tissue function. Thus, we can ultimately say that, based on the canons of wound healing, a therapeutically ideal laser treatment causes acute injury without structural damage. This in turn generates the desirable endpoint of complete repair without scar tissue formation, thus restoration and normalization of tissue function. LIRD violates this maxim.

This new understanding holds that any degree of LIRD lethal to the target RPE is not only undesirable but a complication counterproductive and detrimental to the goal of therapeutically effective retinal laser treatment. "Non-damaging" laser can thus only properly refer to the complete absence of LIRD at the histopathologic level at any point postoperatively, as the RPE is affected but not killed by laser exposure. Functional retina is lost, RPE cells, the mediators of laser response, are destroyed rather than revitalized and the therapeutic response thus diminished. Finally, as the previously discussed clinical studies illustrate, violation of tissue integrity, no matter how small, can "light the fuse" for the eventual development of CNV by promoting angiogenesis and/or compromising the natural barrier to vascularization presented by the healthy and intact RPE/Bruch's membrane complex [39–42, 44].

30.7 Laser: Mechanism of Action

As stated, laser efficacy derives from its ability to generate a sublethal injury to the RPE leading to repair [8]. At the cellular level, this results in normalization of RPE function, or "homeotrophy." By improving RPE function, retinal function and autoregulation are improved via normalized expression of, and response to, RPE-derived factors such as cytokines and interleukins. Photoreceptor toiletry and waste processing are improved and thus debris accumulation diminished [26, 29, 30, 33–35, 93–96]. At the tissue level, this leads to improved retinal and visual function via activation of reparative laser-induced acute inflammation which is inherently antagonistic to disease-driving chronic inflammation. Therefore, for the laser to be therapeutically effective, it must cause an acute, brief, and once-off "injury" to the RPE to activate tissue repair and to be maximally beneficial, the laser must be "tissue-sparing" and thus sublethal to the RPE. MPL such as panmacular SDM stands alone in its ability to predictably and reliably fulfil both criteria [8]. So, in the absence of LIRD, how does laser work to elicit retinal repair and functional restoration?

Heat shock proteins (HSPs) are a family of proteins that are constitutively expressed in all cells, having critical roles in maintaining homeostasis and normal cell function, but, as noted above, are also significantly upregulated in response to acute insults, such as heat and oxidative stress, perceived by the cell to be existential threats [97]. HSPs are typically grouped into different subfamilies according to their molecular weights in kilo Daltons (hsp100, hsp90, hsp70, hsp60, hsp40, and small HSPs (sHSP), which includes α-crystallins). Each has a particular role. The hsp 70 family is of particular relevance to the current discussion [98]. HSP activation is especially sensitive to the acuity and severity of a cellular threat. Thus, the insidiously progressive dysfunctions of chronic disease are poor triggers of HSP-mediated repair [18, 22, 23, 49, 57, 58, 62, 63]. In chronic disease, the homeostatic functions of HSPs may become taxed to the point of failure, leading to failure of the HSP system itself and further accumulation of damage, debris, chronic inflammation, cell death, and tissue failure [49, 99–103].

As noted above, thermal laser exposure is an effective trigger of HSP activation [49, 97, 104]. The attributes of SDM which are ideal in this regard arise from the facility of SDM to controllably photocoagulate only a small fraction of intracellular proteins sufficient to activate HSP-mediated cellular repair, but insufficient to cause cell death [8, 105]. Most importantly, this laser-induced HSP activation response (salvific and homeotrophic, rather than baseline and homeostatic) results in the repair of not only the acute laser-induced damage but also proceeds to indiscriminate repair of the accumulated damage from the underlying chronic disease process that has escaped HSP surveillance and would otherwise lead to progressive cellular dysfunction and ultimate death. Independence of the salvific HSP repair process from the cause(s) of the accumulated cell damage and resultant dysfunction particular to the underlying disease process makes the reset phenomenon both powerful and elegant, and the basis for the description of retinal laser in chronic retinopathies as a "non-specific trigger of disease-specific repair" [49, 100–103].

30.8 Laser and AMD-Biologic Effects

Laser activation of RPE HSPs triggers a cascade of reparative and modulated inflammatory effects, factors, and processes that improve cell and retinal function. These include decreased expression of angiogenesis promoters VEGF, TGF-β, and bFGF; increased angiogenesis inhibitor pigment epithelial-derived factor expression; improved mitochondrial function; increased retinal nitrous oxide levels; inhibition of apoptosis; modulation of tissue matrix metalloproteinases; reduced free radical species and increased superoxide dismutase activity; increased mRNA expression of cytokine markers of reparative acute inflammation and decreased markers of chronic inflammation; local and systemic immunomodulation including local stem cell activation and monocyte and hematopoietic progenitor cell recruitment to the retina; and improved retinal macro- and microglial function [8, 22, 23, 47, 58, 63, 106–116]. Absent compromise of the RPE/Bruch's membrane complex integrity and tissue scarring from LIRD that increase the risk of CNV in AMD, any or all of the above responses to laser treatment sublethal to the RPE such as SDM may contribute to a reduced risk of age-related CNV.

As noted, a characteristic abnormality in AMD is the accumulation of metabolic by-products such as lipofuscin, damaged organelles, and nonfunctioning or toxic proteins [117]. This informs us that the RPE in AMD is functioning in an environment of chronic oxidative stress, while still managing to maintain relatively normal visual cycle metabolism and upkeep of Bruch's membrane. With aging the normal level of homeostatic HSP function is insufficient to maintain repair. This oxidative stress-induced cellular damage also contributes to increased protein misfolding and formation of detrimental protein aggregates within the cytosol, further compromising cell function [118, 119]. Here, activation of additional compensatory processes may mitigate HSPs failure. Two that are particularly important are the proteasome and autophagy pathways. The first involves tagging misfolded proteins with ubiquitin and transferring them to the proteasome degradation pathway, which is a multicatalytic proteolytic complex that recognizes and selectively degrades oxidatively damaged and ubiquitinated proteins. The second, the autophagy pathway is in itself an inbuilt intracellular waste disposal system [120–124].

30.9 Why Drusen Elimination Might Be Undesirable

HSPs, the proteasome, and cellular autophagy are the three key intracellular pathways that maintain RPE homeostasis. In aging, all are increasingly compromised leading to activation of the nuclear factor-kappaB (NF-kappaB) signalling pathway. NF-kappaB, a transcription factor that plays a critical role in diverse cellular processes associated with proliferation, cell death, and development; as well as innate and adaptive immune responses, is normally sequestered in the cytoplasm by a family of inhibitory proteins known as inhibitors of NF-kappaB. Activation of NF-kappaB leads to the assembly of the NLRP3 inflammasome and activation of a tissue repair response [119].

Clinically, we recognize this stage of the immune response to aging as the typical inflammaging-associated AMD phenotype of soft drusen and pigmentary alterations at the macula. In other words, these clinical characteristics are key biomarkers of what is happening at the cellular and molecular level. As biomarkers they are important because they inform us that the RPE is chronically stressed and functionally compromised, but still viable. From a natural history perspective, the disappearance of these lesions is often associated with the death of RPE leading to ARGA and visual loss [125]. Once begun, the process of ARGA is progressive [96].

Although drusen are a sign of impaired autophagy and inflammaging (and indirectly of impaired proteasomal degradation and HSP function), their presence nonetheless indicates that these pathways are still functional [93]. SDM appears to reduce the risks of visual loss in high-risk AMD from both ARGA and CNV by improving, rather than further stressing and decompensating RPE function; and by preserving the integrity of the RPE/Bruch's membrane complex [11, 26, 56].

As noted above, the NF kappaB pathway, resulting in the assembly of the NLRP3 inflammasome, appears to be crucial to the pathogenesis of AMD [126]. The biological significance of NLRP3 inflammasome activation is the release of active IL-1β and IL-18 into the extracellular space. The secreted IL-1β facilitates the chronic inflammatory response in the tissues while IL-18 promotes caspase-3 dependent RPE apoptosis, both hallmarks of AMD [65]. Inhibition of IL-1β and IL-18 expression via RPE HSP activation is thus yet another point in the disease process where retinal laser sublethal to the RPE may reduce the risk of CNV in AMD by inhibiting chronic inflammation [127].

Finally, at the tissue level, retinal laser-induced inflammatory recalibration in the direction of restoration and repair and away from progressive degeneration has local microglial and systemic components. These include activation of resident retinal stem cells and recruitment of bone marrow-derived stem cells, a potent combination that can foster repair, regeneration, and functional restoration [54, 55, 111].

While difficult to demonstrate clinically in dry AMD, the images in Figs. 30.1, 30.2, 30.3, 30.4, 30.5 illustrate the anti-inflammatory effects of panmacular and total retinal SDM as monotherapy in various other clinical settings described above. Note also the complete absence of LIRD in each case.

30.10 Summary

In summary, as the most important cause of CNV and related visual loss, AMD is a complex web of dysfunctional intracellular and extracellular events involving hundreds, if not thousands, of signalling molecules in innumerable interrelations. At our current level of understanding it is hard to envisage a targeted therapy, acting on a specific molecule(s) at a particular point in a particular pathway(s), that might singularly modulate a disease process of such complexity. The complexity of targeted therapeutic alteration of cell physiology dwarfs the comparative simplicity of binding VEGF in the extracellular space accounting for the failure of targeted drug therapy to prevent AMD—and thus CNV—to date. Yet the judicious application of light seems to do exactly that. Rather than attempting to selectively manipulate cell chemistry, retinal laser awakens powerful and fundamental mechanisms of cellular repair and functional restoration harnessing this same biologic complexity to advantage. Acting on a fraction of proteins in a single cell via HSP activation, laser is a catalyst launching a multitude of cascading effects within and far beyond the cell, resulting in physiologic—and thus ideal—functional normalization, "resetting" the RPE. The resultant reversal of the chronic disease process reduces the risks of visual loss—including the development of CNV. Absent LIRD, the benefits of modern laser are unopposed by adverse treatment effects and are greatest in eyes with the highest risks of age-related visual loss [11, 56]. Conversely, LIRD is adverse to retinal integrity and retinal and visual function. In AMD, LIRD may accelerate retinal degeneration, further increasing the risk of visual loss from ARGA and CNV, especially in the sickest, most compromised and vulnerable eyes [44, 52, 53]. Thus drusen elimination requiring LIRD appears undesirable, especially in the most functionally compromised high-risk eyes, and of uncertain long-term benefit in eyes with early AMD. In contrast, retinal laser treatment sublethal to the RPE, and thus wholly therapeutic, appears to hold great promise in the prevention of visual loss from chronic progressive retinopathies in general, and from CNV in AMD in particular. Further study will be illuminating.

Key Learning Points

1. While CNV may result from focal damage to the macula from a number of causes, the main cause is chronic progressive disease, principally age-related macular degeneration.
2. All chronic progressive retinopathies (CPRs) are neurodegenerations, and as such have much in common despite disparate etiologies and phenotypes.
3. Dysfunction of the retinal pigment epithelium is a key commonality of all CRPs, leading to the second key commonality of chronic, self-perpetuating, degenerative inflammation. These are the key predisposing factors to CNV in AMD.
4. The therapeutic effects of retinal laser treatment improve RPE and thus retinal function, and are antagonistic to chronic inflammation, resulting in repair and functional restoration.
5. Laser-induced retinal damage (LIRD) is the cause of all adverse treatment effects and compromises the therapeutic benefits of laser treatment while offering no unique benefits over modern retinal laser therapy which is reliably sublethal to the RPE. LIRD increases

AMD progression and the risks of visual loss, including CNV, particularly in high-risk eyes.

6. By eliminating LIRD and maximizing therapeutic laser effects, modern retinal laser, epitomized by low-intensity/high-density subthreshold diode micropulse laser (SDM), safely slows disease progression, reducing the risks of visual loss and CNV in AMD, especially in the highest risk eyes.
7. By addressing the commonalities of retinal neurodegenerations via non-targeted, pathoselective disease-specific repair, SDM may offer similar benefits in other retinopathies that predispose to macular CNV.

Financial Disclosures

Dr. Luttrull:

Ojai Retinal Technologies, LLC—Management, Patent, Equity.

Retinal Protection Sciences, LLC—Management, Equity.

Replenish, Inc.—Patent, Equity.

Dr. Kent:

None.

References

1. Jepson CN, Wetzig PC. Photocoagulation in disciform macular degeneration. Am J Ophthalmol 1969;67(6):920–930. Epub 1969/06/01. PubMed PMID: 5785852.
2. Argon laser photocoagulation for senile macular degeneration. Results of a randomized clinical trial. Arch Ophthalmol 1982;100(6):912–918. Epub 1982/06/01. PubMed PMID: 7046707.
3. Avila MP, Weiter JJ, Jalkh AE, Trempe CL, Pruett RC, Schepens CL. Natural history of choroidal neovascularization in degenerative myopia. Ophthalmology 1984;91(12):1573–1581. Epub 1984/12/01. PubMed PMID: 6084222.
4. Francois J, De Laey JJ, Cambie E, Hanssens M, Victoria-Troncoso V. Neovascularization after argon laser photocoagulation of macular lesions. Am J Ophthalmol 1975;79(2):206–210. Epub 1975/02/01. PubMed PMID: 1167736.
5. Recurrent choroidal neovascularization after argon laser photocoagulation for neovascular maculopathy. Macular Photocoagulation Study Group. Arch Ophthalmol 1986;104(4):503–512. Epub 1986/04/01. PubMed PMID: 2420315.
6. A randomized, placebo-controlled, clinical trial of high-dose supplementation with vitamins C and E, beta carotene, and zinc for age-related macular degeneration and vision loss: AREDS report no. 8. Arch Ophthalmol. 2001;119(10):1417–36. Epub 2001/10/23. PubMed PMID: 11594942; PubMed Central PMCID: PMC1462955.
7. Heier JS, Antoszyk AN, Pavan PR, Leff SR, Rosenfeld PJ, Ciulla TA, et al. Ranibizumab for treatment of neovascular age-related macular degeneration: a phase I/II multicenter, controlled, multidose study. Ophthalmology. 2006;113(4):633.e1–4. Epub 2006/02/18. https://doi.org/10.1016/j.ophtha.2005.10.052. PubMed PMID: 16483659.
8. Chhablani J, Roh YJ, Jobling AI, Fletcher EL, Lek JJ, Bansal P, et al. Restorative retinal laser therapy: present state and future directions. Surv Ophthalmol. 2017. Epub 2017/10/11. https://doi.org/10.1016/j.survophthal.2017.09.008. PubMed PMID: 28987614.
9. Guymer RH, Brassington KH, Dimitrov P, Makeyeva G, Plunkett M, Xia W, et al. Nanosecond-laser application in intermediate AMD: 12-month results of fundus appearance and macular function. Clin Exp Ophthalmol 2014;42(5):466–479. Epub 2013/10/15. https://doi.org/10.1111/ceo.12247. PubMed PMID: 24118741.
10. Jobling AI, Guymer RH, Vessey KA, Greferath U, Mills SA, Brassington KH, et al. Nanosecond laser therapy reverses pathologic and molecular changes in age-related macular degeneration without retinal damage. FASEB J 2015;29(2):696–710. Epub 2014/11/14. https://doi.org/10.1096/fj.14-262444. PubMed PMID: 25392267.
11. Luttrull JK, Sinclair SH, Elmann S, Glaser BM. Low incidence of choroidal neovascularization following subthreshold diode micropulse laser (SDM) in high-risk AMD. PLoS One 2018;13(8):e0202097. Epub 2018/08/24. https://doi.org/10.1371/journal.pone.0202097. PubMed PMID: 30138455.
12. Friedman DS, O'Colmain BJ, Munoz B, Tomany SC, McCarty C, de Jong PT, et al. Prevalence of age-related macular degeneration in the United States. Arch Ophthalmol 2004;122(4):564–572. Epub 2004/04/14. https://doi.org/10.1001/archopht.122.4.564. PubMed PMID: 15078675.
13. Wong WL, Su X, Li X, Cheung CM, Klein R, Cheng CY, et al. Global prevalence of age-related macular degeneration and disease burden projection for 2020 and 2040: a systematic review and meta-analysis. Lancet Glob Health 2014;2(2):e106–e116. Epub 2014/08/12. https://doi.org/10.1016/s2214-109x(13)70145-1. PubMed PMID: 25104651.
14. Molnar I, Pournaras CJ, Tsacopoulos M, Gilodi N, Leuenberger PM. [Panphotocoagulation. Mechanism of action and early indications]. Ophtalmologie: organe de la Societe francaise d'ophtalmologie 1987;1(4):449–452. Epub 1987/10/01. PubMed PMID: 3153915.

15. Shimizu K. Light coagulation in diabetic retinopathy and the mechanism of its effect. Ganka Ophthalmol 1971;13(11):1001–1006. Epub 1971/11/01. PubMed PMID: 5169175.
16. Stefansson E. Oxygen and diabetic eye disease. Graefes Arch Clin Exp Ophthalmol 1990;228(2):120–123. Epub 1990/01/01. PubMed PMID: 2186971.
17. Brader HS, Young LH. Subthreshold diode micropulse laser: a review. Semin Ophthalmol 2016;31(1–2):30–39. Epub 2016/03/10. https://doi.org/10.3109/08820538.2015.1114837. PubMed PMID: 26959127.
18. Chen G, Tzekov R, Li W, Jiang F, Mao S, Tong Y. Subthreshold micropulse diode laser versus conventional laser photocoagulation for diabetic macular Edema: a meta-analysis of randomized controlled trials. Retina 2016;36(11):2059–2065. Epub 2016/10/25. https://doi.org/10.1097/iae.0000000000001053. PubMed PMID: 27096529.
19. Luttrull JK, Musch DC, Mainster MA. Subthreshold diode micropulse photocoagulation for the treatment of clinically significant diabetic macular oedema. Br J Ophthalmol 2005;89(1):74–80. Epub 2004/12/24. https://doi.org/10.1136/bjo.2004.051540. PubMed PMID: 15615751; PubMed Central PMCID: PMC1772486.
20. Luttrull JK, Musch DC, Spink CA. Subthreshold diode micropulse panretinal photocoagulation for proliferative diabetic retinopathy. Eye (Lond) 2008;22(5):607–612. Epub 2007/02/13. https://doi.org/10.1038/sj.eye.6702725. PubMed PMID: 17293791.
21. Luttrull JK, Spink CJ. Serial optical coherence tomography of subthreshold diode laser micropulse photocoagulation for diabetic macular edema. Ophthalmic Surg Lasers Imaging 2006;37(5):370–377. Epub 2006/10/05. PubMed PMID: 17017196.
22. Luttrull JK, Chang DB, Margolis BW, Dorin G, Luttrull DK. Laser resesitization of medically unresponsive neovascular age-related macular degeneration: efficacy and Implications. Retina 2015;35(6):1184–1194. Epub 2015/02/05. https://doi.org/10.1097/iae.0000000000000458. PubMed PMID: 25650711.
23. Luttrull JK, Margolis BW. Functionally guided retinal protective therapy for dry age-related macular and inherited retinal degenerations: a pilot study. Invest Ophthalmol Vis Sci 2016;57(1):265–275. Epub 2016/01/29. https://doi.org/10.1167/iovs.15-18163. PubMed PMID: 26818793.
24. Luttrull JK. Improved retinal and visual function following panmacular subthreshold diode micropulse laser for retinitis pigmentosa. Eye (Lond). 2018;32(6):1099–110. Epub 2018/02/17. https://doi.org/10.1038/s41433-018-0017-3. PubMed PMID: 29449615; PubMed Central PMCID: PMCPMC5997672.
25. Luttrull JK, Samples JR, Kent D, Lum BJ. Panmacular subthreshold diode micropulse laser (SDM) as neuroprotective therapy in primary open-angle glaucoma. In: Samples JR, Kneppper PA, editors. Glaucoma research 2018–2020. Amsterdam: Kugler Publications; 2018. p. 281–94.
26. Abdelsalam A, Del Priore L, Zarbin MA. Drusen in age-related macular degeneration: pathogenesis, natural course, and laser photocoagulation-induced regression. Surv Ophthalmol 1999;44(1):1–29. Epub 1999/08/31. PubMed PMID: 10466585.
27. Bressler NM, Munoz B, Maguire MG, Vitale SE, Schein OD, Taylor HR, et al. Five-year incidence and disappearance of drusen and retinal pigment epithelial abnormalities. Waterman Stud Arch Ophthalmol 1995;113(3):301–308. Epub 1995/03/01. PubMed PMID: 7534060.
28. Bressler SB, Maguire MG, Bressler NM, Fine SL. Relationship of drusen and abnormalities of the retinal pigment epithelium to the prognosis of neovascular macular degeneration. The Macular Photocoagulation Study Group. Arch Ophthalmol 1990;108(10):1442–1447. Epub 1990/10/01. PubMed PMID: 1699513.
29. Chamberlin JA, Bressler NM, Bressler SB, Elman MJ, Murphy RP, Flood TP, et al. The use of fundus photographs and fluorescein angiograms in the identification and treatment of choroidal neovascularization in the Macular Photocoagulation Study. The Macular Photocoagulation Study Group Ophthalmology 1989;96(10):1526–1534. Epub 1989/10/01. PubMed PMID: 2479899.
30. Smiddy WE, Fine SL. Prognosis of patients with bilateral macular drusen. Ophthalmology 1984;91(3):271–277. Epub 1984/03/01. PubMed PMID: 6201789.
31. Ho AC, Maguire MG, Yoken J, Lee MS, Shin DS, Javornik NB, et al. Laser-induced drusen reduction improves visual function at 1 year. Choroidal Neovascularization Prevention Trial Research Group. Ophthalmology 1999;106(7):1367–1373.; discussion 74. Epub 1999/07/16. PubMed PMID: 10406624.
32. Olk RJ, Friberg TR, Stickney KL, Akduman L, Wong KL, Chen MC, et al. Therapeutic benefits of infrared (810-nm) diode laser macular grid photocoagulation in prophylactic treatment of nonexudative age-related macular degeneration: two-year results of a randomized pilot study. Ophthalmology 1999;106(11):2082–2090. Epub 1999/11/26. https://doi.org/10.1016/s0161-6420(99)90487-6. PubMed PMID: 10571341.
33. Dithmar S, Pollithy S, Ach T. Disappearance of central confluent soft drusen following vitrectomy and ILM peeling. Eye (Lond). 2013;27(6):779–81. Epub 2013/04/06. https://doi.org/10.1038/eye.2013.35. PubMed PMID: 23558209; PubMed Central PMCID: PMCPMC3682349.
34. Lim LT, Holicki J, Walker JD. Disappearance of extramacular drusen after chronic retinal detachment. Oman journal of ophthalmology. 2012;5(1):67.

Epub 2012/05/05. https://doi.org/10.4103/0974-620x.94793. PubMed PMID: 22557885; PubMed Central PMCID: PMCPMC3339683.

35. Duvall J, Tso MO. Cellular mechanisms of resolution of drusen after laser coagulation. An experimental study. Arch Ophthalmol 1985;103(5):694–703. Epub 1985/05/01. PubMed PMID: 4039560.

36. Argon laser photocoagulation for neovascular maculopathy. Three-year results from randomized clinical trials. Macular Photocoagulation Study Group. Arch Ophthalmol. 1986;104(5):694–701. Epub 1986/05/01. PubMed PMID: 2423061.

37. Treatment techniques and clinical guidelines for photocoagulation of diabetic macular edema. Early Treatment Diabetic Retinopathy Study Report Number 2. Early Treatment Diabetic Retinopathy Study Research Group. Ophthalmology. 1987;94(7):761–74. Epub 1987/07/01. PubMed PMID: 3658348.

38. Akduman L, Olk RJ. Subthreshold (invisible) modified grid diode laser photocoagulation in diffuse diabetic macular edema (DDME). Ophthalmic Surg Lasers 1999;30(9):706–714. Epub 1999/11/26. PubMed PMID: 10574491.

39. Laser treatment in patients with bilateral large drusen: the complications of age-related macular degeneration prevention trial. Ophthalmology. 2006;113(11):1974–86. Epub 2006/11/01. https://doi.org/10.1016/j.ophtha.2006.08.015. PubMed PMID: 17074563.

40. Owens SL, Bunce C, Brannon AJ, Wormald R, Bird AC. Prophylactic laser treatment appears to promote choroidal neovascularisation in high-risk ARM: results of an interim analysis. Eye (Lond) 2003;17(5):623–627. Epub 2003/07/12. https://doi.org/10.1038/sj.eye.6700442. PubMed PMID: 12855972.

41. Owens SL, Bunce C, Brannon AJ, Xing W, Chisholm IH, Gross M, et al. Prophylactic laser treatment hastens choroidal neovascularization in unilateral age-related maculopathy: final results of the drusen laser study. Am J Ophthalmol 2006;141(2):276–281. Epub 2006/02/07. https://doi.org/10.1016/j.ajo.2005.08.019. PubMed PMID: 16458680.

42. Kaiser RS, Berger JW, Maguire MG, Ho AC, Javornik NB. Laser burn intensity and the risk for choroidal neovascularization in the CNVPT Fellow Eye Study. Arch Ophthalmol 2001;119(6):826–832. Epub 2001/06/19. PubMed PMID: 11405833.

43. Rodanant N, Friberg TR, Cheng L, Aurora A, Bartsch D, Toyoguchi M, et al. Predictors of drusen reduction after subthreshold infrared (810 nm) diode laser macular grid photocoagulation for nonexudative age-related macular degeneration. Am J Ophthalmol 2002;134(4):577–585. Epub 2002/10/18. PubMed PMID: 12383815.

44. Virgili G, Michelessi M, Parodi MB, Bacherini D, Evans JR. Laser treatment of drusen to prevent progression to advanced age-related macular degeneration. The Cochrane database of systematic reviews. 2015;(10):Cd006537. Epub 2015/10/24. https://doi.org/10.1002/14651858.CD006537.pub3. PubMed PMID: 26493180; PubMed Central PMCID: PMCPmc4733883.

45. Dorin G. Subthreshold and micropulse diode laser photocoagulation. Semin Ophthalmol 2003;18(3):147–153. Epub 2004/10/30. https://doi.org/10.1076/soph.18.3.147.29812. PubMed PMID: 15513476.

46. Luttrull JK, Sramek C, Palanker D, Spink CJ, Musch DC. Long-term safety, high-resolution imaging, and tissue temperature modeling of subvisible diode micropulse photocoagulation for retinovascular macular edema. Retina 2012;32(2):375–386. Epub 2011/10/06. https://doi.org/10.1097/IAE.0b013e3182206f6c. PubMed PMID: 21971077.

47. Lavinsky D, Wang J, Huie P, Dalal R, Lee SJ, Lee DY, et al. Nondamaging Retinal Laser Therapy: Rationale and Applications to the Macula. Invest Ophthalmol Vis Sci. 2016;57(6):2488–500. Epub 2016/05/10. https://doi.org/10.1167/iovs.15-18981. PubMed PMID: 27159441; PubMed Central PMCID: PMCPMC5995023.

48. Roider J, Brinkmann R, Wirbelauer C, Laqua H, Birngruber R. Subthreshold (retinal pigment epithelium) photocoagulation in macular diseases: a pilot study. Br J Ophthalmol. 2000;84(1):40–7. Epub 1999/12/28. PubMed PMID: 10611098; PubMed Central PMCID: PMCPMC1723228.

49. Sramek C, Mackanos M, Spitler R, Leung LS, Nomoto H, Contag CH, et al. Non-damaging retinal phototherapy: dynamic range of heat shock protein expression. Invest Ophthalmol Vis Sci 2011;52(3):1780–1787. Epub 2010/11/20. https://doi.org/10.1167/iovs.10-5917. PubMed PMID: 21087969.

50. Sramek CK, Leung LS, Paulus YM, Palanker DV. Therapeutic window of retinal photocoagulation with green (532-nm) and yellow (577-nm) lasers. Ophthalmic Surg Lasers Imaging 2012;43(4):341–347. Epub 2012/05/17. https://doi.org/10.3928/15428877-20120426-05. PubMed PMID: 22589338.

51. Roider J, Brinkmann R, Wirbelauer C, Birngruber R, Laqua H. Variability of RPE reaction in two cases after selective RPE laser effects in prophylactic treatment of drusen. Graefes Arch Clin Exp Ophthalmol 1999;237(1):45–50. Epub 1999/02/10. PubMed PMID: 9951641.

52. Guymer RH, Wu Z, Hodgson LAB, Caruso E, Brassington KH, Tindill N, et al. Subthreshold nanosecond laser intervention in age-related macular degeneration: the LEAD randomized controlled clinical trial ophthalmology 2018. Epub 2018/09/24. https://doi.org/10.1016/j.ophtha.2018.09.015. PubMed PMID: 30244144.

53. Prahs P, Walter A, Regler R, Theisen-Kunde D, Birngruber R, Brinkmann R, et al. Selective retina therapy (SRT) in patients with geographic atrophy due to age-related macular degeneration. Graefes Arch

Clin Exp Ophthalmol 2010;248(5):651–658. Epub 2009/12/22. https://doi.org/10.1007/s00417-009-1208-1. PubMed PMID: 20024687.
54. Midena E, Pilotto E. Emerging Insights into Pathogenesis. Dev Ophthalmol 2017;60:16–27. Epub 2017/04/21. https://doi.org/10.1159/000459687. PubMed PMID: 28427061.
55. Vujosevic S, Micera A, Bini S, Berton M, Esposito G, Midena E. Proteome analysis of retinal glia cells-related inflammatory cytokines in the aqueous humour of diabetic patients. Acta Ophthalmol 2016;94(1):56–64. Epub 2015/08/14. https://doi.org/10.1111/aos.12812. PubMed PMID: 26268591.
56. Luttrull JK. Slowed progression of age-related geographic atrophy following subthreshold diode micropulse laser—in review. 2019.
57. Luttrull JK, Sinclair SH. Safety of transfoveal subthreshold diode micropulse laser for fovea-involving diabetic macular edema in eyes with good visual acuity. Retina 2014;34(10):2010–2020. Epub 2014/05/20. https://doi.org/10.1097/iae.0000000000000177. PubMed PMID: 24837050.
58. Luttrull JK, Dorin G. Subthreshold diode micropulse laser photocoagulation (SDM) as invisible retinal phototherapy for diabetic macular edema: a review. Curr Diabetes Rev 2012;8(4):274–284. Epub 2012/05/17. PubMed PMID: 22587512; PubMed Central PMCID: PMC3412206.
59. Lavinsky D, Cardillo JA, Melo LA, Jr., Dare A, Farah ME, Belfort R, Jr. Randomized clinical trial evaluating mETDRS versus normal or high-density micropulse photocoagulation for diabetic macular edema. Invest Ophthalmol Vis Sci 2011;52(7):4314–4323. Epub 2011/02/25. https://doi.org/10.1167/iovs.10-6828. PubMed PMID: 21345996.
60. Franceschi C, Campisi J. Chronic inflammation (inflammaging) and its potential contribution to age-associated diseases. J Gerontol A Biol Sci Med Sci 2014;69 Suppl 1:S4–S9. Epub 2014/05/17. https://doi.org/10.1093/gerona/glu057. PubMed PMID: 24833586.
61. Howcroft TK, Campisi J, Louis GB, Smith MT, Wise B, Wyss-Coray T, et al. The role of inflammation in age-related disease. Aging (Albany NY). 2013;5(1):84–93. Epub 2013/03/12. https://doi.org/10.18632/aging.100531. PubMed PMID: 23474627; PubMed Central PMCID: PMC3616233.
62. Baldwin RL. Energetics of protein folding. J Mol Biol 2007;371(2):283–301. Epub 2007/06/22. https://doi.org/10.1016/j.jmb.2007.05.078. PubMed PMID: 17582437.
63. Kregel KC. Heat shock proteins: modifying factors in physiological stress responses and acquired thermotolerance. J Appl Physiol (1985). 2002;92(5):2177–86. Epub 2002/04/19. https://doi.org/10.1152/japplphysiol.01267.2001. PubMed PMID: 11960972.
64. Medzhitov R. Origin and physiological roles of inflammation. Nature 2008;454(7203):428–435. Epub 2008/07/25. https://doi.org/10.1038/nature07201. PubMed PMID: 18650913.
65. Ambati J, Atkinson JP, Gelfand BD. Immunology of age-related macular degeneration. Nat Rev Immunol 2013;13(6):438–451. Epub 2013/05/25. https://doi.org/10.1038/nri3459. PubMed PMID: 23702979; PubMed Central PMCID: PMC3941009.
66. Xu H, Chen M, Forrester JV. Para-inflammation in the aging retina. Prog Retin Eye Res 2009;28(5):348–368. Epub 2009/06/30. https://doi.org/10.1016/j.preteyeres.2009.06.001. PubMed PMID: 19560552.
67. Doyle SL, Campbell M, Ozaki E, Salomon RG, Mori A, Kenna PF, et al. NLRP3 has a protective role in age-related macular degeneration through the induction of IL-18 by drusen components. Nat Med 2012;18(5):791–798. Epub 2012/04/10. https://doi.org/10.1038/nm.2717. PubMed PMID: 22484808; PubMed Central PMCID: PMC3984677.
68. Hollyfield JG, Bonilha VL, Rayborn ME, Yang X, Shadrach KG, Lu L, et al. Oxidative damage-induced inflammation initiates age-related macular degeneration. Nat Med 2008;14(2):194–198. Epub 2008/01/29. https://doi.org/10.1038/nm1709. PubMed PMID: 18223656; PubMed Central PMCID: PMC2748836.
69. Kaneko H, Dridi S, Tarallo V, Gelfand BD, Fowler BJ, Cho WG, et al. DICER1 deficit induces Alu RNA toxicity in age-related macular degeneration. Nature 2011;471(7338):325–330. Epub 2011/02/08. https://doi.org/10.1038/nature09830. PubMed PMID: 21297615; PubMed Central PMCID: PMC3077055.
70. Tarallo V, Hirano Y, Gelfand BD, Dridi S, Kerur N, Kim Y, et al. DICER1 loss and Alu RNA induce age-related macular degeneration via the NLRP3 inflammasome and MyD88. Cell 2012;149(4):847–859. Epub 2012/05/01. https://doi.org/10.1016/j.cell.2012.03.036. PubMed PMID: 22541070; PubMed Central PMCID: PMC3351582.
71. Tseng WA, Thein T, Kinnunen K, Lashkari K, Gregory MS, D'Amore PA, et al. NLRP3 inflammasome activation in retinal pigment epithelial cells by lysosomal destabilization: implications for age-related macular degeneration. Invest Ophthalmol Vis Sci 2013;54(1):110–120. Epub 2012/12/12. https://doi.org/10.1167/iovs.12-10655. PubMed PMID: 23221073; PubMed Central PMCID: PMC3544415.
72. Anderson DH, Radeke MJ, Gallo NB, Chapin EA, Johnson PT, Curletti CR, et al. The pivotal role of the complement system in aging and age-related macular degeneration: hypothesis re-visited. Prog Retin Eye Res 2010;29(2):95–112. Epub 2009/12/08. https://doi.org/10.1016/j.preteyeres.2009.11.003. PubMed PMID: 19961953.
73. Clark SJ, Perveen R, Hakobyan S, Morgan BP, Sim RB, Bishop PN, et al. Impaired binding of the age-

related macular degeneration-associated complement factor H 402H allotype to Bruch's membrane in human retina. J Biol Chem 2010;285(39):30192–30202. Epub 2010/07/28. https://doi.org/10.1074/jbc.M110.103986. PubMed PMID: 20660596; PubMed Central PMCID: PMC2943316.
74. Johnson PT, Betts KE, Radeke MJ, Hageman GS, Anderson DH, Johnson LV. Individuals homozygous for the age-related macular degeneration risk-conferring variant of complement factor H have elevated levels of CRP in the choroid. Proc Natl Acad Sci USA 2006;103(46):17456–17461. Epub 2006/11/03. https://doi.org/10.1073/pnas.0606234103. PubMed PMID: 17079491; PubMed Central PMCID: PMC1859950.
75. Khandhadia S, Cipriani V, Yates JR, Lotery AJ. Age-related macular degeneration and the complement system. Immunobiology 2012;217(2):127–146. Epub 2011/08/27. https://doi.org/10.1016/j.imbio.2011.07.019. PubMed PMID: 21868123.
76. Lachmann PJ. The amplification loop of the complement pathways. Adv Immunol 2009;104:115–149. Epub 2009/01/01. https://doi.org/10.1016/s0065-2776(08)04004-2. PubMed PMID: 20457117.
77. Laine M, Jarva H, Seitsonen S, Haapasalo K, Lehtinen MJ, Lindeman N, et al. Y402H polymorphism of complement factor H affects binding affinity to C-reactive protein. J Immunol 2007;178(6):3831–3836. Epub 2007/03/07. PubMed PMID: 17339482.
78. Richards A, Kavanagh D, Atkinson JP. Inherited complement regulatory protein deficiency predisposes to human disease in acute injury and chronic inflammatory states the examples of vascular damage in atypical hemolytic uremic syndrome and debris accumulation in age-related macular degeneration. Adv Immunol 2007;96:141–177. Epub 2007/11/06. https://doi.org/10.1016/s0065-2776(07)96004-6. PubMed PMID: 17981206.
79. Sjoberg AP, Trouw LA, Clark SJ, Sjolander J, Heinegard D, Sim RB, et al. The factor H variant associated with age-related macular degeneration (His-384) and the non-disease-associated form bind differentially to C-reactive protein, fibromodulin, DNA, and necrotic cells. J Biol Chem 2007;282(15):10894–10900. Epub 2007/02/13. https://doi.org/10.1074/jbc.M610256200. PubMed PMID: 17293598.
80. Tuo J, Grob S, Zhang K, Chan CC. Genetics of immunological and inflammatory components in age-related macular degeneration. Ocul Immunol Inflamm 2012;20(1):27–36. Epub 2012/02/14. https://doi.org/10.3109/09273948.2011.628432. PubMed PMID: 22324898; PubMed Central PMCID: PMC3292785.
81. Clark RA. Basics of cutaneous wound repair. J Dermatol Surg Oncol 1993;19(8):693–706. Epub 1993/08/01. PubMed PMID: 8349909.
82. Singer AJ, Clark RA. Cutaneous wound healing. N Engl J Med 1999;341(10):738–746. Epub 1999/09/02. https://doi.org/10.1056/nejm199909023411006. PubMed PMID: 10471461.
83. Hageman GS, Anderson DH, Johnson LV, Hancox LS, Taiber AJ, Hardisty LI, et al. A common haplotype in the complement regulatory gene factor H (HF1/CFH) predisposes individuals to age-related macular degeneration. Proc Natl Acad Sci USA 2005;102(20):7227–7232. Epub 2005/05/05. https://doi.org/10.1073/pnas.0501536102. PubMed PMID: 15870199; PubMed Central PMCID: PMC1088171.
84. Haines JL, Hauser MA, Schmidt S, Scott WK, Olson LM, Gallins P, et al. Complement factor H variant increases the risk of age-related macular degeneration. Science 2005;308(5720):419–421. Epub 2005/03/12. https://doi.org/10.1126/science.1110359. PubMed PMID: 15761120.
85. Klein RJ, Zeiss C, Chew EY, Tsai JY, Sackler RS, Haynes C, et al. Complement factor H polymorphism in age-related macular degeneration. Science 2005;308(5720):385–389. Epub 2005/03/12. https://doi.org/10.1126/science.1109557. PubMed PMID: 15761122; PubMed Central PMCID: PMC1512523.
86. Bonafe M, Storci G, Franceschi C. Inflamm-aging of the stem cell niche: breast cancer as a paradigmatic example: breakdown of the multi-shell cytokine network fuels cancer in aged people. BioEssays 2012;34(1):40–49. Epub 2011/11/17. https://doi.org/10.1002/bies.201100104. PubMed PMID: 22086861.
87. Varadhan R, Yao W, Matteini A, Beamer BA, Xue QL, Yang H, et al. Simple biologically informed inflammatory index of two serum cytokines predicts 10 year all-cause mortality in older adults. J Gerontol A Biol Sci Med Sci 2014;69(2):165–173. Epub 2013/05/22. https://doi.org/10.1093/gerona/glt023. PubMed PMID: 23689826; PubMed Central PMCID: PMC4038244.
88. Tobe T, Ortega S, Luna JD, Ozaki H, Okamoto N, Derevjanik NL, et al. Targeted disruption of the FGF2 gene does not prevent choroidal neovascularization in a murine model. Am J Pathol 1998;153(5):1641–1646. Epub 1998/11/12. https://doi.org/10.1016/s0002-9440(10)65753-7. PubMed PMID: 9811357; PubMed Central PMCID: PMC1853405.
89. Kent D, Sheridan C. Choroidal neovascularization: a wound healing perspective. Mol Vis. 2003;9:747–55.
90. Clark RAF. Wound repair: overview and general considerations. In: Clark RAF, editor. The molecular and cellular biology of wound repair. Second ed. New York: Plenum; 1996. p. 1–50.
91. Hunt TK. Basic principles of wound healing. J Trauma 1990;30(12 Suppl):S122–S128. Epub 1990/12/01. PubMed PMID: 2254971.
92. Nathan C, Sporn M. Cytokines in context. J Cell Biol. 1991;113(5):981–6.

93. Blasiak J, Pawlowska E, Szczepanska J, Kaarniranta K. Interplay between Autophagy and the Ubiquitin-Proteasome System and Its Role in the Pathogenesis of Age-Related Macular Degeneration. International journal of molecular sciences. 2019;20(1). Epub 2019/01/11. https://doi.org/10.3390/ijms20010210. PubMed PMID: 30626110; PubMed Central PMCID: PMCPMC6337628.
94. Bornstein P. Diversity of function is inherent in matricellular proteins: an appraisal of thrombospondin 1. J Cell Biol. 1995;130(3):503–6.
95. Mones J, Garcia M, Biarnes M, Lakkaraju A, Ferraro L. Drusen Ooze: a novel hypothesis in geographic atrophy. Ophthalmol Retina 2017;1(6):461–473. Epub 2017/01/01. https://doi.org/10.1016/j.oret.2017.02.006. PubMed PMID: 31047436.
96. Schmitz-Valckenberg S, Sadda S, Staurenghi G, Chew EY, Fleckenstein M, Holz FG. Geographic atrophy: semantic considerations and literature review. Retina. 2016;36(12):2250–64. Epub 2016/08/24. https://doi.org/10.1097/iae.0000000000001258. PubMed PMID: 27552292; PubMed Central PMCID: PMCPMC5115977.
97. Pockley AG. Heat shock proteins, inflammation, and cardiovascular disease. Circulation 2002;105(8):1012–1017. Epub 2002/02/28. PubMed PMID: 11864934.
98. Fort PE, Lampi KJ. New focus on alpha-crystallins in retinal neurodegenerative diseases. Exp Eye Res. 2011;92(2):98–103. Epub 2010/12/01. https://doi.org/10.1016/j.exer.2010.11.008. PubMed PMID: 21115004; PubMed Central PMCID: PMCPmc4454605.
99. Dudeja V, Vickers SM, Saluja AK. The role of heat shock proteins in gastrointestinal diseases. Gut. 2009;58(7):1000–9. Epub 2009/06/13. https://doi.org/10.1136/gut.2007.140194. PubMed PMID: 19520890; PubMed Central PMCID: PMCPMC2896385.
100. Lu RC, Tan MS, Wang H, Xie AM, Yu JT, Tan L. Heat shock protein 70 in Alzheimer's disease. BioMed research international. 2014;2014:435203. Epub 2014/11/29. https://doi.org/10.1155/2014/435203. PubMed PMID: 25431764; PubMed Central PMCID: PMCPMC4241292.
101. Morimoto RI, Santoro MG. Stress-inducible responses and heat shock proteins: new pharmacologic targets for cytoprotection. Nat Biotechnol 1998;16(9):833–838. Epub 1998/09/22. https://doi.org/10.1038/nbt0998-833. PubMed PMID: 9743115.
102. Srivastava K, Narang R, Bhatia J, Saluja D. Expression of heat shock protein 70 gene and its correlation with inflammatory markers in essential hypertension. PLoS One. 2016;11(3):e0151060. Epub 2016/03/19. https://doi.org/10.1371/journal.pone.0151060. PubMed PMID: 26989902; PubMed Central PMCID: PMCPMC4798713.
103. Xu Q, Metzler B, Jahangiri M, Mandal K. Molecular chaperones and heat shock proteins in atherosclerosis. Am J Physiol Heart Circ Physiol. 2012;302(3):H506–14. Epub 2011/11/08. https://doi.org/10.1152/ajpheart.00646.2011. PubMed PMID: 22058161; PubMed Central PMCID: PMCPMC3353778.
104. Santoro MG. Heat shock factors and the control of the stress response. Biochem Pharmacol 2000;59(1):55–63. Epub 1999/12/22. PubMed PMID: 10605935.
105. Lanneau D, de Thonel A, Maurel S, Didelot C, Garrido C. Apoptosis versus cell differentiation: role of heat shock proteins HSP90, HSP70 and HSP27. Prion. 2007;1(1):53–60. Epub 2007/01/01. PubMed PMID: 19164900; PubMed Central PMCID: PMCPmc2633709.
106. De Cilla S, Vezzola D, Farruggio S, Vujosevic S, Clemente N, Raina G, et al. The subthreshold micropulse laser treatment of the retina restores the oxidant/antioxidant balance and counteracts programmed forms of cell death in the mice eyes. Acta Ophthalmol. 2018. Epub 2018/12/27. https://doi.org/10.1111/aos.13995. PubMed PMID: 30585429.
107. Gao X, Xing D. Molecular mechanisms of cell proliferation induced by low power laser irradiation. Journal of biomedical science. 2009;16:4. Epub 2009/03/11. https://doi.org/10.1186/1423-0127-16-4. PubMed PMID: 19272168; PubMed Central PMCID: PMCPMC2644974.
108. Iwami H, Pruessner J, Shiraki K, Brinkmann R, Miura Y. Protective effect of a laser-induced sub-lethal temperature rise on RPE cells from oxidative stress. Exp Eye Res 2014;124:37–47. Epub 2014/05/08. https://doi.org/10.1016/j.exer.2014.04.014. PubMed PMID: 24800654.
109. Karu TI, Kolyakov SF. Exact action spectra for cellular responses relevant to phototherapy. Photomed Laser Surg 2005;23(4):355–361. Epub 2005/09/08. https://doi.org/10.1089/pho.2005.23.355. PubMed PMID: 16144476.
110. Lund DJ, Sliney DH. A new understanding of multiple-pulsed laser-induced retinal injury thresholds. Health Phys 2014;106(4):505–515. Epub 2014/02/25. https://doi.org/10.1097/HP.0b013e3182a2a837. PubMed PMID: 24562071.
111. Caballero S, Kent DL, Sengupta N, Li Calzi S, Shaw L, Beli E, et al. Bone marrow-derived cell recruitment to the neurosensory retina and retinal pigment epithelial cell layer following subthreshold retinal phototherapy. Invest Ophthalmol Vis Sci. 2017.
112. Flaxel C, Bradle J, Acott T, Samples JR. Retinal pigment epithelium produces matrix metalloproteinases after laser treatment. Retina 2007;27(5):629–634. Epub 2007/06/15. https://doi.org/10.1097/01.iae.0000249561.02567.fd. PubMed PMID: 17558327.

113. Hattenbach LO, Beck KF, Pfeilschifter J, Koch F, Ohrloff C, Schacke W. Pigment-epithelium-derived factor is upregulated in photocoagulated human retinal pigment epithelial cells. Ophthalmic Res 2005;37(6):341–346. Epub 2005/09/15. https://doi.org/10.1159/000088263. PubMed PMID: 16158012.
114. Inagaki K, Shuo T, Katakura K, Ebihara N, Murakami A, Ohkoshi K. Sublethal photothermal stimulation with a micropulse laser induces heat shock protein expression in ARPE-19 cells. J Ophthalmol 2015;2015:729792. Epub 2015/12/24. https://doi.org/10.1155/2015/729792. PubMed PMID: 26697211; PubMed Central PMCID: PMC4677213.
115. Karu T. Photobiology of low-power laser effects. Health Phys 1989;56(5):691–704. Epub 1989/05/01. PubMed PMID: 2651364.
116. Midena E, Bini S, Martini F, Enrica C, Pilotto E, Micera A, et al. Changes of aqueous humor muller cells' biomarkers in human patients affected by diabetic macular edema after subthreshold micropulse laser treatment. Retina. 2018. Epub 2018/10/10. https://doi.org/10.1097/iae.0000000000002356. PubMed PMID: 30300267.
117. Kaarniranta K, Tokarz P, Koskela A, Paterno J, Blasiak J. Autophagy regulates death of retinal pigment epithelium cells in age-related macular degeneration. Cell biology and toxicology. 2017;33(2):113–28. Epub 2016/12/03. https://doi.org/10.1007/s10565-016-9371-8. PubMed PMID: 27900566; PubMed Central PMCID: PMCPMC5325845.
118. Kaarniranta K, Elo M, Sironen R, Lammi MJ, Goldring MB, Eriksson JE, et al. Hsp70 accumulation in chondrocytic cells exposed to high continuous hydrostatic pressure coincides with mRNA stabilization rather than transcriptional activation. Proc Natl Acad Sci USA. 1998;95(5):2319–24. Epub 1998/04/16. PubMed PMID: 9482883; PubMed Central PMCID: PMCPMC19331.
119. Kaarniranta K, Salminen A, Eskelinen EL, Kopitz J. Heat shock proteins as gatekeepers of proteolytic pathways-Implications for age-related macular degeneration (AMD). Ageing Res Rev 2009;8(2):128–139. Epub 2009/03/12. PubMed PMID: 19274853.
120. Buchner J. Supervising the fold: functional principles of molecular chaperones. FASEB J 1996;10(1):10–19. Epub 1996/01/01. PubMed PMID: 8566529.
121. Johnson LV, Leitner WP, Rivest AJ, Staples MK, Radeke MJ, Anderson DH. The Alzheimer's a beta-peptide is deposited at sites of complement activation in pathologic deposits associated with aging and age-related macular degeneration. Proc Natl Acad Sci USA 2002;99(18):11830–11835. Epub 2002/08/22. https://doi.org/10.1073/pnas.192203399. PubMed PMID: 12189211; PubMed Central PMCID: PMC129354.
122. Kopito RR. Aggresomes, inclusion bodies and protein aggregation. Trends Cell Biol 2000;10(12):524–530. Epub 2000/12/21. PubMed PMID: 11121744.
123. Ryhanen T, Hyttinen JM, Kopitz J, Rilla K, Kuusisto E, Mannermaa E, et al. Crosstalk between Hsp70 molecular chaperone, lysosomes and proteasomes in autophagy-mediated proteolysis in human retinal pigment epithelial cells. J Cell Mol Med. 2009;13(9b):3616–31. Epub 2008/11/20. https://doi.org/10.1111/j.1582-4934.2008.00577.x. PubMed PMID: 19017362; PubMed Central PMCID: PMCPMC4516511.
124. Ryhanen T, Viiri J, Hyttinen JM, Uusitalo H, Salminen A, Kaarniranta K. Influence of Hsp90 and HDAC inhibition and tubulin acetylation on perinuclear protein aggregation in human retinal pigment epithelial cells. J Biomed Biotechnol. 2011;2011:798052. Epub 2010/10/29. https://doi.org/10.1155/2011/798052. PubMed PMID: 20981255; PubMed Central PMCID: PMCPMC2963810.
125. Mones J, Garcia M, Biarnes M, Lakkaraju A, Ferraro L. Drusen Ooze: a novel hypothesis in geographic atrophy. Ophthalmol Retina. 2017;1:461–73.
126. Gao J, Liu RT, Cao S, Cui JZ, Wang A, To E, et al. NLRP3 inflammasome: activation and regulation in age-related macular degeneration. Mediators Inflamm. 2015;2015:690243. Epub 2015/02/24. https://doi.org/10.1155/2015/690243. PubMed PMID: 25698849; PubMed Central PMCID: PMCPMC4324923.
127. Martine P, Chevriaux A, Derangere V, Apetoh L, Garrido C, Ghiringhelli F, et al. HSP70 is a negative regulator of NLRP3 inflammasome activation. Cell Death Disease. 2019;10(4):256. Epub 2019/03/16. https://doi.org/10.1038/s41419-019-1491-7. PubMed PMID: 30874540; PubMed Central PMCID: PMCPMC6420651.

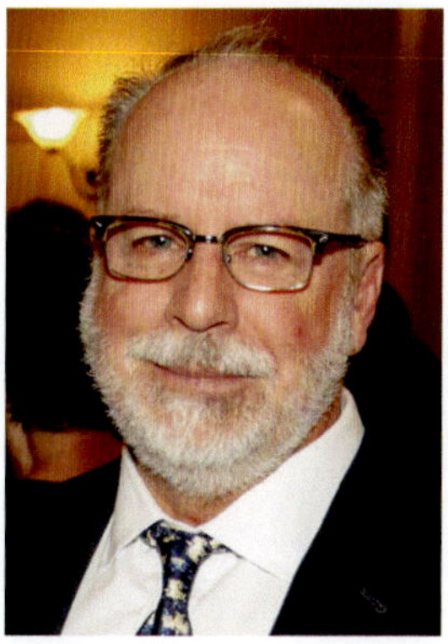

Jeffrey K. Luttrull, MD, is a vitreoretinal surgeon and clinical researcher practicing in Ventura, California. His interests and publications include medical and surgical retina, with a special interest in retinal laser therapy. He is the founder and director of LIGHT: The International Retinal Laser Society.

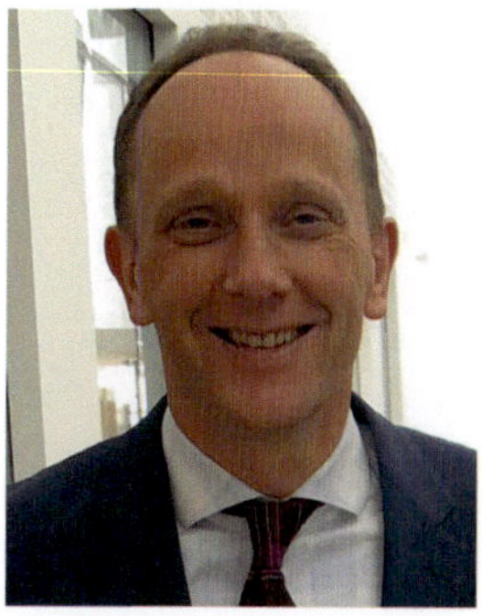

David Kent FRCOphth is a vitreoretinal surgeon practicing in The Vision Clinic, Kilkenny, Ireland. His research interests include the experimental investigation and therapeutic use of light to modulate and promote repair in the aging retina. He has been a member of the RPE Cell biology section of ARVO since 1996 and currently serves as a director of LIGHT: The International Retinal Laser Society.

31 Choroidal Neovascularization: Newer Molecules

Aamir A. Aziz, Ibrahim Khanani, Fawwaz A. Siddiqui, Ryan N. Constantine, and Arshad M. Khanani

31.1 Introduction

Over the past two decades the treatment for neovascular age-related macular degeneration (NVAMD) has undergone significant improvements. No longer are patients destined for blindness, but rather, efficacious therapies are now enabling patients to maintain vision as well as improve visual outcomes following the onset of symptoms. By highlighting the development of current therapies for NVAMD, one can gain insight into the direction the field is headed in the future [1].

With the elucidation of direct scientific evidence supporting the role of vascular endothelial growth factor (VEGF) in ocular angiogenesis, development and administration of anti-VEGF therapies aimed at treating NVAMD, was established as the primary therapeutic avenue. The first antiangiogenic molecule approved by the U.S. Food and Drug Administration (FDA) for the treatment of ocular neovascularization was pegaptanib. It is an RNA aptamer that binds VEGF165 and was shown in Phase II and III clinical trials to decrease visual loss associated with NVAMD [2].

Prior to the development of pegaptanib, Genentech (South San Francisco, CA) developed bevacizumab, a humanized anti-VEGF antibody aimed at blocking VEGF-A. Bevacizumab initially entered Phase I clinical trials for cancer. With results indicating its efficacy and minimal toxicity profile, it was subsequently approved for the co-treatment with chemotherapy of colon cancer by the FDA in 2004 [3]. However, increasing evidence showing the role of VEGF in ocular angiogenesis as noted above led to the off-label use of intravenous bevacizumab for the treatment of NVAMD [4]. Shortly thereafter, off-label intravitreal injections of bevacizumab for the treatment of NVAMD were shown to be effective with minimal systemic side effects [5].

Ranibizumab is also developed by Genentech (South San Francisco, CA) and received FDA approval in 2006. Ranibizumab is a monoclonal antibody fragment that inhibits angiogenesis by inhibiting vascular endothelial growth factor A. Two pivotal Phase III trials; ANCHOR and MARINA established efficacy and safety of ranibizumab in patients with NVAMD [6, 7].

A third molecule, aflibercept, developed by Regeneron Pharmaceuticals (Tarrytown, NY) employs a different anti-VEGF strategy. Aflibercept functions as a VEGF-trap, acting as a receptor decoy to sequester VEGF. Aflibercept is a recombinant fusion protein consisting of vascular endothelial growth factor (VEGF)—binding portions from the extracellular domains of human VEGF receptors 1 and 2 that are fused to the Fc portion of human IgG1 [8]. Aflibercept was

A. A. Aziz · I. Khanani · F. A. Siddiqui
R. N. Constantine · A. M. Khanani (✉)
Sierra Eye Associates, Reno, NV, USA

J. Chhablani (ed.), *Choroidal Neovascularization*, https://doi.org/10.1007/978-981-15-2213-0_31

approved by the FDA in 2011 following the Phase III results from the two pivotal trials: VIEW 1 and VIEW 2. These trials indicated that aflibercept dosed every two months was not inferior to monthly ranibizumab dosing [3].

Despite the effectiveness of the current therapies available for patients with NVAMD, there continues to be a need for treatment options with increased durability. Achieving this goal is not easy and significant effort has been invested in discovering new efficacious targets and molecules aimed at decreasing the treatment burden that patients with NVAMD face. The remainder of this chapter focuses on new molecules that are in clinical development for the treatment of NVAMD.

31.2 Brolucizumab

Brolucizumab is a single-chain antibody fragment with a molecular weight of 26 kDa. This molecule is considerably smaller than any other available anti-VEGF agent [9]. This results in concentrated molar dosing and potent VEGF-A inhibition. The 6 mg dose of brolucizumab is equivalent to approximately 11–12 times higher molar dose than 2 mg aflibercept. Preclinical studies have shown that the smaller molecular size results in increased ocular tissue penetration, increasing localized concentrations of the molecule in deeper levels of the retina.

During animal studies, brolucizumab showed a fourfold lower systemic exposure in comparison to ranibizumab while also showing tolerability to higher doses and a high affinity to VEGF [10]. Early human studies also exhibited positive results, where a single dose of brolucizumab was shown to be more potent and longer lasting than a single dose of ranibizumab.

The Phase II (OSPREY) study met its primary endpoint and confirmed non-inferiority of brolucizumab to aflibercept in terms of mean change in best-corrected visual acuity (BCVA) from baseline to weeks 12 and 16. The study also showed that eyes treated with brolucizumab had more stable central subfield reductions, received fewer unscheduled treatments, and had higher rates of fluid resolution [11]. This led to the initiation of pivotal Phase III HAWK and HARRIER studies which looked at 1825 patients with treatment-naïve NVAMD that were either treated with brolucizumab or aflibercept. In HAWK and HARRIER, patients received three monthly doses of brolucizumab and then received either a dose every 8 weeks or every 12 weeks based on disease activity assessment. Patients in the aflibercept arm received three monthly doses and then a dose every 8 weeks per the label. The studies met the primary endpoint of non-inferiority of brolucizumab compared to aflibercept in mean change in best-corrected visual acuity from baseline to week 48 [12]. Patients gained +6.6 (6 mg) and +6.1 (3 mg) letters with brolucizumab versus +6.8 letters with aflibercept in HAWK and +6.9 (6 mg) letters with brolucizumab versus +7.6 letters with aflibercept in HARRIER. The other key endpoints were patients maintained on every 12-week dosing till week 48 as well as anatomic outcomes at week 16 and week 48. Fifty-six percent of eyes in HAWK and 51% in HARRIER were maintained on every 12-week dosing till week 48. As far as anatomic outcomes, patients treated with brolucizumab 6 mg had significantly less intraretinal fluid (IRF), subretinal fluid (SRF), and subretinal pigment epithelium (Sub-RPE) fluid at week 16 and week 48 [13]. Brolucizumab treatment resulted in an additional 30–40% of patients with no fluid compared to aflibercept at those time points. The overall safety of brolucizumab was comparable to aflibercept. Based on the data from HAWK and HARRIER, Brolucizumab received FDA approval in the United States in October 2019.

31.3 Abicipar

Abicipar is a novel designed ankyrin repeat protein (DARPin) which functions by binding to targeted proteins with increased precision and affinity [14]. A new agent functioning against choroidal neovascularization, abicipar pegol targets the VEGF-A_{165} isoform, which is primarily expressed in humans and associated with pathologic angiogenesis [14]. Abicipar has a small molecular weight of 32 kDa with a polyethylene tail, which effectively increases the drug's intravitreal half-life. Abicipar 2 mg dose is equal to approximately 3.4 times the 2 mg aflibercept dose and demonstrates an increased period of effectiveness when compared to ranibizumab at equal molar doses. When comparing abicipar to ranibizumab or aflibercept, abicipar has a 100-fold increased affinity for VEGF-A_{165}.

In the Phase II REACH study, abicipar demonstrated BCVA and CRT improvements that were similar between abicipar and ranibizumab at weeks 16 and 20. This was 8 and 12 weeks after the last abicipar injection and 4 weeks after the last ranibizumab injection, confirming a durability effect [15].

In the Phase III CEDAR and SEQUOIA studies, 1885 treatment-naïve NVAMD eyes were randomized to abicipar or ranibizumab. Patients received either 0.5 mg ranibizumab monthly, 2.0 mg abicipar pegol every 8 weeks after 3 monthly doses, or 2.0 mg abicipar pegol every 12 weeks after doses at baseline, week 4, and week 12. The primary endpoint at week 52 of non-inferiority to ranibizumab was met. 91.2% and 96% of each abicipar arm lost less than 15 letters at week 52 compared to baseline [16]. Looking at the ocular safety, approximately 15% of patients in the abicipar treatment groups experienced inflammatory events [17]. More information is needed to understand these events better, but the current hypothesis is that this could be related to the manufacturing process. The company is working on a better purification and manufacturing process. The open-label safety Phase III MAPLE study was conducted with the improved manufacturing process in an effort to increase safety. Results from MAPLE has shown improvements in these inflammatory event rates at 8.9%, a reduction from the 15% experienced by patients in CEDAR and SEQUOIA [18].

31.4 Faricimab

Faricimab (formerly RG7716) is the first bispecific antibody that is designed for intravitreal use. It has been developed using CrossMAb technology to bind VEGF-A on one arm and angiopoietin-2 (Ang2) on the other. Preclinical studies have shown that Ang-2 levels are elevated in patients with AMD [19–22] and blocking Ang-2 reduces VEGF-induced endothelial barrier breakdown [23]. Animal studies have also shown that combined VEGF-A/Ang-2 inhibition reduces CNV lesion number and area, inhibits retinal leukocyte infiltration, and prolongs anti-leakage effect. Phase I study results confirmed faricimab was safe and well-tolerated with improvements in BCVA and anatomic parameters for patients with difficult-to-treat neovascular AMD [24], leading to Phase II AVENUE and STAIRWAY studies.

AVENUE confirmed the efficacy and safety of faricimab every 4 and 8 weeks in patients with treatment-naïve NVAMD compared to monthly doses of ranibizumab. STAIRWAY was designed to evaluate the efficacy and durability of faricimab in treat-naïve patients with NVAMD. Patients were treated with four monthly doses of faricimab and then treated every 16 week or every 12 weeks based on disease activity compared to ranibizumab monthly. The primary endpoint was efficacy of faricimab given every 16 weeks and every 12 weeks as assessed by BCVA [24]. Prespecified disease activity was performed at week 24, which was 12 weeks after the last faricimab dose. Sixty-five percent of patients treated with faricimab had no disease activity 12 weeks after the last injection. Vision gains were similar between all three treatment groups and were fully maintained through week 52. Patients treated with every 16-week faricimab gained +11.4 chart letters from baseline, compared to +10.1 letters in 12-week faricimab and +9.6 letters in every 4-week ranibizumab group. All three treatment regimens showed a similar proportion of patients gaining +15 chart letters and avoiding a loss of more than −15 letters. Anatomic outcomes were also similar among three groups as evaluated by change in central subfield thickness as well as reduction in CNV lesion size from baseline to week 52. There were no new safety signals and the overall safety profile of faricimab was similar to ranibizumab. Based on the data from the AVENUE and STAIRWAY studies, faricimab holds the potential of extended durability in patients with NVAMD. Therefore, Phase 3 TENAYA/LUCERNE studies were initiated in 2019 and are currently ongoing.

31.5 Nesvacumab

Nesvacumab is a fully human monoclonal antibody and effectively inactivates Ang2. When combining nesvacumab with an anti-VEGF agent, the potential for preventing the pathological processes of angiogenesis in neovascular AMD is greatly increased.

The Phase I study combined nesvacumab and aflibercept, while evaluating safety and tolerance in 20 patients with neovascular AMD and DME. The reported results exhibited that visual and anatomical improvement at all dose levels, with no reported dose-limiting toxicities, ocular inflammation, or any unexpected systemic effects [25].

The Phase II study, ONYX, evaluated patients with wet AMD, using a combination of nesvacumab and aflibercept. The results of this study did not provide sufficient differentiation between the combination therapy and independent aflibercept to support a Phase III study [26].

31.6 Squalamine Drops

Developed by OHR Pharmaceutical, squalamine is a topical antiangiogenic ophthalmic eye drop that functions by inhibiting multiple growth factors, such as VEGF, platelet-derived growth factor (PDGF) and basic fibroblast growth factor (bFGF) [27, 28].

In the Phase III study, squalamine drops were given topically in conjunction with ranibizumab injections ($n = 119$), compared to an independent treatment of just ranibizumab ($n = 118$). Patients with the squalamine/ranibizumab combination experienced an average of an +8.33 chart letter improvement from baseline visual acuity, while the ranibizumab monotherapy patients experienced a +10.58 chart letter improvement. Although there was no difference in the safety profile of both therapy groups, the difference in mean improvement of acuity using squalamine failed expected efficacy results, ending the hope for squalamine as a topical therapy for NVAMD.

31.7 Fovista

Fovista is an aptamer directed against platelet-derived growth factor (anti-PDGF). PDGF functions by recruiting pericytes to neovascular complexes and once there, they supply VEGF and additional growth factors necessary for endothelial cells to build new blood vessels [29]. Both cell culture and animal models showed that overexpression of PDGF resulted in an increased proliferation of pericytes and tumor growth [30–32]. By inhibiting PDGF, Fovista indirectly decreases the VEGF load, thus inhibiting neovascularization within the retina.

After positive Phase II trials, Fovista was tested in combination with ranibizumab compared to ranibizumab monotherapy in two separate Phase III trials. No significant improvements in visual acuity were reported with the combination therapy when compared to patients treated with ranibizumab monotherapy [33]. Therefore, the Fovista development program has been terminated.

31.8 KSI-301

KSI-301 is an antibody biopolymer conjugate developed by Kodiak Sciences [34]. KSI-301 also targets VEGF and in vitro assays demonstrate that the molecule has increased potency when compared to bevacizumab, ranibizumab, and aflibercept. The molecular weight is 950 kDa, as a result of its phosphorylcholine biopolymer. This biopolymer leads to increased ocular tissue bioavailability in both the retina and the choroid when compared to aflibercept (approximately a 30-day increase in both cases).

The Phase 1a trial met safety outcomes and improvements in vision and retinal thickness in heavily previously treated patients with diabetic macular edema. All dose levels were well-tolerated without any drug-related adverse events. Twelve weeks after the single dose, median vision gain from baseline was +9 letters, and median OCT improvement of −121 microns were observed across all three dose levels.

Phase 1b trials recently began in 2019 with safety, efficacy and durability as the key endpoints. The 1b trials tested multiple doses of KSI-301 in treatment-naïve patients with NVAMD, diabetic macular edema, and retinal vein occlusions. Interim data from the trial revealed that the wAMD cohort gained an average of +8 letters from baseline and showed a −96 micron improvement in median retinal thickness [35]. The positive results influenced both an extension of the 1b trial and the Phase 2 trial DAZZLE, which began in Q3 of 2019. DAZZLE is a randomized trial comparing KSI-301 to aflibercept and seeks to extend injection intervals for KSI-301 after 3 loading doses to up to 20 weeks, greatly reducing the treatment burden of afflicted patients.

31.9 Sunitinib

Sunitinib malate is a multiple receptor tyrosine kinase inhibitor that is approved as an oral agent for solid tumors including renal cell carcinoma, imatinib-resistant gastrointestinal stromal tumor, and pancreatic neuroendocrine tumors. Whereas bevacizumab, ranibizumab, and aflibercept all function to inhibit VEGF-receptors 1 and 2 (VEGFR), sunitinib selectively inhibits VEGFR-1, -2, -3, platelet-derived growth factor receptors (PDGFR-α, -β), stem cell growth factor receptor (KIT), colony-stimulating factor receptor (CSFR-1), and Fms-related tyrosine kinase receptor (FLT3). Sunitinib is formulated as injectable intravitreal poly-(lactic-co-glycolic acid) (PLGA) molecules that aggregate to form a depot in the inferior vitreous out of the visual axis. The depot allows sunitinib to be regarded with the potential of only two injections per year, a massive decrease for patients receiving monthly injections.

Preclinical animal studies support biannual dosing following a single intravitreal injection of sunitinib [36]. A Phase 1/2a study of a single injection of sunitinib with dose-escalating cohorts showed that sunitinib maintained BCVA and CST that was equivalent to patients receiving standard of care intravitreal anti-VEGF agents with 6-week dosing. The majority of the adverse events noted in the Phase 1/2a study were the result of the migration of the bio-absorbable particles into the anterior chamber due to incomplete aggregation into a depot. These events were described as self-limited and reversible as the formulation biodegrades within the eye and at month 6 there were no observed sequelae.

A new optimized version of sunitinib has been manufactured to eliminate particle dispersion for Phase 2b NVAMD study, which was initiated in Q3 of 2019. The study ALTISSIMO compares 1 mg and 2 mg doses of sunitinib biannually to a 2 mg dose of aflibercept administered every 2 months. Sunitinib is also currently being tested for its safety and efficacy in RVO and DME, along with NVAMD.

31.10 Conbercept

Conbercept is a recombinant fusion protein targeting VEGF-R-1 and -2 [37]. Conbercept is composed of the second IgG domain of VEGF-R-1 and the third and fourth domains of VEGF-R-2 to the Fc region of human IgG. The agent has a molecular weight of 143 kDa and in-vitro assays revealed that the drug has a 30-fold increased affinity for VEGF than ranibizumab or bevacizumab. The biochemical functionality of conbercept allows it to target both VEGF-A, -B, and -C, along with placental derived growth factors (PIGF).

In the trial AURORA, patients were randomized 1:1 to either a 0.5 mg dose or 2.0 dose. After three monthly doses, patients were randomized to either a prn treatment schedule or continued monthly, with no changes to their initial dosage randomization. At month 3, mean BCVA improvement in the 0.5 mg cohort was +8.97 letters, while the 2.0 mg cohort had an increase of +10.43 letters. At the month 12 evaluation, mean BCVA improvement was +14.31 letters for the 0.5 mg prn cohort and +9.31 for the 0.5 mg monthly cohort. At the same checkpoint, BCVA improvements for the 2.0 mg cohort were +12.42 for the 2.0 mg prn cohort, and +15.43 for the 2.0 mg monthly cohort, respectively. Statistically significant reductions in central retinal thickness (CRT) were also found. At month 12, CRT reduction was −119.8 microns for the 0.5 mg prn cohort, −129.7 microns for the 0.5 mg monthly cohort, −152.1 microns for the 2.0 mg prn cohort, and −170.8 microns for the 2.0 mg monthly cohort. Two serious adverse events were recorded in this trial, a case of endophthalmitis associated to the injection procedure, and cataract development associated to the study drug.

The subsequent trial PHOENIX randomized patients 2:1 to two cohorts: treatment and delayed treatment [38]. In the treatment cohort, patients were given monthly injections of conbercept 0.5 mg for 3 months, then extended to quarterly injections of the same dosage. In the delayed treatment cohort, patients received sham injections monthly for 3 months, then moved to conbercept 0.5 mg injections monthly for 3 months, then extended to quarterly injections at the 0.5 mg dosage. By month 12, the treatment group showed a +9.9 letter gain in BCVA, while the delayed treatment group showed a +8.8 letter improvement. Both groups showed reductions in CRT with no statistical significance between the two cohorts. No ocular serious adverse events were noted in relation to the study drug.

Currently, conbercept is being studied at the global level in two masked, randomized studies known as PANDA-1 and PANDA-2. Both trials have three cohorts in a 1:1:1 randomization, of 0.5 mg conbercept every 8 weeks, 1.0 mg conbercept every 12 weeks, and 2.0 mg aflibercept every 8 weeks. All three cohorts received 3 monthly loading doses and were then extended to their respective intervals. PANDA-2 differs at week 40, where all patients then begin a capped (max interval of 16 weeks) prn treatment of their cohort. Both studies are ongoing and follow patients through 96 weeks, with the hopes that conbercept proves itself as non-inferior to aflibercept.

31.11 OPT-302

OPT-302 is a soluble form of VEGF-R-3 and functions as a "trap" molecule that blocks VEGF-C and VEGF-D [39]. When an anti-VEGF agent such as ranibizumab blocks VEGF-A, the proteins VEGF-C and VEGF-D are noted to be upregulated. OPT-302 is designed to work in conjunction with an anti-VEGF-A agent and provides a more complete inhibition of the four classes of VEGFs by also inhibiting VEGF-C/-D.

OPT-302 recently completed its Phase 2b trial and met its primary endpoints [40]. Combined OPT-302 and ranibizumab treatment had increased vision gains compared to ranibizumab monotherapy. Along with these results, OPT-302/ranibizumab also showed anatomical improvements, including a reduced central subfield thickness (CST), a decrease in choroidal neovascularization (CNV) lesion size and decreases in intra-/subretinal fluid. Patients in the 2.0 mg OPT-302/ranibizumab therapy gained +14.2 letters, while the low-dosage cohort of 0.5 mg OPT-302/ranibizumab gained +9.4 letters. The ranibizumab monotherapy group showed an improvement of +10.8 letters. By week 24, the 2.0 mg OPT-302/ranibizumab cohort showed a mean CST reduction of −147 microns, from baseline. The ranibizumab monotherapy showed a −134 micron reduction at the same checkpoint. OPT-302 is currently in preparation for Phase 3 studies as the Phase 2a study for DME nears completion.

31.12 Conclusions

Despite currently available efficacious vision saving therapies for NVAMD, including bevacizumab, ranibizumab, and aflibercept, significant efforts continue to be made toward developing novel therapies for patients suffering from NVAMD. The current treatment regime for those afflicted with NVAMD, typically the aging population, is burdensome. To maintain visual acuity, Q4 weekly to Q8 weekly office visits are the norm and for an elderly patient population, can pose several challenges including cost, transportation, and postinjection pain and discomfort. As outlined in this chapter, the focus is to develop new molecules with increased durability as compared to current therapies. These longer lasting treatments for NVAMD carry the hope of decreasing treatment burden and improving visual acuity outcomes in the real world.

References

1. Holz FG, Tadayoni R, Beatty S. Multi-country real-life experience of anti-vascular endothelial growth factor therapy for wet age-related macular degeneration. Br J Ophthalmol. 2015;99:220–6.
2. Gragoudas ES, Adamis AP, Cunningham ET Jr, Feinsod M, Guyer DR. VEGF inhibition study in ocular neovascularization clinical trial group pegaptanib for neovascular age-related macular degeneration. N Engl J Med. 2004;351:2805–16.
3. Kim LA, D'Amore PA. A brief history of anti-VEGF for the treatment of ocular angiogenesis. Am J Pathol. 2012 Aug;181(2):376–9.
4. Michels S, Rosenfeld PJ, Puliafito CA, Marcus EN, Venkatraman AS. Systemic bevacizumab (Avastin) therapy for neovascular age-related macular degeneration: twelve-week results of an uncontrolled open-label clinical study. Ophthalmology. 2005;112:1035–47.
5. Rosenfeld PJ, Moshfeghi AA, Puliafito CA. Optical coherence tomography findings after an intravitreal injection of bevacizumab (Avastin) for neovascular age-related macular degeneration. Ophthalmic Surg Lasers Imaging. 2005;36:331–5.
6. Rosenfeld PJ, Brown DM, Heier JS, Boyer DS, Kaiser PK, Chung CY, Kim RY. MARINA study group ranibizumab for neovascular age-related macular degeneration. N Engl J Med. 2006;355:1419–31.
7. Brown DM, Kaiser PK, Michels M, Soubrane G, Heier JS, Kim RY, Sy JP, Schneider S. ANCHOR study group ranibizumab versus verteporfin for neovascular age-related macular degeneration. N Engl J Med. 2006;355:1432–44.
8. Semeraro F, Morescalchi F, Duse S, Parmeggiani F, Gambicorti E, Costagliola C. Aflibercept in wet AMD: specific role and optimal use. Drug Des Devel Ther. 2013;7:711–722. Published 2013 Aug 5. https://doi.org/10.2147/DDDT.S40215
9. Positive phase II data highlights benefits of Alcon's RTH258 for patients with neovascular (wet) age-related macular degeneration [Internet]. Alcon. Alcon; 2015 [cited 2019Feb13]. Available from https://www.alcon.com/media-release/positive-phase-ii-data-highlights-benefits-alcons-rth258-patients-neovascular-wet-age
10. Dugel P. Results of ESBA 1008, a single-chain antibody fragment for the treatment of neovascular AMD. Paper presented at: Annual meeting of the American Society of Retina Specialists; San Diego, CA; August 9–13, 2014.
11. Dugel PU, Jaffe GJ, Sallstig P, Warburton J, Weichselberger A, Wieland M, Singerman L. Brolucizumab versus aflibercept in participants with neovascular age-related macular degeneration: a randomized trial. Ophthalmology. 2017 Sep;124(9):1296–1304. https://doi.org/10.1016/j.ophtha.2017.03.057. Epub 2017 May 24.
12. Dugel P.U., Koh A., Ogura Y., Jaffe G., Schmidt-Erfurth U., Brown D. HAWK and HARRIER: phase 3, multicenter, randomized, double-masked trials of brolucizumab for neovascular age-related macular degeneration. Ophthalmology. 2019 Apr 12. pii: S0161-6420(18)33018-5. https://doi.org/10.1016/j.ophtha.2019.04.017. [Epub ahead of print].
13. Novartis. Two-year data for Novartis brolucizumab reaffirm superiority versus aflibercept in reducing retinal fluid in patients with nAMD [Press Release] (2018 Oct 27) [cited 2019Feb13]. Available from https://novartis.gcs-web.com/Two-year-data-for-Novartis-brolucizumab-reaffirm-superiority-versus-aflibercept-in-reducing-retinal-fluid-in-patients-with-nAMD
14. Gerard A. Rodrigues, Matthew Mason, Lori-Ann Christie, Candice Hansen, Lisa M. Hernandez, James Burke, Keith A. Luhrs, Thomas C. Hohman; Functional Characterization of Abicipar-Pegol, an Anti-VEGF DARPin Therapeutic That Potently Inhibits Angiogenesis and Vascular Permeability. Invest Ophthalmol Vis Sci. 2018;59(15):5836–5846. https://doi.org/10.1167/iovs.18-25307
15. Callanan D, Kunimoto D, Maturi RK, Patel SS, Staurenghi G, Wolf S, Cheetham JK, Hohman TC, Kim K, López FJ, Schneider S, and for the REACH Study Group. Double-masked, randomized, phase 2 evaluation of abicipar pegol (an anti-VEGF DARPin therapeutic) in neovascular age-related macular degeneration. J Ocular Pharmacol Therapeutics. Dec 2018. https://doi.org/10.1089/jop.2018.0062 [Epub ahead of print].
16. Khurana R. Phase 3 CEDAR and SEQUOIA clinical trial results. Presentation at; 2018; American Academy of Ophthalmology, Chicago, IL.
17. Allergan and molecular partners announce two positive phase 3 clinical trials for abicipar pegol 8 a [Internet]. Allergan. Allergan; 2018 [cited 2019 Feb 13]. Available from https://www.allergan.com/news/news/thomson-reuters/allergan-and-molecular-partners-announce-two-posit.aspx

18. Molecular Partners. Allergan and Molecular Partners Announce Topline Safety Results from MAPLE Study of Abicipar pegol [Press Release] (2019 Apr 2) [Cited 2019 June 02]. Available from https://www.molecularpartners.com/allergan-and-molecular-partners-announce-topline-safety-results-from-maple-study-of-abicipar-pegol/
19. Thurston G, Daly C. The complex role of angiopoietin-2 in the angiopoietin-tie signaling pathway. Cold Spring Harbor Perspectives in Medicine. 2012;2(9).
20. Khanani AM. The Tie2 activator AKB-9778, used in combination with ranibizumab, enhances reduction of diabetic macular edema compared to ranibizumab monotherapy. Invest Ophthalmol Vis Sci. 2016;57(12); no pagination specified. http://iovs.arvojournals.org/article.aspx?articleid=2560785 Accessed May 15, 2017.
21. Campochiaro PA, Khanani AM. Enhanced benefit in diabetic macular edema from AKB-9778 Tie2 activation combined with vascular endothelial growth factor suppression. Ophthalmology. 2016;123:1722–30.
22. Chakravarthy U, Bailey C, Brown D, Campchiaro P, et al. Phase I trial of anti-vascular endothelial growth factor/anti-angiopoietin 2 bispecific antibody RG7716 for neovascular age-related macular degeneration. Ophthalmol Retina [Internet]. 2017 Nov–Dec [cited 2019 Jun 1]: 1(6); 474–485. Available from https://doi.org/10.1016/j.oret.2017.03.003.
23. Regula JT, Lundh von Leithner P, Foxton R, Barathi VA, Cheung CM. Targeting key angiogenic pathways with a bispecific CrossMAb optimized for neovascular eye diseases. EMBO Mol Med. 2016 Nov 2;8(11):1265–88. https://doi.org/10.15252/emmm.201505889. Print 2016 Nov.
24. Khanani AM, et al. Simultaneous inhibition of VEGF and Ang-2 with faricimab in neovascular AMD: STAIRWAY phase 2 results. Presented at the 2018 American Academy of Ophthalmology (AAO) Annual Meeting; 2018 Oct 26; Chicago, United States.
25. Brown DM. Phase 1 study of combination therapy with nesvacumab and aflibercept for neovascular AMD and diabetic macular edema. Presented at: American Academy of Ophthalmology annual meeting; Oct. 14–18, 2016; Chicago, IL.
26. Regeneron Provides Update on EYLEA® (aflibercept) Injection and Nesvacumab (Ang2 Antibody) Combination Program [Internet]. Regeneron Pharmaceuticals Inc. Regeneron Pharmaceuticals Inc.; 2017 [cited 2019 Mar 1]. Available from https://newsroom.regeneron.com/news-releases/news-release-details/regeneron-provides-update-eylear-aflibercept-injection-and
27. OHR Pharmaceutical provides update on ongoing squalamine clinical trial in wet-AMD [press release]. New York, NY: OHR Pharmaceutical; April 10, 2017. Available from http://www.ohrpharmaceutical.com/media-center/press-releases/detail/482/ohr-pharmaceutical-provides-update-on-ongoing-squalamine.
28. OHR-102 Squalamine [Internet]. OHR Pharmaceutical, Inc. (OHRP). OHR Pharmaceutical, Inc.; 2018 [cited 2019 Mar 12]. Available from https://www.ohrpharmaceutical.com/product-portfolio/squalamine
29. Reinmuth N, Liu W, Jung YD, et al. Induction of VEGF in perivascular cells defines a potential paracrine mechanism for endothelial cell survival. FASEB J. 2001;15(7):1239–41.
30. Benjamin LE, Hemo I, Keshet E. A plasticity window for blood vessel remodelling is defined by pericyte coverage of the preformed endothelial network and is regulated by PDGF-B and VEGF. Development. 1998;125(9):1591–8.
31. Lindahl P, Johansson BR, Levéen P, Betsholtz C. Pericyte loss and microaneurysm formation in PDGF-B-deficient mice. Science. 1997;277(5323):242–5.
32. Furuhashi M, Sjöblom T, Abramsson A, et al. Platelet-derived growth factor production by B16 melanoma cells leads to increased pericyte abundance in tumors and an associated increase in tumor growth rate. Cancer Res. 2004;64(8):2725–33.
33. Elvidge S. Opthotech's Fovista crashes out in wet AMD [Internet]. BioPharma Dive. Industry Dive; 2017 [cited 2019 Mar 14]. Available from https://www.biopharmadive.com/news/opthotech-fovista-phase-3-failure-setback-novartis/449248/
34. Do D. Phase 1 first-in-human study of KSI-301: a novel anti-VEGF antibody biopolymer conjugate with extended durability. Presentation presented at: 2019; Angiogenesis, Exudation, and Degeneration Symposium, University of Miami – Miller School of Medicine; February 9, 2019.
35. Antibody biopolymer conjugates: a novel scientific approach and platform for extended-durability retinal medicines – first results from a phase 1b Proof of Concept Study of KSI-301, an anti-VEGF ABC" presented by Pravin U. Dugel, MD at American Society of Retina Specialists 2019 on July 27, 2019.
36. Peterson WM, Yang M. GB-102 for Wet AMD: a novel injectable formulation that safely delivers active levels of sunitinib to the retina and RPE/choroid for over four months. Poster presented at; ARVO; 2016 May 1–5; Seattle, WA, USA.
37. Sharma, Priya, Jeffrey S Heier. The Phase 3 clinical trial of conbercept for exudative AMD. Retinal Physician, PentaVision, Inc., 1 Apr. 2019.
38. Liu K, et al. Conbercept for treatment of neovascular age-related macular degeneration: results of the randomized phase 3 PHOENIX study. Am J Ophthalmol. 2019;000(197):156–67.
39. Opthea presents phase 1/2a data of OPT-302 in wet AMD at the Retina Society 2018 Annual Meeting. GlobeNewswire News Room, "GlobeNewswire", 14 Sept. 2018,
40. https://www.opthea.com/wp-content/uploads/2019/08/OPT.-2019_08_07_ASX_Ph2b-wAMD-Results_Final.pdf

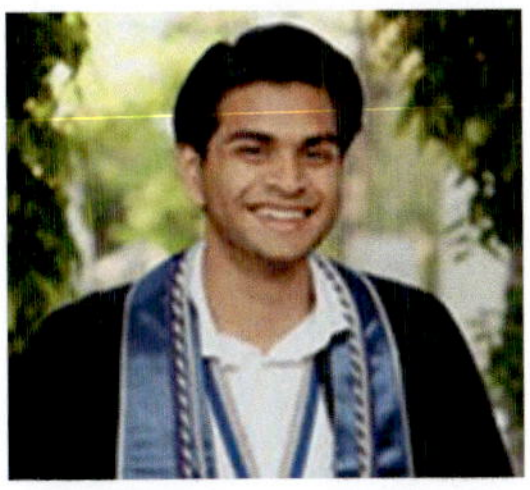

Aamir A. Aziz, B.S. is a clinical research coordinator under Arshad Khanani, M.D., M.A. at Sierra Eye Associates in Reno, NV. His degree is in Biochemistry and Molecular Biology from the University of Nevada, Reno, for which he completed a research thesis focused on muscle fatigue regulated by potassium channels in peripheral Schwann cells. Aamir is currently pursuing a career in medicine as a retina surgeon.

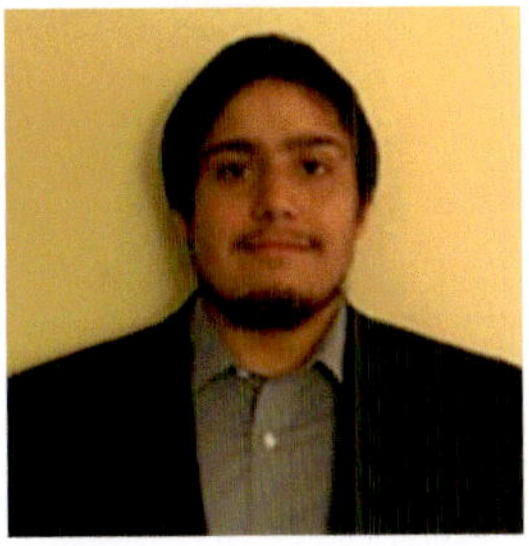

Ibrahim Khanani is an incoming freshman at Duke University studying computer science. His interests lie in artificial intelligence and applications of machine learning.

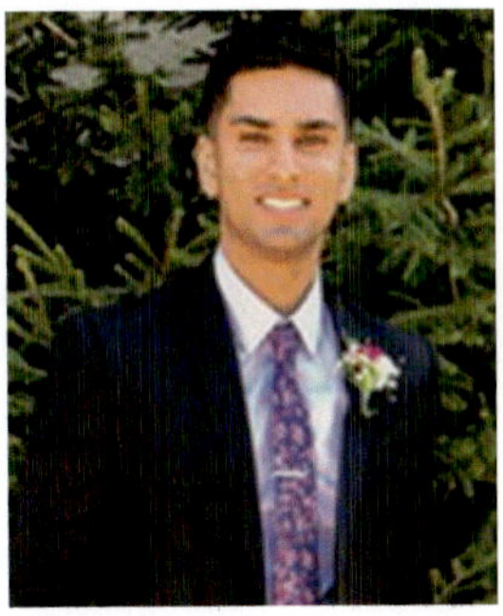

Fawwaz A. Siddiqui, B.S. currently works as a Clinical Research Coordinator for Dr. Arshad Khanani at Sierra Eye Associates. Born and raised in Reno, Nevada, Fawwaz graduated with a Bachelor's in Biochemistry and Molecular Biology from the University of Nevada-Reno in Spring 2019. Fawwaz is pursuing a career in medicine and research.

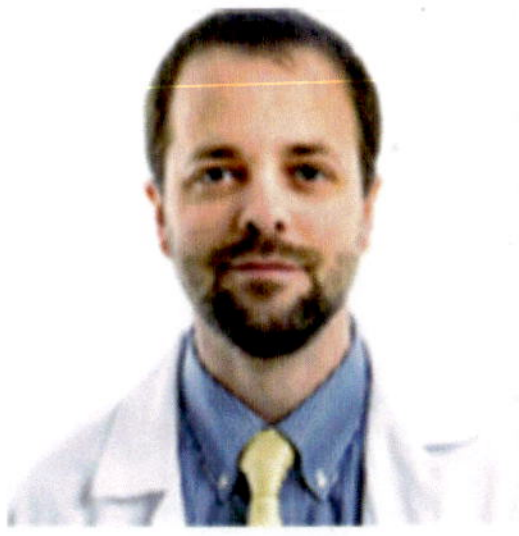

Ryan N. Constantine, M.D., Ph.D. completed his M.D., Ph.D. and intern year at the University of Utah. He then completed his ophthalmology residency at the highly regarded Duke Eye Center in Durham, North Carolina. After finishing his vitreoretinal fellowship at Sierra Eye Associates in Reno, Nevada, Dr. Constantine has accepted a position as a retina surgeon with the Orion Eye Center in Bend, Oregon.

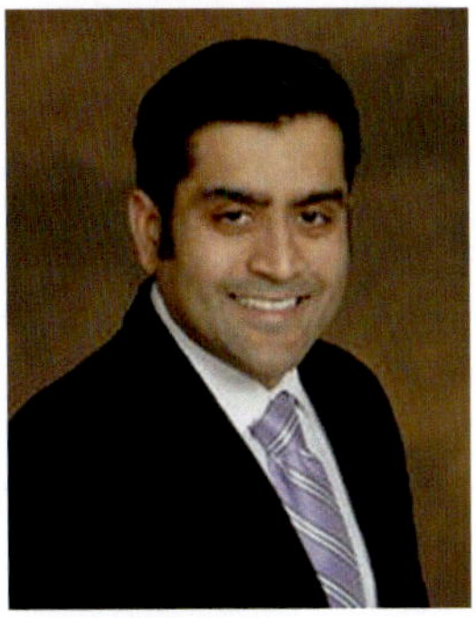

Arshad M. Khanani, M.D., M.A. is a fellowship-trained vitreoretinal specialist and is certified by the American Board of Ophthalmology. As an undergraduate, Dr. Khanani was honored twice with the Howard Hughes Medical Institute Research Award. During his medical training, he received several research awards and designed multiple prospective clinical trials, leading to publications in major ophthalmology journals. Due to his strong interest in clinical research, Dr. Khanani founded the clinical research section at Sierra Eye Associates. He has been a principal investigator for over 50 clinical trials and has been a top enroller in the country for multiple Phase 1–3 trials. He also serves as a member of clinical trial steering committees and scientific advisory boards for multiple companies. His articles have been published in top ophthalmology journals. Dr. Khanani has also presented his work at major ophthalmology meetings worldwide and has been invited multiple times as a guest speaker nationally and internationally. Dr. Khanani has received numerous awards of distinction including the Patients' Choice Award, the Compassionate Doctor Recognition Award, and the Top 10 Doctor—State Award. He has been named in Marquis Who's Who in the World and has received the Albert Nelson Marquis Lifetime Achievement Award. Dr. Khanani has also received the Honor Award and the Senior Honor Award from the American Society of Retina Specialists for his contributions. He has also been consistently named one of America's Top Ophthalmologists and has also been included in The Leading Physicians of the World publication. In 2019, he received the Nevada Business Magazine "Healthcare Heroes—Physician of the Year" award for his continued dedication to the field of ophthalmology.